BSAVA Manual of Canine and Feline Emergency and Critical Care

Editors:

Lesley King
VB DipACVECC DipACVIM MRCVS
School of Veterinary Medicine,
University of Pennsylvania,
3900 Delancey Street,
Philadelphia, PA 19104, USA

and

Richard Hammond
BVetMed BSc CertVA MRCVS
Royal Veterinary College,
University of London,
Hawkshead Lane,
North Mymms,
Hatfield, Herts AL9 7TA

Published by:

British Small Animal Veterinary Association
Kingsley House, Church Lane
Shurdington, Cheltenham
GL51 5TQ, United Kingdom

A Company Limited by Guarantee in England.
Registered Company No. 2837793.
Registered as a Charity.

Copyright © 1999 BSAVA

Figures 22.3 and 22.20 were designed and created by
Vicki Martin Design and are printed with their permission.

A catalogue record for this book is available from the British Library

ISBN 0 905214 40 4

The publishers and contributors cannot take responsibility for information
provided on dosages and methods of application of drugs mentioned in this
publication. Details of this kind must be verified by individual users from the
appropriate literature.

Typeset and printed by: Lookers, Upton Poole, Dorset, UK

Other Manuals

Other titles in the BSAVA Manuals series:

Manual of Canine and Feline Gastroenterology
Manual of Canine and Feline Nephrology and Urology
Manual of Canine and Feline Wound Management and Reconstruction
Manual of Canine Behaviour
Manual of Companion Animal Nutrition and Feeding
Manual of Exotic Pets
Manual of Feline Behaviour
Manual of Ornamental Fish
Manual of Psittacine Birds
Manual of Raptors, Pigeons and Waterfowl
Manual of Reptiles
Manual of Small Animal Anaesthesia and Analgesia
Manual of Small Animal Arthrology
Manual of Small Animal Clinical Pathology
Manual of Small Animal Dentistry, 2nd edition
Manual of Small Animal Dermatology
Manual of Small Animal Diagnostic Imaging
Manual of Small Animal Endocrinology, 2nd edition
Manual of Small Animal Fracture Repair and Management
Manual of Small Animal Neurology, 2nd edition
Manual of Small Animal Oncology
Manual of Small Animal Ophthalmology
Manual of Small Animal Reproduction and Neonatology

Contents

Contributors

Janet Aldrich DVM
Emergency and Critical Care Services, Veterinary Medical Teaching Hospital,
School of Veterinary Medicine, University of California, Davis, CA 95616, USA

Frances Barr MA VetMB DVR PhD DipECVDI MRCVS
University of Bristol, Department of Clinical Veterinary Science, Langford House, Langford, Bristol, BS40 5DU

Dawn M. Boothe DVM PhD DipACVIM DipACVP
Dept of Physiology & Pharmacology, Texas A&M University, School of Veterinary Medicine, College Station, TX 77843, USA

Dorothy Brown DVM DipACVS
School of Veterinary Medicine, University of Pennsylvania, 3900 Delancey Street, Philadelphia, PA 19104, USA

Kenneth Drobatz DVM DipACVIM DipACVECC
Section of Critical Care, Department of Clinical Studies, School of Veterinary Medicine, University of Pennsylvania, 3900 Delancey Street, Philadelphia, PA 19104, USA

Gary England BVetMed PhD DVetMed CertVA DVR DVRep DipACT FRCVS
Royal Veterinary College, Hawkshead Lane, North Mymms, Hatfield, Herts AL9 7TA

Reid Groman DVM
Department of Small Animal Medicine, College of Veterinary Medicine, Texas A&M University, College Station, TX 77843, USA

Tim Hackett DVM DipACVECC
Department of Clinical Sciences, School of Veterinary Medicine, Colorado State University, Fort Collins, CO 80523, USA

Susan Hackner BVSc DipACVIM DipACVECC MRCVS
VCA Veterinary Referral Associates, 15021 Dufief Mill Road, Gaithersburg, MD 20878, USA

Richard Hammond BSc BVetMed CertVA MRCVS
Royal Veterinary College, University of London, Hawkshead Lane, North Mymms, Hatfield, Herts AL9 7TA

Daniel J. Holden BVetMed DVA MRCVS
Division of Companion Animals, Department of Clinical Veterinary Science, University of Bristol, Langford House, Langford, Bristol, BS40 5DU

David Holt BVSc DipACVS
Section of Surgery, School of Veterinary Medicine, University of Pennsylvania, 3900 Delancey Street, Philadelphia, PA 19104, USA

Dez Hughes BVSc DipACVECC MRCVS
Section of Critical Care, Department of Clinical Studies - Philadelphia School of Veterinary Medicine, University of Pennsylvania, 3850 Spruce Street, Philadelphia, PA 19104-6010, USA

Karyl Hurley BSc DVM DipACVIM DipECVIM
Waltham Centre for Pet Nutrition, Freeby Lane, Waltham on the Wolds, Near Melton Mowbray, Leicestershire, LE14 4RT

Lesley King MVB DipACVECC DipACVIM MRCVS
Section of Critical Care, Department of Clinical Studeis, School of Veterinary Medicine, University of Pennsylvania, 3900 Delancey Street, Philadelphia, PA 19104, USA

Sorrel Langley-Hobbs BVetMed DSAS(Orth) MRCVS
Queen's Veterinary School Hospital, Department of Clinical Veterinary Medicine, University of Cambridge,
Madingley Road, Cambridge CB3 0ES

Deborah Mandell VMD DipACVECC
VCA Veterinary Referral Associates, 15021 Dufief Mill Road, Gaithersburg, MD 20878, USA

Karol A. Mathews DVM DVSc DipACVECC
Service Chief, Emergency and Critical Care Medicine, Ontario Veterinary College, University of Guelph,
Guelph, Ontario, CANADA, N1G 2W1

Kathryn Michel DVM MS DipACVN
School of Veterinary Medicine, University of Pennsylvania, 3900 Delancey Street, Philadelphia,
PA 19104, USA

William W. Muir DVM PhD DipACVA DipACVECC
Ohio State University, College of Veterinary Medicine, Department of Clinical Sciences, 1935 Coffey Road,
Columbus, OH 43210, USA

Matthew J. Pead BVetMed PhD CertSAO MRCVS
Department of Small Animal Medicine and Surgery, The Royal Veterinary College, University of London,
Hawkshead Lane, North Mymms, Hatfield, Herts AL9 7TA

Elisa Petrollini CVT
Emergency Service, School of Veterinary Medicine, University of Pennsylvania, 3900 Delancey Street,
Philadelphia, PA 19104, USA

Robert Poppenga DVM PhD
Toxicology Laboratory, New Bolton Center, University of Pennsylvania, 382 West Street Road,
Kennett Square, PA 19348, USA

Petra Roosje
Institut für Tierpathologie, Länggasstrasse 122, CH-3012 , Berne, Switzerland

Sheldon A. Steinberg DVM DipACVIM(Neurology)
Section of Neurology, School of Veterinary Medicine, University of Pennsylvania, 3900 Delancey Street,
Philadelphia, PA 19104, USA

Rebecca L. Stepien DVM MS DipACVIM
School of Veterinary Medicine, University of Wisconsin - Madison, 2015 Linden Drive West, Madison,
WI 53706, USA

Charles H. Vite DVM DipACVIM(Neurology)
Section of Neurology, School of Veterinary Medicine, University of Pennsylvania, 3900 Delancey Street,
Philadelphia, PA 19104, USA

Lori Waddell DVM
Intensive Care Unit, School of Veterinary Medicine, University of Pennsylvania, 3900 Delancey Street,
Philadelphia, PA 19104, USA

Clare Walters BVetMed CertVA MRCVS
Department of Clinical Veterinary Medicine, University of Cambridge, Madingley Road,
Cambridge CB3 0ES

Robert N. White BSc BVetMed CewrtVA DipECVS MRCVS
Davies White, Manor Farm Business Park, Higham Gobion, Hitchin, Herts SG5 3HR

Foreword

This Manual marks a further momentous step in the international collaboration of Editors and authors, under the BSAVA banner, in order to produce the finest text possible. Nineteen authors based in America, Canada and Switzerland have combined with eight home-based contributors to provide a book which collates and expands the current knowledge in this field.

As the expectations of the pet-owning public increase, partly as a result of increasing exposure of veterinary medicine in the media, so practitioners continually strive to provide better services. The concept of emergency medicine for animals is only now becoming a realistic part of the small animal clinical repertoire.

This Manual breaks new ground by discussing the veterinary treatment of emergencies ranging from shock to sustained trauma in a wide variety of organ systems. It deals comprehensively with critical care and the nursing and monitoring requirements involved, without which any attempts to provide intensive care would be futile. I am confident that both practitioners and nurses will find this Manual of immense value to them as they strive to push back the barriers of clinical possibility.

John F.R. Hird
BSAVA President 1998-99

Preface

Critically ill patients are among the most stressful cases seen in veterinary practice. These are the animals that keep us awake at night and pull us from our homes and families on holiday weekends. These are the animals for whom decisions must be made NOW – not on Monday morning when it may be too late to make a difference in their survival. For the owners of these pets, the sudden onset of critical illness often represents a catastrophic crisis. As veterinary surgeons, we must take care of both the critically ill pet and the distressed owner. It is vital that we have a logical and thoughtful understanding of the disease process, combined with the ability to act quickly and decisively in an emergency.

In addition, in order to optimize our management of these challenging cases, we must also be able to retrieve practically applicable information in a timely way. This Manual is intended as a resource for every veterinary surgeon who cannot predict what crisis will be faced the next time the door opens or the telephone rings. It represents the current 'State-of the Art' in practical management of critical patients, written by experts who daily manage these dogs and cats in their clinical practice.

Our knowledge of the specialty of small animal emergency and critical care has grown exponentially in the last 20 years, partly in response to the expanding availability of sophisticated monitoring and management techniques, and partly in response to an increased demand for higher quality care from pet owners. The survival of critically ill animals can now be improved by our knowledge of these dynamic disorders, and by application of the fundamental principles of emergency and critical care. But it's important to recognize that this specialty is still in its infancy – there is so much that we don't know, and so much left to learn. We hope that this text may also serve to generate interest and excitement among its readers, so that more veterinary surgeons will choose to specialize in this dynamic, frustrating, challenging and fascinating field of veterinary medicine.

The editors would like to dedicate this book to our families, in recognition of their love and support. Without them we could not do what we do.

Lesley G. King MVB DipACVECC DipACVIM MRCVS
Philadelphia, Pennsylvania, USA

Richard Hammond BVetMed BSc CertVA MRCVS
London, England

March 1999

CHAPTER ONE

Triage and Initial Assessment

Kenneth J. Drobatz

INTRODUCTION

Triage can be defined as the evaluation of and allocation of treatment to patients according to a system of priorities designed to maximize the number of survivors.

All stages of emergency evaluation are important to the successful management of the critically ill patient — telephone triage, waiting room triage, primary survey and treatment, secondary survey and the emergency plan. Critically ill patients have little physiological reserve to tolerate mistakes of omission or commission. Anticipation and prevention of problems before they occur is one of the cornerstones of optimal emergency and critical care medicine. Always assume the worst and treat for it, while maintaining the philosophy 'above all, do no harm'.

TELEPHONE TRIAGE

The initial contact between a client and the veterinary surgery or hospital is often via the telephone. The information obtained from this conversation may allow for triage of the patient, may help in diagnosis, and may provide information regarding first aid treatment for the pet.

The immediate aim of telephone triage is to determine whether the patient needs to be examined by the veterinary surgeon immediately and what the owner should do for the pet before coming to the surgery. The owner should be calmed if necessary, so that concise and accurate information can be obtained. Questions should be directed at determining:

- The nature of the injury
- How the animal is breathing
- The colour of the mucous membranes
- The level of consciousness
- The presence and severity of bleeding
- The heart rate
- The presence and severity of wounds
- The ability of the animal to ambulate
- The presence of obvious fractures
- The severity of vomiting and diarrhoea if present
- The ability to urinate
- The degree of abdominal distension
- Whether there is coughing.

Patients with the following should be brought to the hospital without delay:

- Respiratory distress
- Neurological abnormalities
- Protracted vomiting
- Slow or rapid heart rate
- Bleeding from body orifices
- Weakness, pale mucous membranes
- Rapid and progressive abdominal distension
- Inability to urinate
- Severe coughing
- Toxin ingestion
- Extreme pain.

Transport and preparation

Owners often want to administer first aid to their pets. In instances where the problem is clearly determined and is relatively simple, advice can often be given over the telephone. Relying on an owner's interpretation of the animal's problems can be risky, however. If there is any doubt about what is occurring, the owner should be advised to bring the pet to the clinic for definitive evaluation.

If trauma has occurred, the patient should be placed on a board or some type of support structure. Fractured limbs can sometimes be stabilized for transport by wrapping a roll of newspaper around the limb or taping or tying a board or piece of cardboard to the leg. The joints above and below the fracture should be stabilized. Splints should be applied with care, since it is often difficult for the owner to determine the location of the fracture; if done incorrectly, splinting has the potential to cause further damage. If doubt exists, the animal should be placed in a confined space or in an area where movement is minimized. Direct pressure or careful application of a tourniquet can control active haemorrhage. Owners should be warned that animals that are in pain, traumatized, neurologically damaged or frightened should be carefully approached and muzzled if possible. Even the friendliest of pets can become aggressive under these circumstances.

Clients may be extremely upset and should be calmed prior to bringing their pet in. Clear directions should be given to the owner for the drive to the clinic, and time of arrival should be estimated. The hospital personnel should be notified about the nature of the emergency and the estimated time of arrival, so that any special preparations may be undertaken if necessary.

TRIAGE AND INITIAL ASSESSMENT

Triage is the sorting out and classification of patients to determine priority of need and the optimal order in which they should be treated. Upon arrival at the veterinary clinic, every animal should be quickly evaluated by a member of the medical team to determine whether it requires immediate treatment or it is stable enough to wait if necessary (Figure 1.1). During the triage, a brief history is obtained about the nature of the primary complaint and its progression. Animals that are in containers or blankets should be taken out and examined. Four major organ systems should be assessed: (1) respiratory, (2) cardiovascular, (3) neurological and (4) renal. Dysfunction in any one of these systems can become life-threatening and should be addressed as rapidly as possible.

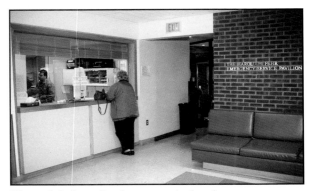

Figure 1.1: Immediately upon arrival at the emergency clinic, every owner should be questioned regarding their pet's condition.

Respiratory rate, rhythm and effort should be determined. Signs of respiratory distress include loud airway sounds, increased breathing rate, abducted elbows, extended head and neck, flaring of the nares, open mouth breathing and paradoxical respiration (see Chapter 5). Cardiovascular system assessment includes mucous membrane colour, capillary refill time and pulse quality and rhythm. Signs of cardiovascular compromise include pale, grey or hyperaemic mucous membranes, very rapid or prolonged capillary refill time, weak or bounding pulse, very rapid or slow pulse rate and irregular or asynchronous pulse rhythm. Immediate neurological assessment should include evaluation of mentation and ability to ambulate. Neurological abnormalities that should be addressed quickly include severe changes in mentation such as

stupor, coma, hyperexcitability, delirium and seizures. Finally, immediate evaluation of the renal system should include assessment of the ability to urinate and palpation of the urinary bladder. Animals with dysfunction in one of the four major organ systems should be brought immediately to the treatment area for further evaluation and treatment (Figure 1.2).

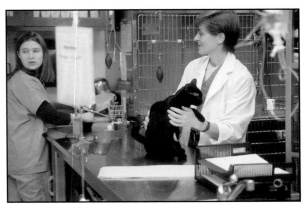

Figure 1.2: Following triage evaluation, animals that are thought to be unstable are brought to the treatment area.

Conditions affecting other body systems are generally not immediately life-threatening in themselves but their effects on the four major organ systems can result in death. For example, a fracture of the femur is not life-threatening by itself, but the resultant blood loss into the thigh musculature may result in hypovolaemia and cardiovascular compromise. Problems that do not immediately affect the four major organ systems, but require that the animal be immediately brought back to the treatment area, include:

- Recent ingestion of, or topical exposure to, a toxin
- Recent seizures
- Trauma
- Excessive bleeding
- Prolapsed organs
- Snake bite
- Hyperthermia
- Open wounds
- Fractures
- Burns
- Dystocia
- Death.

Also, if an owner is overly concerned, even if the animal appears physiologically stable it should be brought to the treatment area for observation.

Emergency assessment of patients conveyed directly to the treatment area includes the primary survey and the secondary survey.

Primary survey

The primary survey amplifies the information obtained during triage. The purpose of the primary survey is to determine further the stability of the patient and to identify and treat any immediate life-threatening conditions. The primary survey includes evaluation and support of the airway, respiratory system, cardiovascular system (poor tissue perfusion, control of haemorrhage) and central nervous system (level of consciousness). Evaluation of these parameters allows the clinician to classify the patient as stable or unstable. Any patient that cannot be clearly classified into either category should be considered unstable.

The primary survey includes evaluation of the same physical parameters as triage. Evaluation of the respiratory system includes determination of: whether the upper airway is patent; mucous membrane colour; and respiratory rate, rhythm and effort. Auscultation of the trachea and all areas of the thorax should be performed. More objective information regarding respiratory function can be obtained from pulse oximetry, arterial blood gas analysis and end tidal CO_2 measurement. Hypoxaemia can result in pansystemic problems due to poor oxygen delivery to the tissues, and requires immediate correction. Oxygen supplementation should be provided to any emergency patient if respiratory compromise is evident, and definitive treatment for the cause of the respiratory compromise should be provided as soon as possible (see Chapter 5).

Assessment of tissue perfusion includes evaluation of mucous membrane colour, capillary refill time, core body temperature to toe web temperature gradient, auscultation of the heart and palpation of pulse rate, rhythm and quality. More in-depth and objective evaluation of tissue perfusion could include arterial blood pressure measurement, central venous pressure determination, blood lactate concentration, pulmonary artery catheter placement and measurement of oxygen delivery and oxygen consumption. Clinical recognition of poor tissue perfusion, such as pale or grey mucous membranes, prolonged or rapid capillary refill time and/or abnormalities of cardiac rate or rhythm, warrants rapid identification of the underlying cause and definitive treatment (see Chapter 3). Prolonged hypoperfusion can cause changes in cellular energetics that result in intracellular sodium and calcium accumulation, cell swelling, cell membrane damage, lipid peroxidation, release of detrimental oxygen free radicals and cell death.

Extreme changes in the patient's mentation such as stupor, coma, or seizures require rapid assessment for the underlying cause, and immediate treatment to prevent any irreversible changes from occurring. Prolonged seizures or hypoglycaemia causing CNS dysfunction can result in irreversible changes if not treated rapidly. Similarly, increased intracranial pressure causing stupor or coma may progress, resulting in herniation of the brain through the foramen magnum.

In summary, the primary survey assures identification and immediate treatment of conditions that are life-threatening. It also allows identification of unstable patients so that appropriate monitoring and potential problems can be anticipated and prevented.

Secondary survey

After the primary survey and stabilization of immediate life-threatening conditions, the secondary survey is performed. This includes a full physical examination, obtaining a detailed history from the owner, assessment of the response to initial therapy and more in-depth diagnostics, including clinical pathology and imaging procedures. It is during this time that a comprehensive diagnostic and therapeutic plan can be made and a cost estimate as well as prognosis can be formulated.

VASCULAR ACCESS AND THE EMERGENCY DATABASE

Intravenous access should be obtained in any critically ill patient for administration of intravenous fluids and drugs (Figure 1.3). Peripheral veins, such as the cephalic or lateral saphenous vein, are the most common vessels utilized for intravenous catheterization, mainly due to their accessibility and familiarity to most emergency personnel. Central venous access using the jugular or medial femoral vein allows higher drug concentrations to be achieved in the coronary vessels (important in cardiopulmonary resuscitation) and allows placement of a larger diameter catheter, facilitating more rapid fluid administration. Central vessels are more difficult to access compared to the peripheral vessels, and this is particularly important in an emergency situation where vascular access must be rapid. In neonates, the easiest and most expeditious way to obtain vascular access is via intraosseous catheter placement. Absorption of drugs via this route is almost as fast as central venous administration.

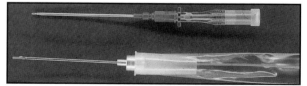

Figure 1.3: *Intravenous access must be established as quickly as possible in the critical emergency patient. Short 'over-the-needle' catheters (top) placed in peripheral veins are best, as the flow rate is optimal in a short, wide-bore catheter. Long 'through-the-needle' catheters (bottom) placed in central veins are ideal for longer periods of hospitalization.*

THE EMERGENCY DATABASE

Measurements of packed cell volume (PCV), total protein (TP), glucose by dipstick and blood urea nitrogen (BUN) by dipstick, plus a blood smear should be obtained in any critically ill patient. Assessment of urine specific gravity prior to fluid therapy and of serum sodium and potassium levels can provide valuable information for use in diagnosis and facilitate appropriate therapy. Blood samples for the emergency database can be collected from the hub of the intravenous catheter as it fills with blood, or obtained from the hub of a 25-gauge needle placed into a peripheral blood vessel (Figure 1.4). The PCV, TP, dipstick glucose, dipstick BUN and blood smear can all be obtained from three heparinized microhaematocrit tubes.

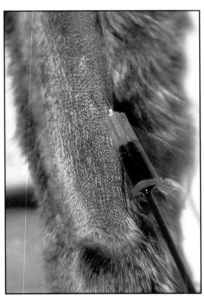

Figure 1.4: Blood samples for the emergency database can be obtained by filling a micro-haematocrit tube from the hub of a 25-gauge needle placed in a peripheral blood vessel, in this case the cephalic vein.

PCV and TP provide information regarding hydration status as well as an estimate of red cell content in the blood. A large buffy coat indicates a high white blood cell count. The colour of the serum may provide clues to the disease process. Icterus may be due to pre-hepatic, hepatic or post-hepatic problems. Lipaemic serum may be due to pancreatitis, post-prandial lipaemia or may be associated with hyper-adrenocorticism. Haemolysed serum may be due to the collection technique or intravascular haemolysis. Increased blood glucose may be due to stress (particularly in cats), head trauma, insulin resistance or diabetes mellitus. Hypoglycaemia is caused by insulin-secreting tumours, insulin-like factor-secreting tumours, sepsis, heatstroke, juvenile hypoglycaemia, storage diseases, severe hepatic dysfunction and insulin overdose. Increased BUN may result from pre-renal, renal or renal causes. The white blood cells, red blood cells and platelets should be evaluated from a properly prepared blood smear. The number and morphology of each cell type should be evaluated and recorded.

The amount of information that can be obtained from a simple emergency database can be tremendous and should not be underestimated. The information gained combined with a thorough history and physical examination can often provide a diagnosis as well as prognosis.

THE EMERGENCY PLAN

The emergency plan depends upon the presenting problem and stability of the patient and the level of nursing and technical support available. A medical problem list should be generated and the problems prioritized from the most to the least life-threatening. The problems should then be addressed in that order, making a diagnostic, therapeutic and monitoring plan for each one. The plans for each problem should be collated and a comprehensive, concise and clearly written hospital order list should be formulated. Categories that should be covered include fluid therapy, medications to be administered, diagnostics to be performed, parameters to be monitored and nursing orders.

Fluid therapy
Fluid therapy orders should include the type of fluid to be administered, the rate of infusion and the route by which the fluid should be given. The frequency of reassessment of the fluid orders depends upon patient stability, and how rapidly the fluid requirements change. In very unstable patients, fluid therapy may require re-evaluation every 30–60 minutes, as the response to therapy is determined. Relatively stable patients, where fluid deficits are being replaced over 24 hours, require less frequent reassessment of fluid orders, perhaps as infrequently as every 12–24 hours. Fluid rate and type are determined not only by cardiovascular status but also by sodium and potassium concentrations. Type of fluid and rate of infusion become very important with extremes of sodium concentrations such as severe hyponatraemia or hypernatraemia. In these cases, fluid therapy orders may need to be changed hourly depending upon the desired rate of sodium concentration changes and response to therapy.

Medication
The types of medication and the dose, route, rate and frequency of administration should be clearly written and reviewed with the individual that will be administering the drugs. All drugs that are being administered should be reviewed for incompatibility with each other, as well as potential adverse effects in specific patients or disease processes. If side effects of a certain drug are of particular concern, specific information about the side effects should be noted in the treatment orders, and the parameters to monitor and therapy for adverse reactions should also be included in the record.

Diagnostic plan
The diagnostic plan should be written and tests listed in priority of importance for the emergency care of the

patient. The stability of the patient as well as the importance of the information that the test will provide should all be considered when requesting a diagnostic test. The question that should be asked for each test should be 'Will the information that I obtain make a difference to what I do on an emergency basis?' If the answer to this question is 'no', then the test should not be done.

Monitoring

Monitoring procedures should be listed and clinician notification criteria should be clearly communicated and reviewed with the nursing personnel. Often, the trend of change in a parameter is more important than the absolute value. Monitoring trends of change allows anticipation of problems before they occur. Monitoring parameters may be divided into physical examination evaluation, clinicopathological data and electronic evaluation.

Physical examination parameters should include:

- Mucous membrane colour
- Capillary refill time
- Pulse rate and quality
- Lung sounds
- Respiratory rate and effort
- Neurological function
- Urination
- Defecation
- Vomiting
- Rectal temperature
- Abdominal pain
- Observation of skin and mucous membranes for petechiations and ecchymoses.

The most common clinicopathological parameters monitored in the emergency room include:

- PCV
- TP
- Dipstick glucose
- Dipstick BUN
- Serum sodium concentration
- Serum potassium concentration
- Blood gas analysis
- Urinalysis
- Blood smear
- Activated clotting times.

Electronic monitoring may include:

- Measurement of central venous pressure
- Continuous electrocardiography
- Blood pressure measurement (Doppler, oscillometric, or direct methods)
- Pulse oximetry
- End-tidal capnography
- Cardiac output
- Oxygen delivery
- Oxygen consumption.

Nursing orders

Nursing orders should be tailored to the needs of each individual patient. The specific disease process, the severity of the patient's condition and the level of staffing should all be considered when orders are written. For example, one nurse cannot provide comprehensive nursing care to a comatose, 50 kg large breed dog that is being mechanically ventilated and receiving peritoneal dialysis.

The emergency plan must take into account the needs of the patient, the client's needs and financial capabilities, the immediate and overall prognosis, and the capabilities of the emergency staff and facility. If it is recognized that the best emergency plan cannot be accommodated by the facility and staff, referral of the patient to a tertiary facility that can provide optimal care should be considered.

CHAPTER TWO

Fluid Therapy

Dez Hughes

INTRODUCTION

It is helpful conceptually to divide fluid therapy into two arbitrary categories: acute and chronic. Acute fluid therapy refers to the treatment of the emergency patient to replace absolute or relative plasma volume deficits within a period of minutes to a few hours. Conversely, chronic fluid therapy refers to the treatment of the haemodynamically stable patient to re-establish and maintain normal water, electrolyte and acid–base balance on a day-to-day basis. In assessing the fluid therapy requirements of an animal, it is extremely important to separate those patients requiring life-saving volume expansion from those requiring a more gradual correction of fluid and electrolyte balance. Central to this goal is an appreciation of the difference between hypoperfusion and dehydration.

Hypoperfusion refers to a local or generalized deficit in tissue blood flow, which results in inadequate oxygen and nutrient delivery and failure to remove metabolic byproducts from the tissues. Global hypoperfusion can occur due to hypovolaemia (a reduction in the effective circulating intravascular volume), reduced cardiac function or the maldistribution of blood flow seen in the systemic inflammatory response syndrome (SIRS). Most animals exhibiting signs of SIRS have some combination of sepsis, pancreatitis, metastatic neoplasia or other causes of severe tissue injury. Hypovolaemia is the most common cause of hypoperfusion and most animals with SIRS and many animals with cardiogenic shock also have concurrent reductions in effective circulating plasma volume. Common causes of hypovolaemia include: haemorrhage; extracellular fluid losses in excess of fluid and solute intake, such as vomiting, diarrhoea and polyuria; and internal losses of plasma volume due to exudation or transudation of fluid from the intravascular space.

Dehydration is strictly defined as a net reduction in the free water content of the body; however, it is often used to refer to combined water and solute loss in excess of intake. Dehydration may lead to hypovolaemia and hypoperfusion depending upon the volume and nature of the fluid which is lost; however, the terms are not synonymous. Unfortunately, the most widely used method for assessment of hydration status combines hydration parameters (moisture of the mucous membranes, skin turgor, presence or absence of retraction of the globe) with perfusion parameters (heart rate, pulse quality, mucous membrane colour and capillary refill time). This combination of hydration and perfusion parameters has compounded the confusion between the terms.

To illustrate the difference, one may consider a dog hit by a car 1 hour previously, which has suffered a fractured spleen and bled half of its blood volume into its abdomen. This animal would have no net change in the water content of its body; however, it would be severely hypovolaemic. In contrast, the geriatric cat with anorexia, hypodipsia and chronic renal failure, with net water loss in excess of intake, may be severely dehydrated but often has surprisingly good perfusion status. The former animal would require rapid intravascular volume replacement to re-expand effective blood volume and thereby preserve perfusion to the major body systems. In the latter, with adequate perfusion of major organs, more conservative fluid therapy over 24–48 hours to re-establish normal fluid and electrolyte balance would be more appropriate. A clear understanding of the distinction between dehydration and hypovolaemia and the clinical assessment of both conditions is therefore necessary to ensure appropriate fluid therapy.

EXTRACELLULAR FLUID HOMEOSTASIS

To understand the choice of intravenous fluids, it is necessary to appreciate how fluids are normally distributed within the body and the factors that control movement of fluid between different compartments. Three major fluid compartments make up the total body water: the intracellular fluid within cells; the interstitial fluid between cells; and the intravascular fluid within blood vessels (Figure 2.1). Together the intravascular fluid and interstitial fluid comprise the extracellular fluid. Total body water is approximately 60% of total body weight; however, this may vary depending upon such factors as the species, age of the animal and the body composition (mainly the fat content). Movement of fluid between compartments depends upon the permeability of the relevant barrier and the concentration of molecules contained within each compartment. For example, the capillary membrane is freely permeable to water and electrolytes, whereas the cell membrane is only freely permeable to water. Movement of water across the cell membrane depends upon the relative concentration of molecules within cells compared to the concentration around the cell. Net movement of water will occur by osmosis into an area with a higher concentration of molecules.

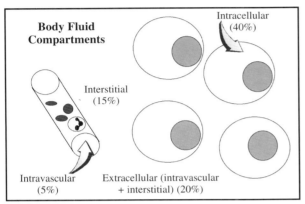

Figure 2.1: Major fluid compartments of the body.

Maintenance of intravascular volume

Capillaries are freely permeable to water and small solutes and are relatively (but not completely) impermeable to macromolecules. This means that a protein concentration gradient exists from the vasculature to the interstitium. The higher concentration of impermeant solutes within the capillaries exerts an osmotic pressure (termed the capillary colloid osmotic pressure) which acts to retain fluid. Fluid exchange between the vasculature and the interstitium is governed by the balance between hydrostatic and osmotic pressure gradients throughout the intravascular compartment and the interstitium. A hydrostatic pressure gradient, in excess of the osmotic gradient at the arterial end of the capillary bed results in a net transudation of fluid into the interstitium. At the venous end of the capillary bed, plasma proteins exert an osmotic force in excess of the hydrostatic gradient, resulting in a net fluid flux into vessels. Although the microvascular barrier greatly restricts macromolecular flux, capillaries are permeable to protein. Of the total quantity of albumin present in the body, 40% is intravascular and 60% is extravascular. Furthermore, all of the albumin present in plasma circulates through the interstitium every 24 hours. The microvascular barrier of skeletal muscle or subcutaneous tissue is relatively impermeable to protein, whereas the pulmonary capillary endothelium is more permeable. Different plasma proteins or artificial colloid molecules may differ in their rate of efflux from a vessel depending upon such factors as their molecular radius, shape and charge. For example, smaller plasma

proteins such as albumin can pass through with less impedance than larger plasma proteins. The hydrostatic and osmotic pressure gradients governing transvascular fluid flux and the permeability of the microvascular barrier can vary between different tissues and at different levels of the capillary bed within the same tissue.

By virtue of its relatively high concentration in the vascular space, albumin usually accounts for 60–70% of the plasma colloid osmotic pressure, with globulins making up the remainder. The variation in colloid osmotic pressure (COP) in dogs is due to differences in globulin concentration rather than albumin. Albumin synthesis, which is unique to the liver, appears to be regulated by the hepatic plasma COP. Equations have been calculated to estimate plasma COP from plasma protein concentrations; however, direct measurement is more accurate. Normal COP in dogs is ~16–24 mm Hg.

Three mechanisms guard against accumulation of fluid in the interstitium. First, extravasation of fluid into a relatively non-distensible interstitium results in an increased interstitial pressure which thereby opposes further extravasation. Second, following extravasation of low protein fluid the interstitial COP falls due to dilution and washout of protein, thereby maintaining the COP gradient between the intravascular space and the interstitium. Third, because the interstitium is not compliant, increased interstitial fluid results in an increased driving pressure for lymphatic drainage. These alterations in Starling forces which act to limit interstitial fluid accumulation have been termed the 'tissue safety factors'. Their relative importance varies depending upon the characteristics of the tissue. In a relatively non-distensible tissue such as tendon, a rise in interstitial pressure may be the most important means by which to counteract filtration. In a tissue with moderate distensibility and with a relatively impermeable microvascular barrier, such as skin, the fall in interstitial COP assumes more importance in protecting against interstitial fluid accumulation. In a distensible tissue that is quite permeable to protein, such as the lung, increased lymph flow appears to be the most important safeguard against interstitial oedema.

Because of this marked heterogeneity in Starling forces and transvascular fluid dynamics between tissues, it is a potentially dangerous oversimplification to view the body as the homogenous sum of its individual parts. A great deal of emphasis has been placed on the manipulation of individual Starling forces in isolation, such as the intravascular COP, rather than addressing the system in its entirety. One should carefully consider the effects on different tissues and organ systems, especially if microvascular permeability is likely to be increased. If the increase in microvascular permeability is sufficient to allow significant extravasation of colloid then there may be no benefit in trying to increase intravascular COP. If a COP gradient cannot be maintained between the intravascular and interstitial spaces then the capillary hydrostatic pressure becomes the major determinant of fluid extravasation. Smaller rises in capillary hydrostatic pressure will result in much greater fluid extravasation than when the endothelium remains intact. From a clinical standpoint, the differences between transvascular fluid flux in the lungs compared to the systemic circulation are the most important.

Control of extracellular volume and concentration

Extracellular fluid homeostasis in the normal animal is controlled by two distinct, but intertwined, feedback loops. One system acts to maintain the concentration, or osmolality, of the body and one regulates the volume of the extracellular fluid. No distinction is made between intravascular fluid and interstitial fluid because the capillary membrane is extremely permeable to water and small solutes.

Osmolality is controlled by hypothalamic osmoreceptors that stimulate thirst and the release of antidiuretic hormone (ADH) from the neurohypophysis. If net water loss from the body exceeds net water gain, plasma osmolality will rise and hypothalamic osmoreceptors then stimulate thirst and release of ADH. The augmented water intake and increased reabsorption of water by the kidney combine to decrease plasma osmolality towards normal. Fluctuations in plasma osmolality necessary to stimulate thirst and ADH release are very small (approximately 4 mOsm/kg in the dog, i.e. an increase in plasma sodium concentration of only 2 mEq/l).

Extracellular volume is primarily dependent upon total body sodium content controlled by the renin–angiotensin–aldosterone system and modulated by atrial natriuretic peptide. Sympathetic discharge and decrease in stretch of renal afferent arterioles stimulates renin release from the juxtaglomerular cells. Renin activates angiotensinogen to angiotensin I which is then converted to angiotensin II. Sodium and water reabsorption is increased by angiotensin II in the proximal tubule and angiotensin II-mediated aldosterone release promotes distal tubular sodium reabsorption.

The feedback loops controlling extracellular volume and osmolality overlap with the hypovolaemic stimulus to ADH release and thirst. The latter is mediated, at least in part, by angiotensin II. The renin–angiotensin–aldosterone system, ADH and thirst thereby increase retention of sodium and water to expand extracellular volume. In summary, the concentration of the extracellular fluid is controlled primarily via modulation of water balance, whereas the volume of the extracellular fluid is regulated by changes in sodium and water balance.

Maintenance of arterial blood pressure

With more acute or severe reductions in effective circulating blood volume, the body reacts to maintain arterial blood pressure and effective circulating blood volume to the heart, lungs and brain. With mild to moderate degrees of hypovolaemia, baroreceptor reflexes initiate sympathetic discharge, causing an increase in heart rate and cardiac contractility and, to a lesser degree, vasoconstriction. This is the so-called 'compensatory' or 'hyperdynamic' phase of hypovolaemia, where mean arterial blood pressure is maintained. After moderate to severe reductions in blood volume, cardiac compensatory mechanisms are insufficient to maintain arterial blood pressure, and vasoconstriction in the peripheral and splanchnic circulation increases. Ultimately, despite a maximum response from counter-regulatory mechanisms, progressively falling blood volume results in a fall in arterial blood pressure, the so-called 'decompensatory' or 'hypodynamic' phase of hypovolaemia.

PATHOPHYSIOLOGY OF ABNORMAL FLUID LOSSES

In a normal animal, fluid is lost in urine and faeces and in evaporation from the respiratory tract. Abnormal losses include vomiting and diarrhoea, polyuria, increased body temperature and panting, bleeding, wound exudation, loss from chest or abdominal drainage tubes, and loss into the interstitium or body cavities (often called third body spacing). The effect of fluid loss from the body on intravascular volume depends upon the magnitude of the loss and the water shifts that occur between the extra- and intracellular spaces as a result of changes in extracellular fluid concentration. These water shifts depend upon the tonicity of the extracellular fluid lost relative to the intracellular fluid.

Loss of pure water or hypotonic fluid causes the extracellular fluid to become more concentrated compared to the intracellular space and water moves out of cells thereby supporting extracellular (and therefore intravascular) volume (Figure 2.2). Because the fluid loss is distributed over the total body water, intravascular depletion is a small proportion of the total loss. With loss of isotonic fluid no water movements occur because there is no change in extracellular concentration to create an osmotic gradient.

With hypertonic fluid loss, the extracellular space becomes hypotonic relative to the intracellular space and water moves into cells exacerbating the extracellular fluid deficit and hypovolaemia (Figure 2.3). The very acute and severe haemoconcentration and hypovolaemia seen in haemorrhagic gastroenteritis is probably an example of hypertonic fluid loss, ostensibly due to a secretory diarrhoea.

To illustrate the effects of fluid loss on intravascular volume status, one may consider a dog with dehydration due to water restriction alone. Dehydration of 12% of body weight would imply a free water deficit of 120 ml/kg which would be shared equally between the intravascular, interstitial and intracellular fluid

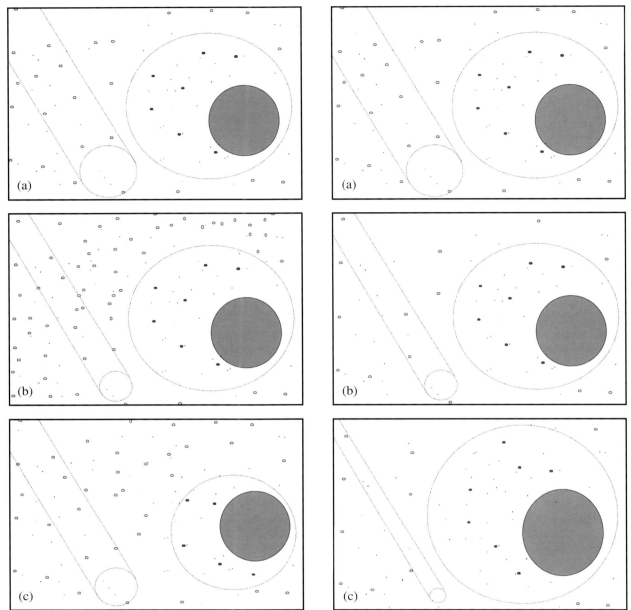

Figure 2.2: *(a) Normal fluid volumes and concentration. The major extracellular cation is sodium (o) and the major intracellular cation is potassium (●). Small dots represent water molecules. (b) Hypotonic fluid loss results in a reduced plasma volume and increased concentration of the extracellular fluid. An osmotic gradient exists which favours the movement of water from the intracellular to the extracellular space. (c) Water moves out of the cells to buffer the reduction in extracellular fluid, thereby supporting the intravascular volume.*

Figure 2.3: *(a) Normal fluid volumes and concentration. (b) Hypertonic fluid loss results in a reduced plasma volume and a reduced concentration of the extracellular fluid. An osmotic gradient exists which favours the movement of water into cells from the extracellular space. (c) Water movement into the cells exacerbates the reduction in intravascular volume.*

compartments (because water moves freely across cell membranes). Assuming that the free water deficit is distributed between these compartments on the basis of their relative size, i.e. 1:3:8 (5, 15 and 40% of body weight, respectively), this would result in a decrease in plasma volume of approximately 10 ml/kg. This is comparable to the volume of blood normally removed from a canine blood donor, usually with little or no untoward effects. Conversely, with loss solely from the intravas-

cular space, i.e. haemorrhage, loss of 5% of body weight (i.e. 50 ml/kg or more than 50% of the blood volume) would result in clinical signs of severe hypovolaemia.

APPROACH TO FLUID THERAPY

The approach to fluid therapy suggested by DiBartola (1992) is helpful when deciding upon a fluid therapy plan.

- Does the animal require fluid therapy?
- What type or types of fluid should be given?
- Which route should be used?
- How much should be given?
- Over what time period should it be administered?
- For how long should therapy be continued?

This approach enables a clear distinction to be made between those animals that require fluid therapy for volume expansion and those that need longer term fluid therapy. Abnormalities of perfusion should always be corrected prior to considering the long term fluid requirements.

Does the animal require fluid therapy?

Clinical assessment of perfusion status

The perfusion status of the animal should be assessed using: mucous membrane colour, capillary refill time (CRT) and vigour, pulse profile (height and width), heart rate, and cardiac auscultation. In uncomplicated hypovolaemia, the clinical perfusion parameters tend to change in a relatively predictable manner; however, these are only intended as approximate guidelines (Figure 2.4). A normal animal should have pink mucous membranes with a vigorous capillary refill which takes 1–1¾ seconds (a 2-second CRT is often prolonged in the setting of a veterinary clinic). Pulses (femoral and metatarsal) should be carefully palpated to allow assessment of the height or amplitude of the pulse (to estimate pulse pressure) and the width or duration. Assessing the height and width of the pulse together allows an estimation of pulse volume and, with careful palpation, a perceptive clinician can almost generate a mental image of the pulse profile (Figure 2.5). One should develop an awareness of the normal variation in pulse profile. A normovolaemic animal which is stressed or in pain will have a slightly higher and narrower pulse profile than a resting animal. The vast majority of unstressed dogs have a heart rate of 80–120 beats per minute in the setting of an emergency clinic

and the effect of body size on heart rate has been somewhat overemphasized in the veterinary literature. Normal heart rate in cats usually varies from 170 to 200 beats per minute. Mucous membranes in normal cats are significantly paler than in dogs and, although it is possible, it is much more difficult to appreciate the pulse profile in a cat.

In the compensatory stages of uncomplicated hypovolaemia, dogs will develop a moderate tachycardia of 130–150 beats per minute. This increase in rate along with the reduced blood volume and increase in cardiac contractility produces a pulse which is narrower and higher than normal (Figure 2.5b). This pulse will also be narrower than the pulse profile of the dog with tachycardia in the absence of hypovolaemia. This pulse profile is often referred to as 'bounding' or 'snappy', but these terms often serve to confuse rather than clarify. In compensatory hypovolaemia metatarsal pulses should still be palpable. Mucous membranes should be pink to pinker than normal with a rapid CRT of less than one second duration.

The increases in heart rate seen in dogs with hypovolaemia are surprisingly independent of body weight, such that severe hypovolaemia results in a heart rate of 170–220 regardless of the body weight. Heart rates in excess of this should raise suspicions of a primary arrhythmia rather than just a sinus tachycardia in response to hypovolaemia. Heart sounds are often very quiet due to the severe hypovolaemia. Mucous membranes have little or no red coloration (white, muddy or grey) and the CRT is prolonged or absent. Femoral pulses are extremely weak (Figure 2.5c) (sometimes referred to as 'thready') and metatarsal pulses are not palpable. While performing the clinical assessment of perfusion, the findings should be continually cross referenced. For example, in a recumbent cat with very weak femoral pulses, pale mucous membranes and a prolonged CRT, the heart rate should be approximately 220 beats per minute. An inappropriately low heart rate should prompt a search for the underlying reason, such as

Clinical sign	Mild (compensatory)	Moderate	Severe (decompensatory)
Heart rate	130–150	150–170	170–220
Mucous membrane colour	Normal to pinker than normal	Pale pink	White, grey or muddy
Capillary refill	Vigorous, <1 second	Reduced vigour, 2 seconds	> 2 seconds or absent
Pulse amplitude	Increased	Moderate decrease	Severe decrease
Pulse duration	Mild decrease	Moderate decrease	Severe decrease
Metatarsal pulse	Easily palpable	Just palpable	Absent

Figure 2.4: *Guidelines for the clinical assessment of uncomplicated hypovolaemia.*

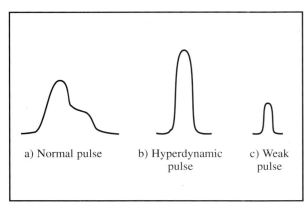

a) Normal pulse
b) Hyperdynamic pulse
c) Weak pulse

Figure 2.5: *Pulse profiles from direct arterial pressure measurement. Assessing the height and width of the pulse together allows an estimation of pulse volume.*

hyperkalaemia associated with the post-renal or renal causes of renal failure.

Lactate

Tissue hypoperfusion results in increased lactate production, and decreased lactate clearance and blood lactate concentration can be used to assess the severity of hypovolaemia. The reference value for plasma lactate concentration in normal dogs in the author's hospital (by direct amperometry) is < 2.5 mmol/l, irrespective of sample site. A blood lactate concentration in the range of 3–5 mmol/l constitutes a mild increase, 5–8 mmol/l is a moderate increase, and >8 mmol/l represents a severe elevation. Clinical experience suggests that lactate concentration accurately reflects the degree of uncomplicated hypovolaemia in dogs. Furthermore, plasma lactate concentrations almost invariably fall with successful fluid resuscitation and can be used to guide fluid therapy in the treatment of hypovolaemia. Failure of plasma lactate concentration to normalize following fluid resuscitation suggests ongoing systemic hypoperfusion or an occult source of lactate production. Lactate can also be used as a prognostic indicator. In one of the landmark studies in people, as lactate concentration increased from 2.1 to 8.0 mmol/l, survival decreased from 90% to 10%. Experimental evidence and clinical experience suggest that similar results will be obtained in canine patients. If plasma lactate concentration fails to fall below 10 mmol/l following appropriate fluid challenge, or if a significant and sustained rise in plasma lactate concentration occurs, the prognosis for survival appears to be grave.

Clinical assessment of hydration status

The widely accepted method for determining hydration status usually involves assessing: the moisture of the gums and cornea, skin turgor, presence or absence of retraction of the globe, and perfusion parameters (Figure 2.6). Dryness of the mucous membranes alone is said to reflect dehydration equivalent to 5% of the body weight and more than 12% dehydration is said to

cause overt signs of shock. Interestingly, there is little or no scientific evidence supporting this scheme. When one considers the variable effect on intravascular volume depending upon the tonicity of fluid losses and the compartments from which the loss occurs, it is apparent that this scheme allows only a rough approximation of fluid deficits.

Clinical signs		Dehydration estimate (% of body weight)
Normal		<5%
Dry mucous membranes only		5%
Reduced skin turgor	Mild	6–8%
Increased heart rate	Moderate	8–10%
Weak pulses	Severe	10–12%
Collapse, shock		12–15%

Figure 2.6: *Guidelines for the clinical assessment of dehydration.*

This scheme will tend to underestimate losses when free water is lost in excess of solute and to overestimate losses of hypertonic fluid. A clinical study performed 20 years ago (Hardy and Osborne, 1979) found that the clinical signs of dehydration due to free water loss were extremely unpredictable. Of the 20 dogs that were deprived of water for periods ranging from 2 to 4 days, 10 showed no clinical signs of dehydration and no dogs exhibited dry mucous membranes or dry or sunken eyes. One dog deprived of water for 4 days lost 16% of its body weight, showed no change in skin turgor, had no change in its packed cell volume and a minimal change in total protein concentration. Despite the limitations of this scheme for assessing replacement fluid requirements, it nevertheless provides a tried and tested starting point on which to base chronic fluid replacement therapy. The tendency to underestimate replacement requirements with increasing free water loss may actually be appropriate because these losses tend to be chronic, requiring more gradual replacement. This scheme should not be used when an animal is showing signs of hypoperfusion, when fluid therapy should be aimed at rapid intravascular volume replacement.

Types of parenteral fluid

Fluids should not be regarded as a single entity; rather, they are a range of pharmacological products each with its own indications and contraindications, much like the choice of antibiotics for different infections or the selection of heart medications for different types of heart disease. The underlying disease processes and fluid deficits will determine which is the most appropriate fluid. The main groups of fluids are: crystalloids, artificial colloids, and blood products. Crystalloids are electrolyte solutions that can pass freely out of the vascular space, whereas colloids contain macromolecules that are retained within the vascular space for a longer time period.

Crystalloids

Crystalloid fluids can be hypotonic, isotonic or hypertonic (Figure 2.7) and the tonicity of the solution will determine its distribution following intravenous infusion (Figure 2.8). Although the osmolality of 5% glucose solution is 252 mOsm/l, the glucose is rapidly taken up by cells and metabolized. Administering glucose solutions is therefore tantamount to giving free water (i.e. water without associated solute). Because free water rapidly passes out of the intravascular space and distributes across the total body water, it is an ineffective intravascular volume expander and should not be used for the treatment of hypoperfusion. Furthermore, rapid infusion of hypotonic solutions can cause severe dilution of serum electrolytes.

The isotonic solutions most commonly available are normal saline, Ringer's solution and Hartmann's solution (lactated Ringer's solution). Following volume expansion with isotonic crystalloids, there is no concentration gradient change between the intracellular and extracellular spaces, therefore no water shifts occur (Figure 2.8c). Intravascular crystalloid equilibrates with the interstitial

space and only 20–25% of the infused volume remains within the intravascular space 1 hour following infusion. Intravenous infusion of hypertonic crystalloid creates a large osmotic gradient (Figure 2.8d) and water is drawn from the interstitial and intracellular compartments producing a rapid expansion of intravascular volume (Figure 2.8e).

Hypertonic saline

Hypertonic saline is most commonly used at a concentration of 7.2–7.5% which, at 2400 mOsm/l, is more than eight times more concentrated than plasma. A dosage of 4–7 ml/kg (dogs) or 2–4 ml/kg (cats) is given over 2–5 minutes and produces a haemodynamic response similar to a crystalloid dose of 60–90 ml/kg. Because the sodium rapidly diffuses out of the vasculature, the effects can begin to wane in as little as 30 minutes following infusion. To prolong the duration of action, hypertonic saline is often constituted with a colloid such as dextran 70 or hetastarch.

Hypertonic solutions have been reported to be safe and effective for the treatment of hypotension in exper-

Fluid	Na$^+$ (mmol/l)	K$^+$ mmol/l	Cl$^-$ (mmol/l)	HCO$_3^-$ precursor	Ca^{2+} (mmol/l)	Osmolality (mOsm/l)	pH
Glucose 5%						252	4
Glucose 5% /NaCl 0.9%	154		154			560	4
NaCl 18% /Glucose 4%	30		30				
NaCl 0.9%	150		150			308	5
NaCl 7.2%	1232		1232			~ 2400	
Ringer's solution	147	4	155		2 (CaCl)	310	5.5
Hartmann's (lactated Ringer's) solution	131	5	111	29 (lactate)	2	272	6.5
*Potassium chloride 0.3%/glucose 5%		40	40				
*Potassium chloride 0.3%/NaCl 0.9%	150	40	190				
*Potassium chloride 15%		2000	2000				
*NaHCO$_3^-$ 8.4%	1000			1000 (HCO$_3^-$)			
*NaHCO$_3^-$ 4.2%	500			500 (HCO$_3^-$)			

Figure 2.7: *Composition of crystalloid fluids for intravenous administration available in the UK. *Not licensed for veterinary use but available on the medical market.*

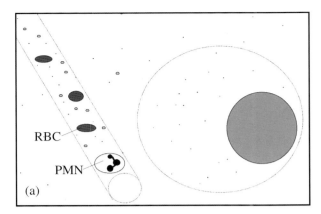

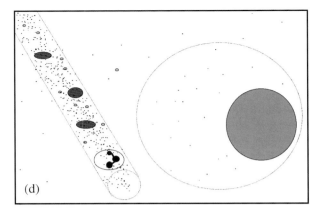

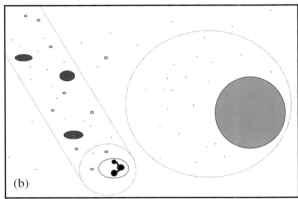

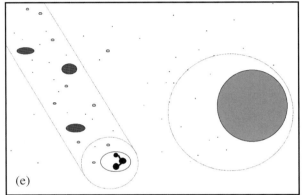

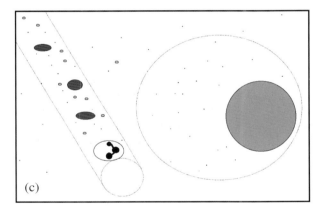

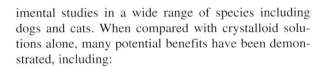

Figure 2.8: *(a) Hypovolaemic shock. Large open dots represent albumin molecules and small dots represent small solutes. (b) Intravascular expansion during infusion of isotonic crystalloid. There is no concentration gradient change between the intracellular and extracellular spaces, therefore no water shifts occur with the intracellular space. (c) Intravascular expansion with isotonic crystalloid. Intravascular crystalloid equilibrates with the interstitial space and intravascular volume falls compared to the initial volume of expansion. (d) Intravascular expansion with hypertonic crystalloid results in a large increase in intravascular sodium concentration and a large osmotic gradient for water flow into the vasculature.*
(e) Intravascular expansion with hypertonic crystalloid. Water passes into the intravascular space from the interstitial and intracellular compartments, producing a rapid, but transient, expansion of intravascular volume.

imental studies in a wide range of species including dogs and cats. When compared with crystalloid solutions alone, many potential benefits have been demonstrated, including:

- A greater, more rapid and sustained restoration of arterial blood pressure
- More rapid, greater and more sustained increment in plasma volume
- Increased cardiac contractility
- Greater and more sustained increment in cardiac output
- Improved oxygen delivery and oxygen consumption
- Improved organ blood flow
- Lower intracranial pressure post-resuscitation

- Improved survival in certain studies
- Lower total volumes of resuscitation fluids required
- Reduction in time taken for resuscitation
- Inexpensive.

Indications: Hypertonic saline is extremely useful when rapid intravascular volume expansion is required, such as the occasional case of severe hypovolaemia when death is imminent. It is also useful in large breed dogs and in hypovolaemic animals when inappropriately small intravenous catheters have been placed. A combination of hypertonic saline and iso- or hyperoncotic colloid appears to be the most appropriate fluid for intravascular volume expansion in the patient at risk for increased intracranial pressure, such as with head trauma. This combination appears to provide the best compromise between raising arterial pressure and minimizing the increase in intracranial pressure, i.e. optimizing cerebral perfusion pressure.

Contraindications: *Dehydration and hyperosmolality:* Animals suffering from dehydration do not have a normal reservoir of interstitial and intracellular fluid for mobilization following infusion of hypertonic saline. Some studies have documented a higher mortality in dehydrated as opposed to euhydrated animals. Similarly, use of hypertonic saline may be contraindicated with hypernatraemia or other hyperosmolal states.

Volume overload: Hypertonic resuscitation has been referred to as small volume resuscitation. Unfortunately, this has led to the mistaken assumption that the magnitude of volume expansion is also small. Volume expansion with hypertonic saline is a very rapid and aggressive method of fluid resuscitation irrespective of the small volume infused. It should be avoided or used with extreme caution in patients in which aggressive volume expansion would be dangerous, such as patients with heart or lung disease. In the author's experience, it can also cause ventricular arrhythmias, especially when given rapidly, so an electrocardiogram should be monitored during infusion of hypertonic saline.

Uncontrolled haemorrhage: Experimental evidence and clinical experience supports the view that aggressive volume expansion in patients with uncontrolled haemorrhage is associated with a higher mortality rate. This is probably due to an increase in the volume of haemorrhage and loss of red blood cells, platelets and clotting factors; however, there are also studies documenting increased mortality with hypertonic saline resuscitation when changes in blood pressure and volume of haemorrhage are taken into account. The most common situation in which uncontrolled haemorrhage is encountered is following a road traffic accident. Intra-abdominal haemorrhage and pulmonary contusions are the most common sites of bleeding. Notably, pulmonary bleeding appears to be exquisitely sensitive to volume expansion. Aggressive fluid resuscitation, such as with hypertonic saline, almost always worsens pulmonary bleeding and this author considers the use of hypertonic saline or any form of aggressive volume expansion, to be absolutely contra-indicated in this patient population.

Artificial colloids

The basis for the use of colloids for volume expansion, as compared to crystalloids, is that they are retained in the intravascular space to a greater degree than crystalloids and are therefore more efficient in maintaining intravascular volume. Colloids also maintain the intravascular COP and the COP gradient between the intravascular and interstitial spaces, thereby reducing the rate of fluid efflux from the vasculature. There is also some evidence that microvascular perfusion may be better following colloid infusion compared to physiologically equivalent volumes of crystalloid. Despite these advantages, it is very important to maintain perspective when assessing the need for colloid therapy. Colloids are not a panacea; rather, they are one more group of drugs with specific indications, contraindications, benefits and risks. Two meta-analyses (Velanovich, 1989; Schierhout and Roberts, 1998) documented a higher overall mortality with colloids compared to crystalloids. The limitations of meta-analyses notwithstanding, one study demonstrated a 12.3% difference in mortality rate in favour of crystalloid therapy in trauma patients and a 7.8% difference in mortality rate in favour of colloid when data from studies that used non-trauma patients were pooled. One of the most interesting conclusions was that colloid therapy appeared to be deleterious in patients with sepsis, capillary leak syndrome and adult respiratory distress syndrome following trauma.

There are three common types of artificial colloid: the gelatins, the hydroxyethyl starches, and the dextrans (Figure 2.9). Gelatins are produced from mammalian collagen, whereas hydroxyethyl starches are derived from amylopectin (the branched form of plant starch). Dextrans are prepared from a macromolecular polysaccharide produced from bacterial fermentation of sucrose. The parent mixtures of macromolecules are separated into fractions according to molecular weight. Artificial colloids are polydisperse, i.e. their molecules vary in molecular weight. Albumin, by comparison, is a monodisperse colloid, with molecules that are all the same size (molecular weight, 69 kD, molecular radius 3.5 nm). The hydroxyethyl starches have a much wider range of molecular weights than dextran 70 or the gelatins. An ideal average molecular weight of 100–300 kD would seem to provide the best compromise between colloid osmotic volume expansion and duration of action. To reduce intravascular hydrolysis of hydroxyethyl starch by amylase, the amylopectin is hydroxyethylated at carbons 2, 3 and 6. The number of hydroxyethyl groups per glucose unit is defined as the molar substitution ratio and the pattern of substitution varies depending upon the synthetic process. Substitution at the 2 carbon position is more effective at reducing intravascular hydrolysis than hydroxyethylation at the other positions. Intravascular persistence of hydroxyethyl starches can therefore be predicted on the basis of their average molecular weight, substitution ratio and C2/C6 hydroxyethylation ratio.

The duration of action of colloids may be expressed in terms of plasma colloid concentrations, measurements of plasma colloid osmotic pressure (COP) or intravascular volume expansion which will all differ to a greater or lesser degree. The initial volume of intravascular expansion is due to the osmotic pressure of the infused colloid which is determined by the number of molecules and not their size. Smaller molecules, which are responsible for a large part of the COP and intravascular volume expansion, are excreted or extravasated within hours. The larger molecules remain in circulation and are enzymatically degraded or

Fluid	Na⁺ (mmol/l)	K⁺ (mmol/l)	Cl⁻ (mmol/l)	Colloid	Ca²⁺ (mmol/l)	pH	COP (mmHg)	Osmolality (mOsm/l)
Gelofusin	77		62.5	Succinylated gelatin (40 g/l) MW 35 kD		7.4	33	279
Haemaccel	145	5.1	145	Degraded gelatin (35 g/l) MW 30 kD	6.25	7.3	25–28	
*Dextran 40 in 5% glucose				Dextran 100 g/l MW 40 kD				
*Dextran 40 in 0.9% NaCl	150		150	Dextran 100 g/l MW 40 kD				
*Dextran 70 in 5% glucose				Dextran 60 g/l MW 70 kD				
*Dextran 70 in 0.9% NaCl	150		150	Dextran 60 g/l MW 70 kD		4.9	40–60	
*Hetastarch 6% in 0.9% NaCl (Hespan)	150		150	Hydroxyethylated amylopectin 60 g/l MW 450 kD		5.5	27	310
*Hetastarch 6% in 0.9% NaCl (eloHAES)	150		150	Hydroxyethylated amylopectin 60 g/l MW 200 kD			30	
*Pentastarch in 0.9% NaCl (HAES-steril 6%)	150		150	Hydroxyethylated amylopectin 60 g/l MW 200 kD			32	
*Pentaspan 10%				Hydroxylated amylopectin 100 g/l MW 250 kD			50	

Figure 2.9: *Composition of artificial colloid fluids for intravenous administration available in the UK. *Not licensed for veterinary use but available on the medical market. MW = average molecular weight*

removed by the monocyte phagocytic system. The rapid initial excretion of small, osmotically active molecules, followed by a gradual elimination of large molecules, results in an exponential decline in intravascular expansion and a narrowing of the distribution of molecular weights. Because the larger molecules will persist longer than the smaller ones, the concentration (i.e. the mass per unit volume) will remain high; however, the COP will decrease more rapidly, hence the COP and degree of volume expansion tend to fall faster than the plasma concentration of colloid. Studies which report the pattern of volume expansion are therefore most applicable to the clinical situation.

Many factors can influence the volume and duration of intravascular expansion associated with artificial colloids, including the species of animal, dosage, the specific colloid formulation, the pre-infusion intravascular volume status and the microvascular permeability. It should be apparent that data from an experimental study in normovolaemic human volunteers given twice the usual dose of a low molecular weight form of hydroxyethyl starch may have little bearing on the effects of high molecular weight hetastarch in a dog with systemic inflammatory response syndrome in hypodynamic septic shock.

Most studies have been performed using high molecular weight hetastarch or dextran 70. Estimates of the initial plasma volume expansion for hetastarch and dextran 70 vary from 70 to 170% of the infused volume, which falls to approximately 50% of the infused volume after 6 hours. Volume expansion with hydroxyethyl starch declines gradually from 60 to 40% of the infused volume over the next 12–18 hours, whereas with dextran 70, it falls from 40 to 20% of the infused volume. In the author's experience, the duration of volume expansion using artificial colloids can be even shorter, especially with capillary leak syndromes. In dogs with hypoalbuminaemia of varying causes receiving hydroxyethyl starch, COP was not significantly different from baseline 12 hours post-infusion (Moore and Garvey, 1996). Gelatins have a shorter duration of action than the other colloids. Following infusion over a 90-minute period, intravascular expansion with polygeline was only 24% of the infused volume. For comparison, as little as 10% of the infused volume of crystalloid may remain in the intravascular space 1 hour following infusion.

Indications: *Volume expansion:* Colloids are the most efficient means of intravascular volume expansion. They are especially useful in disease states associated with an increase in microvascular permeability provided that the increase in permeability is not sufficient to allow significant extravasation of colloid. Because the osmotic effect of the colloid macromolecules is due to the number, rather than the size, if more than 50% leak into the interstitium, there could be a net reduction in intravascular volume as water leaves the intravascular space along with colloid. The dilemma therefore becomes determining the magnitude of the increase in permeability, i.e. how big are the 'gaps' in the microvascular barrier. There is a growing body of evidence which suggests that hydroxyethyl starches can reduce the increases in microvascular permeability seen in several capillary leak states. The optimal molecular weight for this effect appears to be between 100 and 300 kD.

Hypoproteinaemia: It is extremely important to bear in mind that the effective COP acting to retain fluid within the intravascular space is the net difference between the intravascular and interstitial COP. As intravascular COP falls, fluid with a lower COP will pass from the vasculature and dilute the interstitial protein concentration such that the interstitial COP will also fall. Consequently, the gradient between intravascular and interstitial COP will be preserved. This means that a low plasma COP *per se* does not necessitate colloid therapy in the absence of clinical signs such as hypovolaemia or oedema. Indeed, people with a hereditary form of complete albumin deficiency have a plasma COP which is still half of normal due to elevated globulin levels, and affected individuals exhibit minimal peripheral oedema. There are also appear to be no serious clinical signs in an autosomal recessive, hereditary albumin deficiency reported in rats. Interestingly, the affected rats exhibit marked hypercholesterolaemia. In the author's clinical experience and in experimental studies, animals with severe hypoproteinaemia (COP <11 mm Hg) may exhibit peripheral oedema but rarely develop pulmonary edema. In dogs with hypoalbuminaemia, hydroxyethyl starch has been shown to result in clinical

improvement of peripheral oedema or ascites (Smiley and Garvey, 1994). Albumin supplementation has been suggested in people because serum albumin concentration has been shown to be an accurate prognostic indicator. Interestingly, the majority of studies investigating the benefits of albumin supplementation have failed to demonstrate a benefit, indeed some have revealed lower survival rates. The role of albumin in maintaining the selective permeability of the microvascular barrier to macromolecules provides another rationale for the prophylactic use of albumin or artificial colloid. It is most important to diagnose and treat the cause of the hypoproteinaemia, rather than administer palliative colloid therapy, which is unlikely to be successful if the underlying cause is not corrected.

Contraindications and side effects: *Coagulopathy:* Deleterious effects on coagulation can occur with hydroxyethyl starch and dextran when administered at doses above 20 ml/kg/day. The important question is whether these coagulopathies are clinically significant. There are many studies which suggest a lack of clinically significant haemorrhage; however, there is also an overwhelming weight of clinical and experimental evidence revealing serious, potentially life-threatening bleeding. This paradox means simply that the coagulation abnormalities are only clinically significant in some cases. Clinical experience suggests that bleeding complications are relatively uncommon in veterinary patients. The effects on coagulation appear to be directly related to the intravascular concentration of artificial colloid. Higher plasma concentrations of colloid may occur following larger doses, repeated administration or reduced intravascular degradation. Larger colloid molecules have a greater effect on coagulation than small molecules. With repeated administration, the small molecules are constantly excreted and the relative concentration of larger molecules increases. This explains why many studies reporting clinically significant bleeding refer to patients who received repeated administration over a period of days. The exact mechanism of action by which coagulation is affected is still not fully understood. The most repeatable findings are a reduction in factor VIII and von Willebrand factor (greater than expected by dilution alone) and weakened clot formation. Desmopressin has been shown to increase factor VIII:C activity following hydroxyethyl starch infusion and should be considered as an adjunct to fresh frozen plasma administration in high risk patients. Colloid molecules may reduce the action of endothelial adhesion molecules thereby reducing endothelial release of von Willebrand factor. Colloid-induced reduction in adhesion molecule interaction may also reduce neutrophil adhesion in sepsis and explain the higher neutrophil counts observed following dextran 70 infusion in endotoxic shock.

Volume overload: Because colloids are retained

within the vasculature to a greater extent than crystalloids, there is a greater likelihood of volume overload with injudicious administration. Most clinicians are more familiar with crystalloid infusion rates, so a helpful method to ensure a safe colloid infusion rate is to estimate the equivalent crystalloid rate. Approximately 20–25% of crystalloid remains within the intravascular space 1 hour after infusion, compared to 100% of the volume of infused colloid, therefore multiplying the colloid infusion rate by four allows one to conceptualize the volume expanding effects of the colloid in terms of an equivalent crystalloid volume. While this approach can be helpful to limit excessive infusion rates, cases with cardiac or pulmonary disease or oliguria warrant direct monitoring of central venous pressures.

Renal failure: The low molecular weight dextrans such as dextran 40 have been reported to cause renal failure. Glomerular filtration of a high concentration of small dextran molecules is postulated to cause blockage of the renal tubules and/or osmotic nephrosis. Because the major route of excretion for all artificial colloids is via the kidneys, they should be used with caution in patients with oliguric or anuric renal failure. This is in contradistinction to patients with oliguria due to hypovolaemia and hypotension, in which colloids may provide the most effective means of intravascular volume expansion.

Allergic reactions and reticuloendothelial dysfunction: Anaphylactic or anaphylactoid reactions have been reported for dextrans, hydroxyethyl starches and gelatins; however, the incidence of serious complications is extremely low. Recently, hydroxyethyl starch has been associated with pruritus in up to one-third of people treated with long-term infusions. Deposits of hydroxyethyl starch in cutaneous nerves and histiocytic skin infiltrates are thought to be responsible. Interestingly, pruritus has also been reported following infusion of lactated Ringer's solution. Several studies have raised concerns regarding the potential effects of plasma substitutes on reticuloendothelial function. Decreased concentrations of the opsonic plasma factor, fibronectin, have also been reported. These appear to be most significant with the artificial gelatins but have also been noted with hydroxyethyl starch.

Interference with clinical biochemistry: Refractometry does not accurately reflect the concentration of synthetic colloids. High molecular weight hydroxyethyl starch and dextran 70 both yield refractometric total protein concentrations of 45 g/l. As plasma volume is replaced by artificial colloid the measured refractometric total protein concentration tends towards that of the artificial colloid. Hence, administering artificial colloid to an animal with a starting total protein above 45 g/l will reduce the measured total protein concentration, whereas administering artificial colloid to an animal with a total protein concentration less than 45 g/l will increase the measured total protein towards 45 g/l. Failure to appreciate the effect of artificial colloid on refractometric total protein concentration can mislead the clinician to misinterpret the fall in total protein as an indication for more colloid. Because assays for serum colloid concentrations are not readily available, therapy with artificial colloids is best monitored by direct measurement of colloid osmotic pressure with a membrane osmometer. The intravascular expansion due to colloid infusion results in significant dilutional effects. Packed cell volume, albumin concentration and serum potassium concentration seem to be most affected. Serum amylase may be elevated to 200–250% of normal following administration of HES due to complex formation and reduced excretion. Hydroxyethyl starch can also produce predictable, but potentially misleading results in blood typing and crossmatching due to increased rouleaux formation.

Artificial haemoglobin solutions

With the relative scarcity of human blood products and the risks of transmissible diseases, there has been an intense research effort towards the development of artificial haemoglobin solutions. A modified bovine haemoglobin product is now approved for use in dogs in the USA. These solutions can be used instead of red blood cells and have the major advantage of a long shelf life. In addition, the size distribution of the constituent molecules means that they provide effective intravascular volume expansion and increases in colloid osmotic pressure. The main disadvantages are that they are very expensive and relatively short acting.

Blood products

Storage of blood or blood products in the UK is not approved by the RCVS. The following applies where such storage is permitted.

Blood can be used as unseparated fresh or stored whole blood or separated following collection into packed red blood cells and plasma. Fresh whole blood and fresh frozen plasma contain clotting factors, whereas the other stored blood products do not. Separation allows more efficient use of blood products because only the required constituent need be used, e.g. red blood cells for chronic anaemia without hypoproteinaemia or fresh frozen plasma for clotting abnormalities without active bleeding. Obviously, the main disadvantage of blood component therapy is the need for access to animal blood banking facilities and it is often easier to keep canine and feline donors. Blood for transfusion can be collected into syringes containing 3.8% sodium citrate in a ratio of 9 ml blood to 1 ml sodium citrate. A stock solution of 3.8% sodium citrate can be made by mixing 43.68 g of sodium citrate with distilled water then autoclaving in a vented container. Due to the lack of preservative, the solution should not be kept longer than 24 hours after opening.

Indications: Blood transfusions can be given for the acute support of intravascular volume or over a period of 4–6 hours in the anaemic patient without serious hypovolaemia. The decision regarding when to transfuse is often defined as a specific packed cell volume (PCV); however, it is essential to consider the intravascular volume status of the animal. For example, in a dog with extreme hypovolaemia from intra-abdominal haemorrhage following a motor vehicle accident, it may be most appropriate to use fresh whole blood for volume expansion to avoid the potentially life threatening haemodilution of red blood cells and clotting factors that may occur using asanguineous fluids. If this dog is examined shortly after the accident, the PCV may not yet have fallen below the normal range. In contrast, in a dog with chronic anaemia due to reduced red blood cell production the anaemia may have taken months to develop and the animal will often be haemodynamically stable with a PCV as low as 10–15%. A PCV of approximately 30 may be best for tissue oxygen delivery as this appears to be the optimal compromise between haemoglobin concentration and blood viscosity. A PCV of 20 is the level often quoted as that below which oxygen delivery to the tissues is seriously impaired.

Equations have been suggested to estimate the required volume of blood to yield the desired increase in PCV. These expressions all assume a constant intravascular volume, which is usually only present in the chronic, stable anaemic patient that is not hypovolaemic. Hypovolaemic animals are usually volume depleted with peripheral vasoconstriction. Following intravascular volume expansion or in animals with maldistributive shock, inappropriate peripheral vasodilatation may result in a greatly increased intravascular space. Furthermore, these animals often receive a combination of blood products, crystalloids and colloids and may have ongoing haemorrhage. It is therefore often difficult to predict the rise in PCV accurately following transfusion in critically ill patients and transfusion requirements should be titrated to clinical response and PCV in each individual patient.

Abnormalities of coagulation: Acquired abnormalities of coagulation are associated with many disease processes in the critically ill patient, such as liver failure, disseminated intravascular coagulation, dilutional coagulopathy, von Willebrand's disease and anticoagulant rodenticide intoxication. When administering blood products for abnormalities of coagulation, there is a tendency to administer insufficient volume, especially when fresh whole blood is used. In addition, some of the clotting factors are distributed to the interstitium, so very large volumes can be necessary.

In a dog that is bleeding due to anticoagulant rodenticide poisoning it is likely that there are little or no vitamin K-dependent clotting factors remaining. Clinical bleeding appears to correlate roughly with prolongation of the commonly used clotting tests (prothrombin time, activated partial thromboplastin time). These results are not significantly prolonged until clotting factor levels fall to approximately one-third of normal. To ensure an adequate response to therapy, one-third of normal clotting factors must be administered, i.e. one-third of plasma volume. If the PCV is 33%, then plasma volume comprises two-thirds of blood volume. Normal blood volume in a dog is 9% of body weight or 90 ml/kg, which equates to a plasma volume of 60 ml/kg. One third of the plasma volume is therefore 20 ml/kg of plasma or 40 ml/kg of fresh whole blood (assuming a donor PCV of 50%).

In an animal that is not anaemic or hypovolaemic it can be difficult to give sufficient clotting factors using whole blood without causing potentially dangerous polycythaemia.

Blood products for colloid support: Albumin has a molecular weight of approximately 69,000 Daltons and a molecular radius of 3.5 nm. It is a monodisperse colloid, which is to say that all albumin molecules are the same size. In addition to its role in maintaining plasma COP, it also carries a wide range of substances such as bilirubin, fatty acids, metals and other ions, hormones and drugs. Albumin is most commonly given to small animal patients as stored or fresh frozen plasma, stored whole blood or fresh whole blood. Because albumin equilibrates with the interstitial space more rapidly and to a greater extent than artificial colloids, relatively large volumes must be given to achieve a sustained rise in plasma COP. When considering chronic albumin supplementation, as opposed to acute volume expansion with blood products, the amount of albumin required can be estimated using an equation which corrects for the expected volume of distribution across the intravascular and interstitial spaces:

Albumin deficit (g) = 10 x (desired [albumin] (g/dl) – patient [albumin] (g/dl)) x (body weight (kg) x 0.3)

To raise the serum albumin from 1.5 to 2.5 g/dl in a 20 kg dog:

Albumin deficit = 10 x (2.5 – 1.5) x (20 x 0.3) = 60 g

This is equivalent to 2 l of plasma or 4 l of fresh whole blood.

Contraindications and side-effects: *Transfusion reactions:* Although there are naturally occurring red cell antigens in dogs, transfusion reactions which occur to a first transfusion are usually not life-threatening and are usually limited to pyrexia, vomiting, facial oedema and pruritus. In contrast, the transfusion reactions seen in type B cats given type A blood or following a second transfusion in sensitized dogs can be more serious.

Ionized hypocalcaemia: When given rapidly for acute volume expansion, blood products should be given through a large bore catheter to facilitate infusion and avoid haemolysis. With rapid administration of citrated blood products, the risk of ionized hypocalcaemia should be considered. Although the fall in ionized calcium which occurs secondary to complexing of ionized calcium with citrate is transient (usually lasting for 30–60 minutes) it can be potentially dangerous when relatively large volumes are administered over a short time period. Intravenous calcium supplementation can be given (e.g. 10% Ca gluconate, 0.25–0.5 ml/kg at not greater than 1 ml per minute). Calcium should be administered through a different intravenous catheter to avoid the risk of causing clotting of the blood product.

Volume, rate, duration and route of administration of fluid therapy

Acute intravenous fluid therapy to replace absolute or relative, plasma volume deficits in the patient with hypoperfusion is often a life-saving procedure which must be performed over minutes to hours. In contrast, chronic fluid therapy to re-establish and maintain normal water, electrolyte and acid base balance, is not usually an emergency response and is planned and re-evaluated on a daily basis. It is vital that one clearly separates acute volume expansion from chronic fluid therapy to ensure that life-threatening problems are corrected in a timely manner.

Acute fluid therapy

To determine the appropriate fluid dosage, abnormalities of perfusion should be graded as to their severity (see Figure 2.4). Mild hypoperfusion, due to uncomplicated hypovolaemia, usually warrants crystalloid fluid rates of 20–40 ml/kg of isotonic fluids in the first hour. Moderate hypoperfusion requires 40–60 ml/kg/h and animals with severe hypoperfusion should receive 60–90 ml/kg/h. Fluid rates and volumes for cats are reduced by one third to a half. Prior to administering aggressive fluid therapy, one should carefully assess the possible reasons for the hypoperfusion and whether there are any contraindications to rapid fluid therapy. The vast majority of animals with poor perfusion have hypovolaemia, maldistributive shock (sepsis or other causes of the systemic inflammatory response syndrome) or cardiogenic shock. The major contraindications to aggressive fluid therapy are cardiac, respiratory or brain disease. Although anuric renal failure also warrants careful fluid therapy, it is impossible to confirm this diagnosis without an appropriate fluid challenge. Most animals with significant heart disease will have a murmur or gallop rhythm on cardiac auscultation; however, with severe hypovolaemia the heart sounds can be very quiet. Fluids for acute intravascular volume replacement should always be given by the intravenous or intraosseous route. Because flow rate is proportional to the fourth power of the radius of the catheter, the largest bore possible should be used. It is also helpful to place two intravenous catheters to ensure an adequate fluid volume can be administered and to provide a back-up if one catheter does not flow or becomes dislodged. In animals with severe hypoperfusion surgical venous cutdowns may be necessary to establish venous access (see Chapter 22).

Animals receiving intravenous fluids for rapid intravascular volume expansion should be constantly monitored to assess the clinical response to therapy. In general, during successful volume replacement, perfusion parameters will gradually and predictably return to normal through the same stages in reverse. Mental status should also improve and there should be no deleterious effects on the respiratory system. Given a dog of a certain body weight with a given degree of hypovolaemia, one can estimate the expected clinical response from a given volume and type of intravenous fluid. This enables the clinician rapidly to detect an inadequate response to volume resuscitation and pursue the underlying cause (e.g. haemorrhage, sepsis/SIRS), while continuing to reassess the appropriate infusion rate and whether colloid or blood component therapy is necessary.

Chronic fluid therapy

For the animal that is dehydrated but not seriously hypovolaemic, it is more appropriate to correct fluid, electrolyte and acid–base abnormalities over a period of 12–24 hours. Chronic fluid therapy should address pre-existing fluid deficits (replacement requirements), normal maintenance requirements and any ongoing losses (see example below). The volume of fluids required for replacement is estimated as a percentage of the animal's body weight based on the clinical signs of hydration status (see Figure 2.6). As discussed previously, this provides only a rough estimate rather than an accurate guide. Because of the need to expand the intravascular and interstitial compartments effectively, an isotonic fluid is used for replacement of pre-existing deficits. So-called 'replacement fluids' have a high sodium content and a low potassium concentration similar to plasma (see Figure 2.7). Maintenance fluid requirements are simply the water and electrolytes needed on a daily basis in a normal animal. They are estimated empirically at 60 ml/kg/day for small dogs and cats and 40 ml/kg/day for larger dogs. In general, the fluid composition required for maintenance is low in sodium (~0.3–0.45%) and high in potassium (~20 mEq/l). Occasionally ongoing losses such as chest tube drainage or losses in diarrhoea can be measured (or weighed); however, this is also usually another estimate. Increased insensible losses such as panting (especially with pyrexia) can be significant and should be taken into account when planning daily requirements. In practice, in the animal with large replacement needs or ongoing losses, the maintenance volume is relatively small and replacement fluids are used alone.

In animals requiring potassium supplementation, an empirical dose is usually added to the intravenous fluids (see Figure 12.6). Because this supplementation chart does not take the fluid rate into account, the potassium infusion rate should be checked in small animals or in animals receiving high fluid rates. An empirical maximum infusion rate of 0.5 mEq/kg/h is suggested for potassium. Potassium should not be added to fluids that are likely to be used for rapid intravenous infusion. Furthermore, inadequate mixing of intravenous fluids after addition of supplementary potassium can result in potassium concentrations an order of magnitude higher than expected.

SAMPLE CHRONIC FLUID THERAPY PLAN

5-month-old, male entire Labrador Retriever, body weight 20 kg

History
- No vaccinations
- 3 days anorexia, lethargy
- 2 days vomiting and diarrhoea 5–6 times/day, becoming bloody

Physical examination
- Depressed
- Heart rate 140, no adventitious heart or lung sounds
- Pulses weak/moderate
- CRT 2 s
- When raised, the skin over the back of the neck falls back more slowly than normal

Daily fluid requirement

Replacement
Fluid deficit = % dehydration x body weight x 10
= 8 x 20 x 10
= 1600 ml

Maintenance
Maintenance requirement = 50 ml/kg/day
= 50 x 20
= 1000 ml/day

Ongoing losses
Ongoing losses = diarrhoea + vomitus
Estimated diarrhoea volume/episode = 100 ml x 5 episodes/day = 500 ml
Estimated vomitus volume/episode = 50 ml x 5 episodes/day = 250 ml
Total ongoing losses = 500 + 250 = 750 ml/day

Daily fluid requirement = Replacement + Maintenance + Ongoing losses
= 1600 + 1000 + 750
= 3350 ml/day
= 3350/24 ml/h
= 140 ml/h

Fluid requirements should be re-evaluated and adjusted on a daily basis. One of the most common mistakes with continued intravenous fluid therapy is failure to readjust fluid rates as the condition of the animal changes. Prolonged use of a low potassium replacement solution in an anorexic animal will inevitably result in hypokalaemia because urinary potassium losses are usually of the order of 20 mEq/l. There is a tendency to misconstrue the impressive autoregulatory abilities of the body and more specifically the kidney, to imply that the choice of intravenous fluids is somewhat academic. Certainly, the normal kidney often compensates admirably for an inappropriate choice of fluid therapy. In animals with renal dysfunction or failure of the body's normal homeostatic mechanisms for water, electrolyte and acid–base balance, failure to select the appropriate fluid and monitor the effects may result in serious and potentially life-threatening complications.

ACKNOWLEDGEMENT

The author would like to thank Dr J.C. Brearley MA VetMB PhD DVA MRCVS who provided the information in Figures 2.7 and 2.9.

REFERENCES AND FURTHER READING

Aukland K and Reed RK (1993) Interstitial-lymphatic mechanisms in the control of extracellular fluid volume. *Physiological Reviews* **73**, 1–78

Boon JC, Jesch F *et al.* (1976) Intravascular persistence of hydroxyethyl starch in man. *European Surgical Research* **8**, 497–503

Brown SA, Dusza K *et al.* (1994) Comparison of measured and calculated values for colloid osmotic pressure in hospitalized animals. *American Journal of Veterinary Research* **55**, 910–915

Chi OZ, Lu X *et al.* (1996) Hydroxyethyl starch solution attenuates blood-brain barrier disruption caused by intracarotid injection of hyperosmolar mannitol in rats. *Anesthesia and Analgesia* **83**, 336–341

Conroy JM, Fishman RL *et al.* (1996) The effects of desmopressin and 6% hydroxyethyl starch on factor VIII:C. *Anesthesia and Analgesia* **83**, 804–807

Cope JT, Banks D *et al.* (1997) Intraoperative hetastarch infusion impairs hemostasis after cardiac operations. *Annals of Thoracic Surgery* **63**, 78–82

Culp AM, Clay ME *et al.* (1994). Colloid osmotic pressure (COP) and total solids (TS) measurement in normal dogs and cats. *Proceedings of the Fourth International Veterinary Emergency and Critical Care Symposium*, San Antonio, TX, p. 705

Curry FE, Michel CC *et al.* (1987) Effect of albumin on the osmotic pressure exerted by myoglobin across capillary walls in frog mesentery. *Journal of Physiology* **387**, 69–82

DiBartola SP (1992) Introduction to fluid therapy. In: *Fluid Therapy in Small Animal Practice*, ed. SP DiBartola, pp. 321–340. WB Saunders, Philadelphia

Falk JL *et al.* (1989) Colloid and crystalloid fluid resuscitation. In: *Textbook of Critical Care*, eds Shoemaker WC and Ayres S, pp 1055–1073. WB Saunders, Philadelphia

Farrow SP, Hall M *et al.* (1970) Changes in the molecular composition of circulating hydroxyethyl starch. *British Journal of Pharmacology* **38**, 725–730.

Funk W and Baldinger V (1995) Microcirculatory perfusion during volume therapy. A comparative study using crystalloid or colloid in awake animals. *Anesthesiology* **82**, 975–982

Guyton AC and Lindsay NW (1959) Effect of elevated left atrial pressure and decreased plasma protein concentration on the development of pulmonary edema. *Circulation Research* **7**, 649–657

Hardy RM and Osborne CA (1979) Water deprivation test in the dog: Maximal normal values. *Journal of the American Veterinary Medical Association* **174**, 479–483

Jones PA, Tomasic M *et al.* (1997) Oncotic, hemodilutional and hemostatic effects of isotonic saline and hydroxyethyl starch solutions in clinically normal ponies. *American Journal of Veterinary Research* **58**, 541–548

Lamke LO and Liljedahl SO (1976) Plasma volume changes after infusion of various plasma expanders. *Resuscitation* **5**, 93–102

Moore LE and Garvey MS (1996). The effect of hetastarch on serum colloid oncotic pressure in hypoalbuminemic dogs. *Journal of Veterinary Internal Medicine* **10**, 300–303

Navar PD and Narar LG (1977) Relationship between colloid osmotic pressure and plasma protein concentration in the dog. *American Journal of Physiology* **233**, H295–H298

Oz MC, FitzPatrick MF *et al.* (1995) Attenuation of microvascular permeability dysfunction in postischemic striated muscle by hydroxyethyl starch. *Microvascular Research* **50**, 71–79

Pappenheimer JR, Renkin EM *et al.* (1951) Filtration, diffusion and molecular sieving through peripheral capillary membranes. A contribution to the pore theory of capillary permeability. *American Journal of Physiology* **167**, 13–46

Rackow EC, Fein IA *et al.* (1977) Colloid osmotic pressure as a prognostic indicator of pulmonary edema and mortality in the critically ill. *Chest* **72**, 709–713

Ring J (1985) Anaphylactoid reactions to plasma substitutes. *International Anesthesiology Clinics* **23**, 67–95

Rippe B and Haraldsson B (1998) Transport of macromolecules across microvascular walls: the two pore theory. *Physiological Reviews* **74**, 163–219

Schierhout G and Roberts I (1998) Fluid resuscitation with colloid or crystalloid solutions in critically ill patients: a systematic review of randomised trials. *British Medical Journal* **316**, 961–964

Shoemaker WC (1976) Comparison of the relative effectiveness of whole blood transfusions and various types of fluid therapy in resuscitation. *Critical Care Medicine* **4**, 71–78

Smiley LE and Garvey MS(1994). The use of hetastarch as adjunct therapy in 26 dogs with hypoalbuminemia: a phase two clinical trial. *Journal of Veterinary Internal Medicine* **8**, 195–202

Starling EH (1896) On the absorption of fluid from the connective tissue spaces. *Journal of Physiology* (London) **19**, 312–326

Staub NC and Taylor AE (1984) *Edema*. Raven Press, New York

Taylor AE (1990) The lymphatic edema safety factor: the role of edema dependent lymphatic factors (EDLF). *Lymphology* **23**, 111–123

Thomas LA and Brown SA (1992) Relationship between colloid osmotic pressure and plasma protein concentration in cattle, horses, dogs and cats. *American Journal of Veterinary Research* **53**, 2241–2243

Treib J, Haass A *et al.* (1995) HES 200/0.5 is not HES 200/0.5. Influence of the C2/C6 hydroxyethylation ratio of hydroxyethyl starch (HES) on hemorheology, coagulation and elimination kinetics. *Thrombosis and Haemostasis* **74**, 1452–1456

Treib J, Haass A *et al.* (1997) Coagulation disorders caused by hydroxyethyl starch. *Thrombosis and Haemostasis* **78**, 974–983

Velanovich V (1989) Crystalloid versus colloid fluid resuscitation: a meta-analysis of mortality. *Surgery* **105**, 65–71

Villarino ME, Gordon SM *et al.* (1992) A cluster of severe postoperative bleeding following open heart surgery. *Infection Control and Hospital Epidemiology* **13**, 282–287

Wareing TH, Gruber MA *et al.* (1989) Increased plasma oncotic pressure inhibits pulmonary fluid transport when pulmonary pressures are elevated. *Journal of Surgical Research* **46**, 29–34

Weil MH and Afifi AA (1970) Experimental and clinical studies on lactate and pyruvate as indicators of the severity of acute circulatory failure (shock). *Circulation* **41**, 989–1001

Wiig H and Reed RK (1987) Volume–pressure relationship (compliance) of interstitium in dog skin and muscle. *American Journal of Physiology* **253**, H291–H298

Yuan Y, Granger HJ *et al.* (1992) Flow modulates coronary venular permeability by a nitric oxide-related mechanism. *American Journal of Physiology* **263**, H641–H646

Zarins CK, Rice CL *et al.* (1976) Role of lymphatics in preventing hypooncotic pulmonary edema. *Surgical Forum* **27**, 257–259

Zarins CK, Rice CL *et al.* (1978) Lymph and pulmonary response to isobaric reduction in plasma oncotic pressure in baboons. *Circulation Research* **43**, 925–930

Zikria BA, Oz MO, Carlson RW 1994 (eds) *Reperfusion Injuries and Clinical Capillary Leak Syndrome*. Futura Publishing Company, Armonk, NY

CHAPTER THREE

Shock

Janet Aldrich

INTRODUCTION

Shock is a syndrome characterized by severe deterioration in clinical signs, such as mental state, mucous membrane colour, capillary refill time, heart rate and pulse quality. It occurs when a global (but unequal) deficit in tissue perfusion damages cells. In vasoconstrictive shock, profound vasoconstriction of some tissue beds damages cells by depriving them of oxygen and other nutrients. In vasodilative shock, inflammatory mediators damage cells. In most cases, elements of both ischaemic and mediator-induced damage are present. Cell damage by these mechanisms impairs cell function and can result in organ failure and death. Treatment of shock aims to prevent more cell damage and to promote healing by optimizing tissue perfusion. Therapeutic endpoints include improvement in clinical signs and other measured parameters such as base deficit, blood lactate concentration and urine output.

CLASSIFICATION OF SHOCK

Events causing shock do so by decreasing:

- The effective circulating blood volume
- The capacity of blood to deliver oxygen to cells
- The ability of the heart to pump blood

- The ability of the vascular system to maintain appropriate vasomotor tone.

Shock may be classified as primarily hypovolaemic (salt and water loss, or whole blood loss), traumatic, cardiogenic or distributive (sepsis or anaphylaxis), as shown in Figure 3.1. Classification schemes, including this one, tend to be oversimplifications because relatively few global, clinically assessable parameters represent a large number of complex, interacting processes occurring at the cellular level.

Hypovolaemic shock

Hypovolaemic shock occurs when loss of circulating blood volume causes a severe decrease in tissue perfusion. Vasoconstriction is the primary compensation for hypovolaemia. Constriction of venous capacitance vessels improves venous return, while arteriolar constriction in non-essential tissues redistributes blood flow to essential circulatory beds (coronary and cerebral). The effect of this vasoconstrictive compensation is perfusion of some vital areas but deprivation of others, particularly the splanchnic circulation. Cells damaged by ischaemia are likely to release inflammatory mediators, potentially causing more cell damage. Vasoconstriction is a short-term solution to a vascular volume problem and is life saving, provided that volume is restored before irreversible cell damage has occurred.

	Hypovolaemic shock		Traumatic shock	Cardiogenic shock	Distributive shock	
Causes	Salt and water loss	Blood loss	Trauma	Failure of the heart as a pump	Sepsis	Anaphylaxis
Vasomotor tone	Constriction	Constriction	Constriction	Constriction	Dilation	Dilation
Cardiac output	Decreased	Decreased	Decreased	Decreased	Increased	Increased
Systemic vascular resistance	Increased	Increased	Increased	Increased	Decreased	Decreased
Initial mechanism of cell damage	Ischaemia	Ischaemia	Ischaemia	Ischaemia	Inflammatory mediators	Inflammatory mediators

Figure 3.1: Classification of shock.

Salt and water loss

Losses outside the body in urine, faeces or vomitus come from the interstitial compartment and, reflecting the composition of that compartment, predominantly contain sodium chloride (salt) and water. Losses of this type are distributed across the extracellular space. Decreases in skin turgor as well as changes in the cardiovascular parameters (mental state, mucous membrane colour, capillary refill time, heart rate and pulse quality) are expected. Red blood cells and proteins are concentrated in a smaller volume of plasma, as indicated by an increase in packed cell volume and total solids.

Blood loss

Haemorrhage causes shock by a combination of volume loss and a decrease in red cell mass, such that oxygen delivery to cells is critically low. Because the lost fluid has the same composition as the remaining blood, no changes in packed cell volume or total solids are initially expected. Over time, redistribution of salt and water from the interstitium replaces a portion of this loss and dilutes the remaining red blood cells and proteins.

Traumatic shock

In trauma, shock is often due to hypovolaemia secondary to bleeding. Extensive tissue trauma can also cause enough capillary damage to result in substantial loss of plasma into the tissues. Additionally, pain can inhibit the vasomotor centre and interfere with the vasoconstrictive response. Extensive tissue damage activates the inflammatory response, causing release of inflammatory mediators from damaged cells.

Cardiogenic shock

Failure of pump function of the heart causes cardiogenic shock. Ventricular volumes and central venous pressure may be increased, but forward flow is inadequate.

Distributive shock

Distributive shock is characterized by non-uniform loss of adequate peripheral resistance. Resistance in specific tissue beds may be increased, decreased or normal, and the clinical picture is that of vasodilation. With adequate volume resuscitation, tissue perfusion increases. Some areas, such as splanchnic tissues, may continue to be perfused ineffectively or, in spite of adequate perfusion, may be unable to use the substrates presented. These vascular and cellular effects largely result from the global release of inflammatory mediators (see 'The systemic inflammatory response syndrome and multiple organ dysfunction syndrome').

Septic shock

Sepsis is the systemic inflammatory response to severe infection, most commonly caused by bacteria or bacterial toxins. Other causative agents include fungi, protozoans and viruses. When sepsis is combined with clinical signs of shock, septic shock is present.

Anaphylactic shock

Anaphylaxis results from an antigen–antibody reaction occurring immediately after an antigen to which the patient is sensitized enters the circulation. Anaphylactic shock is characterized by venous dilation that increases venous capacitance and decreases venous return, arteriolar dilation that decreases arterial pressure, and increased capillary permeability that results in hypovolaemia due to loss of plasma into tissues. Urticaria, angioedema, laryngeal oedema and bronchospasm may also be present.

CLINICAL SIGNS AND RELATED CARDIOVASCULAR PARAMETERS

The clinical signs of shock and the cardiovascular parameters that these signs represent are shown in Figure 3.2. Correct interpretation of these signs, based on knowledge of their physiology, is of primary importance in the initial management of shock patients. The signs serve both to identify that a state of shock exists and as some of the endpoints of resuscitation.

Clinical signs related to intravascular volume

Mental state

Mental state refers to the level of consciousness and the behaviour of the patient. The brain has a high metabolic rate and low energy reserves, making it dependent on a constant supply of oxygen and glucose. Decreases in brain perfusion cause deterioration in the mental state.

Mucous membrane colour

The amount and the composition (haemoglobin, oxygen) of blood in the underlying capillary beds create the normally pink colour of mucous membranes. Either anaemia or severe vasoconstriction can cause mucous membranes to be pale or white. Vasodilation and venous pooling cause mucous membranes to be excessively red, a condition common in sepsis.

Capillary refill time

Digital pressure applied to a mucous membrane pushes blood out of the underlying capillary bed. Capillary refill time is the time it takes, in seconds, for blood to refill the capillary bed after digital pressure is removed. This is usually about 1 second. The rate of refill is determined by the tone of the precapillary arteriolar sphincters. Vasoconstriction lengthens and vasodilation shortens the capillary refill time. Capillary refill time is *not* a measure of cardiac output; instead, it is a measure of peripheral vasomotor tone.

Clinical signs	Cardiovascular parameters represented by the clinical signs	Changes in clinical signs due to changes in vasomotor tone	
		Vasoconstriction	Vasodilation
Mental state	Perfusion to the brain	Altered mental state	
Mucous membrane colour	Volume and composition (haemoglobin, oxygen) of capillary blood	Pale to white mucous membranes	Hyperaemic (red, injected) mucous membranes
Capillary refill time	Peripheral vasomotor tone	Slow to absent capillary refill time	Fast capillary refill time
Heart rate	Response to vascular volume	Increased heart rate	Increased heart rate
Pulse quality	Pulse pressure (systolic minus diastolic blood pressure)	Poor pulse quality	Bounding pulse quality
Extremity temperature	Perfusion to the extremities	Cool extremities	Warm extremities

Figure 3.2: Clinical signs of shock and related cardiovascular parameters.

Heart rate

Increased heart rate is an early and sensitive indicator of vascular volume loss. If tachycardia is due to volume loss, restoration of an effective circulating blood volume should cause a decrease in heart rate. Other causes of tachycardia, such as pain, fever, hypoxaemia or hypercapnia, should be considered.

Pulse quality

Pulse quality is a subjective impression of the fullness, or amplitude, of the pulse. It is determined by the pulse pressure (difference between systolic and diastolic pressure) and the duration of the pressure waveform. Pulse quality is most indicative of stroke volume and is not well correlated with arterial blood pressure. Vasoconstriction and small stroke volume are the most common causes of poor pulse quality (lack of fullness of the pulse).

Temperature of extremities

Vasoconstriction decreases blood flow to the extremities, causing them to cool. The surface temperature of an extremity can be measured by taping a clinical thermometer between the toes. The core to toe-web temperature difference is normally 4°C. Increases in the gradient indicate peripheral vasoconstriction.

Clinical signs related to interstitial volume

Interstitial volume can be assessed by evaluating skin turgor and mucous membrane moistness. Losses of salt and water (as with severe vomiting, diarrhoea or diuresis) cause loss of both interstitial and intravascular volume. Acute blood loss causes a decrease in vascular volume, but at least in the early stages may leave the interstitial volume unchanged.

Skin turgor

Skin turgor (skin elasticity) causes skin to return to its normal position after being gently lifted into a tented position. The elasticity of the skin and subcutaneous tissues is a measure of the amount of fluid (salt and water) and fat in the interstitial space. Interstitial dehydration causes the skin to remain tented for several seconds. However, the assessment of skin turgor is subject to a fairly large degree of error. In states of normal hydration, thin patients have decreased skin elasticity due to loss of subcutaneous fat. Because of higher subcutaneous stores of fat and water, young patients usually have more skin elasticity than do older patients.

Mucous membrane moistness

The degree of moistness of the mucous membranes reflects the status of the interstitial space. However, other problems such as nausea or oral disease may cause excessive salivation, which may make the membranes appear moist, even in the face of interstitial volume deficits.

Changes in vasomotor tone

Changes in vasomotor tone characterize the shock state and form the basis for its recognition and treatment. Neither vasoconstriction nor vasodilation is uniform across the vascular system, nor throughout the body. Moreover, changes in the tone of arteries have different effects from changes in the tone of veins. Since shock is a cellular event, impairment of adequate blood flow to the capillaries, where oxygen and nutrient transport to the cells occurs, is of primary concern.

The tone of metarterioles determines most (80%) of the systemic resistance, and changes in metarteriolar tone redistribute blood flow. Some organs, particularly brain, heart and kidney, have an intrinsic ability (autoregulation) to regulate their blood flow in the face of changes in arteriolar tone. The capillary beds comprise the largest area of the vascular system and the site of nutrient exchange between blood and cells. Changes in capillary hydrostatic or oncotic pressure cause changes in fluid movement across capillary membranes, with increases in hydrostatic or decreases in oncotic pressures promoting loss of fluid to the interstitium. In shock, arteriovenous connections allow blood to bypass the capillary bed. The venous system normally contains about 65% of the total blood volume, as veins store large quantities of blood that can be made available to the remainder of the circulation. This capacity is exploited in shock therapy when large volumes of fluid are administered rapidly. Venoconstriction causes an increase in venous return to the heart.

Vasoconstriction

Hypotension initiates a vasoconstrictive response within 30 seconds, as sympathetic reflex responses are mediated through baroreceptors in the thorax and central nervous system receptors. Within 10 minutes, angiotensin and vasopressin begin to contribute to vasoconstriction and to conservation of salt and water by the kidneys. Over the next few hours, as capillary hydrostatic pressure decreases, reabsorption of interstitial fluid and stimulation of thirst contribute to complete restoration of vascular volume. The vasoconstrictive response supports life in the short term, but puts some organs at risk. Arteriolar vasoconstriction redistributes flow to the cerebral and coronary circulation, which in combination with intrinsic autoregulation, favours perfusion of the heart and brain. At the same time, it severely decreases flow to splanchnic, muscle and skin vascular beds.

Vasodilation

Infectious agents and/or their toxins, trauma and ischaemia can damage cells. Any severe cellular insult can initiate a systemic inflammatory response in which cells produce mediators that change the extracellular environment. Vasodilation is one sign of the presence of systemic inflammation. Tissue perfusion is compromised and venous return is decreased when blood pools in the capillary beds. Improvement in blood volume can restore tissue perfusion, provided that adequate forward flow is maintained.

IRREVERSIBLE SHOCK

If the state of shock is sufficiently severe and prolonged, irreversible cell damage occurs and treatment will be unsuccessful. Processes contributing to irreversible shock include:

* Decreased coronary blood flow that damages the myocardium and causes decreased cardiac output, further compromising coronary blood flow
* Decreased blood flow to the vasomotor centres in the brain that impairs the vasoconstrictive response, resulting in further decreases in cerebral and coronary circulation
* Release of inflammatory mediators from cells damaged by shock that promote the production of more inflammatory mediators, thus causing more cell damage.

CARDIOVASCULAR ELEMENTS OF TISSUE PERFUSION

Deficits in tissue perfusion have important negative consequences on cell function, including energy deficits and stimulation of systemic inflammation. Restoration and maintenance of tissue perfusion are the primary goals of shock therapy. Figure 3.3 is a schematic representation of the cardiovascular elements that combine to provide adequate blood flow to cells (tissue perfusion). These cardiovascular elements are global parameters taken at one point in time and represent an average measure of multiple, interactive processes.

Cardiac output

Cardiac output is the volume of blood pumped by the heart each minute and is the product of heart rate and stroke volume. In the closed cardiovascular system, cardiac output cannot exceed venous return to the right ventricle.

Stroke volume

Stroke volume is the volume of blood ejected per heartbeat. It depends on preload, contractility and afterload.

Heart rate

Increased heart rates usually produce increased cardiac output. However, excessively fast heart rates allow insufficient time for ventricular filling and can result in decreased cardiac output. When heart rates are slow, cardiac output is partially maintained, as increased time for ventricular filling results in increased stroke volume. Pathologically slow heart rates do not allow sufficient beats per minute to maintain cardiac output.

Preload

Preload refers to the volume of blood in the ventricles at end-diastole. In a physiological sense, it depends on circulating volume, venous tone, atrial contraction and

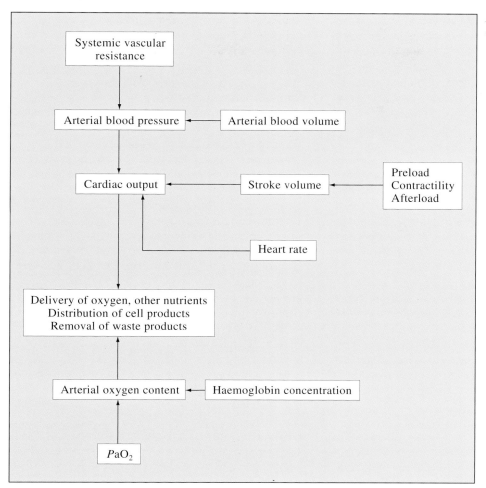

***Figure* 3.3:** *Cardiovascular elements of tissue perfusion.*

intrathoracic pressure. From a clinician's viewpoint, circulating volume and venous return are usually the most important and the most readily treated components of preload. Venous return depends on the state of the systemic venous circulation. Venoconstriction, induced by sympathetic stimulation, increases venous return and preload. Decreased venous tone (increased venous capacitance) reduces venous return.

Contractility
Contractility, the ability of cardiac myocytes to shorten during systole, reflects the ability of the heart to act as a pump. In shock, decreases in myocardial perfusion, sympathetic activation, acidosis and myocardial depressant factors have deleterious effects on contractility.

Afterload
Afterload refers to the forces that oppose myocardial muscle contraction and thereby ejection of blood from the ventricle.

Systemic vascular resistance
Resistance, the relationship between blood pressure and blood flow, is calculated rather than directly measured. Mean arterial pressure (*MAP*) is the arterial pressure,

averaged over time. Central venous pressure (*CVP*) is the pressure measured at the tip of a catheter placed in a jugular vein, usually positioned so that the tip is close to the heart. It represents right atrial pressure and reflects the filling pressure of the right ventricle. Cardiac output (*CO*) is the volume of blood pumped by the heart each minute. Systemic vascular resistance (*SVR*) is calculated as: $(MAP–CVP) \div CO$.

Arterial blood pressure
Cardiac output and systemic vascular resistance create arterial blood pressure. Pressures in the arteries reflect ventricular contractility and arterial resistance, with a small contribution from the viscosity of blood. While adequate blood pressure is required for blood flow, the presence of normal arterial blood pressure does not guarantee that adequate flow is occurring. For example, administration of α-adrenergic agonists to support blood pressure can create extreme vasoconstriction in some vascular beds. The resultant increase in overall vascular resistance can create adequate blood pressure but a decreased total systemic perfusion. On the other hand, low blood pressures do not necessarily mean that flow is not occurring, because tissue perfusion is determined by the difference between arterial blood pressure and intra-organ pressure. If intra-organ pressure is low,

then adequate flow can be obtained even with lower than normal arterial blood pressures. Blood pressure cannot be reliably estimated by digital palpation of the pulse because pulse quality (amplitude) reflects stroke volume and is not well correlated with arterial blood pressure. Arterial blood pressure can be measured by indirect or direct means, but it is often difficult to obtain these measurements in severely vasoconstricted shock patients.

Arterial oxygen content

The purpose of blood circulation is, in large part, to deliver oxygen to the tissues. The amount of oxygen contained in a volume of blood is a total of the oxygen carried bound to haemoglobin and that carried in a dissolved state in plasma. Of the two, by far the largest contribution to arterial oxygen content comes from haemoglobin.

Haemoglobin

Haemoglobin combines reversibly with oxygen. When all of the haemoglobin is combined with oxygen, the blood is fully saturated. The saturation of arterial blood (SaO_2) depends primarily on the partial pressure of oxygen (PaO_2). Under normal conditions arterial blood is about 97% saturated, i.e. 97% of the haemoglobin is combined with oxygen.

PaO_2

PaO_2 measures the tension of oxygen dissolved in physical solution in plasma, irrespective of the haemoglobin concentration. The PaO_2 determines the saturation of the haemoglobin molecule with oxygen. PaO_2 will be normal as long as the respiratory system is working properly. Severely anaemic patients will have a normal PaO_2 but a severely decreased arterial oxygen content, since there is little haemoglobin with which molecular oxygen can associate.

ENERGY DEFICIT IN SHOCK

Energy production

Shock is a cellular event with life-threatening consequences, many of which are due to a cellular energy deficit. Cellular processes depend on a supply of energy obtained from food and transferred to ATP (adenosine triphosphate). ATP is one of the most important molecules in nature, as it is the common currency of energy exchange. ATP provides energy for ion and metabolite transport, cellular motility, muscle contraction and anabolism. Life depends on its continual production and availability for use.

Aerobic metabolism

In aerobic metabolism, cells extract energy by oxidative combustion of foodstuff molecules, using oxygen as an electron acceptor, in a series of enzymatically controlled steps of oxidation–reduction that are built into the cell. Molecular oxygen is a perfect electron acceptor because

it has a high affinity for hydrogen and its electron, thus allowing liberation of the largest amount of free energy. This sequence allows complete oxidation of food and extraction of the maximum amount of energy.

Anaerobic metabolism

In anaerobic metabolism, cells use electron acceptors other than oxygen in the process of extracting energy from foodstuff molecules. Glycolysis is an anaerobic fermentation process that occurs in the cytosol and produces pyruvate or lactate, NADH and ATP. When the oxidative pathways in the mitochondrion have stopped because of lack of oxygen, pyruvate becomes the final electron acceptor and is reduced to lactate. This allows anaerobic glycolysis to proceed but only 2 mmol of ATP (instead of the potential 36 mmol during aerobic metabolism) are formed from each millimole of glucose.

In pathological states of decreased tissue perfusion such as shock, global energy production switches from efficient, mitochondrial based oxidative metabolism to inefficient, oxygen-independent, cytosol based glycolysis. This is a short-term and only partial solution to the problem of inadequate energy production caused by failure of oxygen delivery to cells. Additionally, the increase in lactate production can cause lactic acidosis (see 'Lactic acidosis').

Consequences of an energy deficit

The consequences of an energy deficit include:

*   Failure to maintain ionic gradients across cell membranes
*   Loss of the transmembrane potential
*   Intracellular accumulation of ions and water
*   Cell swelling and eventually, cell death.

Cell membranes are fitted with pumps (e.g. Na^+–K^+-ATPase) that maintain intracellular ionic concentrations and a transmembrane potential. Loss of energy for these pumps allows sodium and water to accumulate intracellularly, while potassium and magnesium are lost to the extracellular space. The transmembrane potential decreases. As sodium and water enter the cells, cell swelling causes changes in microfilament and microtubule function. The energy deficit causes mitochondrial dysfunction and decreased electron transport. As ischaemia persists, mitochondrial swelling worsens and lysosomal breakdown occurs. Terminally, structural integrity of the cell is lost due to breakdown of intracellular structures and the cell membrane.

THE SYSTEMIC INFLAMMATORY RESPONSE SYNDROME (SIRS) AND THE MULTIPLE ORGAN DYSFUNCTION SYNDROME (MODS)

Inflammation is, in general, a beneficial appropriate

response to injury, whether from ischaemia, trauma or infection. The redness, heat, swelling and pain that signal inflammation are caused by vasodilation, increased blood flow, increased capillary permeability and stimulation of nerve endings. These and many other changes are caused by inflammatory mediators that interact with cells to change cell function and intercellular communication. The inflammatory process is normally self-regulating and balanced between pro- and anti-inflammatory processes. It is essential to the control and eventual resolution of tissue damage.

In combination with an appropriately severe insult, tachycardia, tachypnoea, hyper- or hypothermia and leucocytosis or leucopenia indicate the presence of systemic inflammation. This may be an entirely appropriate response and one that is essential to control and resolution of the injury. However, if inflammation becomes excessive, or if the balance between pro- and anti-inflammatory processes is lost, cells distant from the original site can be damaged. Systemic inflammation becomes an amplifying cascade that interferes with the function of various organs, potentially causing their failure. In these circumstances, instead of being the solution, inflammation has become the problem. The same changes that would benefit damaged tissue can, when poorly regulated, cause microvascular injury, cardiac dysfunction, hypotension and shock. Organs distant from the site of original injury fail, a syndrome that has been named the multiple organ dysfunction syndrome (MODS).

Attempts have been made to define types of systemic inflammation with and without infection. The goal is to recognize the progression of systemic inflammation to multiple organ dysfunction, and to allow grouping of patients with similar disease so as to evaluate various therapies. An abbreviated version of those definitions is:

- Systemic inflammatory response syndrome (SIRS) — the systemic inflammatory response to a severe insult, including two or more of the following: tachycardia, tachypnoea, hyper- or hypothermia, leucocytosis or leucopenia
- Sepsis — SIRS with evidence of infection
- Severe sepsis — sepsis with evidence of organ dysfunction and evidence of hypoperfusion that responds to volume loading
- Septic shock — severe sepsis that requires both volume loading and inotropes to restore tissue perfusion
- Non-infectious SIRS progresses through similar stages to those described for severe SIRS and sterile shock.

The clinician concerned with the management of individual patients already recognizes that the sickest patients are the most likely to die. These definitions do not necessarily contribute additional information. However, this author considers the concept of the systemic inflammatory response to be of primary importance in explaining how any severe insult can lead to an amplifying and dysregulated cascade of tissue damaging events that eventually leads to failure of multiple organs and death.

Mediators of inflammation

The inflammatory cascade is a mediator driven, complex, overlapping system with a high degree of redundancy. An inflammatory mediator may induce a cell to:

- Elaborate a receptor
- Shed a receptor
- Secrete a mediator
- Adhere to another cell
- Release an enzyme
- Enhance its usual function
- Perform a new function.

Some mediators induce mostly pro-inflammatory activities, others mostly anti-inflammatory activities. Some mediators may elicit different effects at different times, stimulating or suppressing the same cell depending on circumstances. This effect has been likened to that of a toggle switch. Mediators may suppress, stimulate, or have no effect on their own production or on that of other mediators. Cells once stimulated to produce inflammatory mediators may respond to a second insult with much greater production of these mediators. It is beyond the scope of this chapter to discuss any but a few representative examples of inflammatory mediators. The reader is referred to the list of references at the end of this chapter for a more complete discussion of the inflammatory process.

Cytokines

Cytokines are polypeptides produced by macrophages and many other cells in response to cell injury. Tumour necrosis factor (TNF) and interleukin 1 are major pro-inflammatory cytokines that promote cellular proliferation, endothelial adhesion, vascular permeability and intravascular coagulation, as well as producing clinical signs of anorexia, hypotension and fever. Other members of the large family of interleukins, such as interleukin 10, have anti-inflammatory activity. An important effect of cytokines is their ability to induce activity of other inflammatory mediators, such as eicosanoids and nitric oxide.

Eicosanoids

Prostaglandins, thromboxanes and leucotrienes are produced by the metabolism of arachidonic acid. Thromboxanes produce hypotension but increase pulmonary vascular resistance. Some prostaglandins are required for maintenance of normal vascular tone and the anti-thrombotic state of vascular endothelium. Leucotrienes decrease blood pressure and increase vascular permeability. Understanding the widespread effects of eicosanoids is important in making therapeutic decisions. For example, non-steroidal anti-inflammatory drugs (NSAIDs) decrease production of prostaglandins and can adversely alter renal blood flow and gastric mucosal integrity.

Kinins

Bradykinin is a peptide mediator that promotes nitric oxide-induced hypotension. It also causes a change in shape of vascular endothelial cells and increases vascular permeability. These changes are prominent in anaphylaxis.

Complement

The products of the complement cascade increase vascular permeability and decrease systemic vascular resistance.

Other mediators

Platelet activating factor increases platelet and neutrophil aggregation. Interferon activates B cells, neutrophils and macrophages. Transforming growth factor promotes cell repair.

Adhesion molecules

Intercellular adhesion molecules (ICAM), integrins and selectins mediate the adhesion of endothelial cells and leucocytes. They are important in the delivery of leucocytes to areas of inflammation. However, they can also promote inappropriate aggregation of leucocytes and cause microvascular obstruction.

Nitric oxide

Nitric oxide (NO) is a gas produced by vascular endothelium and is the final mediator of vasodilation and a regulator of normal vasomotor tone. It also inhibits platelet aggregation and contributes to the normal anti-thrombotic property of vascular endothelium. Normally, NO is produced in pulses. Inflammation induces continuous production of large amounts of NO, which can cause excessive vasodilation and vascular hyporeactivity to vasoconstrictors.

Multiple organ dysfunction syndrome

When inflammation becomes systemic, organs, tissues and systems distant from the site of the original insult can be damaged. Commonly involved are the vascular endothelium, lungs, kidney, heart, liver and the blood clotting system. The number of organs that are malfunctioning is inversely correlated with survival in critically ill patients. Prevention, when possible, is preferred over waiting until dysfunction is evident and then attempting to revive a failing organ. Following are three representative examples of organ failure caused by ischaemia and systemic inflammation. Specific management of these and other organ failure syndromes common in emergency patients is discussed in more detail in other sections of this text.

Acute lung injury and acute respiratory distress syndrome

Acute lung injury (ALI) is the clinical state of impairment of pulmonary gas exchange that follows acute injury to the alveolar capillary membrane. In its most severe form, it is called the acute respiratory distress syndrome (ARDS). The pathophysiology of ALI/ARDS is inflammatory mediator-related damage to the capillary membrane that allows exudation of fluid from the vascular space and its accumulation in the alveoli. Clinical indications that ARDS is occurring include:

- Thoracic radiographs showing bilaterally symmetrical alveolar filling without evidence of left heart failure
- PaO_2/FiO_2 ratio of <200, where FiO_2 is the fractional concentration of oxygen in inspired gas.

Shock is a major risk factor for the development of ALI. Treatment of the shock state and any underlying cause of shock are of primary importance in the prevention of ALI.

Acute renal failure

Acute renal failure in shock may be caused by ischaemia secondary to decreased renal perfusion (pre-renal) or by mediator-related damage to renal cells. Drugs that impair renal perfusion also contribute to renal failure. Catecholamines and NSAIDs are commonly implicated. Adrenaline, particularly in high doses, can cause profound renal vasoconstriction. NSAIDs reduce the synthesis of renal vasodilatory prostaglandins. Prevention of acute renal failure by prompt restoration of renal perfusion is of paramount importance. Urine output is a measure of kidney perfusion and should be closely monitored in all shock patients.

Disseminated intravascular coagulopathy (DIC)

The normal anti-thrombotic properties of vascular endothelium can be severely impaired by the actions of inflammatory mediators released in shock. Inappropriate and widespread activation of the coagulation cascade results in the formation of microthrombi that obstruct blood flow and further compromise tissue perfusion. Consumption of platelets and coagulation factors can lead to bleeding. DIC is always secondary to a primary disease and is common in shock patients. Prompt restoration and maintenance of adequate tissue perfusion and treatment of the underlying cause are the best preventive measures.

TREATMENT OF SHOCK

General considerations

The best outcome is achieved by the application of a therapeutic plan that addresses all aspects of the disease.

Treatment is directed toward the underlying cause, as well as the multi-system consequences of the initiating event. In critically ill patients such as shock patients, there are no unimportant problems. Therapy must be directed toward all aspects of the disease, but must be prioritized to manage the most life-threatening aspects first. If the patient is not breathing or the heart is not beating effectively, cardiopulmonary cerebral resuscitation is the first priority (see Chapter 17). If the patient is in shock, but also has life-threatening breathing or airway problems, management of the respiratory emergency takes precedence over volume restoration (see Chapter 5). Pre-existing problems, especially cardiac disease, may limit the ability of volume restoration to improve tissue perfusion. Once initial resuscitation has been achieved, ongoing management and careful monitoring should continue.

Special considerations

Cardiogenic shock
Treatment of cardiogenic shock is directed toward improving myocardial contractility, reducing afterload and/or preload and controlling serious arrhythmias (see Chapter 4). In some patients, heart disease may not be the primary cause of shock, but may compromise the effectiveness of the heart as a pump and limit the application of volume restoration therapy. This is always a concern when applying volume restoration therapy for shock, because the pre-existing status of the heart is usually not known. However, most dogs and cats presented in shock do not have serious pre-existing heart disease. The author usually elects to treat with volume restoration unless there are specific indications (heart murmur, abnormal lung auscultation) that the patient will be volume intolerant. Careful continuous monitoring of cardiovascular and pulmonary status and appropriate adjustment of therapy is fundamental for all shock patients.

Hypovolaemic, traumatic and distributive shock
Treatment of the underlying cause of these types of shock, while beyond the scope of this chapter, is essential to the long-term outcome and, especially regarding control of bleeding, essential to the short-term outcome as well. Resuscitation from these types of shock is primarily directed toward volume restoration.

Endpoints of resuscitation
The goal of shock therapy is to restore tissue perfusion by increasing intravascular volume and consequently increasing venous return, stroke volume, cardiac output and delivery of oxygen and other nutrients to cells (see Figure 3.3). Therefore, therapeutic goals (endpoints) of resuscitation should be readily available observations or measurements that are relevant to tissue perfusion. An ideal endpoint would be a parameter that unequivocally reflected tissue perfusion at every level, was per-

fectly correlated with outcome and could be easily measured in the clinical setting. Such an endpoint has not yet been identified.

Lacking a perfect endpoint, the author uses the following parameters related to cardiovascular status and tissue perfusion.

Clinical signs related to intravascular volume and vasomotor tone (see Figure 3.2):

- Mental state
- Mucous membrane colour
- Capillary refill time
- Heart rate
- Pulse quality
- Extremity temperature.

Parameters related to tissue perfusion:

- Blood lactate
- Urine output
- Base deficit.

There are obviously limits to these parameters, since they are global measurements and can represent a sum of opposing processes. Adequate tissue perfusion at every level may not be achieved even if these global endpoints are met. However, these appear to be the best endpoints available at the current level of knowledge. Other parameters related to tissue perfusion, such as central venous pressure and arterial blood pressure, can also be used as endpoints.

Although not a specific endpoint of resuscitation, treatment of the underlying cause of shock is an essential goal of therapy. Outcome is closely related to the ability of treatment to restore all tissues to normal.

Supranormal oxygen delivery
Some have proposed that one important goal of therapy should be to achieve supranormal oxygen delivery. The justification for this approach is that during the period of shock an oxygen debt accrued, due to mismatch between oxygen delivery and oxygen demand. A period of supranormal oxygen delivery is a means of correcting this debt. This approach resulted in improved survival in some groups of critically ill patients. A recent meta-analysis of seven studies in this area concluded that there was insufficient evidence to recommend this strategy in a group of unselected patients (Heyland *et al.*, 1996). Overall, it appears that survival may be improved in some groups of patients if supranormal oxygen delivery is achieved by optimizing vascular volume, but not if persistent use of vasopressors is required to achieve this goal.

Gastric intramucosal pH
The perfusion of gut mucosa is likely to be decreased in shock, and decreased splanchnic perfusion often persists after apparently adequate resuscitation to global

endpoints. Because gut intramucosal pH (pHi) falls below normal when perfusion is inadequate, a decreased pHi is a potentially valuable tissue-specific marker for perfusion. Published reports have shown variable correlation between pHi (measured by tonometry) and other measures of tissue perfusion. Anecdotal reports indicate that the technique can be moderately difficult to implement in clinical patients. pHi is not commonly measured in veterinary patients at this time.

Endpoints in uncontrolled abdominal bleeding due to trauma

In the special circumstance of uncontrolled abdominal bleeding secondary to penetrating trauma, a delay in volume restoration until bleeding is controlled has been proposed (Bickell *et al.*, 1994a). This approach should be used with caution if control of abdominal haemorrhage cannot be achieved in a short time (less than 1 hour). While a decrease in hydrostatic pressure may decrease blood loss, failure to restore tissue perfusion can damage cells and lead to organ failure and death. Moderate resuscitation (rather than no resuscitation) has been recommended (Smail *et al.*, 1998) and is the author's usual choice in these patients.

Fluid therapy: choosing a fluid

Appropriate fluids for resuscitation of shock are isotonic, or nearly isotonic, crystalloids (Na^+ 130–154 mEq/l) with or without the addition of colloids, or hypertonic saline. Clinically applicable, scientific proof that one of these fluids is better than another would be in the form of prospective, randomized, controlled clinical trials containing large numbers (hundreds) of patients with similar shock states. Many such trials have been done in human patients, particularly in traumatic and haemorrhagic shock. Randomized controlled clinical trials of this scope are uncommon in veterinary medicine. A recent review (Schierhout and Roberts, 1998) of randomized controlled trials in human patients examined the effect of fluid choice (crystalloids or colloids) on mortality. In 19 trials studying over 1300 human patients, the risk of death was slightly higher (24 versus 20%) in the group given colloids. Considering these and other trials, it appears that crystalloids and colloids are nearly equivalent in effect, when titrated to the same endpoints.

Isotonic crystalloids expand the entire extracellular space (intravascular and interstitial). While the intravascular expansion is welcome, the interstitial expansion can sometimes, but certainly not always, be a problem. The interstitium is a compliant structure. Among its many functions is to act as a reservoir from which fluid can be drawn into the vascular space in time of need. Moderate increases in interstitial volume can be a safety factor protecting against post-resuscitation hypovolaemia. Severe interstitial oedema can impair delivery of oxygen and other nutrients to cells by increasing the diffusion distance for these substances.

The pretreatment state of the interstitial volume (decreased, normal or increased) is a guide to fluid selection. Restoration of a depleted interstitial volume with isotonic crystalloids is essential and failure to do so can lead to repeat episodes of hypovolaemia. Expansion of a normal interstitium may, or may not, have adverse effects. Concern is often expressed about expansion of the interstitial space in the lung and resultant alveolar oedema, caused by administration of large volumes of isotonic crystalloids. This has been addressed in a canine shock model, which found that large volume resuscitation with isotonic crystalloid did not increase lung water or impair gas exchange (Bickell *et al.*, 1994a). The normal lung has a large 'oedema safety factor', partly because it is well supplied with lymphatics. Expansion of lung interstitium does not necessarily mean that alveolar flooding will occur. The sudden appearance of alveolar flooding in shock patients is not necessarily due to over-expansion of lung interstitium. It is now recognized to be part of ARDS.

A marked to severe increase in interstitial volume (oedema), or a high risk for developing it, is a specific indication for choosing colloids, or hypertonic saline, for resuscitation. The risk of over-expansion of the interstitium with isotonic crystalloid resuscitation is high in patients with low pretreatment albumin.

As with any drug, clinicians develop preferences based on individual experiences. Such preferences are useful reflections of experience but are also subject to the errors inherent in anecdotal reports. There are probably more differences between patients than between the effects of the commonly used resuscitation fluids. Careful continuous monitoring of the shock patient is the best guide to determining the appropriateness of the fluid selection. A detailed discussion of fluid types is presented in Chapter 2. Some special considerations for fluid use in resuscitation of shock include:

- Isotonic crystalloids
    Readily available, inexpensive
    Repair both intravascular and interstitial deficits
    Large volumes are required
    May cause interstitial oedema if amounts used are excessive relative to the capacity of the interstitial space.
- Colloids
    More expensive than crystalloids
    Primarily repair intravascular, not interstitial, deficits
    Volumes required for equivalent endpoints are less than for isotonic crystalloids
    Specifically indicated if patient has low albumin or over-expansion of the interstitial space
    May cause bleeding disorders if given in large amounts.

- Hypertonic saline
    Inexpensive
    Temporarily redistributes volume from the interstitial and intracellular spaces to the intravascular space
    Very small volumes are required for initial resuscitation
    Isotonic crystalloids and/or colloids are usually also required
    Multiple effects on immune system activity and vasomotor tone.

Fluid therapy: volume and rate

The author's usual starting dose of fluids in treatment of shock is:

- Isotonic crystalloids
    Dog: 45–90 ml/kg
    Cat: 20–40 ml/kg
- Colloids
    Dog: 10–20 ml/kg
    Cat: 5–10 ml/kg
- Hypertonic saline (7.5%)
    Dog or cat: 5 ml/kg

Rate of fluid administration

The desired rate of administration of fluids to treat shock is, quite simply, as rapidly as possible. Intravenous catheters of the largest diameter and shortest length practicable allow for the most rapid flow rates. Additional increases in flow rate can be achieved by enclosing the fluid bag in a pressure bag that is then inflated with air to apply pressure to the fluid delivery system. One litre of fluid can be delivered in approximately 7 minutes with this system. For large patients, multiple peripheral catheters should be placed, so as to maximize the amount of fluid delivered within the initial resuscitation period.

If collapse of veins makes it difficult to place a venous catheter, an intraosseous catheter should be inserted (see Chapter 23). Because it may be difficult to achieve high flow rates through an intraosseous catheter, initial resuscitation with hypertonic saline may be preferred.

If improvement in the endpoints of resuscitation is not achieved at the end of the initial fluid bolus, a repeat bolus of the same amount should be considered. If isotonic crystalloids are used, a decrease in vascular volume is expected following initial resuscitation, as redistribution occurs across the extracellular space. With colloids, a more steady state of vascular volume expansion is expected. Hypertonic saline has only a transitory effect and follow-up therapy with isotonic crystalloid or colloid is usually necessary.

Blood transfusion

Oxygen content and delivery of oxygen to tissues cannot be maintained without adequate haemoglobin concentration. The minimum acceptable packed cell volume (PCV) in shock patients has not been established. If there is no evidence to the contrary, it is safest to assume that the patient is not well adapted to anaemia, and the PCV should be maintained above 18% in cats and above 25% in dogs. It is desirable to administer blood slowly over several hours. However, the author often infuses blood at the fastest rate possible in shock patients, when circumstances demand. Usually the blood transfusion is administered simultaneously with other fluids in order to support vascular volume.

The transition plan

When the initial endpoints of resuscitation have been achieved, these parameters may thereafter oscillate within a range of normal, or deteriorate. Initial success in resuscitation cannot be assumed to be a complete resolution of the problem of shock. Tissue perfusion must not only be restored, it must be maintained. Often the initial resuscitation plan, or a modification of it, must be repeated several times before the patient's condition is stabilized. Close monitoring provides for early detection of deterioration of endpoints, so that therapeutic interventions can be made in a timely manner.

Metabolic acidosis and base deficit

Metabolic acidosis is common in shock patients. Adverse effects of a decrease in pH with particular importance in shock patients include:

- Decreased cardiac contractility and heart rate; arrhythmias
- Arteriolar dilation and venoconstriction
- Increase in rate and depth of respiration (Kussmaul respiration)
- Renal sodium and potassium wasting.

Base deficit is calculated from the arterial blood gas and is an approximation of global tissue acidosis. An increase in base deficit is usually, but not always, associated with increased blood lactate. Both parameters, base deficit and blood lactate, address the same issue of tissue perfusion and therefore their normalization is an appropriate endpoint of resuscitation.

Lactic acidosis

Increased blood lactate concentration is significant in shock patients because it is a marker of decreased tissue perfusion, and because high levels are correlated with decreased survival. Lactate is obtained from anaerobic glycolysis. Lactate and H^+ production can be substantially increased in shock because of the increase in anaerobic glycolysis and ATP hydrolysis. Lactic acid accumulates intracellularly and diffuses out of the cell into the extracellular space where it causes an equimolar decrease in bicarbonate concentration. The resultant acidosis contributes to the metabolic acidosis that is common in shock. There is sometimes a poor correlation between the presence of acidaemia and blood lactate concentration. Simultaneous counteracting processes tending to produce alkalaemia may mask the presence of an acidaemia. Direct measurement of lactate in blood is the best means of detecting lactic acidosis. Limitations of availability and the technical requirements of this test may make this determination difficult to obtain in some circumstances.

When oxygen delivery is restored, the liver can metabolize lactate. A high blood lactate level, that persists after apparently adequate resuscitation, indicates that tissue perfusion has not been restored. This is a legitimate indicator of a poor prognosis in a shock patient. Blood lactate levels should begin to decline within 15–30 minutes after successful resuscitation.

Treatment of metabolic acidosis in shock patients

Metabolic acidosis in shock patients is primarily due to decreased tissue perfusion and is best corrected by directing therapy toward restoration of blood flow to all tissues. Bicarbonate therapy may also be used, especially if acidaemia is severe (see Chapter 12).

Urine output

Since renal vasoconstriction (and decreased urine output) is an appropriate response to hypovolaemia, sufficient preload must be established before the adequacy of urine output can be evaluated. A central venous pressure of about 10 cm H_2O, mean arterial blood pressure >80 mmHg and absence of peripheral vasoconstriction indicate that preload is adequate. Under these conditions, and in the absence of any other source of fluid losses, urine output should be only slightly less than fluid input.

Because urine output is such a good indicator of perfusion of a local, and vital, tissue bed (the kidney), the establishment of adequate urine output is an excellent endpoint of resuscitation. Therefore, urine output should be closely monitored, usually by placing a urinary catheter and closed collection system, in all shock patients.

Vasopressors

The goal of fluid therapy in shock is to support adequate tissue perfusion without the need for vasopressor therapy. Pulse quality, or amplitude of the pulse, is related to stroke volume and is not well correlated with arterial blood pressure. Therefore, blood pressure cannot be reliably estimated from digital palpation of a peripheral artery. In shock patients, vasopressors are usually not administered unless significant hypotension, determined by direct or indirect blood pressure measurement, persists after adequate volume resuscitation. If a vasopressor is needed, an agent that causes minimal peripheral vasoconstriction such as dobutamine (5–15 mg/kg/min) or dopamine (3–10 mg/kg/min)

should be used, monitoring the effect with frequent or continuous blood pressure measurement.

Anaphylactic shock

In addition to fluid therapy, treatment with adrenaline is of proven efficacy in anaphylactic shock. For life-threatening reactions, adrenaline should be given intravenously (0.01–0.02 mg/kg). Further discussion of the use of α-agonists is provided in Chapter 17.

Antibiotic therapy

Specific indications for antibiotics in shock patients include direct evidence of a bacterial infection, such as sepsis and septic shock, or penetrating trauma. Often the clinician simply has a concern that infection, especially of gut origin, might develop. One of the most important barriers to bacterial translocation from the gut to the systemic circulation is the presence of facultative anaerobes on the mucosal surface. These are quite susceptible to antibiotics and their destruction has been shown to promote bacterial translocation. Because of this effect, antibiotics administered for prophylaxis may increase bacterial translocation, possibly predisposing a patient to infection.

Even in the absence of known infection, intravenous broad-spectrum antibiotic therapy is indicated in shock patients who are febrile, have bloody diarrhoea, or have substantially increased or decreased neutrophil counts. The risks and benefits of antibiotic therapy, in the absence of known infection, are very difficult to define in this patient group.

Reperfusion injury

The univalent reduction of oxygen forms reactive oxygen intermediates (ROI) such as superoxide ion, hydrogen peroxide and the hydroxyl radical. Under ischaemic conditions, cells accumulate abnormal concentrations of cytosolic calcium and iron. This provides a source of substrate for the generation of superoxide and hydroxyl radicals when cells are reperfused. The significance of these reactive oxygen intermediates is their reactivity. They damage cell membranes, proteins and nucleic acids. Scavengers of oxygen radicals include mannitol, dimethylsulphoxide (DMSO), superoxide dismutase (SOD), vitamin E and 21 aminosteroids. Other treatments include inhibitors of oxygen radical production such as allopurinol (inhibits xanthine oxidase).

Immunoregulatory and mediator directed therapy

Corticosteroids

Corticosteroids have been extensively studied as therapy for septic shock. Preclinical data in animal models was positive when steroids were given before the shock state was induced. However, the clinical application of this research data has been disappointing, to say the least. Nine randomized controlled clinical trials in human patients have been published. A recent meta-analysis of these trials (Cronin *et al.*, 1995) concluded that there was no benefit to the administration of a short course of steroids (<48 hours) in septic patients. Moreover, there was a trend toward increasing mortality in some treated patients. Interest in the use of steroids in septic patients continues. Currently, studies are addressing the dose and timing of administration (low dose constant rate infusion over 5–10 days) as key issues in finding a place for these agents in the treatment of sepsis and septic shock (Bollaert *et al.*, 1998).

Tumour necrosis factor and interleukins, generated as part of the inflammatory response in shock, activate the hypothalamic–pituitary–adrenal (HPA) axis and cause an increased production of corticosteroids. In spite of the increased endogenous levels of corticosteroids, their effect at the cellular level may be diminished by receptor resistance and decreased extraction from the blood.

Corticosteroids suppress arachidonic acid metabolism and reduce the production of prostaglandins, thromboxane and leucotrienes. Adverse effects of corticosteroids include gastrointestinal ulceration and increased risk of infection. Both are major concerns in shock patients.

Corticosteroids are the most important modulator of the host defence response. At the current level of understanding, we do not know enough about the use of these potent agents in shock patients. The risk:benefit ratio cannot be properly identified without more information. In the absence of adequate data, advice about whether or not to use these drugs is mostly a matter of personal preference. With the exception of using them to counteract a severe allergic reaction in anaphylactic shock, the author's preference is to not use corticosteroids in shock patients.

Mediator directed therapy

The search for more effective therapy for shock, particularly for septic shock, is currently focused on development of therapies that modulate the inflammatory response, usually by suppressing it. Therapy directed against many inflammatory mediators has been studied extensively. The results of clinical trials have been disappointing in that no improvement in survival has been demonstrated when these agents are used. The clinical failures were most likely due to a combination of factors, including:

- Interference with the balance between pro- and anti-inflammatory cytokines
- Selection of patients with heterogeneous disease processes
- Inappropriate endpoint selection (survival may not be the best endpoint for certain therapies)
- Improper dose, route or timing of administration.

The reader is referred to a recent commentary (Vincent, 1998) and two scientific reports (Abraham *et al.*, 1998; van Dissel *et al.*, 1998) that illustrate the current work and challenges in this area of research.

Inflammatory mediators cause a wide variety of changes in cell function that are only crudely represented by clinical signs. The inflammatory process is complex, highly integrated and, at present, incompletely understood. It contains both pro- and anti-inflammatory processes, both of which, when properly regulated, are essential to eventual recovery. Due to the incomplete knowledge in this area, it is not possible to determine the need of an individual for external regulation of the inflammatory response. Therefore, it is also not possible to predict whether a mediator directed therapy will be helpful or injurious. It is most likely that the same therapy might be helpful at one point in time and injurious at another.

REFERENCES AND FURTHER READING

Abraham E *et al.* (1998) Double-blind randomised controlled trial of monoclonal antibody to human tumour necrosis factor in treatment of septic shock. *Lancet* **351**, 929–933

Astiz ME and Rackow EC (1998) Septic shock. *Lancet* **351**, 1501–1505

Bickell WH, Barrett SM, Romine-Jenkins M, Hull SS Jr and Kinasewitz GT (1994a) Resuscitation of canine haemorrhagic hypotension with large-volume isotonic crystalloid: impact on lung water, venous admixture, and systemic arterial oxygen saturation. *American Journal of Emergency Medicine* **12**, 36–42

Bickell WH, Wall MJ Jr, Pepe PE, Martin RR, Ginger VF, Allen MK and Mattox KL (1994b) Immediate versus delayed fluid resuscitation for hypotensive patients with penetrating torso injuries. *New England Journal of Medicine* **331**, 1105–1109

Bishop MH, Shoemaker WC, Appel PL *et al.* (1995) Prospective randomized trial of survivor values of cardiac index, oxygen delivery, and oxygen consumption as resuscitation endpoints in severe trauma. *Journal of Trauma* **38**, 780–787

Bollaert P-E, Charpentier C, Levy B, Debouverie M, Audibert G and Larcan A (1998) Reversal of late septic shock with supraphysiologic doses of hydrocortisone. *Critical Care Medicine* **26**, 645–650

Cronin L, Cook DJ, Carlet J, Heyland DK, King D, Lansang MA and Fisher CJ Jr (1995) Corticosteroid treatment for sepsis: a critical appraisal and meta-analysis of the literature. *Critical Care Medicine* **23**, 1430–1439

Dinarello CA (1997) Pro-inflammatory and anti-inflammatory cytokines as mediators in the pathogenesis of septic shock. *Chest* **112**, 321S–329S

Heyland DK, Cook DJ, King D, Kernerman P and Brun-Buisson C (1996) Maximizing oxygen delivery in critically ill patients: a methodologic appraisal of the evidence. *Critical Care Medicine* **24**, 517–524

Hoyt DB (1998) Immune regulation with hypertonic saline in trauma patients. *Proceedings of the Society of Critical Care Medicine 27th Educational & Scientific Symposium.* Postgraduate Review Course, pp. 32–33

Members of the American College of Chest Physicians/Society of Critical Care Medicine Consensus Conference Meeting (1992) Definitions for sepsis and organ failure and guidelines for the use of innovative therapies in sepsis. *Critical Care Medicine* **20**, 864–874

Schierhout G and Roberts I (1998) Fluid resuscitation with colloid or crystalloid solutions in critically ill patients: a systematic review of randomised trials. *British Medical Journal* **316**, 961–964

Smail N, Wang P, Cioffi WG, Bland KI and Chaudry IH (1998) Resuscitation after uncontrolled venous haemorrhage: does increased resuscitation volume improve regional perfusion? *Journal of Trauma* **44**, 701–708

van Dissel JT, van Langevelde P, Westendorp RGJ, Kwappenberg K and Frolich M (1998) Anti-inflammatory cytokine profile and mortality in febrile patients. *Lancet* **351**, 950–953

Vincent JL (1998) Search for effective immunomodulating strategies against sepsis. *Lancet* **351**, 922–923

CHAPTER FOUR

Cardiovascular Emergencies

Rebecca L. Stepien

Emergencies of the cardiovascular system may involve primary abnormalities of the heart or extra-cardiac abnormalities that have a direct effect on cardiac function. Primary cardiac abnormalities include impaired function or damage to the heart muscle (e.g. cardiomyopathies or thoracic trauma), abnormal flow patterns within the heart (e.g. valvular regurgitation) or primary rhythm abnormalities (e.g. ventricular tachycardia). Extra-cardiac abnormalities affecting cardiac output may include pericardial effusion, systemic hypertension, thrombosis, or metabolic abnormalities, especially those involving electrolyte disorders.

PHYSICAL ASSESSMENT OF THE CARDIOVASCULAR SYSTEM

Emergency presentation of patients with clinical signs of cardiovascular disease usually involves quick but thorough assessment and rapid, decisive action. Recognition of clinical signs and physical findings as typical of various cardiovascular abnormalities should lead to ancillary cardiac testing. Most critically ill patients have changes in cardiovascular findings compared to normal animals, but it is crucial to differentiate whether cardiac abnormalities are the cause or the result of clinical signs. Clinical findings with possible cardiovascular and non-cardiovascular causes are listed in Figure 4.1.

Physical examination
Physical examination of the critically ill cardiac patient involves subjective assessment of physical findings and rapid accumulation of data (Figure 4.2). Typical historical findings include dyspnoea, collapse, syncope, cough, cyanosis or signs of peripheral thromboembolism (primarily in cats). When historical and physical examination findings are supportive of cardiovascular disease, further cardiovascular testing is warranted if the patient is stable enough to tolerate manipulation.

Electrocardiography
Electrocardiograms (ECGs) are crucial in the diagnosis and therapy of cardiac dysrhythmias. All unstable emergency patients should have an ECG recorded as a baseline assessment, regardless of suspected illness. Tachycardia accompanied by weak pulses due to hypovolaemic shock may be indistinguishable from the same findings caused by ventricular tachycardia, yet ventricular tachycardia requires treatment with anti-dysrhythmic medications, whereas sinus tachycardia due to shock-related hypotension usually resolves with therapy of the underlying problem. Animals with accelerated idioventricular rhythm, second degree heart block or junctional tachycardia due to digitalis intoxication may each have heart rates within accepted normal ranges, but recognition of these abnormalities may provide critical information regarding the diagnosis.

In stable patients, a baseline ECG recording is recommended to provide evidence of admission status for comparison in case of later development of dysrhythmias. If cardiovascular disease is suspected, the ECG provides not only a quick assessment of rhythm status, but also provides information regarding conduction abnormalities and cardiac size.

ECG recording in the critically ill patient should involve as little patient stress as possible. Lead 2 ECG recordings are usually adequate for rhythm diagnosis, but multiple leads may be necessary to confirm the presence of P waves, or to better recognize rhythm disorders in patients with smaller complexes than usual. Recordings may be taken with the patient in any position; sternal recumbency is often the most comfortable for dyspnoeic patients. Electrocardiographic coupling gel, rather than alcohol (e.g. spirits), should be used to moisten the lead contact points to avoid inadvertent ignition should emergency use of defibrillation paddles become necessary.

Arterial blood pressure
Arterial blood pressure (ABP) measurement is useful in the initial assessment of cardiovascular function. Methods of blood pressure measurement are discussed in Chapter 16. Indirect blood pressure measurement systems (e.g. Doppler sphygmomanometric or oscillometric methods) are useful to document high blood pressure in patients with systemic hypertension, but are less useful in hypotensive patients where repeatable detection of a distal limb pulse may be difficult. Invasive methods of monitoring blood pressure involve

Clinical finding	Possible cardiac causes	Possible systemic causes
Dyspnoea	Pulmonary oedema Pleural effusion Pericardial effusion	Primary respiratory disease Airway obstruction Pulmonary thromboembolism Acid–base disorders Pain/anxiety
Cough (dogs)	Left atrial enlargement Severe pulmonary oedema	Primary respiratory disease Airway disorders
Cough (cats)	Rarely associated with CHF	Primary respiratory disease Feline asthma
Cyanosis	Severe pulmonary oedema Right-to-left shunt (congenital heart disease)	Airway obstruction Severe respiratory disease Methaemoglobinaemia
Ascites	Right-sided CHF Caudal vena cava obstruction	Hypoproteinaemia Portal hypertension Peritonitis Peritoneal haemorrhage
Heart murmur	Valvular disease Myocardial disease Congenital heart defects	Anaemia (PCV <25%) 'Innocent' murmurs (dogs <16 weeks old) Pyrexia
Sinus tachycardia	Hypotension due to CHF	Dehydration Pyrexia or hyperthermia Anaemia Shock/blood loss Pain/anxiety
Syncope or collapse	Dysrhythmias Inappropriate drug therapy Pericardial effusion	Hypoglycaemia Electrolyte disorders Anaemia Neurological disorders Musculoskeletal abnormalities
Ectopic tachycardias	Primary myocardial disorder/trauma Myocardial hypoxia	Systemic hypoxia Acid–base disorders Electrolyte disorders Sepsis Drug toxicity Autonomic nervous system abnormalities
Bradycardia	Sick sinus syndrome Atrioventricular block	High vagal tone Hyperkalaemia or other electrolyte disturbances
Peripheral paresis	Systemic thromboembolism	Musculoskeletal abnormalities Neurological disorders
Peripheral oedema	Severe right-sided CHF	Hypoproteinaemia Vasculitis Lymphatic disorders

Figure 4.1: Cardiac and non-cardiac causes of abnormal cardiovascular clinical findings. The lists are not all-inclusive. CHF: congestive heart failure, PCV: packed cell volume.

Physical parameter	Cardiovascular disease
Heart rate and rhythm	Tachycardia or bradycardia Irregular rhythm accompanied by pulse deficits
Respiratory rate and character	Increased respiratory rate Dyspnoea or shallow breathing Panting (cats)
Thoracic auscultation — cardiac	Gallop rhythm Heart murmur Muffled heart sounds (pericardial effusion)
Thoracic auscultation — respiratory	Crackles Increased large airway sounds Muffled respiratory sounds (pleural effusion)
Abdominal assessment	Fluid wave or abdominal fluid distension accompanied by jugular distension Hepatomegaly
Peripheral vascular assessment	Weak or bounding pulses Pulse deficits Jugular distension Jugular pulsation Cyanosis Slow capillary refill time
Other	Peripheral paresis accompanied by pulselessness Peripheral oedema accompanied by other signs of right-sided or biventricular CHF

Figure 4.2: *Physical findings associated with cardiovascular disease. CHF: congestive heart failure.*

placement of an arterial catheter and are more accurate than indirect methods when blood pressure is low. The dorsal pedal artery is accessible and catheterizable in most dogs using local anaesthetic infiltration (e.g. lignocaine), while cats may require a femoral arterial surgical 'cut-down' to establish an arterial line. Once arterial access is established, baseline blood pressure is recorded and continuous monitoring can be used to measure blood pressure throughout therapy.

Hypotension may be defined as a *systolic* pressure of less than 90 mm Hg and a *mean arterial pressure* (MAP) below 65 mm Hg, in most dogs and cats. In animals with heart failure, maintenance of MAP in a range between 70 and 80 mm Hg provides decreased afterload, but adequate blood pressure to serve end organs. In the hypotensive heart failure patient, increases in blood pressure may be attained by administration of positive inotropes with or without addition of fluid therapy, while in the hypertensive patient decreases in blood pressure are achieved through the use of vasodilating drugs.

Central venous pressure

Central venous pressure (CVP) is used to estimate filling pressures on the right side of the heart (i.e. right atrial pressure). CVP is measured and monitored via a catheter placed in the cranial vena cava or right atrium via the jugular vein (see Chapter 16). Low CVP usually results from hypovolaemia, but increased CVP may result from increased intravascular volume and/or decreased cardiac output. CVP measurement can also be used to monitor volume status in non-cardiogenic shock patients through the use of an intravenous fluid challenge, but if cardiac disease is suspected or if initial CVP measurements are elevated, fluid boluses should be avoided.

Elevated CVP

Elevated CVP (reflecting elevated right atrial pressure) indicates failure of the right ventricle (RV) to adequately pump the volume of blood presented during ventricular filling. This may be due to increased intravascular volume (e.g. fluid overload) or right-sided cardiac abnormalities. In cardiac patients, elevated CVP may reflect RV inflow abnormalities (e.g. tricuspid valve insufficiency/stenosis or cardiac tamponade due to pericardial disease), primary myocardial disease, or RV outflow obstruction (e.g. pulmonic stenosis, pulmonary hypertension, pulmonary thromboembolism). Some abnormalities are co-existent (e.g. right-sided congestive heart failure (CHF) secondary to severe tricuspid insufficiency). Notably, pulmonary hypertension leading to elevations in CVP may be due to left ventricular failure and elevated left atrial pressure. CVP may therefore be serially monitored to judge the efficacy of therapy for left heart failure. CVP monitoring is not as sensitive to elevations in left atrial pressure as pulmonary capillary wedge pressure monitoring, but is easier to maintain in clinical veterinary patients. In cases of acute CHF, therapy involves controlled volume depletion of the patient; serial CVP measurement allows the clinician to follow decreases in right atrial pressure while avoiding excessive dehydration. Target CVP (in the acute CHF patient) to maintain optimal cardiac output without leading to fluid overload is approximately 10–15 cm H_2O or 7–11 mm Hg.

Decreased central venous pressure

Decreased CVP usually reflects hypovolaemia. When low CVP accompanies signs of low output (e.g. exercise intolerance or collapse, weak pulses, slow capillary refill time) in animals with heart disease but no congestive signs, low filling pressures as a contributing cause of low output is suspected. Serial CVP monitoring is used to document increases in right atrial pressure into the normal to slightly above normal range in response to fluid administration, in order to maximize ventricular filling.

Pulmonary artery wedge pressure

Pulmonary artery wedge pressure is measured using a balloon-tipped catheter in the main pulmonary artery. In veterinary patients, the catheter is usually introduced through a jugular vein and advanced into the right ventricle to the main pulmonary artery using typical pressure tracings or fluoroscopic guidance. When the balloon is deflated, the pressure measured is the main pulmonary artery pressure, but when the balloon is inflated and carried by blood flow to 'wedge' in a smaller pulmonary artery, the 'wedge pressure' recorded is roughly equal to left atrial pressure. Pulmonary artery wedge pressure measurements are an accurate reflection of left ventricular filling pressures and may be used to serially monitor the efficacy of CHF therapy in reducing left atrial pressure. In many clinical cases of acute CHF in veterinary patients, dyspnoea and patient anxiety are limiting factors for patient manipulation. In these cases, fast and accurate placement of a balloon-tipped catheter can be difficult. Since continuous monitoring of pulmonary artery wedge pressure is not commonly available in most veterinary clinics, other methods of monitoring will be emphasized here.

Arterial blood gas

Arterial blood gas analysis is helpful in the respiratory management of patients with dyspnoea due to CHF. Hypoxaemia (PaO_2 <80 mm Hg on room air), arterial desaturation as measured by pulse oximetry (arterial O_2 saturation <90% on room air) and hyperventilation ($PaCO_2$ <35 mm Hg) are consistent with respiratory impairment related to pulmonary oedema. In patients with fulminant pulmonary oedema, PaO_2 is frequently 40–60 mm Hg or less while the patient is breathing room air and hypoxia usually drives respiration, resulting in hyperventilation. Development of hypercarbia ($PaCO_2$ >45 mm Hg) is an ominous sign, reflecting profound (imminently life-threatening) pulmonary dysfunction and/or fatigue of the muscles of respiration. In these cases, assisted ventilation may be necessary.

Thoracic radiographs

Emergency radiography is covered in detail in Chapter 23. Acute pulmonary oedema is generally recognizable based on history and physical examination findings and the stress related to positioning an animal for radiographs may worsen its clinical condition. In most cases, anaesthesia for the purpose of taking radiographs is contraindicated, as most anaesthetic regimens have depressant effects on either the cardiovascular or the respiratory systems. In some cases, marginal amounts of pulmonary oedema can be worsened greatly by use of negatively inotropic anaesthetic regimens. Animals with severe dysrhythmias should never be anaesthetized until the rhythm has been stabilized. In general, while thoracic radiographs contribute greatly to diagnosis of the underlying disease and differentiation of cardiac disease from pulmonary disease, most cases of severe congestive heart failure can be diagnosed without immediate radiographs.

ACUTE HEART FAILURE: RECOGNITION AND MANAGEMENT

Algorithms for emergency patients in heart failure are presented in Figures 4.3 and 4.4. Immediate identification of key clinical signs indicative of pulmonary oedema, pleural effusion, low output failure, cardiac tamponade and severe dysrhythmias may be life-saving. Once the nature of the clinical presentation is recognized, emergency therapy may (and often must) proceed in the absence of an anatomical diagnosis of the underlying heart disease. Once the patient's condition is stable, further diagnostic testing may be used to establish the underlying cause and develop a definitive treatment plan. If signs of cardiogenic shock (i.e. tachycardia, cool extremities, weak pulses, prolonged capillary refill time) are present but congestive signs (e.g. pulmonary oedema or ascites) are not, low filling pressures secondary to hypovolaemia may be complicating the underlying cardiac disease.

Most animals presented to the emergency service do not arrive with a previous diagnosis and the unstable nature of many cardiovascular emergencies makes extensive diagnostic testing dangerous. The following

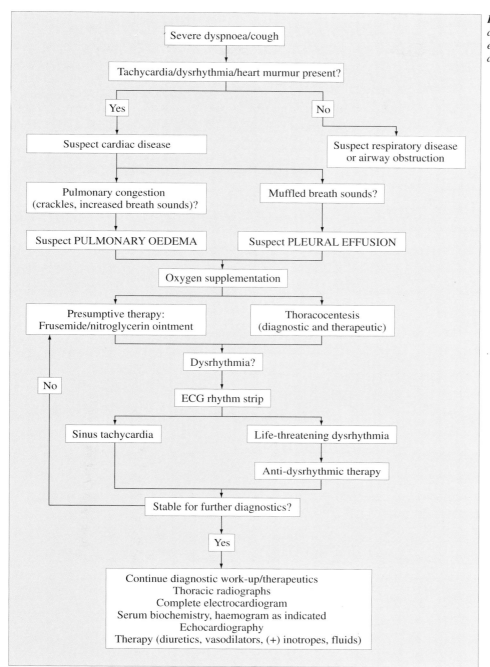

discussion outlines general approaches to the major presenting signs of dogs and cats with cardiovascular emergencies. Dosing regimens for commonly used drugs are outlined in Figure 4.5. Systemic hypertension (hypertensive crisis) and systemic thromboembolism are addressed separately.

Severe pulmonary oedema: recognition and emergency stabilization

Key points

- Recognition
    Dyspnoea ± gagging cough
    Pulmonary crackles/increased breath sounds on auscultation
    Other physical findings typical of cardiac disease.
- Therapy
    Oxygen supplementation
    Frusemide administration
    Vasodilator administration (with some exceptions)
    Opioid sedation
    Low stress environment.
- Typical underlying cardiac conditions
    Dilated cardiomyopathy (dog/cat)
    Mitral insufficiency secondary to progressive

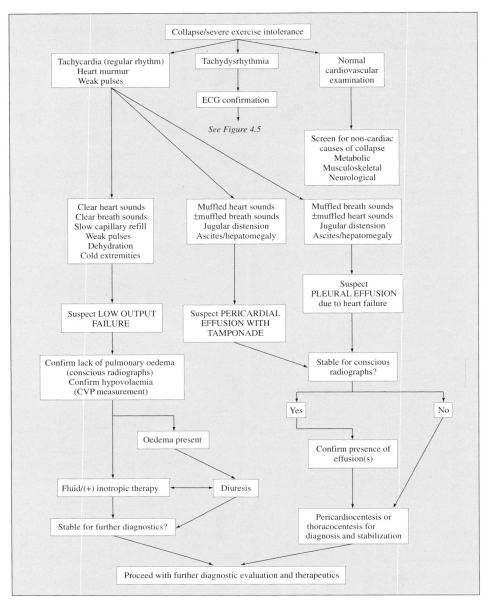

Figure 4.4: *Emergency diagnostic/therapeutic evaluation of the collapsed patient.*

endocardiosis or acute chordae tendineae rupture (dog)
Hypertrophic or restrictive cardiomyopathy (cat)
Decompensated congenital heart disease (e.g. patent ductus arteriosus, ventricular septal defect, mitral dysplasia, mitral stenosis (dog/cat)).

In dogs, pulmonary oedema commonly results in respiratory difficulty and gasping, often associated with a gagging cough that may produce white or blood-tinged foam. Cats with severe pulmonary oedema often pant, but seldom cough until oedema fluid begins to fill the main airways. In both species, severe dyspnoea is accompanied by cyanosis, abdominal contraction with respiration and signs of anxiety, including dilated pupils and resistance to restraint. Recognition of harsh or loud breath sounds on auscultation, usually with pulmonary crackles, in association with other clinical findings of cardiac disease (see Figure 4.2), should lead to a tentative diagnosis of pulmonary oedema and institution of treatment (Figure 4.6).

Oxygen supplementation

The most important component of therapy for acute pulmonary oedema is oxygen supplementation. Supplemental oxygen should be provided immediately upon recognition of dyspnoea or cyanosis and continued throughout stabilization. Initially, oxygen may be supplied via facemask, oxygen cage or nasal insufflation; the choice of modality is dependent on availability, the patient's toleration of administration and manipulation requirements with regard to further diagnostic testing. If arterial blood gas analysis is available, confirmation of any level of hypoxaemia should lead to at least temporary supplementation, but a PaO_2 of <60 mm Hg or oxygen saturation of <90% warrants aggressive oxygen

Diuretics
Frusemide (D) 2–6 mg/kg i.v., i.m., s.c. every 6–12 h, orally every 8–24 h, (C) 1–4 mg/kg i.v., i.m., s.c., orally every 12–48 h

Vasodilators
Acepromazine: (D, C) 0.03–0.05 mg/kg i.m., s.c. no more than every 6 h
Hydralazine: (D) 1–3 mg/kg orally every 12 h
Nitroglycerin ointment (2% = 15 mg/inch): 1.25–2.5 mg/5 kg body weight, cutaneously every 6–12 h
Nitroglycerin patch: (D) 2.5–10 mg/24 h as patch, 24 h on, 24 h off, (C) 2.5–5 mg, patch as dog
Sodium nitroprusside: (D) 1–5 µg/kg/min (start low and titrate up while monitoring blood pressure)
Amlodipine besylate: (D) 0.05 mg/kg orally once daily, (C) 0.625 mg per cat orally once daily

Inotropes
Digoxin (i.v. dosing for dogs only): (D) 0.01–0.02 mg/kg i.v. divided into 2–4 doses over 4 h; each dose given over 15 min
Dobutamine: (D) 2–15 µg/kg/min (start low and titrate up)
Dopamine: (D) 2–10 µg/kg/min (start low and titrate up)
Isoprenaline: (D, C) 0.04–0.08 µg/kg/min i.v.

Antidysrhythmics
Diltiazem: (D): 0.25 mg/kg i.v. (over 3 min)
Esmolol: (D, C) 0.5 mg/kg i.v. bolus, 25–200 µg/kg/min
Lignocaine: (D) 2–4 mg/kg i.v. bolus, 30–80 µg/kg/min, (C) 0.2–0.4 mg/kg i.v. slow bolus
Procainamide: (D) 5–15 mg/kg i.v., i.m. every 6 h, 10–20 mg/kg orally every 6 h, 10–40 µg/kg/min
Propranolol: (D) 0.1–2 mg/kg orally every 8 h, start low/titrate, 0.04–0.06 mg/kg i.v. slowly, (C) 2.5–5 mg total dose every 8 h, start low/titrate
Verapamil: (D, C) 0.05 mg/kg every 30 min up to 0.15–0.5 mg/kg total

Sedatives
Morphine: (D) 0.05–0.1 mg/kg i.v. repeated every 10 min until effects are seen (up to 0.4 mg/kg total), dose repeated every 1–4 h
Butorphanol: (D, C) 0.2–0.4 mg/kg i.v., i.m., s.c. every 1–4 h as needed for sedation
Buprenorphine: (D, C) 0.005–0.01 mg/kg i.v., i.m., s.c. every 4–6 h as needed for sedation

Other
Aspirin (for antithrombotic therapy): (C) 80 mg/cat every 48 h
Atropine: (D, C) atropine response test: 0.04 mg/kg i.m., emergency therapy of bradycardia: 0.02–0.04 mg/kg s.c., i.m., i.v. every 6–8 h
Calcium gluconate (for therapy of hyperkalaemia): (D,C) 2–10 ml of a 10% solution slowly i.v.
Dextrose (for therapy of hyperkalaemia): (D, C) 5–10% dextrose-containing fluids i.v., or 1–2 ml/kg 50% dextrose i.v. (may administer with insulin, see Insulin, below)
Glycopyrrolate: (D, C) 0.005–0.01 mg/kg s.c., i.m., i.v.
Insulin (for therapy of hyperkalaemia): (D, C) 0.55–1.1 IU/kg regular insulin in parenteral fluids with 2 g dextrose per unit of insulin administered
Sodium heparin (for antithrombotic therapy): 100–300 IU/kg s.c. tid
Warfarin: (C) 0.25–0.5 mg/cat/day
Sodium bicarbonate (for therapy of hyperkalaemia): (D, C) 1–2 mEq/kg i.v.

Figure 4.5: *Drugs used in therapy of cardiovascular emergency patients. Ranges are approximate; clinical evaluation of the patient dictates dosage of drug administered. (D:Dog, C:Cat)*

therapy. Clinical status of the patient must be monitored closely; evidence of progressive respiratory fatigue, lack of PaO_2 response to oxygen supplementation or progressive hypercapnia are all indications for mechanical ventilation.

Diuretic therapy

After oxygen supplementation has been established, aggressive diuretic therapy provides the next compo-

nent of stabilization. Loop diuretics are the most potent and fast-acting diuretics available in veterinary practice, and immediate administration of 2–8 mg/kg (use lower end of the dosage range in cats) of frusemide intravenously usually results in increased urine flow within approximately 30 minutes. Animals who have never received frusemide are more sensitive to its effects; patients who have received large oral doses of frusemide over the course of chronic heart failure

Medication	Action	Contraindications	Monitoring concerns	Onset of action
Butorphanol	Opioid sedative Sedative effects in depressed animals	Altered level of consciousness	Over-sedation	Onset of action: 5–10 min (i.v.)
Buprenorphine	Opioid sedative Sedative effects in depressed animals	Altered level of consciousness	Over-sedation	Onset of action: 5–10 min (i.v.)
Dobutamine	Catecholamine Positive inotrope	Dysrhythmias	Dysrhythmias (continuous ECG) Blood pressure	CRI: 1–2 min
Dopamine	Catecholamine Positive inotrope Renal vasodilator (at low doses)	Dysrhythmias Hypertension at doses >10 µg/kg/min	Dysrhythmias (continuous ECG) Blood pressure	CRI: 1–2 min
Frusemide	Loop diuretic Acute vasodilation (i.v. route only) Preload reduction through diuresis	Hypovolaemia	Dehydration Hypokalaemia Hypomagnesaemia	i.v.: 5–10 min
Hydralazine	Arterial dilator Decrease afterload by direct arterial dilation	Hypotension Hypovolaemia Fixed or dynamic LV outflow obstruction Inability to swallow Oral medication	Hypotension	Oral: 30–60 min
Morphine	Opioid sedative Decrease sensation of dyspnoea (CNS effect) Decrease vasoconstriction by decreasing SNS tone (decreases preload) Antianxiety effects	Hypercapnia (hypoventilation)	Hypoventilation Over-sedation Altered level of consciousness **Do not use in cats**	i.v.: 5–10 min
Nitroglycerin ointment (2%)	Venodilator Decrease preload by systemic and pulmonary venous dilation	None	Use gloves when in contact with ointment	Peak effect: 1 h
Sodium nitroprusside	Arterial/venous dilator Decrease preload and afterload by direct vasodilation	Hypotension Hypovolaemia Fixed or dynamic LV outflow obstruction	Acute hypotension (use invasive ABP monitoring) Thiocyanate or cyanide toxicity if administered for >48 h	CRI: 1–2 min

Figure 4.6: *Medications commonly used in therapy of acute congestive heart failure. ABP: arterial blood pressure, CNS: central nervous system, LV: left ventricle, SNS: sympathetic nervous system.*

therapy may need higher doses to induce emergency diuresis. Response to frusemide administration (e.g. urination) should occur within 60–90 minutes of intravenous administration. Cats and some fastidiously trained dogs may not urinate in the cage and the provision of litter boxes (cats) and occasional removal from the cage to urinate (dogs) reduces additional stress in these animals. If urination or a palpable increase in bladder size does not occur in response to frusemide

administration, the initial diagnosis should be reconsidered. If CHF is still deemed likely, additional doses of frusemide (2–4 mg/kg i.v.) can be administered. Water should be available at all times.

Vasodilators

Vasodilators, especially arterial dilators, provide rapid 'off-loading' of the ventricle and are indicated in patients with pulmonary oedema due to impaired left ventricular function, or mitral insufficiency, and those with severe systemic hypertension. By decreasing the resistance to left ventricular ejection, cardiac function is improved and the regurgitant fraction is decreased. In order to obtain this response, the left ventricle must be able to sustain adequate stroke volume. Consequently, marked arterial vasodilation is contraindicated in animals with fixed left ventricular stroke volume (e.g. hypertrophic cardiomyopathy, mitral stenosis, aortic stenosis, many causes of right ventricular failure). Severe pulmonary oedema in these animals must be managed primarily by preload reduction (e.g. frusemide, low salt diet, venodilators) and judicious use of angiotensin converting enzyme inhibitors.

Venodilators, such as nitroglycerin ointment, are often recommended as adjunctive therapy for acute pulmonary oedema. Dermally applied nitroglycerin ointment (2%) or nitroglycerin-impregnated skin patches have been used to effect systemic and pulmonary venodilation and reduce preload. Although the efficacy of dermally applied nitroglycerin ointment in the dog has been questioned (DeLellis and Kittleson, 1992), use of this medication remains common due to ease of application and lack of serious side effects. Angiotensin converting enzyme inhibitors are important in the therapy of chronic congestive heart failure but are less helpful for management of acute pulmonary oedema. The slower onset of action, oral route of administration and relatively mild arterial dilation produced by this family of drugs as compared with other, more potent vasodilators makes them less useful in acute emergencies.

Sodium nitroprusside (SN) and hydralazine remain the most commonly used and most effective acute arteriodilators for veterinary medicine. The relative advantages and disadvantages of either drug must be weighed in an individual patient. The potent effects of these medications make close monitoring of blood pressure mandatory during administration, and patients with acute pulmonary oedema must be continuously reassessed for moment-to-moment changes in cardiovascular status. Evidence of effective vasodilation includes bright pink mucous membranes with rapid capillary refill time, palpably warm ears and lips and gradual decreases in dyspnoea, anxiety and pulmonary oedema, as assessed by resolution of pulmonary crackles. Signs of hypotension include collapse, tachycardia, weak pulses, decreased urine output and worsening renal biochemistry values.

Sodium nitroprusside: SN is a rapidly acting and potent 'mixed' vasodilator, causing both preload and afterload reduction. It is administered intravenously as a continuous infusion and with a half-life of minutes, can be titrated to effect. SN is used less frequently than other vasodilators in veterinary patients due to perceived monitoring problems. With careful blood pressure monitoring however, SN can be used effectively to decrease both afterload and preload and provide rapid

relief of acute pulmonary oedema and acute hypertension. Contraindications for use of SN are listed in Figure 4.6.

Indications for use are:

- Acute pulmonary oedema due to CHF when normal to elevated systemic vascular resistance is present
- Acute pulmonary oedema secondary to mitral valve chordae tendineae rupture
- Acute hypertensive crisis.

Animals with CHF typically have low or normal measured arterial blood pressure, but in an animal with compromised myocardial function (e.g. dilated cardiomyopathy), normal blood pressures may represent elevated systemic vascular resistance. Known hypotension is a contraindication for SN administration, but normal to mildly elevated arterial blood pressure, accompanying low cardiac output and congestive signs, is an indication for its use.

Direct arterial blood pressure monitoring should ideally be established prior to administration of SN. Doppler or oscillometric methods can be used to monitor patients receiving SN, but the tendency of these methods to be inaccurate at low ABP limits their usefulness in this setting. Once a direct ABP tracing is obtained, a continuous rate infusion (CRI) of SN can be initiated, beginning with an infusion rate of 1 µg/kg/min and titrating up at intervals of 5–10 minutes to a target mean ABP of approximately 70–80 mm Hg. SN is light-sensitive and should be prepared in relatively high concentrations to provide for low fluid administration rates compatible with CHF. Any additional fluid therapy or medication infusions should be given separately to allow independent changes in administration rate. Because of the potency of SN, a fluid or syringe pump is mandatory to precisely control infusion rate. When an effective dose is ascertained, SN can be administered continuously for 48–72 hours with minimal risk of toxicity. Rapid improvement in clinical signs is usually noted in the first 3–6 hours when SN is administered concurrently with frusemide and other adjunctive therapies.

Hydralazine: Hydralazine is a potent oral arterial dilator. It has been used extensively in veterinary patients for both acute and chronic heart failure. The indications for use of hydralazine in the therapy of acute pulmonary oedema are the same as those for SN. Hydralazine may be chosen for acute therapy if SN is not readily available, invasive ABP monitoring or use of an infusion pump is not possible or monetary concerns preclude the use of a CRI. If the animal is too unstable for oral medications, SN should be considered instead of hydralazine. Contraindications for use of hydralazine are similar to SN and are listed in Figure 4.6.

ABP should be measured prior to therapy to exclude hypotension, as hydralazine should not be used if blood pressure is low. Animals with fulminating pulmonary oedema are usually given a higher initial dose of hydralazine than patients with more chronic signs. In acute CHF, the first dose of hydralazine may range from 1–2 mg/kg orally. Blood pressure is assessed approximately one hour post-dosing. Target response is a mean (if measured invasively or by oscillometric methods) or systolic (if measured by Doppler sphygmomanometry) ABP decrease of 20–40 mm Hg. If such a decrease is not achieved with the initial dose, an additional 1 mg/kg is administered orally, resulting in a cumulative dose of 2 mg/kg. This may be repeated up to a cumulative dose of 3 mg/kg in most dogs. When an effective dose has been documented, that dose is repeated at 12 hour intervals.

Sedatives and stress reduction

Opioid sedatives are used to treat acute CHF in human and veterinary patients. Morphine is the prototypical opioid for use in the setting of acute pulmonary oedema, providing both sedative and vasodilating effects. Morphine may be given intramuscularly or subcutaneously, but the intravenous route is preferred, in order to speed onset of action and assure absorption. Morphine has central respiratory depressant effects, but these effects are believed to be advantageous in CHF therapy. By blunting ventilatory reflexes, morphine lessens the sensation of dyspnoea and decreases anxiety associated with increased work of breathing. Administration also leads to vasodilation, resulting in a decrease in preload. These effects are specific to morphine; the common synthetic opioids butorphanol and buprenorphine provide variable degrees of sedation, but have no vasoactive properties. Intravenous oxymorphone is not recommended for patients with cardiogenic pulmonary oedema due to the increased pulmonary venous pressure associated with its administration.

Provision of a *low stress environment* is a basic but often challenging component of therapy of acute pulmonary oedema. Most animals arriving at the veterinary surgery with pulmonary oedema have endured a car ride and multiple episodes of being coaxed, prodded, lifted and carried. Several minor interventions may limit additional stress and allow for a faster and more comfortable evaluation of the patient:

- Provide oxygen immediately and supplement throughout the evaluation process, but avoid struggling with the patient who resists a facemask (consider an oxygen cage, 'flow-by' oxygen, or nasal supplementation for these patients)
- Gather vital signs and perform a limited physical examination with minimal manipulation of the patient
- Attempt to leave the patient in sternal recumbency whenever possible, including during thoracocentesis
- If multiple medications are to be given, organize

them in advance to administer with minimal manipulation
- Give as many medications as possible parenterally
- Postpone radiographs until patient is stable
- Once medications are administered, maintain the patient with minimal handling while drug therapy takes effect
- Do not 'overwarm' the patient (no additional heat supplementation if body temperature is >38°C).

Pleural effusion: recognition and emergency stabilization

Key points

- Recognition
    Dyspnoea with muffled heart/breath sounds, especially the ventral thorax
    Jugular distension
    Ascites
    Other physical findings typical of cardiac disease
- Therapy
    Oxygen supplementation
    Low stress environment
    Thoracocentesis
    (Opioid sedation)
- Typical underlying cardiac conditions
    Hypertrophic or restrictive cardiomyopathy (cat)
    Thyrotoxic heart disease (cat)
    Dilated cardiomyopathy (dog/cat)
    Pericardial effusion (dog, various aetiologies)
    Decompensated congenital heart disease (e.g. atrial septal defect, atrioventricular canal defect, pulmonic stenosis, tricuspid stenosis)
    Severe tricuspid insufficiency secondary to endocardiosis (dog).

Cats may develop pleural effusion with severe left-sided disease only, but in dogs, pleural effusion that is not associated with pericardial effusion usually indicates biventricular heart failure. The occurrence of right-sided heart failure secondary to left-sided failure may actually result in resolution of pulmonary oedema, such that patients with severe left-sided heart disease and a history of pulmonary oedema may be presented with pleural effusion and ascites as their predominant clinical signs.

Once significant pleural effusion has accumulated, full expansion of the lungs is difficult and patients eventually become overtly dyspnoeic. Cats may function quite well with significant amounts of pleural effusion but decompensate suddenly as fluid accumulation exceeds critical levels. Pulmonary oedema may accompany pleural effusion in patients with biventricular failure; in these cases, mechanical removal of fluid must be accompanied by medical therapy for pulmonary oedema.

Pleural effusion that leads to clinical signs of dyspnoea and discomfort is best treated by mechanical removal. Frusemide administration with sodium restriction may be successful in reducing effusions in chronic cases, but the effect of medical therapy on cavitary effusions is not rapid enough to be life-saving. In severely dyspnoeic animals suspected of having significant pleural effusion, a diagnostic thoracic aspiration should be performed prior to radiographic confirmation of the presence of fluid. If a technically adequate aspiration is achieved and no pleural fluid is obtained, other diagnoses should be considered.

Thoracocentesis may require sedation in animals who are anxious or fractious. Most animals with profound dyspnoea will tolerate thoracocentesis with minimal restraint if supplemented with oxygen, maintained in sternal recumbency and given a local anaesthetic. Rapid and deft aspiration of pleural fluid leads to immediate relief of dyspnoea. In contrast to abdominocentesis, as much fluid as possible should be removed. Continual ECG monitoring during the procedure is recommended, and any necessary treatments can be continued during thoracocentesis (e.g. oxygen supplementation). Thoracic radiographs after thoracocentesis are more helpful than prior to the procedure, when large amounts of fluid are likely to obscure intrathoracic structures.

LOW OUTPUT FAILURE AND CARDIOGENIC SHOCK: RECOGNITION AND EMERGENCY STABILIZATION

Key points

- Recognition
    Collapse or weakness with tachycardia, weak pulses, slow capillary refill, cold extremities
    Low or normal ABP
    May be accompanied by pulmonary oedema
    May be accompanied by significant dehydration
- Therapy
    Aggressive invasive monitoring (ABP and CVP)
    Positive inotropes administered via CRI
    Fluid therapy/electrolyte management
    Cautious vasodilation
    Frusemide, if needed
- Typical underlying cardiac conditions
    Dilated cardiomyopathy (dog/cat)
    Mitral insufficiency with dehydration (dog)
    Hypertrophic or restrictive cardiomyopathy (cat).

Low output cardiac failure is one of the most problematic emergency presentations associated with cardiac disease. This clinical presentation may occur with concurrent pulmonary oedema, necessitating simultaneous CHF management, or may occur in chronic CHF patients who are experiencing complications of therapy (i.e. digoxin toxicity, or when azotaemia and electrolyte imbalances have resulted in decreased intake, vomiting and eventually debilitating dehydration).

Recognition of cardiogenic shock should be followed by rapid assessment for underlying causes. History and physical examination findings, results of quick 'bench-top' tests (e.g. PCV, total protein concentration, labstick assessment of renal function) and analysis of the ECG add crucial information. This allows the clinician to divide low output failure patients into those with concurrent congestive signs, those who are markedly hypovolaemic with or without drug toxicity and those who are experiencing significant dysrhythmias as the basis for low output signs.

Low cardiac output with pulmonary oedema

This clinical presentation is typical of dogs or cats with dilated cardiomyopathy or cats with hypertrophic cardiomyopathy (HCM). In the case of dilated cardiomyopathy, poor systolic function is accompanied by increased filling pressures, but cardiac output is still inadequate. This combination of physiological events is manifested clinically as a dog or cat with clinical weakness, collapse or signs of shock accompanied by pulmonary oedema, with or without dysrhythmias. These animals most often are normotensive or mildly hypotensive, with MAP in the range of 60–90 mm Hg. Cats with HCM have low cardiac output due to diastolic dysfunction and are treated differently (see below).

Clinical approach to severe systolic dysfunction

Therapy of critically low cardiac output with pulmonary oedema consists of maximizing forward blood flow while limiting elevations in left atrial pressure needed to accomplish ventricular filling. Dysrhythmias may need to be managed immediately, or concurrently with other therapies (see section on Dysrhythmias later).

Cardiac output depends on maintaining sufficient preload and heart rate (with minimal dysrhythmias) while encouraging cardiac output with positive inotropic drugs and arterial vasodilators. Use of potent arterial dilators without inotropic and preload support frequently leads to hypotension; invasive monitoring is very helpful to 'balance' therapy in these patients.

After physical examination is complete and baseline data has been gathered (e.g. ECG, any blood tests), an arterial catheter and a jugular catheter should ideally be placed for measurement of ABP and CVP, respectively. Baseline measurements are recorded. Therapeutic goals consist of a mean ABP of 70–80 mm Hg with CVP between 5 and 15 cm H_2O or 3 and 11 mm Hg.

Arterial blood pressure is reduced through the cautious use of arterial dilators as described earlier. Decreases in blood pressure are offset by encouraging contractility with positive inotropic drugs. Both types of medications are simultaneously titrated, using ABP, heart rate and CVP, as well as the physical condition of the patient, to guide dosing. The combination of arterial dilators and positive inotropes often increases cardiac output enough to decrease left atrial pressures and relieve pulmonary oedema, making heroic doses of frusemide unnecessary. If relief of oedema does not occur rapidly enough for patient comfort, low to moderate doses of frusemide may be used to decrease preload. Rapid, aggressive diuresis should not be employed unless oedema is life-threatening, to avoid dehydration and worsening of low output signs.

Dobutamine is the positive inotrope recommended for most cases of CHF therapy; this selective ß$_1$ agonist increases contractility with minimal increases in heart rate. It is delivered via CRI and titrated to effect. Higher doses of dobutamine may result in supraventricular or ventricular dysrhythmias, but these usually respond to decreases in infusion rate or cessation of the infusion. *Dopamine* is the alternative positive inotrope often used in veterinary patients. The effects of dopamine are similar to those of dobutamine, but dopamine may be slightly more dysrhythmogenic and higher doses may result in increased systemic vascular resistance (see Figure 4.6).

Clinical approach to severe diastolic dysfunction

Acute low cardiac output due to diastolic dysfunction (e.g. hypertrophic or restrictive cardiomyopathy) is usually accompanied by pulmonary oedema. In diseases typified by diastolic dysfunction, systolic function is normal or increased. Relief of pulmonary oedema is achieved by administration of diuretics and venodilators as outlined above, but care must be taken to avoid over-diuresis.

Arterial vasodilation and positive inotropic drugs are contraindicated in acute heart failure due to diastolic dysfunction, as their use may result in tachycardia and hypotension. When pulmonary oedema has been relieved with diuretic and venodilating therapy, cautious administration of calcium channel blockers or ß-blockers may slow heart rate and improve diastolic function. Note that calcium channel blockers and ß-blockers are contraindicated when overt CHF is present.

Low cardiac output with hypovolaemia

The combination of low cardiac output with a hypovolaemic state is usually the result of complications of CHF therapy (e.g. over-diuresis or digoxin toxicity leading to dehydration). In some cases, systemic effects of non-cardiac disease (e.g. chronic renal failure) cause decreased intake and eventual dehydration, leading to cardiac decompensation. The therapeutic plan includes rehydration and adjustment of any electrolyte disturbances while encouraging cardiac output with positive inotropic medications.

Clinical approach

Initial assessment of the hypovolaemic patient with low cardiac output includes serum biochemical analysis to document evidence of dehydration, organ failure and any electrolyte imbalances. Serum digoxin concentrations are measured. Most animals with clinical signs of hypovolaemia and no evidence of CHF benefit from reduction or temporary discontinuation of diuretic therapy. Discontinuation of vasodilators must be approached with more caution, as rebound hypertension may occur if vasodilators are discontinued abruptly. In many cases, once diuretics are withdrawn, vasodilator doses are decreased but not completely discontinued.

Intravenous fluid administration should precede positive inotropic therapy, or at minimum, be administered concurrently. Traditionally, lower sodium fluids are recommended (0.45% NaCl with 2.5% dextrose) and are supplemented with potassium and magnesium based on measured blood concentrations of these electrolytes. In most cases, 'maintenance' fluid administration rates (2–3 ml/kg/day) are sufficient for initial supplementation and use of fluid pumps for administration is highly recommended. As rehydration is accomplished (documented through monitoring of physical examination, weight and blood tests), positive inotropic drugs are added to encourage increases in cardiac output. Continuous ABP and CVP monitoring allows rough assessment of cardiac output. Rehydration at maintenance or slightly above maintenance rates continues until CVP approaches 12–15 cm H$_2$O; if hypotension exists when CVP is normal, increased rate of infusion of positive inotropic drugs is warranted.

CARDIAC TAMPONADE: RECOGNITION AND EMERGENCY STABILIZATION

Key points

- Recognition
    Collapse or weakness with tachycardia, weak pulses, slow capillary refill, cold extremities
    Muffled heart sounds ± muffled breath sounds
    Jugular distension
    Ascites
    Low or normal ABP
    Small QRS complexes on ECG
    Dyspnoea with normal pulmonary auscultatory findings
- Therapy
    Pericardiocentesis
    Fluid therapy support if hypovolaemia is present
    Frusemide therapy to relieve ascites after pericardiocentesis
- Typical underlying cardiac conditions
    Idiopathic (dog, cat)
    Cardiac neoplasia (e.g. haemangiosarcoma (dog), lymphosarcoma (dog/cat))
    Extracardiac neoplasia (e.g. mesothelioma (dog))

Infection (e.g. feline infectious peritonitis (cat), bacterial (dog)).

Pericardial effusion and tamponade may be one of the most underdiagnosed causes of collapse and ascites in dogs. Paradoxically, pericardial effusion may be one of the most over-treated abnormalities once diagnosed, when pericardiocentesis is often performed regardless of the haemodynamic need for this procedure.

Pericardial effusion may accumulate in dogs and cats due to identifiable causes (e.g. infection or neoplasia) or may be idiopathic. Pericardial effusion is associated with acute clinical signs when tamponade occurs. 'Tamponade' may be defined as the presence of pericardial fluid at increased pressure, leading to compression of the heart and right-sided heart failure. When accumulation of fluid is gradual, the pericardium stretches to accommodate it, and compression of the heart does not occur until large amounts of fluid have accumulated. If effusion is acute (e.g. acute haemorrhage into the pericardium), much smaller amounts of fluid are required to substantially raise intrapericardial pressure. In most cases of pericardial effusion, underlying cardiac function is normal. Therefore, the emphasis is on immediate relief of tamponade, if present, and subsequent pursuit of underlying causes of the effusion.

If clinical signs of tamponade are not present, pericardial effusion may not need to be treated as an emergency. Clinical recognition of pericardial effusion can be difficult if it is not causing tamponade and requires a high index of suspicion. In many cases, pericardial effusion is identified on echocardiographic examination when no outward clinical signs are detected. Other indicators of the presence of small-to-moderate amounts of pericardial fluid include cardiomegaly on radiographs, or attenuated QRS voltages on the ECG.

The emergency presentation of cardiac tamponade typically involves evidence of cardiogenic shock (i.e. weakness, tachycardia, pallor, slow capillary refill time and weak pulses) accompanied by jugular distension, hepatomegaly and variable amounts of ascites. Cardiac tamponade should top the differential diagnosis list for animals lacking a heart murmur that have the combination of ascites and jugular distension, especially if muffled heart sounds are noted. Pleural effusion is also commonly seen in conjunction with pericardial effusion. Documenting the presence of pericardial effusion in animals with pleural effusion helps distinguish right heart failure due to primary cardiac disease from tamponade, but may not be immediately possible (see below). Animals with cardiac tamponade are frequently tachypnoeic even though pulmonary infiltrates or pleural effusion are not present. Tachypnoea probably reflects decreased respiratory movement of the chest wall and diaphragm due to ascites and pleural effusion.

If the patient is stable enough for thoracic radiography, pericardial effusion can be suspected based on the presence of an enlarged heart with a crisp silhouette border and the absence of indentations demarcating chambers ('globoid' heart). Pulmonary perfusion is usually decreased and smaller than normal pulmonary arteries may be noted. The presence of pulmonary infiltrates with uncomplicated pericardial effusion is unusual and should lead the clinician to look for other causes of clinical signs, or factors complicating pericardial effusion. In some cases, large amounts of pleural effusion obscure the cardiac silhouette and radiographic analysis cannot definitively establish the diagnosis of pericardial effusion.

Emergency echocardiography is extremely useful to establish the diagnosis in cases of suspected pericardial disease. In most cases, a complete echocardiographic examination can be postponed until the animal's condition is stabilized, but a brief echocardiographic examination with the animal in sternal recumbency can confirm the presence of a large echo-free space surrounding the heart. When tamponade is present, the right atrium and/or right ventricular wall may collapse in early diastole. Echocardiographic examination can also be used to determine the most advantageous area on the thorax from which to perform the pericardiocentesis. An area with a large amount of fluid and no interfering structures (especially lung) is chosen.

If echocardiography is not available and the animal is not stable enough for conscious radiography, presumptive pericardiocentesis may be life-saving. The procedure for pericardiocentesis is described in Chapter 22. Patients with cardiogenic shock should receive intravenous fluid support as the effusion is relieved, in order to increase their cardiac output. In most cases, local anaesthesia is sufficient for the procedure and a continuous ECG is recommended to monitor for centesis-related dysrhythmias. Samples of the fluid are saved for fluid analysis and cytology. Packed cell volume of the fluid and peripheral blood can be compared to establish the diagnosis of intrapericardial haemorrhage.

Withdrawal of pericardial effusion continues until no more can be easily withdrawn, the heart is detected 'bumping' on the centesis needle or catheter, or concurrent echocardiographic imaging establishes a significant reduction in fluid amount. In some cases, attempts at pericardiocentesis yield only small amounts of fluid, yet the clinical signs may be relieved. If removal of a small amount of fluid decreases the intrapericardial pressure enough to re-establish right-sided filling, temporary relief is anticipated. Occasionally, attempted pericardiocentesis leads to laceration of the pericardium. In these cases, the effusion is released into the pleural space and clinical signs of tamponade are relieved for longer periods of time.

Moderate doses of frusemide with concurrent cage rest frequently leads to resolution of ascites over the first few days after pericardiocentesis. Once the tamponade has been relieved, further diagnostic testing to establish the cause of the pericardial effusion can be pursued. A complete echocardiographic examination can be used to screen for obvious right atrial masses indicative of haemangiosarcoma, but lack of an identifiable mass in the right atrium does not rule out other types of neoplasia (e.g. mesothelioma) or small masses below the size identifiable with ultrasound technology. Abdominal ultrasound is recommended in animals with pericardial effusion with no identifiable right atrial mass, to look for other sites of primary neoplasia. In many cases, however, diagnosis of the cause of pericardial effusion relies on excluding as many causes as possible with diagnostic imaging, then monitoring the patient's progress. Idiopathic pericardial effusions may be recurrent until palliative pericardiectomy is performed, but survival for longer than 8 months after pericardiectomy usually indicates non-neoplastic causes for the effusion (Stepien *et al.,* 1997).

A special case of pericardial effusion occurs as a result of left atrial rupture. This situation is rare but life-threatening. Left atrial rupture in the dog is usually the result of acute elevations in left atrial pressure secondary to chordae tendineae rupture related to chronic mitral endocardiosis. Typically, the patient has a chronic history of mitral valve insufficiency but has acutely collapsed. Signs of cardiogenic shock are common, as is jugular distension and fulminant, life-threatening pulmonary oedema. If thoracic radiographs and an echocardiogram are obtained, pericardial effusion may be documented. In these cases, pulmonary oedema is usually the life-limiting problem and aggressive therapy of the oedema with diuretics and vasodilators is life-saving. The pericardial effusion should not be removed, as decreasing the intrapericardial pressure will allow further leakage from the left atrial rupture. If the animal survives the acute stages of CHF, left atrial tears may heal spontaneously. Occasionally, healed but previously undiagnosed left atrial ruptures are documented as an incidental finding in dogs that have died from other causes.

DYSRHYTHMIAS: RECOGNITION AND MANAGEMENT

Dysrhythmias are a common finding in emergency and critically ill patients. When other overt signs of CHF are not present, it may be difficult to differentiate dysrhythmias caused by intrinsic cardiac disease from those resulting from severe traumatic or metabolic derangements. Nonetheless, rapid diagnosis and therapy of emergency dysrhythmias is of paramount importance and most dysrhythmias respond to appropriate antidysrhythmic therapy regardless of their aetiology. Once the dysrhythmia has been controlled, the underlying cause(s) can be addressed.

Underlying causes of dysrhythmias generally fall into one of several general categories (Figure 4.7). Many of these causes can be ruled out based on history, clinical examination findings, blood chemistries and

Intrinsic cardiovascular disease
Myocardial disease
    Cardiomyopathies
    Infiltrative (e.g. neoplasia, fibrosis)
Pericardial disease/neoplasia
Ischaemia
Hypotension
Hypertension
Disorders of sinoatrial function
Conduction disorders
Congenital heart disease
Acquired valvular diseases (e.g. endocardiosis, endocarditis)

Hypoxia Systemic (e.g. pulmonary disease, anaemia, anaesthesia) Local (myocardial infarction)
Infection Sepsis Septic shock Severe pyrexia
Metabolic disease Acid–base disorders Electrolyte disorders Neurological disease Organ failure Endocrine disorders
Autonomic nervous system disorders/imbalances Vagal disorders (situational or pathological) Sympathetic nervous system stimulation (e.g. stress, drugs, pain)

Drugs/toxins
Direct effects
    Prodysrhythmic medications
    Most antidysrhythmic medications
    Methylxanthines
    Anaesthetic and sedative agents
    Toxic plants
    Autonomic nervous system alteration (e.g. anticholinergics)
Indirect effects
    Medications that alter acid–base/electrolyte status
        Diuretics
        Angiotensin-converting enzyme inhibitors

Figure 4.7: *Potential causes of dysrhythmias*

other routine diagnostic tests. The presence of documented cardiac disease does not rule out other causes of dysrhythmias, especially when the patient has been receiving medications that may alter electrolyte and acid–base status. Medical therapy of CHF may alter sodium and potassium balance or affect renal function. Electrolyte imbalance can directly cause or worsen pre-existing dysrhythmias and alterations in renal function may lead to decreased elimination of medications and accumulation of toxic plasma drug concentrations.

Key points

- Detect dysrhythmia during examination
- Diagnose dysrhythmia based on ECG

- Determine haemodynamic significance of dysrhythmia
- Begin therapy while searching for underlying causes (see Figure 4.7)
- In cases of probable hyperkalaemia, immediate therapy is mandatory regardless of haemodynamic status.

Suspicion of dysrhythmia in a critically ill patient is the most important step toward therapy. Detection of an inappropriately rapid or slow rhythm, especially if irregular, should prompt the clinician to examine the patient more closely for additional compatible signs of cardiac dysfunction. Although sinus arrhythmia is a commonly recognized cause of irregular cardiac rhythm, this variation of normal rhythm is associated with resting vagal tone and is therefore not commonly seen in severely ill emergency patients. If present, a normal sinus arrhythmia may be clinically differentiated from a pathological dysrhythmia through a combination of auscultation and palpation of peripheral pulses, then confirmed as benign with a lead 2 ECG recording.

Identification of a dysrhythmia based on a lead 2 ECG recording must be rapid and accurate. Frequently, measurement of individual wave sizes (e.g. P and R wave height and width) adds little diagnostic information in acute emergencies, but recognition of the presence or absence of individual waves and recognition of interval variations (e.g. P–Q or Q–T intervals) are an important component in rapid diagnosis. After the patient is stabilized, closer scrutiny of the ECG and exact measurements may be performed.

Stepwise emergency ECG analysis is outlined in Figures 4.8 and 4.9. Once the rhythm is identified, appropriate therapy can be instituted. Lack of response to appropriate therapy should prompt re-evaluation of the rhythm diagnosis and initiate a search for complicating issues. Hypokalaemia or hypomagnesaemia may decrease the efficacy of some antidysrhythmic medications and should be identified and rectified as soon as

Diagnosis	ECG findings	Typical clinical findings	Suggested therapy
Sinus bradycardia	Regular rhythm P waves associated with every QRS	No pulse deficits May be no clinical signs	Rule out vagal involvement with atropine response test Acute: dobutamine or isoprenaline CRI, temporary pacemaker Chronic: permanent pacemaker
Sinus arrest	Sinus bradycardia with irregular pauses >3 s Pauses ended by ectopic complexes (escape complexes)	Irregular Usually no pulse deficits May be associated with syncope Pulses variable in strength; pulses following pauses are typically strong	As above
Bradycardia–tachycardia (associated with sick sinus syndrome)	Very irregular rhythm Sinus bradycardia, sinus pauses interspersed with paroxysmal SVT	Often associated with syncope Pulse deficits present	Permanent pacemaker implantation precedes therapy of SVT Post-pacemaker, treat SVT as needed
Atrial asystole (atrial standstill)	No P waves Normal or wide QRS complexes T waves tall or deep, often symmetrical ('tented')	Associated with hyperkalaemia (e.g. urinary obstruction, acute renal failure, hypoadrenocorticism) Pulses usually weak Shock may be present	Check potassium concentration Treat presumptively if compatible disease is present and no potassium testing available EMERGENCY THERAPY FOR HYPERKALAEMIA: sodium bicarbonate OR dextrose OR insulin + dextrose OR calcium gluconate
Second degree atrioventricular block	Normal P waves Some P waves are not associated with QRS complexes, creating a pause in rhythm Pauses may be ended by escape complexes	No pulse deficits Irregular rhythm on auscultation May be associated with syncope	Atropine response test Acute: if no response to atropine, intravenous dobutamine or isoprenaline OR temporary pacemaker Chronic: permanent pacemaker implantation
Third degree atrioventricular block	Normal P waves Wide and bizarre QRS complexes at rate <P wave rate No relationship between P waves and QRS complexes	Strong pulses No pulse deficits May be associated with collapse	Immediate temporary or permanent pacemaker implantation Multiform escape QRS complexes or irregular escape rhythm: increased risk of sudden death

Figure 4.8: *Diagnosis and therapy of bradydysrhythmias (heart rate < 60 bpm in dogs and < 120 bpm in cats). In critically ill animals, the presence of a normal heart rate may be inappropriate and indicate dysfunction. CRI: continuous rate infusion, SVT: supraventricular tachycardia.*

Diagnosis	ECG findings	Typical clinical findings	Suggested therapy
Sinus tachycardia	Regular rhythm P waves associated with every QRS complex	No pulse deficits Ausc: regular rhythm	Treat underlying condition
Atrial premature depolarizations	Single, tall narrow premature ectopics Ectopic depolarizations have normal or abnormal P waves	Pulse deficits Ausc: irregular rhythm	No direct treatment unless CHF present or rate of premature depolarizations >20–30/min May resolve with therapy of underlying problem Digoxin therapy if CHF present ß-blockers or calcium-channel blockers if no CHF
Atrial tachycardia OR supraventricular tachycardia	Paroxysmal or sustained tachycardia, usually >250 bpm (dogs), >300 bpm (cats) Complexes tall and narrow in lead II Negative or no P waves associated with ectopic complexes	Rapid, weak pulses Pulse deficits common Ausc: irregular rhythm if paroxysmal, regular if sustained May be associated with syncope	Attempt vagal manoeuvre (e.g. ocular and carotid sinus massage) Intravenous propranolol or esmolol or verapamil or diltiazem
Atrial fibrillation	Irregularly irregular rhythm Tall, narrow complexes No P waves	Pulse deficits Ausc: irregular rhythm with variation in pitch of heart sounds	In CHF: digoxin No CHF: ß-blockers or calcium-channel blockers
Ventricular premature depolarizations	Wide, bizarre-appearing premature QRS complexes Ectopics have no P waves Underlying rhythm usually sinus in origin	Pulse deficits Ausc: irregular rhythm 'dropped beats'	Acute: intravenous lignocaine or procainamide
Accelerated idioventricular rhythm (slow ventricular tachycardia)	Intermittent occurrence of ectopic rhythm at rate similar to sinus rate Ectopic complexes are wide and bizarre Ectopic complexes have no P waves	Ectopic depolarizations are associated with palpably weaker pulses No pulse deficits Ausc: regular or mildly irregular	No direct therapy if mean arterial pressure is normal and rate of ectopic rhythm is <160 bpm Usually resolves with resolution of underlying problems
Ventricular tachycardia	Paroxysmal or sustained tachycardia, often >220 bpm (dogs), >250 bpm (cats) Complexes wide and bizarre in lead II No P waves associated with ectopic complexes	Weak pulses Pulse deficits Ausc: irregular rhythm with variation in pitch of heart sounds	Intravenous lignocaine or procainamide (dogs) Intravenous ß-blockers (cats) Check potassium concentrations if rhythm is non-responsive to lignocaine

Figure 4.9: *Diagnosis and therapy of tachydysrhythmias (heart rate >140 bpm in dogs and >200 bpm in cats). In critically ill animals, presence of sinus tachycardia is a frequent finding and usually resolves with therapy of underlying problem. In all cases, diagnostic work-up including measurement of electrolytes should be performed as soon as feasible. Ausc: auscultation, CHF: congestive heart failure.*

possible. Hypoxaemia and acidaemia may also limit antidysrhythmic drug efficacy and are identifiable based on blood gas analysis.

The haemodynamic significance and electrical instability of the dysrhythmia should be evaluated before therapy and if treatment is instituted, re-evaluated throughout therapy. The haemodynamic significance of a dysrhythmia depends on the impact of the dysrhythmia on cardiac output. During tachydysrhythmias, premature contractions of the ventricle related to supraventricular or ventricular premature depolarizations are associated with decreased stroke volume due to incomplete diastolic ventricular filling and abnormal patterns of ventricular contraction. This decreased stroke volume is detected clinically as a 'pulse deficit', an ausculted contraction that is not followed by a palpable

peripheral pulse. If heart rate is within the normal range and few pulse deficits are detected, a dysrhythmia may not need to be treated directly (see 'accelerated idioventricular rhythm', below). If pulse deficits are present, the ECG should be evaluated carefully to determine if direct antidysrhythmic therapy is warranted. Sinus bradycardia and sinus arrest are associated with normal to slightly augmented stroke volume, due to prolonged diastolic filling times, but patients with these dysrhythmias have decreased overall cardiac output due to limited heart rate. Thus, even though pulses may be palpably normal and no pulse deficits may be detected, cardiac output may be compromised to a critical level in some patients with profound sinus bradysrhythmias. Similarly, the combination of decreased stroke volume (due to abnormal ventricular contraction) and bradycardia associated with third degree atrioventricular block (AVB) may contribute to haemodynamic compromise. As in other bradycardic patients, acceptable peripheral pulse strength does not guarantee adequate cardiac function.

The choice of an antidysrhythmic medication or procedure is based on the clinician's knowledge of which agent or treatment modality is appropriate, effective, available, practical to administer and affordable. The clinician should always have several therapeutic options in mind when choosing an antidysrhythmic regimen, then tailor the regimen to fit the patient. Most dysrhythmias are treated according to their origin (e.g. supraventricular versus ventricular) and some are treated based on the proposed mechanism of the dysrhythmia (e.g. re-entry versus increased automaticity). Some dysrhythmias are treated by palliative methods that control the clinical signs without attempting to address the origin of the dysrhythmia directly (e.g. pacemaker implantation for third degree AVB).

Dysrhythmias and shock

A common clinical dilemma involves the presence of a severe tachy- or bradydysrhythmia in a collapsed or shocked patient. In the ideal situation, both abnormalities would be treated simultaneously, but in many cases, the clinician must immediately weigh the relative contributions of both abnormalities to clinical signs and treat accordingly. Guidelines for determining the course of therapy in dysrhythmic shock patients must allow for patient variation, but some general guidelines may be followed (specific therapeutic recommendations appear in subsequent sections).

Bradydysrhythmias and shock

Sinus bradycardia, sinus arrest, or bradycardia associated with second or third degree AVB is an inappropriate response to shock. An abnormally low heart rate in a patient with signs of poor cardiac output should lead the clinician to suspect primary cardiac disease (e.g. abnormal sinus node function or AVB), profound electrolyte disturbances (e.g. hyperkalaemia or hypocalcaemia), drug toxicity (e.g. digoxin), or neurological disorders, especially intracranial space-occupying lesions or cerebral oedema. When atrial standstill (also termed atrial asystole or sinoventricular rhythm) is present, hyperkalaemia should be ruled out as quickly as possible. Presumptive therapy for hyperkalaemia should be administered prior to confirmation of potassium concentrations if the patient is bradycardic with an appropriate clinical disease (e.g. urinary obstruction, acute renal failure or hypoadrenocorticism) and ECG findings (Figure 4.10). If third degree block is present with an escape rhythm that is excessively slow (i.e. <30 bpm), irregular or multiform in appearance, intravenous catecholamine support should be initiated immediately and a temporary or permanent pacemaker implanted as soon as possible (Figure 4.11).

Supraventricular tachycardias and shock

Supraventricular tachycardia (SVT) associated with signs of cardiogenic shock may be the cause of the low output signs, or result from whatever cardiac insult led to the signs of shock. In some cases, SVT will spontaneously resolve when the patient has been stabilized. Unfortunately, it is often difficult to discern which patients will revert to sinus rhythm without direct antidysrhythmic therapy. In general, if the patient has no other signs of primary cardiac disease and is in shock (e.g. hypovolaemic or toxic shock), aggressive therapy for shock usually results in slowing or conversion of the abnormal rhythm, but the patient should be monitored closely for development of pulmonary oedema during rapid fluid infusions. If SVT persists despite

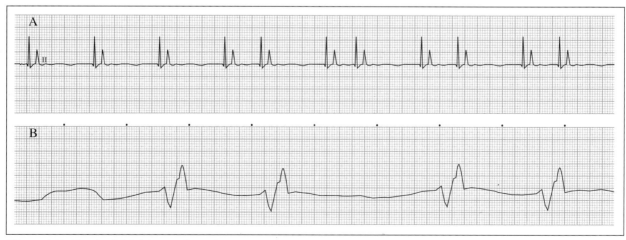

Figure 4.10: Two lead 2 ECG recordings (25 mm/s, dots indicate 1 sec markers) from (A) a dog with hypoadrenocorticism and (B) a cat with aortic thromboembolism. Despite similar serum concentrations of potassium (approximately 10 mmol/l in both cases), the appearance of the ECG differs. In both cases, bradycardia is present and P waves are not identifiable. Normal width QRS complexes with tall T waves are noted in strip (A), but abnormal intraventricular conduction is diagnosed based on the wide and bizarre appearance of the QRS complexes in strip (B). Immediate therapy of hyperkalaemia is indicated.

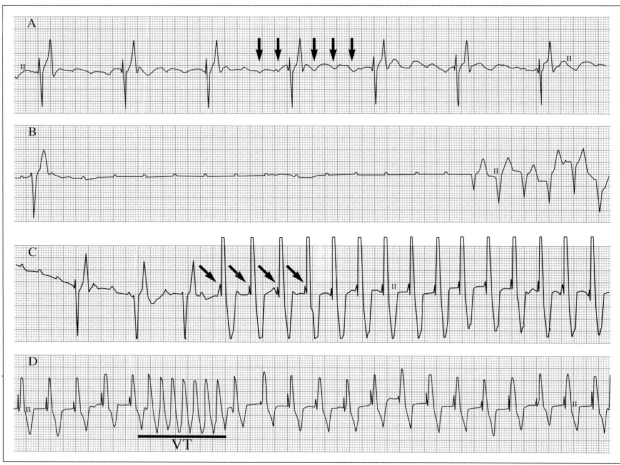

Figure 4.11: *Lead 2 ECG recorded from a 12-year-old Chesapeake Bay Retriever with acute collapse. (A) Third degree heart block is present. Unconducted P waves (arrows) are noted with unrelated ventricular escape complexes at a ventricular rate of 40 bpm. (B) Failure of the escape focus leads to intermittent ventricular asystole and clinical collapse; these asystolic periods are terminated by a rapid ventricular rhythm at a rate of 100 bpm. (C) Successful 'capture' of the ventricular rhythm is achieved via insertion of a temporary pacing lead into the right ventricle via the jugular vein. Arrows identify pacing spikes. (D) Migration of the temporary pacing lead to the right ventricular outflow tract is associated with paroxysms of ventricular tachycardia (VT). The ventricular tachycardia resolved with repositioning of the lead wire. All strips are recorded at 25 mm/s.*

appropriate fluid therapy, direct antidysrhythmic therapy may be instituted. In either case, vagal manoeuvres may be attempted to convert the SVT to sinus rhythm.

Atrial fibrillation (AF) is seldom found in patients free of cardiac disease. When AF is present in a patient with cardiogenic shock, signs of CHF are treated first, especially if pulmonary oedema is present. Once CHF is stabilized, therapy of AF is pursued, with the goal of limiting ventricular response rate to less than approximately 160 bpm in dogs or >180 bpm in cats. A special case exists when catecholamines must be administered for positive inotropic effects. In these situations, administration of drugs like dopamine or dobutamine may increase ventricular response rate to atrial fibrillation to markedly rapid rates (>250 bpm). Simultaneous intravenous use of digoxin may be advisable in these cases to limit unacceptable heart rate response to catecholamine stimulation.

Ventricular tachycardia and shock

Ventricular tachycardia (VT) should be treated directly with intravenous antidysrhythmic medications if the rate of depolarization is greater than 160 bpm. At increasing rates of depolarization, especially those greater than 240 bpm (Figure 4.12B), VT may be electrically unstable and must be addressed immediately to support cardiac output and avoid ventricular fibrillation. Frequent (>20–30/min) VPDs, especially if multiform in appearance, or repetitive VPDs occurring in pairs or paroxysms are often treated directly (Figure 4.12A), but in some cases may resolve with therapy of the underlying disease. In cases where the chances of adverse drug effects are low (e.g. use of lignocaine in dogs), administration of antidysrhythmic medication may be advisable until the patient's haemodynamic situation is improved.

Therapy of bradydysrhythmias

Bradydysrhythmias may be relatively benign or life-threatening. The primary focus of evaluation of the bradycardic emergency patient is the differentiation of vagally mediated bradydysrhythmias from pathological

25mm/s, 0.25cm : 1mV

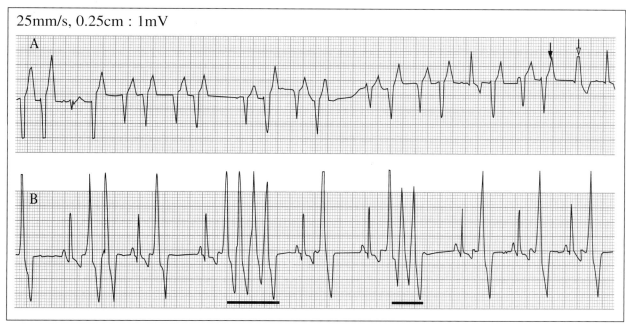

Figure 4.12: *Lead 2 ECG recordings (25 mm/s) from two dogs with ventricular tachycardia. (A) Repetitive, multiform ventricular premature depolarizations occur at a rate of approximately 120 VPD/min. Closed and open arrows identify two differing ventricular complex configurations. (B) Uniform ventricular ectopics occur at an overall rate of 120 per minute, but the rate of ventricular depolarization during paroxysms of ventricular tachycardia (marked by bars) exceeds 300 bpm. In both cases, immediate therapy is recommended.*

dysrhythmias. In a patient with low cardiac output, elimination of bradydysrhythmias but continued signs of low cardiac output after vagolytic therapy implies that the slow heart rate is not the cause of clinical signs.

Sinus bradycardia, sinus arrest, sick sinus syndrome

Sinus bradycardia with or without sinus arrest may reflect a primary problem with sinus node function or reflect systemic abnormalities, especially those which enhance vagal activity. Sinus bradycardia may be associated with some sedatives, anaesthetic agents, antidysrhythmic medications and medications or conditions that alter electrolyte balance. These bradycardias are usually self-limiting and resolve with removal of the underlying cause. Clinical signs that may be attributed to bradycardia include exercise intolerance, weakness, lethargy and, if periods of sinus arrest occur, syncopal episodes. In some cases, sinus node disease may be suspected if 'inappropriate' bradycardia is present in a critically ill patient. Sick sinus syndrome is a clinical syndrome consisting of variable combinations of sinus bradycardia, sinus arrest and SVT (Figure 4.13). Affected animals occasionally show no clinical signs but often exhibit lethargy, exercise intolerance and syncope. Although death as a result of this dysrhythmia is rare, clinical signs may severely affect quality of life in affected animals.

All animals presented for emergency examination and found to have bradycardia should have an ECG recorded to diagnose the dysrhythmia. Dogs with sinus rhythms at rates below 'normal range' but no clinical signs or other ECG abnormalities should be monitored as they are treated for their underlying disease. Dogs and cats that show clinical signs of exercise intolerance, weakness, lethargy, syncope or other 'collapse' behaviours and have sinus bradycardia should be further evaluated following administration of atropine or glycopyrrolate. Vagally mediated (physiological) sinus bradycardia will be abolished by administration of such vagolytic drugs and bradycardia as an aetiology for clinical signs may be ruled out.

If administration of vagolytic drugs is unsuccessful in converting sinus bradydysrhythmias to a sinus rhythm at an appropriate rate and clinical signs appear to be associated with poor cardiac output, positive chronotropic drugs may be administered as temporary support until a temporary or permanent pacemaker can be implanted. Dopamine, dobutamine or isoprenaline may be used to support heart rate in affected animals. These drugs are administered via CRI and dosed 'to effect'; continuous ECG and invasive blood pressure monitoring are used to document the response, while monitoring for dysrhythmias that may be caused by these catecholamines. If periods of sinus arrest alternate with SVT on the pre-treatment ECG, concurrent therapy for the SVT may be needed once blood pressure has been supported with the catecholamines. Temporary pacing with an intravenous pacing lead, if available, may be used to support heart rate until a permanent pacemaker can be implanted. Short-term catecholamine support may be necessary to maintain blood pressure during placement of the temporary pacing lead.

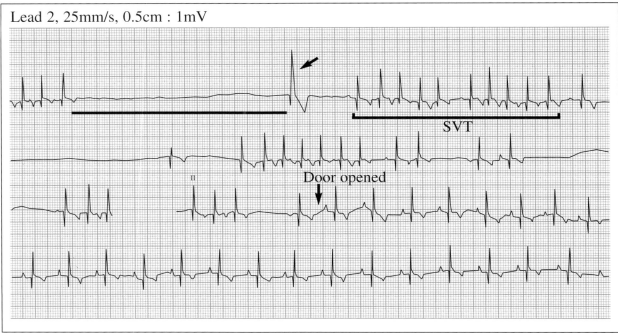

Lead 2, 25mm/s, 0.5cm : 1mV

Figure 4.13: Lead 2 ECG recording (25 mm/s, 0.5 cm:1 mV) from a Miniature Schnauzer with sick sinus syndrome. Sinus rhythm is apparent intermittently, alternating with periods of sinus arrest (bar) terminated by a ventricular escape complex (arrow). Paroxysmal supraventricular tachycardia (SVT) is intermittently present. When the dog is stimulated ('door opened'), a normal sinus rhythm resumes. No emergency therapy for the arrhythmia was indicated, but a permanent transvenous pacemaker was successfully implanted the following day.

Atrial standstill (atrial asystole)

Atrial standstill may be a primary problem (associated with atrial myopathies) or occur as a result of systemic abnormalities such as hyperkalaemia or digitalis intoxication. When hyperkalaemia is the underlying cause, anticholinergic drugs may increase the heart rate minimally, but immediate definitive therapy of the hyperkalaemic state is necessary to prevent ventricular asystole and death of the patient. If increased potassium concentrations are acute, serum potassium concentrations >6.5 mmol/l should be treated immediately and the underlying cause (e.g. urethral obstruction) should be addressed. In severe cases (potassium >8 mmol/l), the hyperkalaemia should be treated prior to any other therapy, and if typical ECG abnormalities are noted in a patient with compatible underlying disease, presumed hyperkalaemia must be treated even if measured serum potassium concentrations are not immediately available. Acute hyperkalaemia may be treated with intravenous calcium gluconate, intravenous glucose with or without insulin, or intravenous sodium bicarbonate (see Figure 4.5). If atrial standstill is persistent and due to pathological changes in the atrium itself, it is treated as AVB (below). Bizarre escape rhythms (see Figure 4.10) may develop in response to hyperkalaemia-associated or persistent atrial standstill; it is imperative to recognize escape rhythms as such and avoid suppressing these life-sustaining rhythms.

Atrioventricular block

High vagal tone and drug-related slowing of nodal conduction are the most common causes of first or second degree AVB. First degree AVB (i.e. prolonged P–Q interval) may occur as a physiological slowing mechanism during episodes of SVT and is not treated under this clinical circumstance. First degree AVB seldom leads to clinical signs in itself but may reflect metabolic abnormalities (e.g. hyperkalaemia) or drug toxicities (e.g. digoxin toxicity) that may be associated with clinical signs.

Vagally mediated second degree AVB is usually abolished by exercise, excitement or stress and therefore is rarely seen in emergency patients. Second degree AVB resulting from AV nodal pathology is permanent, non-responsive to vagolytic drugs and may lead to clinical signs of low cardiac output, especially during exercise. True syncope may occur if second degree AVB results in long periods of ventricular asystole.

Third degree AVB is manifest as P waves (usually occurring at a normal or increased sinus rate) with no relation to QRS complexes (see Figure 4.11). In most cases, the escape rhythm is ventricular in origin and discharges at a slow rate (25–40 bpm), but escape rhythms may originate in the AV node or Bundle of His, leading to a faster escape rhythm (i.e. 60–100 bpm). If clinical signs of low cardiac output are present in association with second or third degree AVB, temporary or permanent pacemaker implantation is warranted. Catecholamines may be administered to support heart rate, but may result in serious dysrhythmias without increasing ventricular escape sufficiently to support blood pressure. In some cases, second or third degree

AVB may be unassociated with clinical signs. This is frequently the case when third degree AVB is diagnosed in cats. In these cases, therapy of other diseases precedes further consideration of the bradycardia, but patients should be closely monitored for development of signs of fluid overload if aggressive fluid therapy is administered.

Therapy of tachydysrhythmias

Classification of antidysrhythmic agents into those used to treat supraventricular tachydysrhythmias, ventricular tachydysrhythmias, or both is helpful when choosing drugs in an emergent situation. Division of tachydysrhythmias into supraventricular and ventricular categories allows rational selection of a hierarchy of medications. In most cases, first line or standard drug therapy is successful for dysrhythmia management. If unsuccessful, or contraindicated in an individual patient, 'second' or 'third line' drugs may be the most appropriate therapy.

Supraventricular tachydysrhythmias

Supraventricular tachydysrhythmias can be divided into sinus rhythms (sinus tachycardia) and non-sinus rhythms (atrial, junctional and nodal re-entry rhythms).

Medications commonly used for therapy of ectopic supraventricular dysrhythmias (e.g. atrial tachycardia, atrial fibrillation) include digitalis glycosides (DG), ß-blocking agents (BB) and calcium channel blocking agents (CCB) (Figures 4.14 and 4.15). Other medications that have been used when dysrhythmias are refractory to these medications or when side effects limit their use include quinidine, procainamide and amiodarone. These drugs may be administered to treat both supraventricular and ventricular dysrhythmias, but because of more frequent side effects with use of these drugs, other antidysrhythmic medications are usually preferred as 'first line' agents for therapy of supraventricular dysrhythmias.

Sinus tachycardia: Sinus tachycardia may be associated with many systemic abnormalities and is treated by rectifying the underlying abnormality (e.g. dehydration, hyperthermia, infection). Sinus tachycardia is often associated with cardiac disease, especially in the presence of CHF. Under these circumstances, control of CHF usually results in resolution of the tachycardia.

Atrial premature depolarizations: Single atrial ectopic depolarizations may not require therapy if they occur at

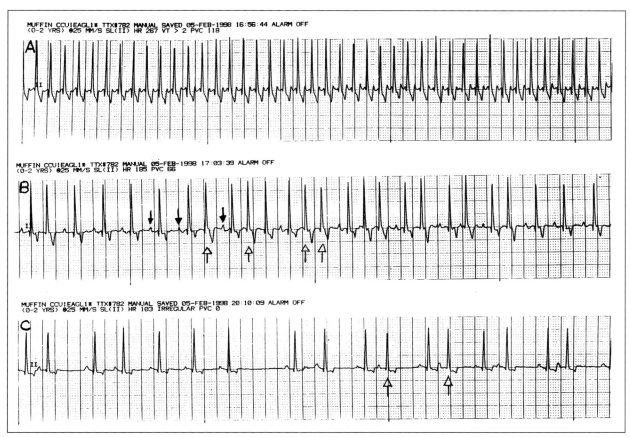

Figure 4.14: *Lead 2 ECG recordings (25 mm/s) from a dog with severe pancreatitis but no primary cardiac disease. (A) Atrial tachycardia at a rate of approximately 270 bpm is present. Vagal manoeuvres were unsuccessful in converting the atrial tachycardia to sinus rhythm. (B) Four minutes following administration of propranolol intravenously, sinus beats conducted with first degree atrioventricular block are present (closed arrows). Frequent atrial premature depolarizations (open arrows) remain (C) Four hours later, a sinus rhythm is present at a heart rate of 110 bpm, but occasional atrial premature depolarizations remain (open arrow).*

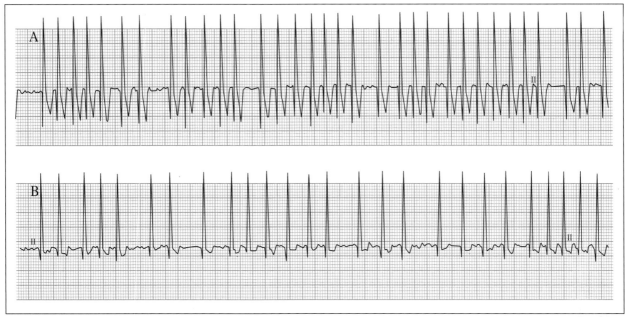

Figure 4.15: Lead 2 ECG recordings (25 mm/s) from a dog with dilated cardiomyopathy and atrial fibrillation (A) Untreated, the ventricular response rate to atrial fibrillation exceeds 220 bpm. (B) 24 hours after initiation of therapy with diltiazem, ventricular response to atrial fibrillation is approximately 140–160 bpm.

low frequency, are not related to CHF or known structural heart disease or failure and are not associated with clinical signs. Occasionally, single atrial ectopics in an animal with a history of syncope may reflect undetected paroxysmal supraventricular tachycardia (SVT). It is not usually necessary to treat isolated atrial ectopics on an emergency basis.

Supraventricular tachycardias: SVT, atrial tachycardia or nodal re-entry tachycardias are not always associated with clinical signs, but if paroxysms of SVT are frequent, sustained SVT is present, or the dysrhythmia is associated with signs of overt heart failure or hypotension, emergency therapy may be required prior to definitive aetiological diagnosis. Emergency therapy for SVT includes augmentation of vagal tone via ocular pressure or carotid sinus stimulation ('vagal manoeuvre'). This procedure may abruptly abolish the tachycardia (suggesting that the dysrhythmia was SVT) or transiently slow the rate of discharge (suggesting sinus tachycardia). If these manoeuvres are unsuccessful initially, they may be successful after supraventricular antidysrhythmic medications have been administered (e.g. ß-blocking agents). Vagal manoeuvres are frequently unsuccessful in conversion of SVT associated with primary cardiac disease. Intravenous administration of BB (propranolol or esmolol) or CCB (verapamil or diltiazem) can be used on an emergency basis to convert persistent SVT to normal sinus rhythm (Figure 4.14). Each of these medications may have significant negative inotropic and hypotensive effects and must be administered as a slow intravenous bolus to avoid precipitation or exacerbation of clinical signs.

Junctional tachycardia: Junctional tachycardias are usually not life-threatening and if the rate of depolarization allows for adequate ventricular filling (i.e. heart rate <140 bpm with no pulse deficits), junctional tachycardia is not usually treated directly. The presence of junctional tachycardia may reflect systemic metabolic derangements (e.g. electrolyte imbalance) or drug toxicity (e.g. DG toxicity). Detection of this dysrhythmia should prompt investigation of drug and metabolic status of the patient even when direct antidysrhythmic therapy is not needed.

Atrial fibrillation: Atrial fibrillation is most frequently diagnosed in emergency patients as a complication of severe cardiac disease. Acute occurrence of AF in previously stable CHF patients may be associated with sudden decompensation, but conversion of AF to a normal sinus rhythm is usually not feasible due to the presence of severe underlying cardiac disease. Atrial fibrillation results in a high rate of atrial depolarization and a rapid and irregular ventricular response. The therapeutic goal for most cases of atrial fibrillation is to control the ventricular response rate. In severe heart failure, the patient may be dependent on an elevated heart rate to support cardiac output, so decreasing the rate of ventricular response must be approached with caution. Antidysrhythmic drugs used for this purpose are often 'titrated' to the desired clinical effect. Digitalis glycosides may be administered intravenously to treat AF with rapid ventricular response when extreme tachycardia is limiting resolution of CHF or when catecholamines must be administered for inotropic support. Gastrointestinal and dysrhythmic side effects of DG are common when the drug is given intravenously, so close monitoring of ECG and frequent patient evaluation must be performed during therapy. Acute oral administration of the CCB diltiazem occasionally results in conversion of acute AF to sinus rhythm, but even when conversion does not occur, ventricular response to AF may be slowed with this medication (see Figure 4.15). Negative inotropic effects of diltiazem may lead to worsening of CHF signs, so patients should be monitored closely for signs of worsening or lack of resolution of pulmonary oedema. Acute administration of ß-blockers will slow the ventricular response rate in atrial fibrillation, but negative inotropic effects make these drugs contraindicated in CHF patients. Atrial flutter is a rare dysrhythmia that involves very high rates of atrial depolarization and very rapid ventricular response and is treated similarly to atrial fibrillation.

Ventricular dysrhythmias

Ventricular antidysrhythmics may be divided into medications used intravenously (e.g. lignocaine, procainamide) and those used chronically (usually orally) to treat various types of ventricular ectopy (quinidine, procainamide, propranolol, mexiletine).

Ventricular premature depolarizations: may or may not require direct intervention. In veterinary emergency cases, VPDs should be treated directly under the following circumstances:

- If the patient is symptomatic for the dysrhythmia (e.g. syncope, weakness, hypotension)
- If paroxysmal or sustained ventricular tachycardia ('VT', three or more ventricular depolarizations in a row with a rate higher than 160 bpm) is present

In addition, direct therapy of single VPDs should be considered if multiform VPDs are present. Invasive blood pressure measurement may confirm hypotension in questionable cases. Hypotension in the presence of ventricular dysrhythmias warrants antidysrhythmic therapy in addition to therapy for blood pressure support.

Ventricular tachycardia: Ventricular tachycardia is treated with parenteral ventricular antidysrhythmic medications. Lignocaine is the first line drug of choice for dogs with VT and administration of one to three boluses of lignocaine intravenously will convert the majority of VT to sinus rhythm. Lignocaine is rapidly acting and may be given as a constant rate infusion; the infusion must be preceded by a loading dose to rapidly achieve therapeutic blood levels. Additional boluses of lignocaine may be necessary to control tachycardia until therapeutic levels are reached and maintained. Lignocaine toxicity is enhanced when there is hepatic compromise and when lignocaine is administered in the presence of several common medications, including BB and cimetidine. The dose of lignocaine should be halved and titrated to effect when these medications are used, or intravenous procainamide may be substituted as emergency therapy. Common signs of lignocaine toxicity include depression, nystagmus, head-bobbing, salivation, vomiting or seizures. If any signs of toxicity occur after bolus administration, further administration should be avoided and intravenous diazepam may be used to temporarily control seizures. Ultimately, neurological side effects related to lignocaine administration cease with discontinuation of the drug. Lignocaine is less effective in the presence of hypokalaemia; normal potassium balance should be restored to allow maximal beneficial effect of lignocaine administration.

If lignocaine administration fails to control ventricular tachycardia, procainamide is recommended as a 'second line' drug. Other possibilities include quinidine, BB or other antidysrhythmic agents, or combinations of these medications. Procainamide or quinidine may be administered parenterally, but in practice, procainamide appears to be associated with fewer side effects and is recommended over quinidine if lignocaine is ineffective. Intravenous quinidine has significant myocardial depressant and hypotensive effects and this route of administration is usually not recommended unless other less hypotensive drugs have failed to control the arrhythmia and acute therapy is required. Intramuscular procainamide is often used as a 'bridge' between intravenous lignocaine therapy and oral procainamide therapy. Intramuscular administration of procainamide is begun as lignocaine is gradually reduced, until oral administration of procainamide can be established. Refractory ventricular tachycardia may respond to synchronized DC cardioversion if this modality is available.

Cats with ventricular dysrhythmias are treated differently than dogs. In cases where ventricular tachycardia is present in hypoxic patients, resolution of hypoxia may lead to resolution of the dysrhythmia. If VT must be treated directly, ß-blocking agents (BB) are the ventricular antidysrhythmic agents of choice. Intravenous propranolol (non-selective BB) or esmolol (cardioselective BB) is given as a slow bolus and esmolol is continued as a CRI if required. Oral BB (e.g. propranolol, atenolol) may be administered as needed to control dysrhythmias if intravenous access is not available, but the onset and effects may be less predictable. Procainamide may be also be used as a ventricular antidysrhythmic in cats, but quinidine may not be tolerated due to frequent gastrointestinal side effects. Lignocaine is tolerated by cats if given slowly at doses much lower than those recommended for dogs; toxicity usually results in neurological signs.

Accelerated idioventricular rhythms (idioventricular tachycardias): Accelerated idioventricular rhythms are slower ventricular rhythms with a rate close to the sinus rate. In some cases, the accelerated idioventricular

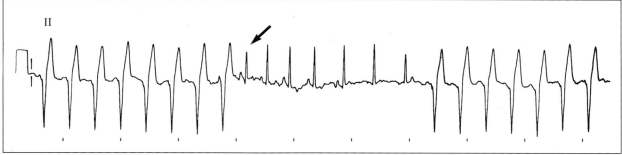

Figure 4.16: *Lead 2 ECG (25 mm/s, dots along the bottom are 1 second markers) recorded from a systemically ill dog with no evidence of primary cardiac disease. An accelerated idioventricular rhythm is noted at the beginning of the recording, with a ventricular rate of approximately 140 bpm. When the sinus rate exceeds the ventricular depolarization rate (instantaneous heart rate approximately 160 bpm at arrow), the sinus node resumes control of the heart rate. When the sinus node slows, the ventricular rhythm is again apparent. Mean arterial pressure remained normal throughout the recording. No direct antidysrhythmic medications were indicated; this rhythm abnormality resolved within 24 hours.*

rhythm will become manifest intermittently when the sinus rate slows slightly due to respiratory sinus arrhythmia (Figure 4.16). These rhythms are usually diagnosed in patients with significant systemic disease, hypoxia or trauma and are thought to be related to changes in autonomic tone or myocardial perfusion (Abbott, 1995). ECG characteristics of idioventricular tachycardia include a rate of depolarization of <160 bpm (usually <140 bpm) with a regular and uniform appearance. Initial ventricular ectopics in a 'run' usually occur late in diastole and may be fusion beats. The rhythm disappears when sinus rate increases (e.g. excitement or administration of vagolytic drugs), but does not typically respond to lignocaine administration. Clinical characteristics of idioventricular rhythms include no overt signs of hypotension. Although qualitative decreases in pulse pressure may be detectable, significant pulse deficits are usually not present. Direct therapy of idioventricular tachycardia in an animal with no signs of primary cardiac disease is often unnecessary, as the rhythm will resolve with resolution of the underlying systemic abnormalities. Direct antidysrhythmic therapy may become necessary if idioventricular tachycardia is complicated by other ventricular ectopics and detection of frequent pulse deficits should lead to reconsideration of a previous decision not to treat. If ventricular tachycardia exceeds 160 bpm, antidysrhythmic therapy should be initiated.

VASCULAR EMERGENCIES

Hypertension: recognition and emergency stabilization

Key points

- Systemic hypertension in veterinary patients is usually secondary to metabolic disease
- Acute blindness due to retinal detachment may be the only presenting sign of systemic hypertension

- Hypertensive crisis may result in neurological signs
- Aggressive vasodilating therapy is indicated to prevent permanent debilitation.

Recognition and management of systemic hypertension is a relatively recent development in clinical veterinary medicine and little clinical literature is available addressing therapy of acute, naturally occurring hypertension in dogs and cats. Management of hypertension is complicated by lack of agreement regarding methods of measurement and 'cut-off' values for diagnosis (Henik, 1997). 'Hypertensive crisis' in humans refers to clinical circumstances requiring rapid reduction of blood pressure. Clinical abnormalities may include acute damage to retinal vessels (haemorrhage, exudates, oedema or detachment), encephalopathic signs, cerebral infarction, acute aortic dissection and acute CHF. In dogs and cats, acute ocular signs are the most frequent indicator of malignant hypertension, but neurological signs (e.g. seizures, ataxia) may be seen (Littman *et al.*, 1988; Snyder, 1991; Littman, 1994). Congestive heart failure is a rare presentation of systemic hypertension in veterinary medicine, but cardiac murmurs are common in hypertensive animals. Acute retinal detachment, especially with hyphaema, or the coincidence of compatible ocular signs with neurological signs should lead the clinician to suspect hypertensive crisis and act quickly to diagnose and treat the abnormality.

Diagnosis
Systemic hypertension must be suspected before it can be diagnosed. Animals presented for acute blindness, intraocular haemorrhage or epistaxis should have their blood pressure assessed at initial presentation. In addition, animals noted to have signs associated with hypertensive retinopathy (e.g. tortuous retinal vessels, retinal haemorrhage, papilloedema) on routine fundic examination, especially if concurrent neurological abnormalities are present, should have their blood pressure assessed immediately. Several systemic diseases are

known to be associated with hypertension in dogs (e.g. hyperadrenocorticism, protein-losing nephropathy) and cats (e.g. chronic renal disease, thyrotoxicosis). Routine blood pressure assessment should be part of the routine diagnostic testing and monitoring of these diseases.

Several methods have been used clinically to measure blood pressure in veterinary patients. The goal of any method is to produce repeatable results with minimal stress to the patient, but the usefulness and repeatability of each method is user-dependent. In some cases, more invasive methods are less stressful if an arterial catheter is placed. Once the catheter is in place in the artery, repeated manipulation of the animal is unnecessary. Direct or Doppler-measured values are recommended in cases of suspected hypertension. Oscillometric methods, while useful for monitoring trends, often are time-consuming and unreliable as single-assessment measurements and may underestimate values at higher pressures (Binns *et al.*, 1995; Henik 1997). Normal values for direct arterial blood pressure and Doppler sphygmomanometry are outlined in Figure 4.17. Oscillometric measurement values are similar to Doppler-measured values.

The rapidity with which a patient's blood pressure has increased is more important in the generation of clinical signs than the absolute value of the blood pressure. Animals with rapidly developing increases in blood pressure show signs at values slightly higher than the normal range, while some animals with chronically high pressures show no outward clinical signs. When associated with any measured elevation in blood pressure, any combination of the following signs are indicative of hypertensive crisis and warrant aggressive interventional therapy:

- Acute blindness, hyphaema or visible retinal detachment
- Acute onset of intracranial neurological abnormalities (e.g. seizures, nystagmus, head-pressing, circling, mentation changes, focal cranial nerve abnormalities)
- Epistaxis.

Therapy (hypertensive crisis)

Acute therapy of hypertension is based on aggressive use of vasodilating drugs. Blood pressure should be monitored frequently throughout initial therapy. Frusemide may be a useful adjunct to vasodilation in the hypertensive crisis, especially when hypertensive encephalopathy is present. Care is taken not to cause dehydration with overzealous use of diuretics. The target blood pressure range for treatment of the hypertensive crisis is a reduction of blood pressure by 25%, rather than immediate reduction to normal levels. In patients with hypertension associated with renal failure, urine output should be closely observed during therapy, as reduction of blood pressure may cause decreases in glomerular filtration, and anuria.

Sodium nitroprusside: Intravenous SN is the drug of choice for rapid reduction of critical hypertension. Continuous rate infusion of SN allows rapid titration of blood pressure to desired levels. Continuous invasive blood pressure monitoring is required when using SN for this purpose. SN should only be used for 48–72 hours to avoid toxicity, and chronic oral antihypertensive therapy should be initiated as soon as possible.

Hydralazine: As a directly acting arterial dilator, hydralazine causes reliable decreases in blood pressure within 1–2 hours after oral administration. Patients must be monitored for side effects such as tachycardia or inappetence. Concern regarding neurohumoral activation after hydralazine administration has led to concurrent administration of frusemide or angiotensin-converting enzyme inhibitors in some cases.

Angiotensin-converting enzyme inhibitors: Angiotensin-converting enzyme inhibitors may be administered as a single therapy or as adjunctive therapy with other vasodilators to animals in hypertensive crisis. The unreliable and sometimes delayed response to these medications makes them less effective than other vasodilators in an acute crisis.

Method of measurement	Canine BP values consistent with hypertension	Feline BP values consistent with hypertension
Arterial puncture	Systolic: >170–180 mm Hg Diastolic: >100–105 mm Hg	Systolic: >200 mm Hg Diastolic: >145 mm Hg
Doppler sphygmomanometry	Systolic: >180–200 mm Hg Diastolic: >100–115 mm Hg	Systolic: >170 mm Hg Diastolic: >100 mm Hg

Figure 4.17: *Criteria for diagnosis of hypertension in dogs and cats. Even though a wide range of normal values exists depending on the technique used and operator-dependent effects, clinical signs of hypertension are usually associated with values well above normal ranges. Abnormal elevation in either systolic pressure, diastolic pressure or both should be considered consistent with hypertension. Stated values are approximate, based on normal values in the author's clinic and published ranges (Dukes, 1992). BP: blood pressure.*

Calcium-channel blockers: Amlodipine besylate, a long-acting CCB, has been advocated for chronic therapy of systemic hypertension (Henik and Snyder, 1997). The slow onset of action of this drug makes it less useful for acute therapy of hypertension, but it may be administered simultaneously with faster-acting agents, then continued chronically once blood pressure is controlled.

A typical therapeutic protocol for hypertensive crisis includes documentation of elevated blood pressure, placement of an intra-arterial catheter for continuous blood pressure monitoring if needed and administration of intravenous or oral vasodilators. Clinical signs of hypertensive encephalopathy should subside rapidly when blood pressure decreases, but ocular signs may take days to weeks to resolve. In many cases, retinal detachment is permanent, but some animals regain some visual ability. Rapid and consistent control of blood pressure is necessary to prevent permanent neurological and renal damage and underlying causes of systemic hypertension should be addressed as soon as feasible. In cases of endocrine-related hypertension (e.g. hyperadrenocorticism or thyrotoxicosis), adequate control of the underlying disease allows reduction or discontinuation of antihypertensive medications.

Thromboembolism: recognition and emergency stabilization

Key points

*   Thromboembolism in cats is usually associated with primary cardiac disease
*   Thromboembolism in dogs is usually secondary to systemic disease
*   Aortic thromboembolism should be suspected in any case of sudden lameness in cats
*   Diagnosis is based on physical findings
*   Analgesia is a mainstay of emergency management
*   Careful fluid therapy is recommended to support perfusion.

Aortic thromboembolism (ATE) is a common and serious complication of the feline cardiomyopathies. Thromboembolic events may occur in dogs but are usually associated with systemic illness (e.g. hyperadrenocorticism, neoplasia) rather than primary cardiac disease. In cats, acute decompensation of cardiac disease may occur due to the pain and stress of ATE.

Many ATE patients are humanely destroyed due to the severity of the signs, severity of concurrent heart disease or overall guarded prognosis for return to function, but some animals can survive to live comfortably for many additional months. Patients who are systemically stable or can be rapidly stabilized often exhibit slow, steady progress toward function of the affected limbs. Improvement in motor function of affected limbs may be seen as early as 3 days after ATE and support-

ive care at home can result in gradual return to function over a period of weeks. If absolutely no improvement is seen in the first week, or if the limb itself deteriorates (cutaneous oedema formation, gas gangrene), full recovery of limb function is unlikely, but amputation of the affected limb is a viable possibility in stable patients.

Diagnosis

Diagnosis of ATE or thromboembolism of other sites is based on physical examination, compatible history and physical evidence of cardiac disease (especially cardiomyopathy). Physical findings in cases of peripheral thromboembolism are specific. Affected limbs are paretic or paralysed; there is pallor of the affected footpads or nailbeds and the affected leg(s) lack an arterial pulse. The leg(s) are cool to the touch and may be stiff if contracture of major muscle groups is present. Since complete paralysis may not occur, peripheral pulses should be carefully evaluated in any case of acute lameness in cats. Affected animals are usually in pain and may vocalize. Cats with ATE related to cardiomyopathy are frequently in CHF at the time of presentation and may be markedly dyspnoeic. Dysrhythmias may be detected on auscultation and confirmed with an ECG recording. Life-threatening CHF and dysrhythmias are treated acutely, before management of ATE begins.

Angiography or echocardiography may confirm the diagnosis and document underlying disease, but are not usually necessary for initial management. Extensive testing may add unacceptable stress to hospitalization and pose a significant risk to the patient. If biochemical evaluation is performed, abnormalities may include evidence of severe muscle injury and organ damage including metabolic acidosis, elevations in lactate dehydrogenase, creatine kinase, creatinine, aspartate aminotransferase and alanine aminotransferase. Evidence of disseminated intravascular coagulation (DIC) may be present on a haemostasis screen. Hyperkalaemia and hypermagnesaemia are occasionally noted, reflecting acidosis, muscle damage, acute renal failure or reperfusion phenomena.

Therapy of ATE

Therapy of CHF, if present, is the highest priority in the management of ATE patients. Some therapies (e.g. acepromazine maleate) may be of benefit for therapy of CHF and ATE simultaneously. Acute CHF therapy, consisting of diuretics, vasodilators and, if needed, antidysrhythmic agents, is administered. Specific therapy for ATE may consist of surgical removal of the thrombus, administration of thrombolytic drugs (e.g. tissue plasminogen activator (t-PA), streptokinase), or supportive medical therapy. Surgical removal of the thrombus, while a possibility in stable patients, is contraindicated in patients with unstable CHF or metabolic status.

Thrombolytic therapy: Despite hopes for thrombolytic drugs as acute therapy for ATE in cats, consistent success with this mode of therapy has been elusive. While t-PA or streptokinase have been used in cats with acute ATE, the unfavourable side effects and high mortality associated with use of these drugs is discouraging. Acute reperfusion of ischaemic tissue may lead to hyperkalaemia, hypermagnesaemia and acidosis (i.e. 'reperfusion syndrome'). Successful treatment of peripheral thrombosis in dogs has been described (Ramsey *et al.*, 1996; Clare and Kraje, 1998), but at this time, acute administration of thrombolytic drugs should be considered experimental and, in general, is not recommended for cats with ATE.

Medical therapy: Pre-treatment neurological, muscular and vascular function is assessed and metabolic status is established via biochemical analysis and blood gas measurements. Stabilization of CHF is an important first step, but care must be taken to avoid dehydration, which may make recovery from metabolic and thromboembolic problems more difficult. The goals of emergency medical therapy for ATE include alleviation of pain, support of collateral circulation to affected muscles and ultimately, prevention of further embolization.

Alleviation of pain associated with acute muscle ischaemia is a major goal of therapy of ATE patients. Analgesics recommended for use in cardiac patients include morphine, butorphanol, buprenorphine, fentanyl or oxymorphone. Each of these opioids has advantages and disadvantages and clinicians should use an available opioid with which they are familiar. The importance of aggressive analgesic therapy cannot be over-emphasized, as pain itself and the stress related to pain are severely debilitating. Since there is little doubt that even quiet-appearing animals are in pain if major muscle groups have become acutely ischaemic or are reperfusing, analgesic drugs should be administered on a strict schedule rather than 'as needed'.

Support of collateral circulation may be achieved through the use of vasodilators. Acepromazine maleate is the drug most often recommended because of its vasodilating and sedating effects. The effect of angiotensin converting-enzyme inhibitors (ACEIs) on perfusion in cases of ATE is unknown, but if ACEIs are used to treat concurrent CHF, hydration and renal function must be closely monitored. Hydration is maintained with controlled delivery of intravenous fluids.

Prevention of further embolization is unreliable at best. Current recommendations consist of administration of sodium heparin to decrease the probability of additional clot formation. Although the success of heparin therapy in this regard is unproven, its use is typically associated with minimal side effects. Some clinicians advocate simultaneous use of warfarin in cats with acute ATE, but extensive clinical data regarding this use have not been published. Aspirin administration, while sometimes recommended for prevention of ATE, is not recommended in the acute therapy of an existing thrombus.

REFERENCES

Abbott JA (1995) Traumatic myocarditis. In: *Current Veterinary Therapy XII: Small Animal Practice*, ed. RW Kirk and JD Bonagura, pp. 846–850. WB Saunders, Philadelphia
Binns SH, Sisson DD *et al.* (1995) Doppler ultrasonographic, oscillometric sphygmomanometric and photoplethysmographic techniques for noninvasive blood pressure measurement in anesthetized cats. *Journal of Veterinary Internal Medicine* **9**, 405–414
Clare AC and Kraje BJ (1998) Use of recombinant tissue-plasminogen activator for aortic thrombolysis in a hypoproteinemic dog. *Journal of the American Veterinary Medical Association* **212**, 539–543
DeLellis LA and Kittleson MD (1992) Current uses and hazards of vasodilator therapy in heart failure. In: *Kirk's Current Veterinary Therapy XI: Small Animal Practice*, ed. RW Kirk and JD Bonagura, Dukes (1992) pp. 700–708. WB Saunders, Philadelphia
Dukes J (1992) Hypertension: a review of the mechanisms, manifestations and management. *Journal of Small Animal Practice* **33**, 119–129
Henik RA (1997) Systemic hypertension and its management. *Veterinary Clinics of North America: Small Animal Practice* **27**, 1355–1372
Henik RA and Snyder PS (1997) Treatment of systemic hypertension in cats with amlodipine besylate. *Journal of the American Animal Hospital Association* **33**, 226–234
Littman MP (1994) Spontaneous systemic hypertension in 24 cats. *Journal of Veterinary Internal Medicine* **8**, 79–86
Littman MP, Robertson JL *et al.* (1988) Spontaneous systemic hypertension in dogs: five cases (1981–1983). *Journal of the American Veterinary Medical Association* **193**, 486–494
Ramsey CC, Burney DP *et al.* (1996) Use of streptokinase in four dogs with thrombosis. *Journal of the American Veterinary Medical Association* **209**, 780–785
Snyder PS (1991) Canine hypertensive disease. *Compendium on Continuing Education for the Practicing Veterinarian* **13**, 1785–1792
Stepien RL, Whitley NT *et al.* (1997) Canine idiopathic pericarditis versus pericardial mesothelioma: comparison of survival in 14 cases (abstract). World Small Animal Veterinary Association World Congress, Birmingham, United Kingdom, p. 320.

CHAPTER FIVE

General Approach to Dyspnoea

Lori Waddell and Lesley King

DEFINITION AND DIAGNOSIS

Dyspnoea may be defined as the sensation of difficulty in breathing that is experienced by patients with compromised respiratory function. This sensation is initiated by either a low partial pressure of oxygen (PaO_2) (hypoxaemia) or high partial pressure of carbon dioxide ($PaCO_2$) (hypercapnoea) in arterial blood. Both hypoxaemia and hypercapnoea may lead to an increased ventilatory drive which produces clinical signs of respiratory distress. Normally, ventilation is stimulated by increases in arterial carbon dioxide concentration, hypoxia only acting as a stimulus when PaO_2 falls below 50 mm Hg. In these circumstances, hypoxic drive will override the effects of any hypocapnoea that may be present due to hyperventilation. Severe hypoxia may produce a paradoxical reduction in ventilatory drive due to depression of brainstem ventilatory motor centres.

It is essential that patients in respiratory distress are recognized immediately. In the emergency room, observation of the patient and a detailed physical examination of the respiratory system are the most important tools for diagnosis and treatment, often providing clues about the causes of dyspnoea when more stressful diagnostic procedures are not possible. The clinician attempts to localize the disease process to the airways, lungs or pleural space. Since dyspnoea is often a life-threatening emergency, this facilitates immediate steps to stabilize the patient.

Observation of respiratory patterns in the dyspnoeic patient

Dogs and cats with dyspnoea may be recognized by an increase in respiratory rate and effort. Increased respiratory effort is a manifestation of recruitment of the secondary muscles of respiration. This includes the scalene and sternomastoid muscles of the neck and chest, the alae nasae which dilate the nostrils, and the muscles of the abdominal wall, which contract when exhalation becomes an active rather than a passive process. Recruitment of the secondary muscles of respiration is a non-specific response to increased respiratory drive and does not necessarily confirm the presence of dyspnoea or hypoxia. Normal respiration is characterized by concurrent outward movement of both the chest and abdomen during inhalation. 'Paradoxical respiration' is recognized by a lack of synchronous movement of the chest and abdominal walls — the diaphragm and caudal intercostal and abdominal muscles tending to collapse inwards and forwards during inhalation. Unlike increased respiratory effort alone, paradoxical respiration is a specific indication of dyspnoea, increased work of breathing and the presence of respiratory muscle fatigue.

Postural adaptations are common in patients with respiratory distress, minimizing resistance to air flow. Many patients in severe respiratory distress breathe through an open mouth to remove the resistance to airflow offered by the nasal turbinates. Similarly, the neck is often extended and the head lifted to straighten the trachea. Most dyspnoeic patients demonstrate some degree of orthopnoea, preferring to stand or lie in sternal recumbency, abducting their elbows to minimize compression of the chest wall (Figure 5.1). Lateral recumbency may limit air flow by reducing the ability to abduct one side of the chest wall during inspiration. Any restraint that limits postural adaptations may lead to further hypoxaemia and decompensation of the patient, a fact that must be borne in mind when restraining these animals for diagnostic procedures such as radiography.

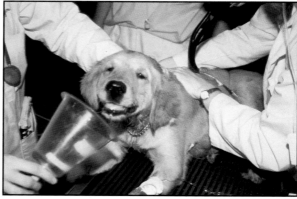

Figure 5.1: *Severe respiratory distress due to neurogenic pulmonary oedema after a choking incident in a 6-month-old Golden Retriever. Notice the pale mucous membranes, extended neck, abducted elbows and reluctance to have an oxygen mask placed over the face.*
Courtesy of Dr Ken Drobatz, University of Pennsylvania.

Physical examination of the dyspnoeic patient

Mucous membrane colour and capillary refill time can yield important information about the functional status of the respiratory system. Owing to the shape of the oxyhaemoglobin dissociation curve, cyanosis only occurs with severe hypoxaemia (less than 80% saturation of arterial blood). Presence of cyanosis therefore indicates the need for immediate oxygen supplementation. In addition, at least 5 g/dl of desaturated haemoglobin must be present for the blue colour of cyanosis to be detectable. When moderate hypoxia is present, the mucous membranes may still be pink (Figure 5.2). Clinicians should therefore not be lulled into a false sense of security by pink mucous membranes. In addition, anaemia or peripheral vasoconstriction may lead to pale mucous membranes and inability to detect cyanosis. In all these cases, use of a pulse oximeter (see Chapter 16) can rapidly and easily confirm the presence or absence of hypoxia without stress to the animal. This method is not affected by moderate anaemia or vasoconstriction. Cherry red or muddy chocolate mucous membranes can indicate the presence of toxins such as cyanide and paracetamol, respectively. Carbon monoxide can also cause bright red mucous membranes (carboxyhaemoglobin). These toxicities all cause respiratory distress by interfering with haemoglobin binding and release of oxygen.

A limited physical examination of the respiratory and cardiovascular systems can be performed rapidly and can be very rewarding. Auscultation of the chest and cervical trachea may detect wheezes, crackles, harshness or increased bronchovesicular sounds, as well as areas of dullness (dorsal, ventral, unilateral). Wheezes are musical or squeaky sounds associated with narrowing of the airways by inflammation, mucosal oedema, mucus or masses. If they occur during inspiration, upper airway pathology should be suspected, whereas disease of the small bronchi or lower airways, such as feline asthma, usually produces expiratory wheezes. Crackles are discontinuous popping sounds that indicate the presence of fluid in the alveoli and airways. They are caused by air bubbling through fluid, or by the opening and closing of small bronchi and alveoli. Crackles occur with parenchymal disease processes and often indicate pulmonary oedema, haemorrhage or purulent exudate in the alveoli. If the lung or heart sounds are dull, muffled or difficult to hear, pleural space disease should be considered. The most common pleural abnormalities include pneumothorax, pleural effusion, diaphragmatic hernia and neoplastic masses. In cats, diminished chest compressibility can be a suggestive finding when an effusion or mediastinal mass is suspected.

Auscultation of the heart and simultaneous palpation of the pulses help to determine whether cardiovascular system disease is contributing to respiratory dysfunction. In dogs with congestive heart failure, a mitral murmur or supraventricular dysrhythmia (often atrial fibrillation) is usually heard. In the absence of these findings, heart failure as a cause of dyspnoea is

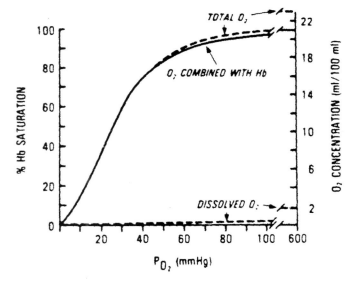

Figure 5.2: *The oxygen–haemoglobin dissociation curve demonstrates the relationship between partial pressure of oxygen dissolved in the blood and the saturation of haemoglobin with oxygen. The sigmoid shape of the curve occurs as a result of a conformational change in the haemoglobin molecule following binding of the first molecule, allowing binding of the remaining three molecules to occur more rapidly. This facilitates both oxygen uptake in the lungs and oxygen release to the tissues. The plateau of >90% haemoglobin saturation also provides a wide margin of safety — lung disease may result in significant decreases in PaO_2 without a concurrent decrease in saturation. Desaturation can occur rapidly, however, once the PaO_2 decreases to a value of <60 mm Hg.*

Reproduced from West JB (1985) Respiratory Physiology — The Essentials, 5th edn, p.69, with permission of Williams & Wilkins, Baltimore.

extremely unusual. Elimination of the presence of cardiovascular disease by auscultation may be more difficult in cats, since they usually suffer from myocardial rather than valvular diseases. Murmurs and dysrhythmias may be absent or intermittent in cats with congestive heart failure.

EMERGENCY STABILIZATION

Initial stabilization of a patient with severe respiratory distress should include increasing the inspired oxygen concentration (oxygen therapy). This should be initiated while a rapid but thorough physical examination is performed. Ideally, the patient should be allowed to rest briefly in an oxygen-enriched environment before further diagnostic investigation and manipulation. This is particularly important for cats, as it allows calming and recovery from transport. A more complete examination and further investigations are performed only when tolerated and shown not to exacerbate signs of distress.

Intravenous access
Intravenous access with an indwelling peripheral catheter placed in the cephalic or saphenous vein should be obtained early during the hospitalization of all dyspnoeic patients. The catheter should be placed with minimal restraint and stress. Establishment of intravenous access allows administration of drugs and allows intravenous anaesthesia to facilitate rapid control over the airway should the animal decompensate.

Thoracocentesis
If dullness is suspected on auscultation of the chest either dorsally or ventrally, thoracocentesis should be immediately attempted to remove pleural air or fluid. In animals with severe distress, this procedure should be performed before radiographs are obtained. Such patients may not be stable enough for radiography, and thoracocentesis will not only be diagnostic but potentially therapeutic. Techniques for thoracocentesis are described in Chapter 22.

Oxygen supplementation
Emergency oxygen therapy can be supplied in several ways. Mask oxygen can be used on any patient that is lying still and tolerates the mask. It may be poorly tolerated in distressed patients and persistent attempts to place the mask over the muzzle of the animal can increase stress (see Figure 5.1). With a tight fitting mask at high oxygen flow rates (5–6 l/min), a fractional inspired oxygen concentration (FiO_2; room air FiO_2 = 0.21) of 0.7–0.8 can be achieved. Care must be taken that the mask is not so tight as to cause rebreathing of carbon dioxide and consequent hypercarbia.

Flow-by oxygen is achieved by holding the oxygen supply pipe near the nostrils or mouth of the animal and provides the same effect as a mask with much less stress.

An oxygen pipe from an anaesthetic machine can supply oxygen (5–8 l/min) to an Elizabethan collar covered with Clingfilm, again allowing the animal to be visible and minimizing stress, although some animals will not tolerate this technique.

Oxygen cages are one of the easiest methods of oxygen administration, but they isolate the patient, making it difficult to examine, monitor and treat these dynamic cases (see Figure 5.3). This may be considered an advantage in some stressed and dyspnoeic cats, however, that may benefit from enforced isolation from strange people in a strange environment. Initial crisis management of dyspnoeic animals may require high oxygen concentrations until the patient has been stabilized. The oxygen percentage in the cage is determined by the extent of filling with 100% oxygen. Although it should be possible to reach an FiO_2 of up to 1.0 many oxygen cages cannot raise the FiO_2 above approximately 0.5, which may be too low for severely dyspnoeic animals. Opening the cage door drops the FiO_2 to room air almost immediately. Oxygen cages may also be associated with inappropriate patient warming and consequent hyperthermia. Large dogs may not fit into standard oxygen cages. Despite these limitations, oxygen cages may represent a useful investment for the emergency practice. At present, no commercially available oxygen supplementation cages are available in the UK, although they may be purchased from the USA. Paediatric incubators provide a suitable alternative for cats, small dogs and neonates. These allow good observation of the patients and although expensive when purchased new, are often available second-hand from human hospitals. Oxygen concentrations of 80–90% are easily attainable using paediatric incubators.

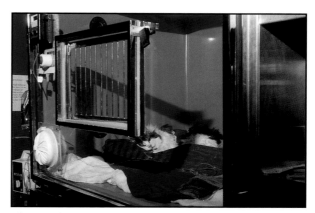

Figure 5.3: *An oxygen cage is an excellent way to provide oxygen supplementation in extremely stressed or fractious animals. Temperature, inspired oxygen concentration and humidity can be controlled in these units.*

For more prolonged oxygen supplementation, nasal oxygen can be provided with nasal oxygen prongs that are manufactured for human patients (Figure 5.4), or by placing a catheter in one or both nostrils and suturing or gluing it in place (Figure 5.5). Nasal prongs penetrate

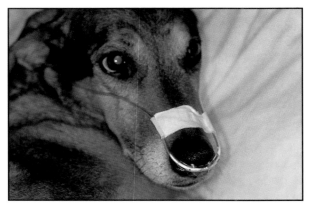

Figure 5.4: Nasal oxygen prongs that are manufactured for human patients can be used in many canine patients to provide oxygen supplementation.

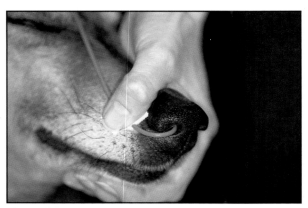

Figure 5.5: Nasal oxygen can also be provided by suturing a red rubber catheter into one nostril and inserting it a pre-measured length equal to the distance from the nostril to the medial canthus of the eye.

approximately 1 cm into both nostrils and usually work well in large breed dogs that are relatively immobile. Nasal catheters can be used in dogs or cats of almost any size. Any type of catheter can be used for this purpose; most commonly 8–12 French red rubber urinary catheters are used. The technique for placement of nasopharyngeal oxygen catheters is described in Chapter 22. Brachycephalic breeds are poor candidates for nasal oxygen supplementation: catheter prongs cannot be adjusted to fit comfortably on their faces; nasal catheters do not stay in place because of the presence of stenotic nares; and these animals may have increased vagal tone, which may be aggravated by the nasal catheter. Animals that are mouth breathing because of dyspnoea or excitement are also poor candidates for this technique, as increased air mixing in the pharynx leads to a reduced effective FiO_2. Generally, nasal oxygen is thought to give an FiO_2 of approximately 0.4 depending on the flow rate of oxygen, the size of the animal and its minute ventilation. The FiO_2 can be increased by placement of a second nasal catheter. Alternatively, a long intravenous catheter can be placed percutaneously into the trachea following the instillation of surface local anaesthetic. Humidified oxygen is

supplied at similar flow rates to those used with the nasal catheter. This system may be especially useful in individuals with laryngeal or upper tracheal obstruction.

Oxygen for long-term therapy should be humidified (saturated with water vapour) to prevent desiccation of the airways, especially if the turbinates are by-passed, as occurs with nasal oxygen catheters. Specially designed units that heat and humidify the inspired air are available for placement in anaesthetic and ventilator circuits, but nasal or cage oxygen humidification can be simply accomplished by bubbling the oxygen through a chamber of distilled water (Figure 5.6).

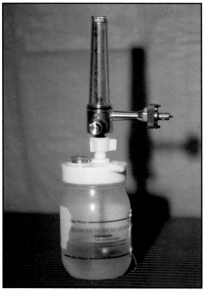

Figure 5.6: Oxygen can be humidified by bubbling it through a chamber filled with distilled water. This reduces airway irritation by preventing desiccation.

Long-term therapy with high concentrations of oxygen (especially at $FiO_2 > 0.6$ for more than 12 hours, or sooner if assisted ventilation is performed) is associated with damage to the lung called oxygen toxicity. Inflammatory injury is caused by toxic metabolites of oxygen, including oxygen free radicals and superoxide molecules. Clinically, oxygen toxicity is rare but may create changes in the lungs that are similar to those seen in the acute respiratory distress syndrome (ARDS). Every effort should be made to minimize the FiO_2 used to maintain critical patients. In the presence of severe dyspnoea, however, it may not be possible to decrease the FiO_2 without provoking severe distress, and the clinician may have to accept the risk of oxygen toxicity in the interests of survival of the patient.

Intubation and positive pressure ventilation

Extremely dyspnoeic animals that cannot adequately ventilate or oxygenate may require anaesthesia and intubation to establish control over the airway and to provide short term positive pressure ventilation (Figure 5.7). This aggressive approach is obviously reserved for the most severe cases of respiratory distress. Clinical parameters indicating that the animal should be intubated include severe distress that is non-responsive to therapy, persistent cyanosis that is not responsive to oxygen supplementation and a fractious patient that cannot be restrained for diagnostics or therapy. In any of these situations, anaesthesia eliminates distress and facilitates handling for diagnostic investigation.

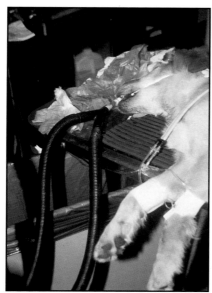

Figure 5.7: *The Golden Retriever puppy pictured in Figure 5.1 after failing to respond to oxygen therapy. He required anaesthesia, intubation and positive pressure ventilation. A large amount of sanguineous fluid has flowed out of his airways and pooled on the table in front of him.*
Courtesy of Dr Ken Drobatz, University of Pennsylvania.

Blood gas analysis, if available, assists in determination of whether positive pressure ventilation should be initiated. General indicators are PaO_2 of 50 mm Hg or less on oxygen supplementation (reference range 90–100 mm Hg) or a $PaCO_2$ greater than 50 mm Hg (reference range 35–45 mm Hg).

Care must be taken when choosing an anaesthetic agent for induction in these patients. Often there is a concurrent cardiovascular system instability and myocardial irritability due to hypoxaemia. Since the clinician will be establishing control over the airway and taking over respiratory function, concerns about ventilatory depression by selected anaesthetic agents are reduced. Intravenous anaesthetic agents are ideal because they allow rapid induction, intubation and therefore airway management. Mask induction or the use of intramuscular agents is associated with a high risk of cardiopulmonary arrest when severe respiratory distress is present.

If upper airway obstruction is suspected, before inducing anaesthesia, the clinician should organize all of the materials required to perform an emergency tracheostomy in the event that endotracheal intubation is not possible. The technique for emergency tracheostomy is described in Chapter 22.

Where there is no evidence of hypovolaemia, propofol may be administered by intravenous injection to effect, although this drug may be associated with vasodilation and production of intrapulmonary arteriovenous shunting. Shunting may severely aggravate a pre-existing hypoxia and, although temporary, is not responsive to increased inspired oxygen concentration or assisted ventilation. Propofol may be used for short-term maintenance of anaesthesia to allow continued intubation. Thiopentone is not associated with intrapulmonary shunting, but may produce ventricular premature contractions where there is myocardial hypoxia and hypotension when there is hypovolaemia. Alternatively, low doses of intravenous opioid analgesics such as fentanyl or morphine, combined with a benzodiazepine sedative agent such as diazepam or midazolam, produce adequate sedation and muscle relaxation to allow endotracheal intubation (for doses see Chapter 18). Respiratory arrest may be temporarily produced with this technique and it is important to immediately ventilate the patient. A method of maintaining anaesthesia to allow continued intubation must therefore be used such as volatile agent inhalation or repeated administration of injectable drugs. Once the animal has been intubated, it should be immediately placed on 100% oxygen and positive pressure ventilation should be initiated by manually bagging the animal until more information is available about respiratory function. The haemodynamic status of the patient should be carefully monitored (see Chapter 16), body temperature measured and supported if necessary and the administration of anaesthetic drugs kept at the minimum required to maintain unconsciousness and lack of response to gentle movement of the endotracheal tube.

Pulmonary function testing in the dyspnoeic patient

Apart from clinical examination, useful methods for pulmonary function testing in the dyspnoeic patient include pulse oximetry, end-tidal capnography and arterial blood gas analysis. These methods are addressed in more detail in Chapter 16. Pulse oximetry is the quickest and least invasive, providing an indirect measure of the saturation of haemoglobin in arterial blood with oxygen. In the awake patient, the small probe is placed on a shaved area of skin on the ear, upper or lower lip, prepuce or vulva, toes, or a skin fold anywhere on the body. In anaesthetized patients, the tongue is the most useful site. Normal haemoglobin saturation is greater than 95% and pulse oximetry readings of 93% or higher are acceptable in non-anaemic critically ill patients breathing room air. Oxygen supplementation should be considered in patients with haemoglobin saturation of less than 93%. Saturation values of 90% correlate with a PaO_2 of approximately 60 mm Hg and indicate severe hypoxaemia. Values less than 90% should be addressed immediately by providing supplemental oxygen or positive pressure ventilation.

End-tidal capnography provides an estimate of the $PaCO_2$ by measuring carbon dioxide in exhaled alveolar gas (see Chapter 16). End-tidal capnography usually is not accurate in tachypnoeic or panting patients. Normal values should be in the 35–45 mm Hg range. Significant respiratory acidosis is associated with $PaCO_2$ of >50 mm Hg requiring measures to improve ventilation. Hypoventilation may be caused by a reduction of ventilatory drive (high doses of opioid analgesics), spinal cord compression, or obstruction of airflow (airway occlusion). These cases should be treated by positive pressure ventilation whilst the underlying cause is determined and managed.

Arterial blood gas analysis is the gold standard for determination of respiratory function. Normal PaO_2 on room air (FiO_2 0.21) is between 85 and 100 mm Hg. Values less than 80 mm Hg are usually treated by increasing the inspired oxygen concentration. When evaluating blood gas samples taken while the patient is receiving supplemental oxygen, normal PaO_2 values must be adjusted to reflect the increased FiO_2. In animals with normal lung function, the PaO_2 is approximately five times the inspired oxygen concentration, so that if a patient is receiving 100% oxygen, the predicted PaO_2 is close to 500 mm Hg. Similarly, an animal with normal lung function receiving 40% oxygen should reach a PaO_2 of about 200 mm Hg. Normal $PaCO_2$ values are approximately 40 mm Hg. Persistent $PaCO_2$ values of greater than 50 mm Hg should be addressed as described above.

Thoracic radiography in dyspnoeic patients

Thoracic radiographs represent one of the most useful diagnostic tools for the clinician faced with a patient in respiratory distress. Detailed information about thoracic radiography is available in Chapter 23.

Although valuable information is provided, radiography is a stressful procedure that can cause significant respiratory decompensation and may not be indicated in patients with severe disease. In these patients, dorsoventral radiographs obtained with the patient restrained in sternal recumbency provide less useful diagnostic information but are likely to produce less compromise of remaining ventilatory function. Alternatively, horizontal beam lateral views may be obtained where suitable radiographic protection protocols are available. The animal should be measured and radiograph settings calculated in advance of radiography. Supplementation of inspired oxygen should be continued during the procedure. If the animal can tolerate the manipulation, it is ideal to obtain at least two and ideally three views of the thorax.

SELECTED RESPIRATORY DISTRESS SYNDROMES

Patient history often provides a significant insight into possible causes of respiratory distress. Trauma and exposure to smoke are two examples of situations in which historical information can be extremely important. Other common presentations, including congestive heart failure or toxicoses such as rodenticide anticoagulant toxicity, are addressed in the relevant chapters of this manual. If no causes for respiratory distress are known, then physical examination findings, their progression and other concurrent problems must be used to form a diagnostic and therapeutic plan.

Trauma

Trauma is a common cause of respiratory distress, most commonly following a road traffic accident (RTA). When a patient is presented with dyspnoea and a history of trauma, the clinician has a limited list of possible differential diagnoses. Specifically, dyspnoea in trauma patients is usually associated with pneumothorax, pulmonary contusions, haemothorax, rib fractures or diaphragmatic hernia. These may occur alone or in any combination.

Pneumothorax

Pneumothorax is the most common result of blunt trauma to the chest. It is caused by leakage of air from the parenchyma or airways into the pleural space, resulting in atelectasis or collapse of the lung lobes (Figure 5.8). Many animals that have sustained trauma have a small air leak that quickly seals over and may not lead to clinical signs. Where clinical signs of dyspnoea are absent and pneumothorax is an incidental finding on a screening radiograph, it is not necessary to remove the air. Air can be left in place and will be gradually absorbed by the body. Tension pneumothorax is a serious condition in which a large pulmonary leak acts as a ball-valve,

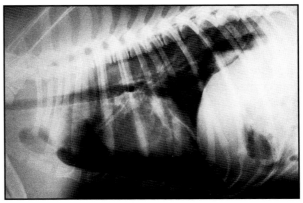

Figure 5.8: *A Pit Bull Terrier after sustaining blunt vehicular trauma to the chest. A pneumothorax can be diagnosed on this lateral thoracic radiograph by elevation of the cardiac silhouette off the sternum and collapse and retraction of the lung lobes. Thoracocentesis resulted in removal of 1500 ml of air.*

allowing air continuously to enter the pleural cavity, but preventing air from leaving. This results in progressively increasing interpleural pressure, resulting in further compression of the lungs and a mediastinal shift away from the pneumothorax.

Animals with pneumothorax present with varying degrees of dyspnoea depending on the amount of air that has leaked into the pleural cavity. Physical examination findings include a rapid shallow respiratory rate, orthopnoea, pale or pink mucous membranes and diminished dorsal lung sounds. Concurrent signs of hypovolaemic shock (tachycardia, poor pulse quality or bounding pulses and delayed or rapid capillary refill time) are common. These may be caused by haemorrhage or by obstruction of venous return to the heart due to the increased interpleural pressure exerted by a tension pneumothorax.

Because pneumothorax is a common finding post-RTA, the first priority for stabilization of any dyspnoeic trauma patient is to perform thoracocentesis, even before radiographs are obtained. Most traumatic pneumothorax patients require thoracocentesis once at presentation, and because the leak seals spontaneously, do not require further treatment for this problem. Some animals have a significant leak of air that continues after the initial thoracocentesis and, although they may show a good initial clinical response, they can become dyspnoeic again within minutes or hours of the procedure, necessitating repeated thoracocentesis procedures. If needle thoracocentesis is required on more than two occasions; if the volumes obtained each time are large; or if the clinician fails to reach a negative pressure endpoint of thoracocentesis (probable tension pneumothorax), placement of chest tubes is indicated. The technique for chest tube placement is outlined in Chapter 22. If considerable volumes of air are leaking into the pleural cavity, management may be facilitated by attachment of the chest tubes to a water-sealed continuous evacuation device. These devices apply a negative pressure of 10–15 cm H_2O to the pleural cavity, simulating normal interpleural pressure, and continuously aspirate air from the chest as it leaks from the lungs. In most cases, the leak seals within 48 hours and no further treatment is necessary. On rare occasions, if the leak fails to seal, exploratory thoracotomy may be required to resolve the problem. Ongoing leaks that have failed to seal spontaneously may represent tears of major airways and are often also accompanied by pneumomediastinum or subcutaneous emphysema.

Pulmonary contusions

Pulmonary contusions are the second most common cause of dyspnoea following blunt thoracic trauma, representing haemorrhage into the pulmonary interstitium and alveoli from ruptured capillaries (Figure 5.9). These animals are often in hypovolaemic (haemorrhagic) shock, combined with respiratory distress and increased bronchovesicular sounds or even crackles.

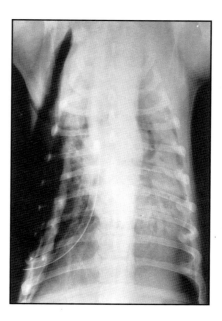

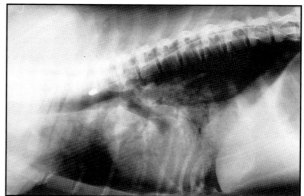

Figure 5.9: *Lateral and ventrodorsal thoracic radiographs of an 11-month-old Basset Hound after sustaining blunt trauma to the chest. A chest tube has been placed in the right side of the chest. Pulmonary contusions are evident in the left lung lobes and several ribs are fractured on that side. A small amount of air remains in the right side of the chest and subcutaneous emphysema is also present on that side.*

Even though these patients are usually in shock, caution should be exercised when resuscitating them, since fluid loading can worsen the severity of pulmonary haemorrhage and can cause accumulation of oedema fluid in addition to blood. Although crackles may sometimes be heard on chest auscultation at presentation, diuretics such as frusemide are contraindicated in the presence of shock. Diuretics do not prevent further haemorrhage into the pulmonary parenchyma and do not promote reabsorption of erythrocytes from the lung. Instead, by causing diuresis, they may exacerbate hypovolaemia.

Pulmonary contusions should be treated by cautious fluid therapy and supportive care (oxygen supplementation) until the lungs have a chance to reabsorb the blood. In severe cases, positive pressure ventilation and/or positive end expiratory pressure may be required to support oxygenation. If pulmonary function deteriorates following fluid therapy, but the cardiovascular system has stabilized, it is likely that pulmonary oedema is present superimposed on the haemorrhage. In this event, judicious use of frusemide can be helpful to resolve the oedema.

Although bacterial pneumonia can be a complication of pulmonary contusions, prophylactic antibiotic therapy is not recommended. Prophylactic antibiotics result in selection for resistant bacterial populations and may not change the incidence of pneumonia. Instead, the patient should be monitored for signs that pneumonia has developed: a productive cough, fever or failure of dyspnoea to resolve within 48–72 hours. If pneumonia occurs, a tracheal wash with culture and sensitivity, followed by appropriate antibiotic therapy, nebulization and coupage are recommended. Techniques for transtracheal and endotracheal washes are described in Chapter 22.

Haemothorax

Serious haemothorax (haemorrhage into the pleural cavity) is an uncommon complication of thoracic trauma. Dull ventral lung sounds may be evident, as well as decreased heart sounds. Patients with significant haemothorax have usually sustained massive trauma to the chest cavity, and other problems, including fractured ribs and pulmonary contusions, should be suspected. If the amount of pleural haemorrhage is small and respiratory distress is believed to be due to other causes such as pulmonary contusions, the blood should not be removed. Minimal invasion of the chest prevents disruption of any clots that have formed and also allows reabsorption of erythrocytes and gradual 'auto-transfusion'. If the animal has significant respiratory compromise because of blood in the pleural space, then thoracocentesis should be performed. In the most severe cases of haemothorax, an emergency thoracotomy may be required to identify and ligate a bleeding vessel.

Rib fractures and flail chest

Rib fractures are another common sequelae of blunt thoracic trauma and are commonly accompanied by pulmonary contusions. Fracture of one or several ribs does not usually require any specific treatment other than rest, pain management and oxygen supplementation (see Figure 5.9). If several ribs are each fractured in more than one place, a flail chest segment can occur. The flail segment is not stabilized by attachment to the spine or sternum and can be observed moving paradoxically relative to the rest of the chest wall during respiration. During inspiration, when the rest of the chest is moving outward, the flail segment is pulled inward by the negative interpleural pressure.

Small to moderate sized sections of flail chest should be managed medically, with oxygen supplementation and analgesia as needed. Dyspnoea in these patients is thought to be primarily caused by contusions. Large flail chest segments can contribute to dyspnoea by preventing effective movement of the chest wall, resulting in hypoventilation. Placing the animal with the affected side down can help stabilize the segment and promote better ventilation. Severe flail segments require surgical stabilization, and some of these animals require postoperative mechanical ventilation if severe pulmonary contusions are also present.

Diaphragmatic hernia

Animals that have sustained trauma may also develop a diaphragmatic hernia: rupture of the diaphragm with penetration of abdominal contents into the thoracic cavity. A variety of organs may be involved in the hernia, including liver, spleen, stomach, omentum and intestines (Figure 5.10). Dyspnoea is caused by the physical presence of these organs, as well as the accumulation of pleural fluid due to inflammation and occlusion of venous return from the viscera. Vascular compromise associated with strangulation may cause tissue necrosis, further compromising organ and pulmonary function. Acute onset of respiratory distress may occur if the stomach herniates and becomes bloated with gas due to occlusion of the cardia. The size of the stomach can increase rapidly due to gas distension. This represents an immediate surgical emergency and the gas distension of the stomach should be relieved by trocharization while the animal is being prepared for surgery.

Diagnosis of diaphragmatic hernia is suggested by clinical findings including diminished lung sounds or auscultation of bowel sounds in the thorax. Some patients may also have signs of dysfunction of the displaced organs such as vomiting or icterus. The diagnosis should be confirmed by plain radiography or by administration of contrast media. If the stomach or intestines are in the chest, they can be easily outlined by

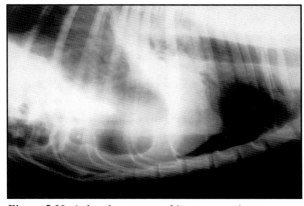

Figure 5.10: *A dog that presented in acute respiratory distress several months after sustaining blunt vehicular trauma to the chest. On this lateral thoracic radiograph, the diaphragm cannot be visualized and abdominal organs, including liver, stomach and loops of bowel, can be seen in the thoracic cavity, indicating that there is a diaphragmatic hernia. This dog underwent an emergency thoracotomy to repair his diaphragmatic hernia.*

a small amount of oral barium. Other techniques, including positional lateral beam radiography or ultrasonography can also provide valuable information.

Diaphragmatic hernias should be repaired surgically as soon as possible. Some patients with diaphragmatic hernia do not have clinical evidence of respiratory distress at the time of trauma and may present years later with their first signs of respiratory compromise. Animals with chronic diaphragmatic hernias may be extremely difficult to treat surgically because of the presence of adhesions and the high likelihood of postoperative re-expansion pulmonary oedema. Thus, early diagnosis and surgical treatment is essential for animals with this problem, even if clinical signs are not initially evident. Thoracic radiography is therefore recommended in all cases of trauma to rule out the presence of an occult diaphragmatic hernia.

Smoke inhalation

Animals that present after exposure to smoke from house fires can have varying degrees of respiratory difficulty. Damage is caused by direct thermal injury and by inhalation of noxious substances produced by combustion. The gases produced in the largest amounts during combustion are carbon monoxide, hydrogen cyanide and carbon dioxide. All three of these gases, combined with low concentrations of oxygen, can cause narcosis. They combine very rapidly with haemoglobin, diminishing its availability and effectiveness for oxygen transfer. Animals that have been exposed to smoke in fires should be immediately treated with a high inspired concentration of oxygen to attempt to displace these gases from haemoglobin. Oxygen therapy should be continued for at least an hour. Other gases produced by combustion vary depending on the materials that have burned and some can be extremely toxic.

The upper airway can become so inflamed and oedematous from thermal burns that obstruction can occur. Patients should be monitored for signs of laryngeal or upper airway obstruction, and tracheostomy or intubation performed if necessary. Airway damage often includes severe necrotizing tracheobronchitis, which is accompanied by exudate and cough. Bacterial pneumonia is a common sequela due to damaged lung defences and proliferation of bacterial pathogens. In worst case scenarios, diffuse inflammatory damage to the lung may be recognized, manifesting as generalized acute lung injury that can progress to ARDS.

Treatment of smoke inhalation should consist of oxygen supplementation, saline nebulization and coupage to promote clearance of material from the airways, bronchodilators and supportive care. Corticosteroids are not recommended in these patients because they are already immunosuppressed. Prophylactic antibiotics should be avoided, as their use prior to the development of pneumonia will only select for resistant bacteria. As with all patients at risk for pneumonia, careful monitoring for signs of pneumonia should be followed by a

tracheal wash for cytology, culture and sensitivity testing before starting antibiotic therapy.

Animals that are caught in fires often suffer skin burns as well as lung injury. Particular attention should be given to the corneas and oronasal mucosa. The corneas should be stained with fluorescein, and ulceration treated if present. Patients with skin burns suffer from profound fluid and protein loss and are among the most critically ill animals, with potential for rapid development of multiple organ dysfunction or failure.

APPROACH TO UNDIAGNOSED RESPIRATORY DISTRESS

When the initial history does not provide specific useful information, the approach to the patient in respiratory distress is one of treatment according to the apparent site of respiratory pathology. The presentation and physical examination, in addition to the history, are often sufficient to determine which areas of the respiratory system are involved. For this purpose, the respiratory tract is divided into the airways (upper and lower), the pulmonary parenchyma and the pleural space. After determining which of these are affected, the clinician can then develop a list of differential diagnoses, diagnostic procedures and therapeutic strategies for the individual patient.

Upper airway disease

Clinical signs of upper airway disease

The clinical signs of disease of the upper airway are listed in Figure 5.11. Because they commonly involve the larynx, upper airway disorders often cause loud stridor that is audible without a stethoscope. On auscultation, upper airway noise is loudest over the trachea. Referred sounds may also be heard on auscultation of the lungs. Most dogs with dynamic upper airway obstructions (such as brachycephalic airway syndrome or laryngeal paralysis) have dyspnoea, primarily heard on inspiration as stridor. The negative forces exerted during inspiration tend to close the upper airway,

---

Dyspnoea

Audible stridor or stertor

Increased inspiratory effort with prolonged inspiratory time (gasping respiration)

Change in vocalization (bark or meow)

Exercise intolerance—clinical signs most severe when stressed or exercising

Excessive panting

Hyperthermia

Figure 5.11: *Clinical and historical signs associated with upper airway or laryngeal obstruction in dogs and cats.*

whereas during exhalation the airway opens. Animals with fixed upper airway obstructions (such as masses or abscesses) tend to have difficulty during both inspiration and expiration.

Dyspnoea in animals with upper airway obstruction is made worse by exercise or excitement and is improved or almost absent at rest. Increased respiratory drive results in enhanced negative inspiratory pressures during exercise, leading to more severe narrowing of the airway. Tests of pulmonary function during dyspnoeic episodes in these patients often reveal a significant hypoxia and hypercarbia, whereas these parameters may become almost normal at rest. This return of pulmonary function to normal at rest is one of the hallmark signs of upper airway obstruction; blood gases usually remain abnormal at rest in animals with parenchymal or pleural disease.

Most dogs with upper airway obstruction suffer from hyperthermia because they are unable to thermoregulate effectively due to an insufficient volume of air passing over the tongue during panting. Hyperthermia starts a vicious cycle, as it stimulates an increased respiration rate and panting, which further narrows the airway.

General approach to management of patients with upper airway obstruction

Management of animals with upper airway obstruction is summarized in Figure 5.12. The most important priority is to encourage the animal to rest quietly in an enriched oxygen environment. Often these animals resist manipulation of the head and neck; therefore, an oxygen cage or intranasal cannula is usually the best approach. Many benefit considerably from sedation. Acepromazine is the drug of choice provided that the animal is not hypovolaemic (phenothiazines may be

associated with vasodilation, which exacerbates signs of hypovolaemia). The dose of acepromazine should be kept at a minimum and may by more effective if combined with a opioid analgesic (neuroleptanalgesia). Opioids may also be used in isolation where there is hypovolaemia, as these agents produce minimal cardiovascular effects. Suggested agents include morphine, pethidine (UK), oxymorphone (USA), butorphanol or buprenorphine. These agents may also be combined with a sedative such as diazepam if they trigger excessive panting. Manipulation and stress should be kept to a minimum, but if the animal is collapsed or sedated, the head and neck should be extended and the tongue pulled out of the mouth to minimize airway resistance. Corticosteroids are often very helpful if significant airway oedema or inflammation is present. They should be initially avoided if neoplasia such as lymphosarcoma is one of the differential diagnoses. Corticosteroids may cause lysis of malignant lymphocytes, thereby making it difficult to confirm the diagnosis. Core body temperature should be monitored carefully and vigorous attempts made to cool the patient with fans, ice, alcohol or cool intravenous fluids if the temperature is greater than 40°C.

Animals that do not respond to this approach should be anaesthetized and intubated, or a tracheotomy performed if necessary (see earlier). Ideally, these animals should not remain intubated through the larynx for more than a few hours, as the tube triggers swelling that may exacerbate the problem following extubation.

In many syndromes of upper airway obstruction, pharyngoscopy and laryngoscopy under general anaesthesia are required to confirm the diagnosis. Following this, steps should be taken to relieve the airway obstruction prior to anaesthetic recovery. Attempts to recover these patients from anaesthesia without supporting the airway are hazardous and often fail. Even if the underlying disease cannot be corrected, a tracheotomy should be performed prior to extubation.

Syndromes of upper airway obstruction

Brachycephalic obstructive airway syndrome (BOAS) is a common cause of respiratory distress in affected breeds of dog (Figure 5.13). Examples include English Bulldogs, Boston Terriers, Boxers, Pekingese and Pugs.

Oxygen supplementation: O₂ cage best

Rest, sedation if necessary

Acepromazine 0.01–0.05 mg/kg i.v. or i.m. if cardiovascularly stable

If collapsed or sedated, extend head and neck and pull tongue out of the mouth

Vascular access

Minimal stress

Anti-inflammatory to immunosuppressive doses of corticosteroids unless contraindicated (Dexamethasone 0.25–0.5 mg/kg i.v. or i.m.)

Monitor temperature, vigorous efforts to cool if needed

Fluid therapy if dehydrated or hypovolaemic

Emergency tracheostomy or intubation if no response to medical management

Figure 5.12: General approach to emergency management of dogs and cats with upper airway obstruction.

Brachycephalic syndrome

Laryngeal paralysis

Tracheal collapse

Nasopharyngeal polyps (feline)

Aspirated foreign bodies

Upper airway neoplasia

Retropharyngeal masses, abscesses or haematomas

Figure 5.13: Common differential diagnoses of upper airway obstruction in dogs and cats.

The components of this syndrome are stenotic nares, redundant pharyngeal soft tissue, excessively long soft palate and hypoplastic trachea (Figure 5.14). Chronic obstruction of the upper airway causes increased negative inspiratory pressure leading to further airway occlusion, inflammation and oedema of the redundant tissue, eversion of the laryngeal saccules and eventually, in end-stage cases, complete laryngeal collapse. In contrast, certain cat breeds (e.g. Persian) often have stenotic nares but do not develop true brachycephalic syndrome. In patients with BOAS, mouth-breathing often improves the clinical signs because some of the airway resistance caused by the stenotic nares is eliminated. These animals also often present with hyperthermia and acute respiratory distress during hot humid weather, after exercise or when extremely excited. Careful questioning of the owners often reveals a history of chronic airway obstruction: snoring and airway noise, which the owners may interpret as 'normal for the breed.'

Treatment is as described above, including oxygen supplementation, sedation, cooling and corticosteroids. Most patients can be managed medically through the presenting crisis, but surgical intervention to prevent future episodes is strongly recommended. Surgical correction of the stenotic nares and the overlong soft palate can greatly improve these patients, especially if performed in young dogs (less than 2 years of age).

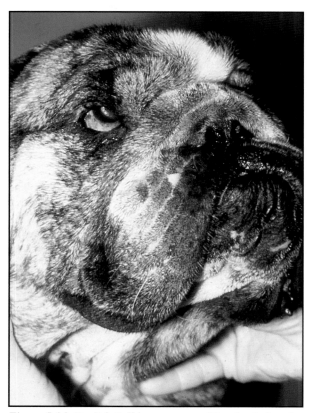

Figure 5.14: *English Bulldogs are one of the classic breeds affected by brachycephalic syndrome. This female required an emergency tracheostomy due to respiratory distress from upper airway obstruction caused by stenotic nares, overlong soft palate, everted saccules and hypoplastic trachea.*

Laryngeal paralysis occurs in dogs and cats due to disruption of innervation of the muscles of the larynx and is classified as either congenital or acquired (idiopathic, traumatic, polyneuropathic or iatrogenic). Idiopathic acquired laryngeal paralysis is the most common form, most often seen in large breed dogs such as Labrador Retrievers, Golden Retrievers and Saint Bernards. Affected dogs can present in severe respiratory distress, cyanosis and collapse. They often have a loud inspiratory stridor and may be hyperthermic. The history may include voice change, gagging while eating and drinking, progressive exercise intolerance and noisy breathing.

Immediate therapy is as described above, with severely affected animals requiring intubation or a temporary tracheotomy. Thoracic radiography should be performed, as aspiration pneumonia and non-cardiogenic pulmonary oedema are common. Definitive diagnosis is made by laryngeal examination on induction of anaesthesia, to determine whether the vocal folds abduct effectively and symmetrically during inspiration. Since anaesthesia affects movement of the larynx, anaesthesia must be light enough that the patient is almost coughing during the laryngeal examination. Paradoxical laryngeal motion is another source of error of interpretation during laryngoscopy. If the larynx is paralysed, inspiration may be accompanied by closure of the larynx owing to negative inspiratory pressures, and exhalation may tend to 'blow the larynx open.' This creates a paradoxical motion of the larynx, which on casual inspection may simulate normal function. Therefore, while performing a laryngeal examination, any observed movement of the larynx must be carefully correlated with the phase of respiration.

Surgical intervention may be delayed until the respiratory crisis has passed, allowing resolution of laryngeal inflammation and oedema. The method of choice is a laryngeal tie-back (arytenoid cartilage lateralization). Postoperative concerns include aspiration pneumonia, laryngeal inflammation and oedema, haemorrhage, or breakdown of the surgical repair. Postoperative complications can be minimized by keeping the animal as quiet as possible and reducing vocalization or coughing in the first 24 hours after surgery.

Tracheal collapse is a common problem in middle-aged to older small breed dogs. These animals often have a progressive history of cough and exercise intolerance. An easily induced cough is commonly found on tracheal palpation. Excitement often triggers a paroxysmal 'honking' cough and dyspnoea. The tracheal rings in these animals are often abnormally C-shaped and fibrodysplastic, and the dorsal tracheal membrane is stretched floppy and weak. Obstruction of the tracheal lumen occurs in the cervical and/or thoracic trachea. Dogs with mitral regurgitation may have enlargement of the left atrium before congestive heart failure occurs. This leads to compression, elevation and collapse of the left mainstem bronchus. Coughing may therefore be triggered which will appear similar to that in patients with primary tracheal collapse and is approached in a similar way, in addition to concurrent management of the primary cardiac disease.

Animals with tracheal collapse can present with varying degrees of dyspnoea. In the most severe cases, complete collapse of sections of the trachea can mimic upper airway obstruction. Other animals can become hypoxic because of spasms of paroxysmal coughing. The diagnosis is difficult to confirm with plain thoracic radiography. Severe collapse can appear radiographically similar to a tracheal soft-tissue mass. One method of clinical diagnosis is by observation of the trachea while coughing under fluoroscopy. The gold standard for diagnosis is bronchoscopy, but this requires anaesthesia, recovery from which is associated with a high degree of risk if surgical correction is not performed at the time of diagnosis.

Management is performed as described above, with the addition of cough suppressants. Opioids, especially butorphanol and with the possible exception of pethidine (meperidine), are antitussive at low doses and are often beneficial. If medical management is ineffective, surgical options are associated with some risk but may produce good results even in patients with end-stage disease. Tracheotomy is usually not of benefit in these patients because the collapse typically occurs throughout the cervical region and intrathoracic trachea or mainstem bronchi. Surgical options currently used in the UK include extraluminal ring prostheses with or without concurrent laryngeal surgery.

Inflammatory nasopharyngeal polyps occasionally cause respiratory stridor and dyspnoea in young, otherwise healthy cats. The polyps are often associated with inflammatory disease of the tympanic bullae or auditory canals. These cats may have an inspiratory stridor, a nasal discharge and otitis externa. The polyp is occasionally visible on oral examination in the awake patient, but sedation is usually required for adequate visualization. The soft palate should be palpated and retracted to detect polyps in the nasopharynx, and a thorough otoscopic examination should be performed. Radiographs of the skull, bullae and nasal cavity should be obtained (Figure 5.15). Polyps may arise from the bullae, ear canals or nasopharyngeal mucosa and must be removed surgically. If there is evidence of otitis, bulla osteotomy may be considered to resolve the underlying cause of the polyp. If the entire polyp is removed, surgery is generally curative.

Aspirated foreign bodies can cause sudden onset of respiratory distress if the foreign body obstructs the airway. Large upper airway obstructions require immediate action, since they may completely obstruct all air flow. The animals often panic and are difficult to restrain, and sedation may be necessary. If possible, vascular access should be established and sedatives or anaesthetics administered intravenously. Because it may be impossible to remove the foreign body fast enough, preparation for an emergency tracheostomy is

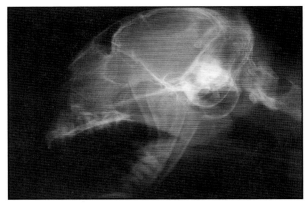

Figure 5.15: *A lateral radiograph of a cat's skull showing an extremely large pharyngeal polyp occluding the pharynx. This cat presented with very loud upper airway stridor.*
Reproduced with permission of Veterinary Learning Systems, Trenton, NJ.

prudent. After expeditious removal of the object, supplemental oxygen should be administered. If the animal is unconscious after foreign body removal, it should be intubated and ventilation assisted until spontaneous breathing and consciousness return.

Upper airway neoplasia also occasionally causes upper airway obstruction. Neoplasia usually causes a slow onset of respiratory distress unless the tumour is very rapidly growing or associated with an abscess. Lymphosarcoma is the most commonly observed neoplasm, especially in cats, but any oral neoplasm may be involved. Oxygen supplementation and sedation may sufficient to improve clinical signs in these animals if they are not too severely affected. If necessary, when the neoplasm is in the proximal trachea or above, emergency tracheostomy can provide an adequate airway until more definitive surgery for the tumour is performed. If the neoplasm is in the thoracic trachea and the patient cannot be stabilized medically, intubation (if possible) or emergency thoracotomy are the only options.

Retropharyngeal masses, abscesses and haematomas are an occasional cause of respiratory distress. The most common retropharyngeal neoplasm is lymphosarcoma, while abscesses can result from haematogenous spread or foreign body penetration. Rapid diagnosis by pharyngoscopy, ultrasound, needle aspiration or even exploratory surgery is essential. These animals can easily progress to complete obstruction of their airway and require emergency tracheostomy. Haematomas can occur secondary to anticoagulant rodenticide ingestion or trauma. In animals with coagulopathies, needle aspiration and surgery are contraindicated. Haemostasis can be difficult, but plasma transfusions and specific antidotes such as vitamin K should eventually stop the haemorrhage.

Lower airway disease

Clinical signs of lower airway disease
Clinical signs of animals with lower airway disease are summarized in Figure 5.16. Disease of the lower airways

Cough

Exercise intolerance

Dyspnoea (severe cases, expiratory dyspnoea in cats with feline asthma)

Increased bronchovesicular sounds

Wheezes

Figure 5.16: Clinical and historical signs associated with lower airway (bronchial) disease in dogs and cats.

usually refers to abnormalities of the small bronchi and is commonly inflammatory in origin. Coughing is the most common historical finding. Typically, the cough is harsh and non-productive and is not beneficial to the patient as it tends to exacerbate inflammation, thereby promoting more coughing. On auscultation, most dogs with lower airway disease have increased bronchovesicular sounds and/or wheezes. Patients with end-stage disease may have significantly increased respiratory rate and effort associated with hypoxia. Thoracic radiographs usually reveal minimal evidence of alveolar disease. Dogs and cats with productive coughing (usually a soft moist sound that is followed by swallowing when the animal expectorates material into the pharynx) should be evaluated for disorders such as pneumonia. In pneumonia, the cough is a necessary part of the clearance mechanism of the lung, rather than being due to bronchial disease alone.

Hypoxia in animals with chronic bronchitis is thought to be attributable to inequality of ventilation and pulmonary perfusion (V–Q mismatch), mainly caused by bronchial obstruction. Bronchial obstruction follows increased mucus production, mucosal hyperaemia and oedema, as well as early collapse of abnormal and weakened small airways. Obesity often contributes to the severity of clinical signs, causing diminished ability to expand the lungs and pressure on the thorax from the chest wall and abdomen. Bronchopneumonia is a common complication because of diminished lung defences. Although some degree of bronchoconstriction can occur, dogs do not suffer from smooth muscle spasm as seen in cats with asthma. Acute severe bronchoconstriction in cats with hyperresponsive airways contributes significantly to dyspnoea in affected animals. Severe cases therefore present with dyspnoea caused by end-stage chronic obstructive pulmonary disease, superimposed bronchopneumonia and, in cats, bronchospasm.

General approach to management of patients with lower airway disease

Priorities for management of lower airway disease are summarized in Figure 5.17. Animals with lower airway disease are usually presented during exacerbations and crises, or when the disease has become end stage. Dyspnoea is a common presentation, especially in cats with feline asthma. As usual, oxygen supplementation

Oxygen supplementation

Rest, sedation not usually required

Minimal stress

Vascular access

Anti-inflammatory to immunosuppressive doses of corticosteroids
    Dexamethasone 0.25–0.5 mg/kg i.v. or i.m. or prednisone 0.5–1 mg/kg i.v., i.m. or orally

Bronchodilators
    Terbutaline 0.01 mg/kg i.v. or i.m. or aminophylline 5.5 mg/kg i.v.

Cough suppressants
    Butorphanol 0.2–0.4 mg/kg i.v. or i.m., 0.5–1.0 mg/kg orally or hydrocodone 1.25–5 mg/kg orally

Antibiotics

Thoracic radiographs to rule out pulmonary alveolar disease

Consider tracheal wash for culture and cytological examination

Figure 5.17: General approach to emergency management of dogs and cats with lower airway disease.

is the first priority. Animals that are extremely distressed may benefit from sedation. Early diagnostic investigation where lower airway disease is suspected should include thoracic radiography. Most patients with bronchial disease have little or no alveolar disease visible on thoracic radiographs. A peribronchial pattern may be present, with 'doughnuts' and 'tramlines,' but alveolar disease should be absent.

If bronchial disease is suspected, corticosteroids can be extremely helpful because of the role of inflammation in the disease process. Initially, high doses are indicated, reducing to the minimal effective dose as soon as possible. Bronchodilators are also considered first-line drugs in these patients. Beta-agonists such as terbutaline have superseded aminophylline in clinical use. Refractory coughing may respond to antitussive drugs such as butorphanol. Since exacerbation of signs may occur due to secondary bacterial infection and even pneumonia, antibiotics may be of value in some cases to diminish exudate production. Ideally, cytology and cultures from the airway (usually obtained by tracheal wash) should be obtained prior to starting antibiotic therapy. Most respiratory crises caused by bronchial disease respond well to medical management, minimal stress and an oxygen-enriched environment.

Syndromes of lower airway disease

Feline asthma, also referred to as allergic bronchitis, is the most common cause of lower airway disease in cats (Figure 5.18). The clinical signs result from bronchial inflammation with peribronchial infiltrates, mucosal

Feline asthma
Chronic bronchitis
Neoplasia
Aspirated foreign body

Figure 5.18: *Common differential diagnoses for lower airway disease in dogs and cats.*

oedema, increased mucus production, bronchiolar smooth muscle hypertrophy and reversible airway obstruction caused by excessive bronchoconstriction. Airway obstruction is most severe during expiration and may lead to air trapping and alveolar hyperinflation. Cats may present with disease at any age, but signs often first appear in young adults. Clinical signs can range from severe dyspnoea to intermittent cough. In severe cases, the cats open-mouth breathe, have pale to cyanotic mucous membranes and may have an abdominal component to respiration. On auscultation, expiratory wheezes are often heard. In the most severe cases, respiratory sounds may be almost absent, as air movement is almost cut off by the severity of bronchial obstruction.

If the cat is in severe distress, obtaining a definitive diagnosis should be delayed until the cat is more stable. The cat should be placed in an oxygen cage, which minimizes stress and allows it to relax after stressful transport. Since bronchoconstriction occurs as a result of inflammation, corticosteroids should be given intravenously if possible (otherwise, intramuscularly). Bronchodilators such as terbutaline have proven to be useful in acute management. In agonal cases, adrenaline should be administered intramuscularly (0.5–0.75 ml of 1:10,000 solution i.m.), for its profound vasoconstrictive, inotropic and bronchodilator effects. If there is no response to medical management and the cat remains in severe distress, anaesthesia and intubation may be required. Occasionally, cats may have pneumothorax secondary to rupture of the hyperinflated alveoli.

Radiographic findings include demonstration of a bronchiolar pattern, collapse of the right middle lung lobe and pulmonary hyperinflation (Figure 5.19). Findings may, however, be normal, especially if radiography is delayed in unstable animals. Definitive diagnosis requires the demonstration of inflammation on analysis of tracheal wash cytology.

Canine chronic bronchitis is recognized as a persistent cough occurring for at least 2 consecutive months in the absence of a specific pulmonary disease. Hyperplasia and hypertrophy of bronchial glands, increased goblet cells, increased airway secretion and increased infiltrates of inflammatory cells are seen. This produces thickened, hyperaemic bronchial walls, obstruction of small airways with mucus and proliferation of epithelial surfaces. The aetiology is uncertain, but environmental factors, allergic disease, inherited

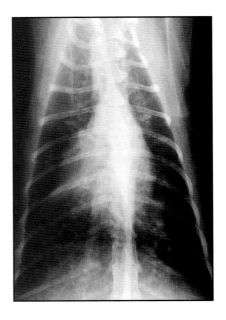

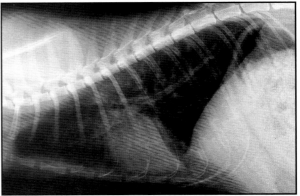

Figure 5.19: *Lateral and ventrodorsal thoracic radiographs of a 3-year-old Domestic Long Hair cat that presented with a 3-month history of coughing and acute respiratory distress. The radiographs show the typical bronchial pattern of feline asthma, often described as 'doughnuts and tramlines', collapse of the right middle lung lobe and pulmonary hyperinflation.*

tendencies and infectious agents may all play a role. Patients with exacerbated or end-stage disease can present with severe distress and cyanosis.

Physical examination findings may include increased airway sounds, wheezes and coarse crackles on chest auscultation caused by opening and closing of small bronchi. Thoracic radiographs usually show a bronchial pattern and the extent of changes does not always correlate with the severity of clinical signs. Immediate management is as described above. In addition, saline nebulization may assist with mobilization of secretions.

Foreign bodies and tumours can also occur in the lower airways. Radiographs may assist in confirming the diagnosis. Chronic bronchial obstruction causes gradual collapse and absorption atelectasis of the affected lung lobe. Even if a foreign body or neoplasm is not suggested on radiographs, the presence of one completely collapsed lung lobe should prompt suspicion of bronchial obstruction. Sudden onset of respiratory distress can be seen after aspiration of a foreign body into the bronchi (Figure 5.20). Foreign bodies may be removed by bronchoscopy or thoracotomy. Neoplasia of the lower airways is usually characterized by a slower, more gradual onset of respiratory distress. Thoracic radiographs and bronchoscopy can aid in the diagnosis, and biopsy assists in its confirmation. Debulking or removal of the mass (often including lung lobectomy) may be necessary, unless the biopsy reveals lymphosarcoma which may respond to chemotherapy.

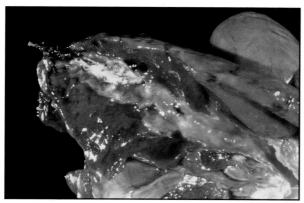

Figure 5.20: *A post-mortem examination of this 4-year-old cat revealed aspirated plant material in a bronchus.*
Reproduced with permission of Veterinary Learning Systems, Trenton, NJ.

Pulmonary parenchymal disease

Clinical signs of pulmonary parenchymal disease
Clinical signs of pulmonary parenchymal disease are summarized in Figure 5.21. Pulmonary parenchymal disease is commonly associated with varying degrees of hypoxia and dyspnoea. Typically, the lungs have decreased compliance. A restrictive pattern of respiration (rapid shallow breathing) is observed and severe hypoxia may be manifested by paradoxical respiration. Hypoxia in patients with pulmonary parenchymal disease is usually caused by ventilation/perfusion mismatch due to filling and collapse of alveoli. Some patients may also have an increased diffusion barrier caused by thickening or infiltration of the alveolar membrane.

Hypoxaemia
Increased respiratory rate or dyspnoea
Restrictive respiratory pattern
Harsh bronchovesicular sounds
Crackles
Nasal discharge
Cough (often productive)

Figure 5.21: *Clinical and historical signs associated with pulmonary parenchymal disease in dogs and cats.*

On auscultation, harsh bronchovesicular sounds and/or crackles are common. Careful auscultation of the heart should be performed to detect the presence of a murmur which might indicate congestive heart failure. Nasal discharge can occur in patients with bronchopneumonia or profound pulmonary oedema. Coughing may be a feature of pulmonary parenchymal disease if there is bronchial irritation or inflammation. Typically, coughing is productive — a soft moist cough that is an important part of clearance of secretions from the pulmonary parenchyma.

Animals with pulmonary parenchymal disease usually have an alveolar pattern on thoracic radiographs. The distribution of the alveolar pattern can give important information about the aetiology of respiratory failure. Occasionally animals may have minor or absent radiographic changes; for example those with pulmonary thromboembolism or interstitial fibrosis.

General approach to management of patients with pulmonary parenchymal disease
The approach to management of animals with pulmonary parenchymal disease is summarized in Figure 5.22. Patients that are dyspnoeic due to suspected pulmonary parenchymal disease should receive oxygen supplementation immediately. Physical examination and historical findings often give an indication of the cause of the dyspnoea. Thoracic radiographs are a valuable diagnostic tool at this stage. If respiratory distress is so severe that thoracic radiographs cannot be safely obtained, the clinician must make a list of the common treatable causes of pulmonary parenchymal disease and treat empirically according to the most likely problems. Often, empirical medical management, combined with oxygen supplementation, can improve the condition of the patient to the point that radiographs can be obtained. If the patient does not improve, or even deteriorates in spite of medical management, an aggressive approach may be required. This usually means anaesthesia and intubation of the patient to facilitate diagnostic testing and therapy. The most common medical problems and their management are described below.

Syndromes of pulmonary parenchymal disease
Pneumonia is one of the most common causes of pulmonary parenchymal disease (Figure 5.23). It is categorized as aspiration, bacterial, viral or fungal, occurring alone or in combination. Pneumonia is more common in dogs than in cats. Physical examination usually reveals increased respiratory rate and effort, pale to cyanotic mucous membranes and harsh lung sounds or crackles. If the animal is stable, the diagnosis is confirmed by radiographic findings of cranioventral alveolar disease (Figure 5.24), cytology showing acute neutrophilic inflammation, and culture and sensitivity testing of airway aspirates obtained by tracheal wash or bronchoalveolar lavage. Serology may be used to assist diagnosis of viral or fungal pneumonia.

Oxygen supplementation

Rest and minimal stress

Vascular access

Thoracic radiographs (if possible)

Medical management according to most likely differential diagnoses:

Bacterial bronchopneumonia
  Tracheal wash for culture and cytological examination
  Stable: amoxicillin/clavulanate 13.75 mg/kg orally bid, enrofloxacin 5 mg/kg orally bid
  Unstable: ampicillin 22 mg/kg i.v. tid with either gentamicin 6 mg/kg i.v. sid (if renal function is normal), or enrofloxacin 5 mg/kg diluted slow infusion i.v. bid
  Nebulization and coupage

Pulmonary oedema
  Frusemide 0.5–2 mg/kg i.v. or i.m.
  Glyceryl trinitrate paste up to 1 inch cutaneously, or nitroprusside 2–10 µg/kg/min (cardiogenic)
  Dobutamine 5 µg/kg/min (cardiogenic)
  Colloids if needed

Haemorrhage
  Fresh whole blood transfusions
  Vitamin K 2 mg/kg s.c. or orally bid

Pulmonary thromboembolism
  Fresh frozen plasma
  Heparin 50–200 units/kg s.c. every 6 hours, or 10–40 units/kg/h i.v. CRI

Pulmonary inflammatory disorders (PIE and LG)
  Dexamethasone 0.25–0.5 mg/kg i.v. or i.m.
  or prednisolone 0.5–1 mg/kg i.v., i.m. or orally

Figure 5.22: General approach to emergency management of dogs and cats with pulmonary parenchymal disease. PIE: pulmonary infiltrate with eosinophils, LG: lymphomatoid granulomatosis.

Pneumonia

Pulmonary oedema (cardiogenic and neurogenic)

Haemorrhage

Pulmonary thromboembolism

Neoplasia: primary or metastatic

Pulmonary inflammatory disease (PIE and LG)

Acute lung injury and ARDS

Figure 5.23: Common differential diagnoses for pulmonary parenchymal disease in dogs and cats. PIE: pulmonary infiltrate with eosinophils, LG: lymphomatoid granulomatosis.

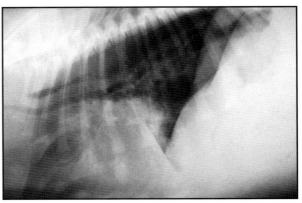

Figure 5.24: Severe aspiration pneumonia in the cranioventral and right middle lung lobes. An alveolar pattern with air bronchograms is present.

Aspiration pneumonia is caused by inhalation of foreign material. This typically comprises oral secretions or gastrointestinal tract contents subsequent to vomiting or regurgitation. Animals with underlying conditions such as pharyngeal/laryngeal dysfunction, megaoesophagus, cleft palate, abnormal mentation, recumbency or debilitation have an increased incidence of aspiration. The acidic pH of gastric reflux material determines the extent of bronchoconstriction and injury to the pulmonary parenchyma. Liquids reach the alveoli within minutes, making attempts to suction the airways futile in most cases. The resultant inflammation impairs lung defences and allows bacteria in the aspirated material to colonize the lungs. By the time most aspiration pneumonia cases are recognized, bacterial infection has occurred. These patients are therefore treated in the same way as those with primary bacterial pneumonia.

Bacterial bronchopneumonia usually occurs as a consequence of bronchogenic invasion (inhalation) of pathogenic bacteria, or occasionally by haematogenous spread. Animals with bronchogenous pneumonia typically have a cranioventral pattern of alveolar disease on radiographs, whereas those with haematogenous pneumonia often have a patchy or nodular distribution. Bacterial pneumonia can be caused by primary respiratory tract pathogens such as *Bordetella bronchiseptica*, or by opportunistic pathogens that proliferate because of suppression of respiratory tract defences. With the exception of animals suspected of *Bordetella* infection, dogs and cats that present with bacterial pneumonia should be carefully evaluated for underlying disorders.

Other causes of pneumonia include viral agents (canine distemper), protozoal organisms (toxoplasmosis), fungal invasion (histoplasmosis, blastomycosis and coccidioidomycosis) and parasitic disease. In addition to general pneumonia management, specific therapy should also be directed against individual organisms.

Bacterial cultures should be obtained before starting antibiotic therapy whenever possible. Gram-negative pathogens and polymicrobial infections are common. Broad-spectrum antibiotic treatment should be started while waiting for the culture results. Oral drugs such as amoxicillin/clavulanate or fluoroquinolones can be used if the animal is not systemically ill. If the patient is hypoxic, dyspnoeic or febrile, intravenous antibiotics must be used until the animal is stable. Combinations of antibiotics that provide broad-spectrum coverage include ampicillin/aminoglycosides, ampicillin/fluoroquinolones, or second-/third-generation cephalosporins. Another potentially valuable therapy is that of nebulization with sterile saline followed by coupage to loosen and mobilize airway secretions, promote coughing and improve airway clearance. Nebulized mucolytic agents are not typically used as they can cause bronchospasm. Oxygen supplementation should be administered as required, and severely affected cases may require positive-pressure ventilation.

Pulmonary oedema is the accumulation of fluid in the alveoli and pulmonary interstitium and is divided by initiating cause into cardiogenic and non-cardiogenic forms. Cardiogenic oedema is the more common and is seen in animals with left-sided heart failure and elevated pulmonary venous pressure. On auscultation, crackles are often evident and may be accompanied by a mitral murmur in dogs or a gallop rhythm in cats. Thoracic radiographs usually reveal cardiomegaly and a peri-hilar alveolar pattern in the dog. In cats, distribution of oedema is less localized. Details of diagnosis and management of cardiogenic pulmonary oedema are available in Chapter 4.

Neurogenic pulmonary oedema can be caused by seizures or head trauma, choking or airway obstruction and electric shock. Although the pathophysiology is not well understood, it is thought that massive sympathetic discharge results in increased peripheral resistance, which raises systemic blood pressure. Blood therefore moves from the systemic circulation into the low pressure pulmonary vasculature. This volume shift dramatically and transiently elevates pulmonary venous pressures. The end result is increased capillary permeability and fluid redistribution to the interstitium and alveoli. The pressures rapidly return to normal, but the changes in permeability remain for several hours.

Affected animals may develop respiratory distress immediately or over several hours after the inciting incident. Varying degrees of respiratory distress occur, and crackles are often heard on auscultation. The diagnosis can be confirmed by thoracic radiography, which reveals an interstitial or alveolar pattern in the dorsocaudal lung fields (Figure 5.25). The extent of lung involvement is determined by arterial blood gas analysis. Typical findings include hypoxia and a $PaCO_2$ that is low, normal or high, depending on the severity of the oedema.

Treatment consists of supportive care, with oxygen supplementation as needed. Diuretics may be administered, but are usually ineffective because the oedema is caused by a vascular permeability change, rather than by a sustained increase in pulmonary venous pressure. The use of corticosteroids in these patients remains controversial and is not currently recommended. Mildly affected animals improve dramatically in 24–48

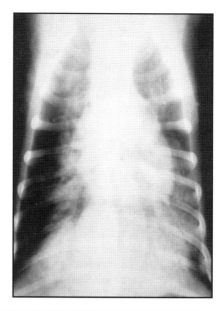

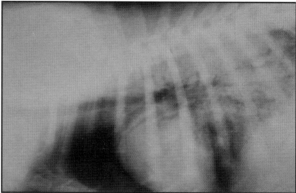

Figure 5.25: *Lateral and ventrodorsal thoracic radiographs of a dog with neurogenic pulmonary oedema following airway obstruction. The typical caudodorsal patchy alveolar pattern is present.*

hours, while the most severely affected animals can have fulminating pulmonary oedema, require positive-pressure ventilation and often do not recover.

Pulmonary haemorrhage can occur secondary to trauma, coagulopathies and neoplasia. Haemorrhage into the parenchyma is most commonly seen following anticoagulant rodenticide ingestion. These animals are presented with coughing (which may include a productive cough with blood-tinged sputum), lethargy or dyspnoea. Varying degrees of anaemia and pale mucous membranes are seen due to blood loss. Radiographs usually reveal a patchy alveolar pattern or pleural effusion. Treatment consists of oxygen support, fresh frozen plasma or fresh whole blood in addition to vitamin K therapy (see Chapters 2 and 15).

Pulmonary thromboembolic disease is caused by pulmonary arterial obstruction by thrombi and results in respiratory distress by the production of severe ventilation/perfusion mismatch. Thrombi form because of systemic hypercoagulability, stasis of blood within vessels or direct endothelial damage. Production of thrombi is seen in disease states such as protein-losing nephropathy, hyperadrenocorticism, immune-mediated haemolytic anaemia, bacterial endocarditis and diro-filariasis, as well as post-surgery. Affected patients often have a sudden onset of respiratory distress, increased respiratory rate and effort, generalized harsh lung sounds and pale to cyanotic mucous membranes. Where thrombus accumulation in the lungs is extensive, an occlusive reduction in venous return to the heart may occur, which will be detected as reduced pulse quality and hypotension. Thoracic radiographs are often normal, but may reveal varying interstitial or alveolar patterns, pleural effusion and dilated or truncated pulmonary arteries (Figure 5.26). The most common clinicopathological finding is thrombocytopenia. A definitive diagnosis can be made using selective or non-selective angiography, but unstable patients may not tolerate this procedure. Ventilation/perfusion scanning with radioisotopes is a non-invasive procedure that can provide useful diagnostic information, but the equipment is not widely available.

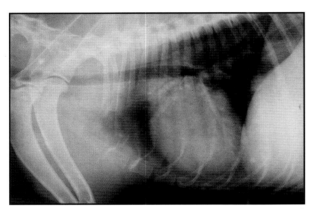

Figure 5.26: A lateral thoracic radiograph of a mixed breed dog with severe, auto-agglutinating haemolytic anaemia that developed acute respiratory distress. A presumptive diagnosis of pulmonary thromboembolism was made based on the severity of the hypoxia and lack of radiographic abnormalities.

The prognosis for thromboembolic disease is fair to guarded, depending on the extent of lung involvement. Oxygen supplementation should be provided, but may not cause dramatic improvement because of pulmonary shunting. Therapy consists of supportive care, treatment of the underlying disease and prevention of further thrombosis using anticoagulants. Heparin can be administered subcutaneously or as an intravenous constant rate infusion. If the predisposing disease is established and considered ongoing, warfarin therapy can also be instituted for long-term maintenance. In such cases, treatment with heparin is tapered and discontinued. Thrombolytic agents such as streptokinase have been used with mixed success in a limited number of patients.

Primary pulmonary neoplasia or metastatic disease can also cause severe respiratory distress. Patient history varies from acute signs to a gradual onset of exercise intolerance and laboured breathing, with or without coughing. Thoracic radiographs and identification of a distant primary neoplasm are often diagnostic. A definitive diagnosis can often be obtained by cytological examination of pleural fluid or fine needle aspiration of the mass. If cytological evaluation and other diagnostics provide equivocal results, exploratory thoracotomy may be required. Supportive care should be provided as needed, but treatment options may be limited. Unless the neoplasm is responsive to chemotherapy, euthanasia is often indicated.

Pulmonary inflammatory disease is an uncommon cause of respiratory distress in small animals. Reported pulmonary inflammatory diseases include pulmonary infiltrate with eosinophils (PIE) and lymphomatoid granulomatosis (LG). In both cases, pulmonary tissue is infiltrated by a non-neoplastic proliferation of eosinophils or lymphocytes. Clinical findings vary from sudden to gradual onset of respiratory distress or coughing. Radiographic findings include mass lesions or infiltration. The diagnosis may be confirmed by a cytological finding of inflammatory cells on samples obtained by tracheal wash or fine needle aspiration. Other underlying causes, such as pulmonary parasites, must also be ruled out. Apart from routine respiratory supportive care, therapy includes immunosuppressive doses of corticosteroids. More aggressive cytotoxic drugs may be required in refractory cases. Many animals respond very well to this therapy.

Acute lung injury (ALI) and ARDS are terms that refer to a syndrome of generalized inflammatory lung injury. Inflammation can be triggered by systemic inflammatory disorders such as septic shock or pancreatitis, or by a severe pulmonary insult such as aspiration pneumonia, pulmonary contusions or smoke inhalation. In ALI, pulmonary inflammation manifests as vasculitis, interstitial and alveolar permeability oedema, and infiltration of inflammatory cells such as neutrophils and macrophages. ARDS is a more severe form, manifested by inflammation as in ALI, accompanied by proliferation of type II pneumocytes, hyaline membranes and interstitial fibrosis. Animals with ALI-like syndrome have mild to moderate degrees of dyspnoea and hypoxia and often respond to fluid restriction, colloid support, low doses of diuretics and treatment of the underlying disease. Despite the fact that this is an inflammatory disease, corticosteroids have been shown to have no effect on mortality rates in human patients with these syndromes, and may be contraindicated because of their immunosuppressive effects. Animals with ARDS have severe pulmonary dysfunction and very poor lung compliance. They usually require positive-pressure ventilation and the prognosis is grave.

Pleural space disease

Clinical signs of pleural space disease
The clinical signs of pleural space disease are summarized

in Figure 5.27. Pulmonary dysfunction can be caused by accumulation of fluid, air or soft tissue within the pleural cavity. Pleural space disease is suggested by physical examination findings that include increased respiratory rate or effort, dyspnoea and auscultation of diminished or dull lung and heart sounds. Depending on the cause, other signs such as fever may also be present. Because the pleural effusion prevents lung expansion, hypoxia is caused by atelectasis and ventilation/perfusion mismatch. Radiographic changes are compatible with increases in either fluid or soft tissue density and may be caused by neoplasia or diaphragmatic herniation into the pleural space.

Increased respiratory rate and effort

Dyspnoea

Cough

Dull or diminished lung and heart sounds on auscultation

Fever

Weight loss and lethargy

Figure 5.27: Clinical and historical signs associated with pleural space disease in dogs and cats.

General approach to management of patients with pleural space disease

The approach to management of patients with pleural space disease is summarized in Figure 5.28. If pleural effusion is suspected and the animal is in severe respiratory distress, routine oxygen supplementation should be provided and thoracocentesis should be performed immediately (before radiographs have confirmed the diagnosis). Thoracocentesis is both a therapeutic and diagnostic procedure and can be life saving in severely compromised patients. The technique is described in Chapter 22. Thoracic radiographs obtained after thoracocentesis has been performed are more valuable than those obtained prior to removal of the fluid. Once the fluid has been removed, radiographs may reveal the cause of the effusion, allowing evaluation of the cardiac silhouette and demonstration of masses.

Pleural effusions are classified according to the type of fluid obtained. Gross examination can identify whether the fluid is haemorrhagic, purulent, chylous or a transudate. Fluid analysis should include protein content, cytology and cell counts. In addition, specific chemical analysis, such as determination of triglyceride concentration, may be indicated. The character of the pleural effusion determines the course of further diagnostic evaluation and the likelihood of recurrence. Specific management will depend on the findings of fluid analysis and presence of underlying disease.

Syndromes of pleural space disease

Pyothorax is the accumulation of a purulent exudate in one or both sides of the pleural space and is more common in cats than in dogs (Figure 5.29). The aetiology includes idiopathic causes, penetrating chest wounds, haematogenous spread, extension from adjacent structures or fascial planes, aspirated foreign bodies, ruptured pulmonary abscesses and ruptured oesophagus. Presenting complaints include lethargy, anorexia, respiratory distress, fever and/or weight loss. The diagnosis is confirmed by high nucleated cell counts in the pleural fluid, with a large number of degenerative neutrophils. Bacteria may be visible, but are not always evident. Both aerobic and anaerobic cultures should be submitted because of the high incidence of anaerobic bacteria in pleural infections. Polymicrobial infections are common.

Treatment should consist of broad-spectrum intravenous antibiotics until the rate of effusion diminishes, followed by oral antibiotics once culture results become available. Since this is a deep tissue infection, prone to recurrence in individual animals, antibiotic therapy is typically continued for 2–3 months. Establishment of thoracic drainage is also important in these patients. Although repeated needle thoracocentesis can be performed, it is a painful procedure that may not be well tolerated. In addition, needle thoracocentesis may not effectively drain the exudate if it is viscous

---

Oxygen supplementation

Rest and minimal stress

Vascular access

Thoracocentesis

Thoracic radiographs (if possible) after thoracocentesis

Fluid analysis:
    Cell counts
    Cytology
    Aerobic and anaerobic culture
    Biochemical analysis if indicated
    (triglycerides)

Figure 5.28: General approach to emergency management of dogs and cats with pleural space disease.

Pleural effusion:
    Pyothorax
    Non-bacterial exudates (FIP or neoplasia)
    Chylothorax
    Transudates (pure or modified)
    Haemothorax
    Sanguineous effusions (lung lobe torsion)
Pneumothorax
Diaphragmatic hernia
Pleural neoplasia or masses

Figure 5.29: Common differential diagnoses for pleural space disease in dogs and cats. FIP: feline infectious peritonitis.

or loculated. Placement of one or more chest drains allows continuous drainage of the fluid as it forms (Figure 5.30 and Chapter 22). Frequency of drainage will depend on the rate of fluid production but is usually performed by gentle aspiration several times daily. Alternatively, the drain may be attached to a pleural suction device which provides gentle continuous negative pressure to the drain (see Chapter 22) and is ideal if large volumes of fluid are produced. Thoracic drainage should continue until the fluid character has changed to a serosanguineous effusion containing non-degenerate neutrophils, and the volume has diminished to 5 ml/kg/day or less. On average, thoracic drainage is required for about 1 week, but the range varies from 2 days to 3 weeks. If patients fail to respond, careful evaluation for underlying causes of pyothorax, such as lung abscesses, should be considered and exploratory thoracotomy may be required.

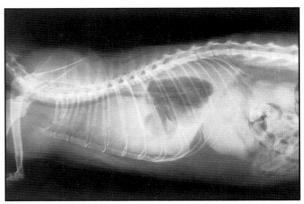

Figure 5.31: A 5-year-old Domestic Long Hair cat that presented for progressive respiratory distress. Thoracic radiographs were taken and show a marked pleural effusion. Thoracocentesis was performed and 150 ml of a chylous effusion were removed.

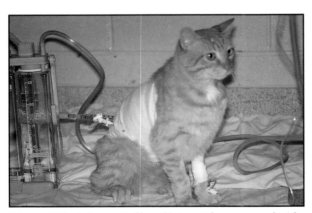

Figure 5.30: A Domestic Short Hair cat that presented with fever, lethargy and dyspnoea. A pyothorax was diagnosed after thoracocentesis, and bilateral chest tubes were placed to allow for continuous drainage.

Non-bacterial exudates also occur. Feline infectious peritonitis virus can cause pleural effusion in affected cats, recognized by a sticky yellow effusion that has a high protein and low cellularity. The prognosis is very poor for affected cats.

Chylothorax is the accumulation of a milky effusion within the pleural space, which has a triglyceride concentration higher than that of a concurrently obtained plasma sample. A true chylous effusion contains chylomicrons, but a pseudochylous effusion, although the same on gross inspection, contains only cholesterol. Chylothorax can occur whenever there is obstruction or leakage of chyle due to disruption of the thoracic duct (Figure 5.31). Common causes include trauma, neoplasia, feline cardiomyopathy and idiopathic disease.

Treatment of chylous effusion aims to remove the underlying cause and decrease the rate of formation. With the exception of chylous effusions caused by heart failure or lymphosarcoma, medical management and low-fat diets are often disappointing. Surgical management is associated with a poor prognosis for complete

correction. Thoracic duct ligation is generally regarded to be the best option, but is associated with a relatively high rate of recurrence. Other alternatives include placement of a pleuroperitoneal shunt device or pleurodesis.

Transudates (pure and modified) are recognized as clear to yellow fluid which has low cellularity and low protein content. The most common cause is right-sided congestive heart failure, management of which is discussed in Chapter 4. A complete cardiac evaluation should be performed, and cardiac disease should be treated appropriately to prevent or reduce recurrence of pleural effusion. Transudates can also develop or be exacerbated by factors such as hypoproteinaemia and low oncotic pressure, or vasculitis. For these reasons, modified transudates in the pleural cavity are common in patients with sepsis or pancreatitis and in patients with pulmonary thromboembolism. Neoplasia may also cause a modified transudate, which may contain exfoliated neoplastic cells. This emphasizes the need for cytological evaluation of all effusions. Thoracic radiographs should be obtained following thoracocentesis to evaluate the cardiac silhouette and to look for evidence of neoplasia. Occasionally, in the absence of cardiac disease, a definitive diagnosis cannot initially be made. As the disease progresses and the effusion returns, the underlying cause can usually be identified.

Haemothorax may be produced following trauma as a result of a coagulopathy or may be caused by neoplasia. Anticoagulant rodenticides are considered the most common non-traumatic cause of haemothorax. Animals with rodenticide poisoning may present in acute respiratory distress with no other obvious signs of bleeding. Treatment requires a source of coagulation factors via fresh whole blood or fresh frozen plasma transfusions as well as vitamin K therapy. Thoracocentesis should only be performed if the animal's respiratory status is severely compromised by the pleural effusion. Congenital coagulopathies such as haemophilia A can also lead to haemothorax, but are less common. Neoplasms such as hemangiosarcoma can also result in a rapidly forming haemothorax, which should also be managed by transfusions and thoracocentesis (with cytological evaluation of the fluid). Patients that do not respond to conservative therapy may require exploratory thoracotomy to establish a diagnosis and to resect bleeding masses.

Sanguineous effusions can be defined as an accumulation of grossly bloody pleural fluid that does not have a high enough packed cell volume to be classified as haemorrhage. The most common causes of sanguineous effusions are lung lobe torsions and neoplasia. Lung lobe torsions are most commonly diagnosed in deep chested dogs, with a predilection for Afghan Hounds and Borzois. Affected animals present with an acute or chronic history of progressive dyspnoea and weight loss. On physical examination, typical findings include dull lung sounds in the ventral portion of the lung fields. Pleural fluid accumulates because of obstruction of venous outflow from the twisted lung lobe, and the fluid is typically bloody with numerous neutrophils on cytology. Chylous effusions are also seen. Thoracic radiographs should be obtained after the fluid has been removed from the pleural cavity. The most common finding is complete collapse of a single lung lobe, which can appear consolidated or with an unusual 'honeycomb' pattern (Figure 5.32). The bronchus of the affected lobe may appear distorted or extend in the wrong direction. Ultrasonography with colour flow Doppler can help confirm the diagnosis by showing lack of blood flow in the torsioned lung lobe. Once a lung lobe torsion is suspected, an emergency thoracotomy is indicated to resect the affected lobe before tissue necrosis triggers the systemic inflammatory response syndrome. If the lobe is resected early in the course of the disease process prognosis is good, but occasionally effusions recur in the days and weeks following surgery. In these cases the character of the effusion may change from sanguineous to chylous. The risk of chylous effusion appears to be particularly high in Afghan Hounds and Borzoi, and in these breeds the prognosis for long-term survival is guarded.

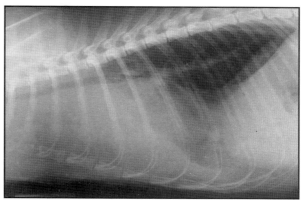

Figure 5.33: *A 9-year-old Siamese cat that presented for increased respiratory rate and effort. Decreased chest compressibility and dull ventral lung sounds were noted on physical examination. This lateral thoracic radiograph shows a marked pleural effusion and elevation of the carina and narrowing of the trachea caused by a large cranial mediastinal mass.*

Neoplastic effusions may also be sanguineous. Exfoliated neoplastic cells may be evident on cytological evaluation of the fluid, but the absence of neoplastic cells does not rule out neoplasia. The most common neoplasm that is easily diagnosed on cytology is lymphosarcoma in cats, which is usually associated with a mediastinal mass that can reduce chest compressibility (Figure 5.33). Other neoplasms that can cause a pleural effusion include carcinomas, chemodectomas, thymomas and mesotheliomas.

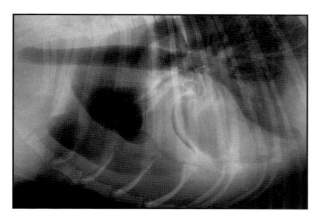

Figure 5.32: *A 3-year-old intact male Afghan Hound presented with acute respiratory distress. Thoracic radiographs revealed a pleural effusion and possible lung lobe torsion. Ultrasonography confirmed this diagnosis and the dog underwent a thoracotomy to remove the right cranial lung lobe.*

FURTHER READING

Berry CR, Moore PF, Thomas WP *et al.* (1990) Pulmonary lymphomatoid granulomatosis in seven dogs (1976–1987). *Journal of Veterinary Internal Medicine* **4**, 157–166

Buback JL, Boothe HW and Hobson HP (1996) Surgical treatment of tracheal collapse in dogs: 90 cases (1983–1993). *Journal of the American Veterinary Medical Association* **208**, 380–384

Drobatz KJ and Concannon K (1994) Noncardiogenic pulmonary edema. *Compendium on Continuing Education for the Practicing Veterinarian* **16**, 333–346

Dye JA, McKiernan BC and Rozanski EA (1996) Bronchopulmonary disease in the cat: historical, physical, radiographic, clinicopathologic and pulmonary functional evaluation of 24 affected and 15 healthy cats. *Journal of Veterinary Internal Medicine* **10**, 385–400

Fossum TW (1993) Feline chylothorax. *Compendium on Continuing Education for the Practicing Veterinarian* **15**, 549–567

Gelzer ARM, Downs MO, Newell SM *et al.* (1997) Accessory lung lobe torsion and chylothorax in an Afghan hound. *Journal of the American Animal Hospital Association* **33**, 171–176

Hackner SG (1995) Emergency management of traumatic pulmonary contusions. *Compendium on Continuing Education for the Practicing Veterinarian* **17**, 677–686

Holtsinger RH and Ellison GW (1995) Spontaneous pneumothorax. *Compendium on Continuing Education for the Practicing Veterinarian* **17**, 197–210

Kapatkin AS, Matthiesen DT, Noone KE *et al.* (1990) Results of surgery and long-term follow-up in 31 cats with nasopharyngeal polyps. *Journal of the American Animal Hospital Association* **26**, 387–392

Keyes ML, Rush JE and Knowles KE (1993) Pulmonary thromboembolism in dogs. *Journal of Veterinary Emergency and Critical Care* **3**, 23–32

King LG and Boothe DM (1997) *Bacterial Infections of the Respiratory Tract in Dogs and Cats.* Bayer, Shawnee Mission, Kansas

Lotti U and Niebauer GW (1992) Tracheobronchial foreign bodies of plant origin in 153 hunting dogs. *Compendium on Continuing Education for the Practicing Veterinarian* **14**, 900–904

Ogilvie GK, Haschek WM, Withrow SJ *et al.* (1989) Classification of primary lung tumours in dogs: 210 cases (1975–1985). *Journal of the American Veterinary Medical Association* **195**, 106–108

Ogilvie GK, Weigel RM, Haschek WM *et al.* (1989) Prognostic factors for tumour remission and survival in dogs after surgery for primary lung tumour: 76 cases (1975–1985). *Journal of the American Veterinary Medical Association* **195**, 109–112

Padrid PA, Hornof WJ, Kurpershoek CG *et al.* (1990) Canine chronic bronchitis: a pathophysiologic evaluation of 18 cases. *Journal of Veterinary Internal Medicine* **4**, 172–180

Parent C, King LG, Walker LM *et al.* (1996) Clinical and clinicopathologic findings in dogs with acute respiratory distress syndrome: 19 cases (1985–1993). *Journal of the American Veterinary Medical Association* **208**, 1419–1427

Parent C, King LG, van Winkle TJ *et al.* (1996) Respiratory function and treatment in dogs with acute respiratory distress syndrome: 19 cases (1985–1993). *Journal of the American Veterinary Medical Association* **208**, 1428–1433

Turner WD and Breznock EM (1988) Continuous suction drainage for management of canine pyothorax — a retrospective study. *Journal of the American Animal Hospital Association* **24**, 486–494

Valentine A, Smeak D, Allen D *et al.* (1996) Spontaneous pneumothorax in dogs. *Compendium on Continuing Education for the Practicing Veterinarian* **18**, 53–62

CHAPTER SIX

Renal and Urinary Tract Emergencies

Karol A. Mathews

Renal emergencies may primarily involve the kidneys (Figure 6.1), or be secondary to pre-renal (Figure 6.2) or post-renal (Figure 6.3) causes. Similarly, lower urinary tract pathology may be primary, or secondary to other initiating factors. A thorough history, physical examination and laboratory information are required to diagnose renal dysfunction or disease, and in many instances diagnostic imaging is necessary to diagnose lower urinary tract injuries or disease accurately. Renal biopsy is required for definitive diagnosis of most renal diseases. Attention to these details will hopefully prevent misdiagnosis and inappropriate prognostication, which may lead to incorrect therapy or euthanasia.

The owner should be questioned regarding:

- Voiding behaviour and frequency
- Urine volume and colour
- Water consumption
- Overall activity
- Appetite
- Vomiting and diarrhoea
- Trauma (within past 7 days)
- Medications, including over-the-counter NSAIDs
- Access to toxins and owner medication
- Acuity of onset of signs
- Previous history of renal or urinary tract disease, cardiac or other system disease
- Recent anaesthesia (surgical, dental or diagnostic procedures)
- Travel history.

The physical examination should include:

- Hydration status
- Mucous membrane colour and capillary refill time
- Presence of pleural or abdominal effusions
- Jugular vein distension
- Heart and respiratory rates
- Pulse pressure and arterial blood pressure
- Abdominal palpation to assess kidney, uterus, prostate size, abdominal masses, fluid or pain
- Body temperature
- Penis, prepuce, scrotum or vulva
- Perineum and anus
- Rectal examination, especially in males and where

Ischaemia
Severe persistent pre-renal causes
Renal vascular thrombosis
Renal parenchymal injury/trauma

Infectious
Bacterial pyelonephritis
Leptospirosis
Lyme nephropathy
Feline infectious peritonitis

Structural
Nephroliths
Polycystic

Immune-mediated
Glomerulonephritis
Amyloidosis
Interstitial nephritis
Systemic lupus glomerulonephritis

Neoplastic
Lymphoma
Haemangiosarcoma

Toxins
Aminoglycosides
Polymyxin B
Sulphonamides
Cephaloridine
Tetracyclines
Amphotericin B
Thiacetarsamine
Non-steroidal anti-inflammatory drugs
Methoxyflurane
Carbon tetrachloride
Ethylene glycol
Heavy metals
Myoglobin
Haemoglobin and red cell stroma
Unknown substances associated with compost ingestion

Figure 6.1: Examples of renal emergencies due to primary renal disease.

pelvic injury is present
- Overall examination to rule out trauma, especially abdomen and pelvis, and to check for enlargement of peripheral lymph nodes.

Inadequate intravascular volume due to fluid translocation or loss
Vomiting
Diarrhoea
Third space losses
Thermal burns
Heatstroke
Blood loss
Hypoadrenocorticism
Hypoalbuminaemia
Vasculitis
Pancreatitis
Shock
Diabetes insipidus (central or renal, e.g. endotoxin)
Diabetes mellitus
Overzealous diuretic use

Increased renal and systemic vascular resistance
Increased circulating catecholamines
Renal sympathetic nervous stimulation
(e.g. unilateral nephrectomy affecting contralateral renal function)
Angiotensin II
Hypothermia

Inadequate intravascular volume due to vasodilation
Anaphylaxis
Inhalational anaesthetics
Sepsis
Heatstroke
Vasodilator therapy

Inadequate cardiac output
Congestive heart failure
Cardiac tamponade
Restrictive pericardial or cardiac disease
Arrhythmias
Positive pressure ventilation
Post-cardiac arrest
Selective anaesthetic protocols

Hyperviscosity
Polycythaemia
Hyperproteinaemia/hyperglobulinaemia

Miscellaneous (reduced urine volume but not necessarily azotaemic)
Antidiuretic hormone (ADH) secretion due to hypotension or hypovolaemia
Opioids (ADH-like effect)
Lung pathology (ADH activity)
Ventilator patients

Figure 6.2: Examples of renal emergencies due to pre-renal disease.

Trauma
Ruptured bladder
Herniated bladder
Ruptured/avulsed ureters
Ruptured/avulsed urethra
Post-traumatic scarring of ureters or urethra
Bladder or urethral haematoma
Iatrogenic ligation of ureters or urethra

Obstruction
Uroliths
Granulomatous urethritis
Neoplasia (extra- or intraluminal or intramural)
Prostatic disease
Stump pyometra
Functional spasm — reflex dysinergia
Urethral inflammation
Herniated, retroflexed bladder
Urethral haematoma
Technical problems associated with an indwelling urinary catheter

Neurological
Spinal injury/disease

Figure 6.3: Examples of renal emergencies due to post-renal disease.

AZOTAEMIA

Definition of terms and concepts related to azotaemia

Azotaemia is defined as an abnormal concentration of urea, creatinine and other nitrogenous substances in blood, and is a laboratory diagnosis. Both urea and creatinine may be increased due to diminished elimination by the kidneys and/or the lower urinary tract. Azotaemia may also occur due to increased production of urea by the liver secondary to gastrointestinal haemorrhage or a high protein meal. Creatinine may be elevated by increased muscle activity. Azotaemia may be transient and therefore does not always imply renal disease, renal failure or insufficiency. Commonly used formulae related to renal function are shown in Figure 6.4.

When azotaemia is associated with metabolic and physiological alterations (depression, anorexia, nausea, vomiting, diarrhoea, melaena, dehydration, stupor, coma or seizures) due to the polysystemic toxic syndrome that occurs as a result of abnormal renal function, the term *uraemia* is used. For uraemia to develop, the function of both kidneys must be reduced by at least 75%. Uraemia may occur in animals with primary renal failure/insufficiency or pre- or post-renal disorders, and may be reversible or irreversible.

Renal disease may not be associated with renal failure, insufficiency or azotaemia and may regress, persist or increase in severity. Renal disease has many aetiologies and may affect the glomeruli, tubules, interstitial tissue, vessels, or a combination of these.

Based on the history and physical findings, immediate and appropriate testing should be performed to evaluate and treat the emergency at hand (trauma and haemorrhage, hyperkalaemia, severe metabolic acidosis or dehydration).

Fractional excretion of sodium

= (Urine [Na$^+$]/Plasma [Na$^+$]) x (Plasma [Cr]/Urine [Cr]) x 100

Normal tubular function or pre-renal disease: <1%

Acute tubular necrosis: >2%

Invalid in such conditions as congestive heart failure, hepatic failure or nephrotic syndrome, as excretion of sodium is impaired and retention of sodium may persist despite renal dysfunction

Anion gap

= ([Na$^+$] + [K$^+$]) - ([HCO$_3^-$] + [Cl$^-$])

Normal value = 15–25

Total CO$_2$ can be used instead of HCO$_3^-$ where venous blood gases cannot be measured

Urine protein:creatinine ratio

Urine protein (mg/dl)/Urine creatinine (mg/dl)

or

Urine protein (g/l)/Urine creatinine (μmol/l) x 8.84

Normal value = <0.5

Average daily maintenance fluid requirements for ill animals (ml)

= 1.5 (70 x $BW^{0.75}$) for all animals

or

= (30 x BW) + 70 for animals between 2 and 40 kg, where BW = body weight in kg

Figure 6.4: Commonly used formulae.

The terms *renal failure* and *renal insufficiency* describe failure of the kidney to concentrate or dilute urine, or to eliminate the products of metabolism appropriately, resulting in azotaemia. Inability to concentrate or dilute the urine usually occurs with approximately 66% reduction in renal function, whereas recognizable failure to eliminate products of metabolism occurs between 66% and 75% reduction in renal function. As a warning, when the creatinine value of a well-hydrated animal lies in the upper end of the normal range, this may suggest more than a 50% reduction in renal function.

A urine sample should be obtained prior to fluid therapy in order to assess the concentrating ability of the kidneys. The urine specific gravity is helpful in localizing the cause of azotaemia (Figure 6.5). Dehydrated azotaemic patients with urine specific gravity >1.030 (in dogs) and >1.045 (in cats) most likely have pre-renal azotaemia. Some cats can effectively concentrate their urine despite significant reduction in renal function, therefore concentrated urine in cats may not exclude renal failure. Azotaemic dehydrated animals that cannot concentrate urine may be receiving medication (e.g. frusemide, corticosteroids) or have an illness (e.g. hypoadrenocorticism, diabetes mellitus, hypercalcaemia, cystitis) that interferes with urine concentrating ability and may not have renal dysfunction.

Cystitis caused by *Escherichia coli* (and possibly other bacteria) can cause a profound polyuria resulting in dehydration, without other typical signs of cystitis. The packed cell volume and plasma total protein in pre-renal azotaemia tend to be increased above normal, unless blood loss or anaemia is present. Response to therapy usually distinguishes between pre-renal and renal azotaemia. Post-renal azotaemia, due to partial or total urinary tract obstruction, is diagnosed on history and physical examination (discussed later) and may be associated with pollakiuria, dysuria, stranguria or polyuria. With pre- and post-renal disease or injury excluded, a presumptive diagnosis of renal failure can be made when azotaemia is associated with isosthenuria (urine specific gravity <1.025 or more commonly 1.008–1.015).

Monitoring and assessment

The diagnostics and treatment for renal or urinary tract emergencies are based on the underlying problem, but patient monitoring is similar in most instances.

Emergency minimum data base

- Serum creatinine and urea, plasma glucose, phosphorus, calcium, electrolytes, packed cell volume (PCV) and total protein (TP), total CO$_2$ or venous blood gases
- Measure serum osmolality if ethylene glycol or salicylate intoxication is suspected
- Urine specific gravity, sediment, protein, glucose, electrolytes, urine culture and sensitivity
- Cytology, urea, creatinine, PCV and TP of abdominal fluid if present
- Abdominal and pelvic radiographs ± abdominal ultrasonography ± contrast studies
- Arterial and central venous blood pressure monitoring.

Additional diagnostic testing

- Complete biochemical profile and complete blood count
- Urine protein:creatinine ratio if indicated
- Urine electrolytes and creatinine if indicated for lesion localization
- Serology if indicated (e.g. *Leptospira*, *Borrelia*)
- Renal biopsy if indicated.

Urine output

Assessment of urine production is one of the most important tools for immediate monitoring of renal function in critical patients. Normal urine production is 1–2 ml/kg/h but may be reduced in dehydrated animals. In all emergency situations, the volume of urine within the bladder should be immediately assessed by abdominal palpation, abdominal radiography or ultrasonography, urinary bladder catheterization or voiding. A urine sample should be obtained for laboratory analysis prior to institution of therapy, via urinary bladder catheterization, cystocentesis or a voided sample. If culture and sensitivity testing are warranted, a sample obtained via

Laboratory test	Pre-renal azotaemia	Parenchymal acute renal failure	Post-renal azotaemia
Urine specific gravity	>1.035 dogs >1.045 cats	1.008–1.029 dogs 1.008–1.034 cats	Variable
Urine to plasma osmolality Urinary sodium concentration Fractional excretion of sodium Urine creatinine:plasma creatinine Urine protein:urine creatinine Urine glucose	>5:1 <20 mEq/l <1% >20:1 <0.5 Absent	> 40 mEq/l >1% <10:1 1 to > 13 Variably present	<0.5
Urine sediment Proteinuria Granular casts Renal epithelial cells Red blood cells >5/hpf Red blood cell ghosts White blood cells >5/hpf Cellular debris Neoplastic cells	Absent/trace Absent Absent Cardiac/emboli Exercise Coagulopathy Cardiac/emboli Absent Absent Absent	Present Present Present Glomerular injury Renal tubular injury Present Present Renal neoplasia	 Absent to many Absent to many Absent/present Absent/present Bladder/urethral neoplasia
Urine colour Dark red/brown Red	 Myoglobin Haemoglobin Blood		 Blood

Figure 6.5: *Differentiation of pre-renal and post-renal azotaemia and parenchymal acute renal failure based on urine analysis. All or individual components of the urine sediment may be present depending on severity, the time from onset of renal injury to presentation and aetiology.*

cystocentesis is recommended. Injury to the urinary system may interfere with urine output. As various problems unrelated to renal function may impair spontaneous voiding, the urinary bladder may require catheterization, palpation or imaging to assess whether urine is being produced over time.

Urine volume can be measured by collection when the animal voids, use of a metabolism cage, by intermittent or continuous urinary bladder catheterization or by placing pre-weighed towels under the vulva or penis and weighing them after voiding. Any increase in towel weight over baseline, unless otherwise soiled, is assumed to be due to urine. Assuming 1000 ml equals 1000 g, the volume of urine voided can be estimated. This technique usually underestimates urine produced, as some urine may remain in the cage. Weighing the animal several times daily assists in estimating urine output. Should the animal's weight decline despite fluid therapy, it is assumed that ongoing losses such as high urine output, vomiting, diarrhoea, salivation, fever or hyperthermia are in excess of fluid administration. A weight loss of 0.1–0.3 kg body weight/1000 kcal energy requirement should be assumed in an anorexic animal.

When the animal is recumbent and monitoring urine output is critically important, most critical care clinicians prefer to use an indwelling urinary catheter attached to a sterile intravenous fluid delivery line and urine collection bag (Figure 6.6). The exterior of the catheter is cleaned several times a day with chlorhexidine. Should the prepuce or vulva become soiled, they are cleaned with chlorhexidine soap and rinsed with warm water. Antibiotics are avoided unless required to treat an existing infection. The urine is cultured after 72 hours, or sooner if indicated. The catheter is removed as soon as possible and the urine cultured upon removal.

Monitoring fluid administration

After urine flow has been established, regardless of the underlying problem, ongoing fluid requirements may be calculated as follows:

- Divide the day into six 4-hour intervals, four 6-hour intervals or three 8-hour intervals, depending on severity of illness and availability of staff
- Determine urine produced during each time interval and add the estimated insensible loss for that period
- Determine ongoing losses in vomitus, diarrhoea and saliva over this same interval
- Determine insensible loss, 20 ml/kg/day, and for each degree Celsius above 38.5 add 10% of normal daily maintenance fluid requirement (if normal daily requirement is 1litre and temperature is 40.5°C

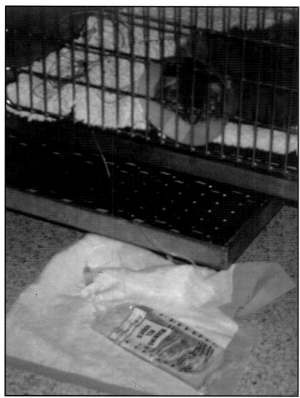

Figure 6.6: A sterile intravenous delivery set and fluid bag is attached to the urinary catheter. The bag may be hooked to a lower cage, or as in this case, placed on a clean barrier on the floor.

then 200 ml should be added). Divide this amount by 6, 4 or 3 depending on intervals selected above
- This total volume of fluid is to be delivered over the next time period.

Any fluid challenge must be monitored closely but if cardiac or pulmonary disease is present, central venous pressure (CVP) monitoring is advised. An increase in CVP > 4 cm H_2O, with a slow decrease to baseline, indicates hypervolaemia or right-sided cardiac disease. Fluid therapy should be discontinued temporarily if the CVP reaches 13 cm H_2O or increases by 2 cm H_2O or more in any 10-minute period. In addition to CVP (or if CVP is not available) the following signs can also indicate overhydration:

- Shivering
- Restlessness
- Serous nasal discharge
- Tachypnoea
- Nausea
- Vomiting
- Tachycardia (followed by bradycardia when severely overloaded)
- Subcutaneous oedema (especially the hock joint and intermandibular space)
- Pulmonary crackles and oedema
- Exophthalmos

- Chemosis
- Cough
- Dyspnoea
- Polyuria
- Diarrhoea
- Depressed mentation
- Ascites.

Monitoring ongoing therapy

The following parameters must be monitored during ongoing patient management, to assess efficacy of therapy and to prevent, identify and treat abnormalities that arise:

- Creatinine or urea or both (daily)
- Urine specific gravity (with urine volume measurement every 1–8 hours)
- Urine sediment (every 48 hours if acute tubular necrosis)
- Weight gain or loss (every 8–24 hours to assess fluid loss/gain)
- Serum electrolytes, specifically potassium (every 4–24 hours with hypo- or hyperkalaemia) and phosphorus
- Venous blood gases, or total CO_2 (every 6–24 hours to assess metabolic status)
- Anion gap (with electrolyte and blood gas or total CO_2 measurements) (see Figure 6.4)
- Urine sodium and creatinine (where indicated to assess pre-renal *versus* renal problem) (see Figure 6.4)
- Urine protein:creatinine ratio (72 hours) to assess therapy and prognosis (see Figure 6.4)
- Urine production (hourly to every 8 hours depending on situation).

The volume of urine output depends on the underlying problem. The goal is to maintain at least 2 ml/kg/h. However, in the presence of renal tubular injury or other causes of loss of concentrating ability, urine output can be extremely high (25–40 ml/kg/h). Hence, the importance of measurement of urinary output and adequate fluid replacement.

APPROACH TO OLIGURIA AND ANURIA

The definition of oliguria is urine production <0.27 ml/kg/h, but if the animal is receiving intravenous fluid therapy, <1–2 ml/kg/h may be oliguric. The cause of decreased urine output should be elucidated, as specific therapy depends on aetiology. The history may reveal a period of polyuria and polydipsia, or an abrupt reduction in urine production (frequently associated with post-renal obstruction). Bradycardia, hypothermia, pale mucous membranes with prolonged capillary refill time, hyperpnoea and halitosis are evident with prolonged anuria and indicate severe metabolic and electrolyte derangements which can occur with pre-, post- or primary renal disease.

Initial treatment

An intravenous catheter is placed and enough blood obtained for a minimum emergency data base and routine minimum data base. Immediate concerns include: the adequacy of circulating volume; hypotension; electrolyte imbalance, especially hyperkalaemia; metabolic acidosis; and the severity of underlying disease. A urine sample should be obtained as soon as possible prior to fluid therapy. Where indicated, a urinary catheter is passed to assess urethral patency, facilitate voiding and measure urine production. Electrocardiographic monitoring is advised to detect cardiac arrhythmias associated with hyperkalaemia, primary cardiac disease or those caused by other metabolic or traumatic disorders. Therapeutic suggestions are outlined below under the specific problems. Guidelines for fluid therapy are described in the section on acute intrinsic renal failure.

APPROACH TO URINE LEAKAGE DUE TO RENAL, URETERAL, BLADDER OR URETHRAL INJURY

Renal parenchymal injury may be due to blunt or penetrating trauma, which may involve one or both kidneys. Renal injury may cause retroperitoneal haemorrhage, haemorrhage into the abdomen or into the parenchyma and pelvis of the kidney, with haematuria and obstruction to urine flow by haematoma formation. Nephroliths may obstruct urine flow from the pelvis of the kidney, causing hydronephrosis with possible traumatic injury and rupture. If the nephrolith is associated with bacterial infection, abscessation and rupture may occur, resulting in peritonitis. *Ureteral obstruction* may also occur with similar consequences. If one kidney or ureter is involved, the other unit may function adequately resulting in normal serum urea and creatinine levels. However, with urine leakage into the peritoneal cavity due to injury, serum urea and creatinine levels will increase. *Bladder rupture* may occur from blunt trauma, erosion of tumour, as a result of cystic calculi obstructing urine flow, aggressive palpation or attempts at unblocking the obstructed urethra.

Urinary tract injury should be suspected in all trauma patients, with a high level of suspicion in patients sustaining abdominal or pelvic injuries. The incidence of urinary tract injury associated with pelvic trauma was 39% in one study (Selcer, 1982). Gentle and thorough palpation of the abdomen and sub-lumbar area should be performed whilst noting areas of tenderness, bladder size, abdominal girth, evidence of free abdominal fluid and injuries to the abdominal wall. Preputial or vulvar bleeding, haematuria, dysuria or anuria are also associated with urinary tract injuries. The inguinal region and perineum should be monitored carefully for swelling or discoloration associated with urine leakage from a ruptured urethra. Repeated physical examination should be performed to detect early signs of intra-abdominal injury. In a study of hospitalized animals only 40% of the diagnoses of ruptured bladder were made within 12 hours after trauma and 22.7% were not diagnosed until necropsy (Burrows, 1974). Injuries or obstruction to any part of the urinary tract may also result from nephroliths, abscesses, neoplasia, perineal, inguinal or abdominal hernias and iatrogenic injuries.

Diagnosis

Diagnosis and localization of urinary tract injury is based on history, physical findings and the emergency minimum data base, continual examination and diagnostic imaging. Metabolic changes associated with urine leakage include increased serum urea and creatinine, increased serum potassium with reduced serum sodium and chloride and a gradually increasing PCV and white blood cell count. Blood bicarbonate and PCO_2 levels gradually decrease as the acidosis worsens. Should vomiting be significant, a mixed metabolic alkalosis and acidosis may be present.

Urinalysis may be abnormal (see Figure 6.5). When haematuria is present, reproductive disease should be ruled out in both males and females, and oestrus and whelping history in bitches and queens should be ascertained. When abdominal distension is noted, or urinary leakage or haemorrhage is suspected, abdominocentesis should be performed. If the fluid is negative for urea nitrogen on a reagent strip, it is not urine. A positive finding, however, may or may not indicate urine, as false positive results may occur. For definitive diagnosis, fluid should be submitted for urea, creatinine and potassium measurements. Values greater than those of peripheral blood indicate that the fluid is urine. Blood easily obtained on abdominocentesis indicates severe haemorrhage, which may be associated with renal parenchymal, blood vessel, liver or splenic injuries.

Diagnostic imaging should be performed in all highly suspect cases of urinary tract trauma. Abdominal radiographs may reveal retroperitoneal changes associated with renal haemorrhage (mass effect with ventral displacement of the colon or streaky increased density in the retroperitoneal space) or a loss of detail within the abdomen indicating free fluid. Non-visualization, displacement or asymmetry of one or both kidneys suggests renal injury. Reduced size or absence of the urinary bladder may indicate rupture or avulsion from the urethra, although a radiographically normal bladder does not rule out rupture. Uroliths (excluding ammonium urate and cystine) may also be visualized within the urinary tract. Ultrasonographic examination of the urinary system may be useful in identifying renal pathology, hydroureter, uroliths, bladder pathology and urethral dilation and obstruction. Excretory urography is required to identify injury, obstruction and perfusion of the kidneys and ureters definitively. Contrast urethrography and cystography, using iodine based contrast material, is extremely useful to identify rupture when leakage of the contrast agent is evident.

Treatment

Renal parenchymal injuries

Renal parenchymal injuries may require surgical treatment if associated with significant haemorrhage or urine leakage. Leakage of contrast during excretory urography, or obstruction of urine flow due to haematoma or other masses, are both indications for laparotomy. Contusions and intracapsular fractures do not require treatment. Renal injuries may be repaired by partial nephrectomy or repair of capsular haemorrhage by deep sutures or omental wrap. If more than 50% of the kidney is destroyed or the pedicle is avulsed, nephrectomy is indicated. A complete examination of both kidneys should be performed prior to surgical intervention unless haemorrhage is occurring.

Ureteral trauma

Ureteral trauma may result in crushing injury, laceration or contusions, usually in the proximal and distal regions. Incomplete tears are debrided and sutured with 5-0 absorbable suture in a simple interrupted pattern. If the ureter is transected, the ends are debrided, spatulated and anastomosed using 5-0 absorbable suture in a simple interrupted pattern. The use of a soft catheter stent, which is placed into the ureter to bridge the anastomotic site, passed into the bladder and exteriorized through the urethra, may facilitate ureteral repair. The catheter is removed after 5–7 days. Ureters avulsed from the bladder can be reimplanted (see further reading). If the ureter is significantly damaged and repair or reimplantation is not an option, renal autograft into the iliac fossa should be considered (Mathews *et al.*, 1994) or nephrectomy should be performed.

Urinary bladder injuries

Urinary bladder contusions result in haemorrhage, which frequently resolves spontaneously. Rupture due to blunt trauma occurs most frequently at the apex. The bladder neck and trigone, urethra or prostate may be lacerated or punctured by pelvic fracture fragments. Since bladder filling and voiding may still be present, frequent examination of the abdomen is necessary to detect uroperitoneum. A urinary catheter may pass easily into the bladder and urethral injury may not be suspected. However, these catheters can be difficult to pass into the bladder and may continue into the peritoneal cavity. Where pelvic injury is severe, it is advisable to take a contrast urethrogram and cystogram to rule out large defects such as complete or partial avulsion of the bladder from the proximal urethra (see Chapter 22).

Surgical approach to the intrapelvic urethra requires osteotomy of the pubis. Debridement and anastomosis of the bladder using 5-0 absorbable suture in a simple interrupted pattern is required. Placement of a urinary catheter may facilitate healing. Small urethral tears can heal over a urinary catheter in 5–7 days without surgical intervention; larger ones, however, require repair. The torn edges of the urethra are debrided and closed with 5-0 absorbable suture in a simple interrupted pattern. If the prostate is injured or opened during the surgical procedure, the capsule is closed. For complete instruction on surgical correction of urological injuries, consult a surgical text (Stone and Barsanti, 1992).

Where urinary leakage is occurring and surgical correction cannot be performed immediately, a urinary catheter can be passed into the bladder and connected to a closed urinary collection system (see Figure 6.6). If a ureteral tear is present, or uroperitoneum persists, it is necessary to place a catheter into the peritoneal cavity to remove urine and prevent peritonitis, uraemia and hyperkalaemia (Figures 6.7 and 6.8).

APPROACH TO ACUTE INTRINSIC RENAL FAILURE

Renal failure is described as acute or chronic. Acute renal failure (ARF) is an abrupt, severe reduction in renal function, commonly caused by ischaemic or toxic insults or infectious agents. Animals may be polyuric, oliguric or anuric, depending on the stage of the disease and the aetiology of the renal insult. The kidneys are either normal in size or large and painful. ARF can occur as a complication in hospitalized animals, especially if high risk patients are not identified and are therefore managed inappropriately. Risk factors are additive: a geriatric patient may be more susceptible to ischaemic or toxic drug injuries than a younger animal. Animals with chronic renal failure usually have a history of polyuria and polydipsia and may have weight loss, reduced exercise tolerance, non-regenerative anaemia and small, irregularly shaped kidneys. Acute-on-chronic renal failure can occur both in and out of the hospital.

Diagnosis of renal failure is based on history, physical examination and laboratory data. ARF occurs in three phases: (1) initial phase, where the insult occurs and oliguria or polyuria and azotaemia are present; (2) maintenance phase, where loss of renal function is established and may progress to irreversible failure; and (3) the recovery phase, where resolution of azotaemia, nephron repair and functional compensation occur. The prognosis for recovery is difficult to define until appropriate therapy has proved unsuccessful.

Diagnostics for acute intrinsic renal failure

The history may reveal exposure to environmental toxins or medications, lack of vaccination for *Leptospira* sp.,

1. Strict aseptic technique is imperative.

2. Place a urinary catheter to remove urine or ensure that the bladder is empty.

3. Clip and surgically prepare and drape the mid-caudal abdomen.

4. Place 1 ml 1% lignocaine into the skin, subcutaneous tissues and abdominal wall on the midline, 1–2 cm caudal to the umbilicus.

5. Make a small incision through skin and subcutaneous tissues to the linea alba if a manufactured peritoneal catheter is used, as the stylet will facilitate passage through the linea alba; or through the linea alba if a sterile feeding tube is used (multiple holes must be made in this tube).

6. Direct the catheter through the incision towards the pelvic inlet. Retract the stylet slightly prior to advancing the catheter. Be sure all holes in the catheter are in the abdomen otherwise urine or dialysate will leak into the subcutaneous tissue. The catheter is secured to the abdominal wall as instructed or with a purse-string and Chinese finger-trap technique.

7. The peritoneal catheter is attached to a three-way stopcock and a sterile intravenous delivery set, with in-line roller clamp; the opposite end of the three-way stopcock is attached to a sterile fluid bag for collection of urine or dialysate.

8. Apply sterile dressing and bandage. All connections should be covered with chlorhexidine or povidine iodine soaked gauze sponges.

Figure 6.7: Peritoneal dialysis: catheter placement.

urinary tract infection or systemic illness. Physical examination should include hydration status, neurological and cardiovascular assessment, temperature, abdominal/bladder palpation, search for systemic illness, body condition and weight. Prior to commencing fluid therapy, blood should be obtained for emergency and routine minimum data bases, and a urine sample should be obtained and tested if possible (Figures 6.5 and 6.9).

Diagnosis is based on serum biochemistry, urinalysis, urine culture, complete blood count, ultrasonography and serology. Leptospirosis may be diagnosed by demonstrating a four-fold rise in agglutination titre over a 1- to 2-week period. A single high titre associated with clinical signs is suggestive of active leptospirosis or ehrlichiosis. Hyperbilirubinaemia and elevations in serum alkaline phosphatase and alanine aminotransferase may be present. Infectious causes are frequently associated with leucocytosis and occasionally non-regenerative anaemia. Thrombocytopenia may be associated with rickettsial disease, vasculitis, disseminated intravascular coagulation, advanced renal disease or ethylene glycol intoxication. Hyperglycaemia has also

1. Commercial dialysate with dextrose 0, 1.5, 2.5 or 4.5% or home-made dialysate using lactated Ringer's solution, or 0.45% saline or 0.9% saline with the appropriate volume of dextrose added. Do not use acetate or gluconate-containing solutions as they are painful when infused. Select 1.5% dextrose if normally hydrated and 4.5% if oedematous, overhydrated or hyperosmolar. The concentration can be reduced as the hydration status and osmolarity improves. The dialysate should be warmed to body temperature.

2. In a small patient where multiple infusions can be obtained from a single dialysate bag, attach the intravenous delivery tubing to one arm of the three-way stopcock and the collection bag to the second arm.

3. Initially infuse 20 ml/kg into the peritoneal space slowly by gravity, while watching the patient's response. Record the volume infused. Overload is detected by an increase in respiratory rate, anxiety, leakage through the insertion site or overly distended abdomen. Close the stopcock. Allow a 45-minute dwell time.

4. If all the dialysate is used, close the roller clamp and place the bag below the patient (on sterile paper or towel). Open the roller clamp to allow slow drainage (over 15 minutes) by gravity. Drain as much as possible. Record the volume and discard.

5. If only a portion of the dialysate is used, close the roller clamp and the stopcock to the dialysate and allow slow drainage by gravity into the collection bag.

6. The dialysate remaining in the bag must be kept warm.

7. Repeat every hour initially. As the patient improves or stabilizes, the procedure can be extended to every 4–6 hours.

8. Initially, volumes of dialysate recovered may be less than infused. Once dehydration is corrected, volumes should equalize or the volume recovered may increase due to ultrafiltration in the oedematous patient.

9. Monitor for fluid overload and assess the patient daily.

10. White blood cell count and Gram staining should be performed on the dialysate daily.

Figure 6.8: Peritoneal dialysis: technique.

Laboratory test	Pre-renal azotaemia	Parenchymal acute renal failure	Post-renal azotaemia
Packed cell volume Total protein	>Normal >Normal	Normal[a] Normal[a]	>Normal[a] >Normal[a]
Serum potassium	Normal High (hypoadrenocorticism) Low (loop diuretic)	Normal or high	Normal or high
Serum sodium	Normal High Low[b]	Normal	Normal
Metabolic acidosis Anion gap	Present Increased	Present Increased	Present Increased

Figure 6.9: Data base, electrolyte and blood gas findings in pre-renal, renal and post-renal azotaemia. [a]Assuming blood loss or anaemia of systemic illness, including chronic renal failure, is not present.
[b]ADH release due to ineffective circulating volume.

been reported in dogs with ethylene glycol intoxication. Hypocalcaemia is a frequent finding in ethylene glycol intoxication and pancreatitis. Hypercalcaemia may be associated with advanced renal disease, cholecalciferol (vitamin D_3) rodenticide intoxication and neoplastic disease. Electrolyte and acid-base information is vital to aid immediate therapy, especially of hyperkalaemia. Hyperkalaemia should be suspected in any patient with a low (or normal) heart rate when in ARF.

The urine protein:creatinine ratio (UP/UC) is a sensitive, rapid and convenient test for the detection and quantification of proteinuria in randomly collected urine samples (see Figure 6.5). UP/UC values <0.5 are normal; values between 0.5 and 1.0 are questionable and values >1.0 are abnormal. There are many causes of increased urine protein, but UP/UC values of 1–5 are usually associated with pre- and post-renal causes or glomerulosclerosis/atrophy, values of 5–13 are associated with non-amyloid glomerulopathy, and values >13 usually indicate severe glomerulopathy or amyloidosis (Lulich and Osborne, 1990).

Treatment

The goals of treatment are to correct fluid, electrolyte and acid–base disorders, establish or maintain urine flow and treat the underlying cause of renal failure. Potentially nephrotoxic drugs must be discontinued. An intravenous catheter is placed using strict aseptic technique, either peripherally for rapid fluid resuscitation or into the jugular vein for fluid therapy and measurement of CVP. If oliguria or anuria are suspected, an indwelling urinary catheter is placed to monitor urine output.

Intravenous fluid therapy is the most important treatment for ARF. An isotonic, alkalinizing, balanced electrolyte solution is preferred to improve acidaemia, which facilitates potassium translocation into cells. If renal failure is associated with hypercalcaemia, 0.9%

sodium chloride is preferred, to enhance calciuresis. Fluids correct dehydration and expand the intravascular space, with subsequent improvement in systemic perfusion. In addition, fluid therapy may overcome some forms of intra-renal vasoconstriction, improve renal perfusion, initiate diuresis and hasten removal of nephrotoxic substances and prevent or correct renal tubular obstruction with cellular debris.

As a guide to the volume of fluid required to rehydrate an animal, calculate hydration deficit and multiply by body weight in kilograms. A 10 kg dog that is 10% dehydrated will require 10 x 10/100 litres = 1.0 litre of fluid to correct the deficit. Ongoing and maintenance losses are calculated (see Figure 6.4) and added to the volume deficit. The rate of administration depends on the acuity of the loss and the volume of urine being produced. In chronic dehydration, when urine is being produced and the patient is not azotaemic, the deficit should be replaced over 24–48 hours. In anuric or suddenly oliguric dogs, regardless of their hydration status, a fluid bolus of 20 ml/kg (dogs) and 10 ml/kg (cats) should be administered over 10 minutes, while monitoring the animal's ability to handle this volume. If urine flow is not established and the animal is showing no signs of fluid overload, the remaining deficit should be administered over the next 1–2 hours. If the animal is judged not to be clinically dehydrated at presentation, it is best to assume 3-5% dehydration and add this volume over 1–2 hours, to ensure volume expansion (e.g. 10 kg x 3–5/100 = 0.3–0.5 l). If more caution is required because of risks of fluid overload, the deficit should be administered over 4 hours and the animal monitored carefully. The goal is to expand the intravascular volume, to replace fluid deficits and to initiate urine production at 1–2 ml/kg/h. Close monitoring is vital to avoid overhydration and to ensure that urine production is maintained.

If an adequate volume of crystalloid has been

administered based on physical examination and appropriate calculation of the deficit, and urine production remains less than 1 ml/kg/h, or the patient is hypotensive, hypoproteinaemic (TP <50 g/l) or anaemic (PCV <25%), further measures are required. Hydroxyethyl starch, pentastarch or oxypolygelatin, plasma, human albumin or whole blood should be administered to increase or maintain oncotic and systemic arterial pressures and to improve renal blood flow and oxygen delivery. If systemic arterial pressures are still unacceptable, dopamine should be added (5–10 µg/kg/min to effect). At this point, hypoadrenocorticism should also be ruled out. Adrenal insufficiency may be primary or secondary and may develop post-trauma or surgery and during sepsis and other critical illness. If cardiac contractility is poor, dobutamine should be added, starting at 5 µg/kg/min (dogs). In cats, dobutamine should be started at 1 µg/kg/min and slowly increased to effect, with a maximum dose of 4 µg/kg/min. Dobutamine and dopamine can be administered simultaneously in dogs. Should hypotension persist, dobutamine should be discontinued and noradrenaline can be used (CRI 0.01–0.1 µg/kg/min) and dopamine can be discontinued or maintained. The goal is to expand intravascular volume, replace fluid deficits and normalize oncotic and blood pressure to initiate urine production at 1–2 ml/kg/h, without overhydration.

Once volume expansion and normotension have been established, if urine production remains less than 1 ml/kg/h, diuretics should be administered. Their use should not be postponed, as renal failure may be difficult to reverse at a later time. Frusemide or mannitol are preferred. If acute tubular necrosis is suspected and the animal is not overhydrated, hyperosmolar (e.g. hypernatraemia, ethylene glycol or salicylate toxicosis, hyperglycaemia), haemorrhaging, has no pulmonary or interstitial oedema and no vasculitis, mannitol may be the better choice. Mannitol produces an osmotic diuresis and reduces cellular oedema and reperfusion injury by scavenging oxygen free radicals. It is given at 0.25 g/kg i.v. over 5–10 minutes and repeated in 30–40 minutes to maintain diuresis. Mannitol should not be repeated if urine flow is <1 ml/kg/h within 60 minutes of the initial bolus.

If there is no response to mannitol, or frusemide is preferred or indicated initially (see contraindications for mannitol above), frusemide should be administered intravenously at 2–4 mg/kg (dog), 2 mg/kg (cat). Frusemide enhances aminoglycoside nephrotoxicity, therefore this combination should be avoided. If no beneficial effect is seen in 30 minutes, the dose should be repeated once in the cat, or once or twice, at 6 mg/kg, in the dog at 1-hour intervals. If mannitol or frusemide are not available, hypertonic dextrose in water (20% solution) at 2–10 ml/min for 1–5 minutes, followed by 1–5 ml/min, for a total daily dosage of 22–66 ml/kg, may establish diuresis. Glucosuria does not necessarily indicate success of diuresis unless urine output approaches 1–4 ml/kg/h.

In anuric or oliguric renal failure, a constant rate infusion of dopamine 1–3 µg/kg/min can be administered in combination with frusemide or mannitol therapy. In dogs, dopamine dilates the afferent arterioles, while in cats dopamine increases cardiac output and decreases sodium reabsorption in the distal tubule and collecting ducts. If tachycardia or an arrhythmia develops during dopamine administration, the drug should be discontinued and re-started at a lower dose. Peritoneal dialysis (see Figure 6.7) or haemodialysis should be considered in the anuric animal when attempts at establishing urine flow have failed.

Metoclopramide (1 mg/kg/24 h CRI, or 0.2 mg/kg every 8 h) for vomiting and H_2 blockers at half the recommended dose, with sucralfate, should be considered for ulcer prophylaxis. Hyperphosphataemia may be treated with phosphate binders or sucralfate. Nutritional support should also be considered. Treatment for specific causes of renal failure should also be pursued.

LOWER URINARY TRACT OBSTRUCTION

Either the bladder or urethra may be obstructed. The history includes stranguria (owners may mistakenly report constipation), dysuria, pollakiuria or anuria, and males are more frequently affected. The clinical condition of a dog or cat with urethral obstruction depends on the duration and severity (partial, total or functional) of the obstruction. Systemic signs are usually not present within 24 hours of obstruction. Post-renal azotaemia develops within 48 hours and then uraemia rapidly develops. With total urethral obstruction no urine is voided, but an occasional drop of urine may drip from the penis or vulva. The abdomen must be palpated gently to avoid more pain and rupture of a large tense urinary bladder. If a bladder cannot be palpated in an animal where urethral obstruction is highly likely, a ruptured bladder should be suspected.

Idiopathic, non-obstructive feline lower urinary tract disease

Diagnosis
Idiopathic, non-obstructive feline lower urinary tract disease, also called 'idiopathic cystitis' (interstitial cystitis in humans), is a diagnosis of exclusion. Suggested pathophysiology and clinical experience is reported elsewhere (Buffington and Chew, 1995). The behaviour of cats with this disease is similar to that of cats with obstructive disease, but physical obstruction is not a feature. Voiding appears painful, and haematuria and pollakiuria may be associated with dysuria. The cat may void in inappropriate places, groom the caudal abdomen and genitals frequently and resent abdominal

palpation. These cats are usually presented as an emergency due to dysuria, inappropriate urination or haematuria. Occasionally the cat cannot void and has a hard, moderately enlarged bladder associated with azotaemia or uraemia. A urinary catheter is passed easily into the urethra and bladder. Crystals and 'mucus-like' material may be present. The urinalysis is usually normal except for the presence of microscopic or grossly visible blood. The pH of the urine is frequently <6.5 and no bacteria are seen. Ultrasonographic and contrast cystography reveals thickening of the bladder wall and contrast material may dissect under the urothelium.

Treatment

If an enlarged bladder is palpated, a urinary catheter should be passed to rule out obstruction and obtain urine for sediment and crystal identification. Urine culture is usually unnecessary, as this disease is not associated with bacteria. If frequent urethral catheterization has been performed, infection may be present and culture is warranted. When cats have been unable to void, presumably due to reflex dysinergia secondary to cystitis, the urinary catheter usually must remain in place for at least 2 days until medical management has taken effect. These cats tend to be azotaemic, requiring fluid therapy (see acute renal failure) to reverse the azotaemia/uraemia. Phenoxybenzamine (0.5 mg/kg orally sid or 0.25 mg/kg orally bid) is administered to reduce urethral spasm but may require 24–48 hours for full effect. Hypotension is a possible but rare side-effect related to alpha-adrenergic blockade, and this drug should not be used in cats with cardiovascular disease. Bethanechol (1.25–5.0 mg orally tid) may be administered, after urethral patency and function have been established, to enhance bladder emptying if detrusor dysfunction is identified. Bethanechol may cause bladder rupture if there is resistance to urine flow. Amitriptyline (2.5–12.5 mg (5 mg typical dose) orally sid at bedtime for 5–7 days), may be used and dosed to produce a barely perceptible calming effect. The analgesic, anti-inflammatory, anticholinergic and reduced adrenergic effects of amitriptyline also contribute to relief of symptoms in these cats. Possible side-effects include urine retention and increased liver enzymes. Increasing water intake, including feeding canned food, reducing stressors in the environment and identifying associated crystalluria, are all necessary to treat the cystitis.

Urethral obstruction

Diagnosis

Urethral obstruction due to uroliths is a common cause of anuria in dogs and cats, but other causes must also be considered. Transitional cell carcinoma and granulomatous urethritis may produce similar clinical signs of obstruction. The animal may appear physiologically normal or may be depressed, vomiting, in shock or coma. A large hard painful bladder may be palpable in the abdomen. Bradycardia, hypothermia, pale mucous membranes with prolonged capillary refill time, hyperpnoea and halitosis may be present. In cats with uroliths, the tip of the penis is often dark red/purple and swollen. In dogs, the urolith may be palpated anywhere from the ischial arch to the os penis and the penis may be discoloured. If uroliths are ruled out, a rectal examination of the prostate and bladder trigone should be performed in the male dog and a vaginal examination for vaginal/urethral masses in the bitch. Ultrasonography and/or contrast urography and cystography, in addition to urine cytology and urethral or bladder biopsy, is required for diagnosis of granulomatous and neoplastic lesions.

Treatment

If the animal is extremely depressed, oxygen should be administered by mask, an intravenous catheter placed, and blood should be obtained for an emergency minimum data base. The degree of dehydration is estimated and an isotonic balanced electrolyte solution is administered over 12 hours if minimally dehydrated, over 4 hours if moderately dehydrated and over 1–2 hours if shock is present. These rates of administration may be modified according to response to therapy, which should be re-assessed every 5–10 minutes. If a bradyarrhythmia is detected, an ECG should be obtained. Hyperkalaemia, if associated with bradycardia, should be treated aggressively (see Chapter 4) prior to relieving the obstruction. If acidosis is present and hyperkalaemia is not associated with life-threatening signs, fluid resuscitation alone will often be sufficient to correct the values.

Relieving the obstruction

If the patient is depressed, sedation is not necessary. If in pain or alert, the dog or cat should be sedated or anaesthetized using one of the following: morphine (0.1–0.3 mg/kg i.m.); butorphanol (0.2–0.4 mg/kg i.v. or i.m.); propofol (2–4 mg/kg i.v.); a short acting thiobarbiturate (5 mg/kg i.v.); mask isoflurane anaesthesia; ketamine (2.5–5.0 mg/kg) mixed with diazepam (0.125–0.25 mg/kg i.v.); or midazolam (0.125–0.25 mg/kg i.v. or i.m.). Caution should be exercised with ketamine combinations if renal compromise is suspected, and vomiting may occur with morphine administration. Prior to anaesthesia, plasma potassium should be estimated where possible and an ECG trace obtained. Severe hyperkalaemia should be addressed. With any medication, the lowest dose possible should be used. If the bladder requires immediate decompression, cystocentesis can be performed prior to relieving the obstruction. A 22 or 20 gauge over-the-needle catheter can be used, the needle removed and an extension with three-way stopcock attached. Care must be taken not to move the catheter and to aspirate carefully, as the bladder might tear. As much urine as possible is removed and then the urethral obstruction can be addressed.

In cats, the penis is gently massaged between the thumb and forefinger and gentle pressure is applied to the bladder. If not immediately relieved, hydropulsion should be attempted, using a polypropylene Tom Cat catheter, an ophthalmic lacrimal duct flush cannula, or a 22 gauge over-the-needle catheter using the needle as a stylet while retracting the point into the catheter. A 12 ml syringe is filled with sterile saline, the penis is extended caudally (making the urethra as straight as possible) and the urethra is flushed while advancing the catheter. When the obstruction is removed, the bladder is pressed gently to empty it, then flushed slowly with warm sterile saline until clear, emptying the bladder each time. In large cats, the Tom Cat catheter may not reach the bladder and a 3.5 Fr. paediatric feeding tube is recommended should the bladder remain catheterized. The catheter is secured to the patient by placing an adhesive tape butterfly around the proximal end of the catheter and suturing it to the prepuce in a horizontal pattern. A sterile intravenous administration set and empty fluid bag are attached to the urinary catheter and then maintained as a closed collection system (see Figure 6.6). The bladder should remain catheterized if relief of the obstruction was difficult, if the urine stream is small, if the bladder was overly distended and detrusor function may be questionable, if the cat is uraemic or markedly azotaemic and diuresis is necessary, or if post-obstructive diuresis is likely and measurement of urine output is necessary.

If a urinary catheter cannot be passed beyond the penile urethra, an emergency urethrostomy or a catheter cystotomy may be required. For emergency decompression of the bladder, a catheter cystotomy is preferred to multiple cystocenteses, while stabilizing the patient for definitive surgical correction. An appropriate analgesic or anaesthetic regimen should be selected and the skin and abdominal wall infiltrated with 1–2 ml of 1% lignocaine. An 8 Fr. Foley urinary catheter is placed into the bladder via a 2–3 cm midline incision through skin and abdominal wall, midway between the umbilicus and pubis. The bladder is exteriorized and stabilized using two retention sutures and a purse-string suture is placed through the serosa and muscular layers of the ventral apical region of the bladder. A stab incision is made within the purse-string suture and the Foley catheter is introduced. The balloon is inflated with sterile saline and the purse-string suture is carefully tightened snugly (avoid tying too tightly or suture line necrosis may occur), after incorporation of omentum. The retention sutures are passed through the linea alba and tied. The midline incision is closed routinely. The catheter is connected to a closed collection system.

In dogs, cystocentesis is performed if necessary, or attempts are made to pass a small gauge catheter beyond the obstruction into the bladder to remove the urine. In males, if the obstruction is due to a urolith (frequently in or behind the os penis), it should be hydropulsed into the bladder using as short a catheter as possible or round-ended teat cannula. Two people are required for this procedure; one occludes the proximal urethra via rectal palpation and compression against the pubic symphysis and the other retracts the penis, cleans the urethral orifice and passes the catheter into the urethra. The urethral orifice is then manually occluded. Using a 35 or 60 ml syringe, half-filled with equal volumes of well mixed sterile saline and sterile aqueous lubricating jelly, the mixture is injected into the urethra (do not use lubricating jelly if there is a tear or deep abrasion in the urethra or bladder) until the urethra is distended. At this point, the proximal occlusion is released while fluid injection is continued to flush the urolith into the bladder. In bitches, a Foley catheter is placed into the urethral orifice and the balloon inflated. The urethra is flushed without proximal occlusion of the urethra. If hydropulsion is not successful in relieving the obstruction, caution must be used to avoid injuring the urethra, and surgical removal is advisable. A cystotomy is then required to remove uroliths retropulsed into the bladder. In some dogs voiding uro-hydropropulsion, a non-surgical technique for removal of urocystoliths (Lulich and Osborne, 1995), may be attempted. A urethrostomy is required to remove uroliths that continue to obstruct the urethra. If attempts to relieve the obstruction fail, emergency decompression of the bladder via catheter cystostomy may be necessary while the patient is stabilized.

If hydropulsion is successful, a urinary catheter is passed into the bladder to remove the urine. The bladder should be gently flushed to remove the lubricating jelly, blood clots or crystals. If the catheter remains in place, it should be attached to a closed urinary collection system. The duration of urinary catheter placement depends on the severity of the problem, but is usually a minimum of 24 hours.

The cause of granulomatous urethritis in bitches is unknown, but it is frequently associated with primary or secondary bacterial cystitis. Catheterization of the urinary bladder is necessary to permit emptying. Immunosuppressive doses of prednisolone (2–3 mg/kg daily) are suggested, with antibiotic therapy based on culture and sensitivity results.

Urethral obstruction due to neoplasia and associated inflammation may be successfully managed with a temporary indwelling urinary catheter, empirical or specific antibiotic therapy based on culture and sensitivity and piroxicam (0.3 mg/kg sid for 3 days, then every 48 h or to effect). If reflex dysinergia is likely, this therapy in addition to phenoxybenzamine (5–15 mg/dog sid for 5–7 days), may be effective.

Haematomas of the bladder or urethra may require hydropulsion and bladder flushing, while maintaining urine flow with an indwelling urinary catheter. If a coagulopathy is present, it should be identified and treated (see Chapter 10) to prevent further bleeding. If the haematoma is due to trauma, the injury should be identified via contrast urography. Inadvertent obstruction of urine flow due to iatrogenic ligation of the urethra may occur after any surgical procedure associated with the urethra (e.g. perineal hernia, castration, urethral surgery) or bladder (e.g. hysterectomy, prostatic surgery).

Perineal hernia with prolapsed urinary bladder may result in anuria and obstructed passage of a urinary catheter. Cystocentesis is required while planning emergency surgical correction. Similarly, prostatomegaly may cause urethral obstruction (see Chapter 11). Inability to void may be associated with spinal disease or injuries, especially those that involve the sacrum (Kuntz, 1995).

After relief of any obstruction, if urine production is <0.5 ml/kg/h and non-responsive to estimated fluid requirements, consider treatment for oliguric/anuric renal failure.

REFERENCES AND FURTHER READING

Binns SH (1994) Pathogenesis and pathophysiology of ischemic injury in cases of acute renal failure. *Compendium on Continuing Education in Small Animal Practice* **16**, 31–40

Bjorling DE (1993) The urinary system. In: *Textbook of Small Animal Surgery, 2nd edn*, ed. D Slatter, pp. 1368–1495. WB Saunders, Philadelphia

Buffington CAT and Chew DJ (1997) Lower urinary tract diseases in cats: the Ohio experience. *Proceedings of the 15th American College Veterinary Internal Medicine Forum, Buena Vista, Florida,* 343–346.

Buffington CAT and Chew DJ (1995) Does interstitial cystitis occur in cats? In: *Kirk's Current Veterinary Therapy Small Animal Practice*, ed. J Bonagura, pp. 1009–1011. WB Saunders, Philadelphia

Burrows CF (1974) Metabolic changes due to experimentally induced rupture of the canine urinary bladder. *American Journal of Veterinary Research* **35**, 1083–1088

Forrester SD (1996) Acute renal failure due to systemic diseases. *Proceedings of the 14th American College of Veterinary Internal Medicine, San Antonio, Texas,* pp. 362–364.

Forrester SD and Brandt KS (1994) The diagnostic approach to the patient with acute renal failure. Symposium on acute renal failure. *Veterinary Medicine* **89**, 212–218

Forrester SD *et al.* (1994) Taking measures to prevent acute renal failure. Symposium on acute renal failure. *Veterinary Medicine* **89**, 231–236

Hitt ME (1986) Hematuria of renal origin. *Compendium on Continuing Education in Small Animal Practice* **8**, 14–19

Kuntz *et al.* (1995) Sacral fractures in dogs: a review of 32 cases. *Journal of the American Animal Hospital Association* **31**, 142–150

Lane IF and Grauer GF (1994) Management of acute renal failure. Symposium on acute renal failure. *Veterinary Medicine* **89**, 319–230

Lane IF *et al.* (1994a) Acute renal failure. Part I. Risk factors, prevention, and strategies for protection. *Compendium on Continuing Education in Small Animal Practice* **16**, 15–28

Lane IF *et al.* (1994b) Acute renal failure. Part II. Diagnosis, management, and prognosis. *Compendium on Continuing Education in Small Animal Practice* **16**, 625–642

Ling GV (1995) Nephrolithiasis: prevalence of mineral type. In: *Kirk's Current Veterinary Therapy Small Animal Practice*, ed. J Bonagura, p. 980. WB Saunders, Philadelphia

Ling GV and Sorenson JL (1995) CVT Update: management and prevention of urate lithiasis. In: *Kirk's Current Veterinary Therapy Small Animal Practice*, ed. J Bonagura, pp. 985–989. WB Saunders, Philadelphia

Lulich JP and Osborne CA (1990) Interpretation of urine protein-creatinine ratios in dogs with glomerular and nonglomerular disorders. *Compendium on Continuing Education in Small Animal Practice* **12**, 59–72

Lulich JP and Osborne CA (1995a) Voiding urohydropulsion: a non-surgical technique for removal of urocystoliths. In: *Kirk's Current Veterinary Therapy Small Animal Practice*, ed. J Bonagura, pp. 1003–1007. WB Saunders, Philadelphia

Lulich JP and Osborne CA (1995b) Canine calcium oxalate uroliths In: *Kirk's Current Veterinary Therapy Small Animal Practice*, ed. J Bonagura, pp. 992–996. WB Saunders, Philadelphia

Mathews KA *et al.* (1994) Renal allograft survival in outbred mongrel dogs using anti-dog thymocyte serum in combination with immunosuppressive drug therapy with or without donor bone marrow. *Journal of Veterinary Surgery* **23**, 347–357

Morgan RV (1982) Urogenital emergencies. Part 1. *Compendium on Continuing Education in Small Animal Practice* **4**, 908–915

Osborne CA (1983) Azotemia: a review of what's old and what's new. Part 1. Definition of terms and concepts. *Compendium on Continuing Education in Small Animal Practice* **5**, 497–510

Osborne CA *et al.* (1995) Feline calcium oxalate uroliths In: *Kirk's Current Veterinary Therapy Small Animal Practice*, ed. J Bonagura, pp. 989–992. WB Saunders, Philadelphia

Osborne CA *et al.* (1995) Canine and feline calcium phosphate urolithiasis In: *Kirk's Current Veterinary Therapy Small Animal Practice*, ed. J Bonagura, pp. 996–1001. WB Saunders, Philadelphia

Pechman RD (1982) Urinary trauma in dogs and cats: a review. *Journal of the American Animal Hospital Association* **18**, 33–40

Selcer BA (1982) Urinary tract trauma with pelvic trauma. *Journal of the American Animal Hospital Association* **18**, 785–793

Stone EA and Barsanti JA (1992) *Urologic Surgery of the Dog and Cat*. Lea and Febiger, Philadelphia

CHAPTER SEVEN

Neurological Emergencies

Charles H. Vite and Sheldon A. Steinberg

CLINICAL EVALUATION OF THE NERVOUS SYSTEM

The neurological examination is a functional examination. Six broad categories of neurological function are assessed:

- Mental status
- Gait
- Postural ability
- Segmental reflexes
- Sensation
- Cranial nerve function.

In each anatomical part of the nervous system, certain signs are recognized that indicate malfunction. The results of examination help to identify which parts of the nervous system are showing evidence of malfunction and help to begin the process of answering the questions:

- Is neurological disease present?
- If so, where is/are the lesion(s)?
- What disease process is likely to be causing the neural dysfunction?

Deficits and clinical signs that may be seen with lesions in specific anatomical sites are listed in Figure 7.1. In general, the likelihood of these deficits and signs occurring increases with the completeness/extent of the lesion. Serious dysfunction may result in dramatic clinical signs. However, serious dysfunction may still be reversible.

SEIZURES AND STATUS EPILEPTICUS

Seizures result from a sudden uncontrolled discharge of neurons in the cerebral cortex or diencephalon. The term 'epilepsy' means recurrent seizures.

Patient assessment and treatment

Recurrent seizures may be classified according to their cause (Podell *et al.*, 1995):

- Reactive seizures occur when the normal brain is

stressed by metabolic or toxic abnormalities caused by extracranial disease. Examples include hepatic encephalopathy, uraemic encephalopathy, hypoglycaemia, hypocalcaemia, polycythaemia and toxins
- Secondary seizures are provoked by structural diseases of the brain. Examples include brain tumours, encephalitis, hydrocephalus and brain trauma
- Idiopathic epilepsy is the consequence of intrinsic chemical abnormality that is not associated with demonstrable intra- or extracranial disease.

When presented with a patient with seizures one should: assess the patient; obtain a good history; place a catheter and draw blood; and administer anticonvulsant medication.

Assessing the patient

Important information may be gained with a 2-minute examination before giving anticonvulsant medication:

- Examine the mucous membranes
- Auscultate the heart
- Determine heart rate
- Assess pulses
- Feel and examine the ears and foot pads for hyperthermia
- Characterize the appearance and duration of the seizure.

An important observation is whether the seizure is generalized or focal. Generalized seizures, characterized by symmetrical involvement of the head and limbs and a loss of consciousness, have little localizing value. Partial seizures occur due to focal, often asymmetrical, disease of the brain and may result in asymmetrical signs such as tonus or clonus of one or more limbs, or turning the head and neck to one side. Partial seizures may also result in complex motor activity including sudden changes in behaviour. Partial seizures may progress to generalized seizures. Idiopathic and reactive epilepsy appear most often as generalized seizures. Secondary epilepsy may appear as: generalized seizures; symmetrical, partial seizures; or asymmetrical,

Location of deficit	Mental status	Gait	Postural ability
Cerebral hemispheres/ diencephalon	Depression, disorientation, stupor, coma; other abnormalities such as aggression and hyperexcitability	Circling (frequently toward the side of the lesion), pacing, or headpressing. Otherwise, gait is normal	Postural reaction deficits contralateral to the side of the lesion
Midbrain	Depression, stupor or coma	Ataxia and spastic tetraparesis/ paralysis. Contralateral spastic hemiparesis/paralysis and ataxia if the lesion is lateralized	Postural reaction deficits contralateral (common) or ipsilateral (less common) to the side of the lesion. Increased extensor tone of the limbs contralateral to the side of the lesion. Decerebrate posture, characterized by opisthotonus with rigid extension of all limbs
Pons/medulla	Depression, stupor or coma	Ataxia and spastic tetraparesis/paralysis. Ipsilateral spastic hemiparesis/paralysis and ataxia if the lesion is lateralized	Postural reaction deficits and increased extensor tone: of the limbs ipsilateral to the side of the lesion; or of all four limbs if lesion involves both sides of the pons/medulla
Cerebellum	Normal	Dysmetria ipsilateral to the side of the lesion. (An over-stepping or goose-stepping gait with a delayed onset of voluntary motion which, when initiated, is exaggerated.) Spasticity ipsilateral to the side of the lesion without paresis/paralysis	A broad-based stance, swaying of body from side to side and a tremor of the head and neck most noticeable when fine movements are required. Dysmetric, spastic postural reactions ipsilateral to the side of the lesion
Cervical spinal cord segments 1–5	Normal	Ataxia and spastic hemi- or tetraparesis/paralysis	Ipsilateral or bilateral postural reaction deficits and increased extensor tone of the limbs
Cervical spinal cord segment 6 to thoracic cord segment 2	Normal	Hindlimbs: ipsilateral or bilateral ataxia and spastic paresis/paralysis Forelimbs: ipsilateral or bilateral flaccid forelimb paresis/paralysis Movement is characterized by scuffing the paws; a stiff, short-strided gait; or inability to support weight	Hindlimbs: ipsilateral or bilateral postural reaction deficits and increased extensor tone of the limbs Forelimbs: ipsilateral or bilateral postural reaction deficits and decreased extensor tone of the limbs
Thoracic spinal cord segment 3 to lumbar cord segment 3	Normal	Hindlimbs: ipsilateral or bilateral ataxia and spastic paresis/paralysis Forelimbs: normal	Hindlimbs: ipsilateral or bilateral postural reaction deficits and increased extensor tone of the limbs Forelimbs: normal
Lumbar cord segment 4 through sacral spinal cord segment 1	Normal	Hindlimbs: ipsilateral or bilateral flaccid paresis/paralysis. Movement is characterized by scuffing the paws; a stiff, short-strided gait; or inability to support weight Forelimbs: normal	Hindlimbs: ipsilateral or bilateral postural reaction deficits and decreased extensor tone of the limbs Forelimbs: normal

Segmental reflexes	**Sensation**	**Cranial nerve function**	**Other**
Normal	Depressed over the face and limbs contralateral to the side of the lesion	Blindness contralateral to the side of the lesion with normal pupillary responses. Bilateral miosis with responsive pupils with diffuse cerebrocortical disease. Dilated pupils, non-responsive to light (fixed) when disease involves the optic chiasm	Seizures. Abnormalities associated with hypothalamic involvement. Cheyne–Stokes respiration
Hyper-reflexia of the limb reflexes contralateral to the side of the lesion	Depressed below the level of this lesion	A dilated and fixed pupil and ventrolateral strabismus ipsilateral to the side of the lesion due to CN III involvement. Bilateral miosis due to CN III stimulation. Dorsolateral rotation of the globe (CN IV)	Hyperventilation
Hyper-reflexia: of the limb reflexes ipsilateral to the side of the lesion; or of all four limbs if lesion involves both sides of the pons/medulla	Decreased over the side of the face ipsilateral to the side of the lesion	Decreased sensation of the face, decreased jaw tone, masticatory muscle atrophy (CN V); decreased palpebral reflex (CN V and VII); medial strabismus, decreased globe retraction (CN VI); drooping lips, inability to blink the eyelids or move the ears (CN VII); nystagmus, head tilt and positional ventral strabismus (CN VIII); dysphagia, dysphonia, decreased gag reflex (CN IX and X); regurgitation, megaoesophagus (CN X); and decreased tongue motion and tongue muscle atrophy (CN XII) ipsilateral to the side of the lesion.	Rapid, shallow breathing; irregular, ataxic breathing; or apnoea
Normal	Normal	An absent menace response, although the eye appears able to see, ipsilateral to the side of the lesion. Off-balance, head tilt, nystagmus and strabismus	Intention tremor. Truncal ataxia
Ipsilateral or bilateral hyper-reflexia of limb reflexes	Decreased at and below the level of the lesion	No abnormalities	Cervical muscle spasms. Horner's syndrome (uncommon). Respiratory muscle paresis/paralysis. Urinary incontinence and decreased ability to express the bladder
Hindlimbs: ipsilateral or bilateral hyper-reflexia of the limb reflexes Forelimbs: ipsilateral or bilateral hyporeflexia of the limb reflexes	Decreased at and below the level of the lesion	No abnormalities	Horner's syndrome ipsilateral to the side of the lesion. Diaphragmatic breathing. Ipsilateral or bilateral depressed cutaneous trunci reflex. Urinary incontinence and decreased ability to express the bladder
Hindlimbs: ipsilateral or bilateral hyper-reflexia of the limb reflexes Forelimbs: normal	Decreased at and below the level of the lesion	No abnormalities	Schiff–Sherrington posture. Urinary incontinence and decreased ability to express the bladder
Ipsilateral or bilateral hyporeflexia of the hindlimbs	Decreased at and below the level of the lesion	No abnormalities	Schiff–Sherrington posture. Urinary incontinence and decreased ability to express the bladder

Figure 7.1 *(continued over page)*

Location of deficit	Mental status	Gait	Postural ability
Sacral spinal cord segments	Normal	Hindlimbs: normal gait or ipsilateral or bilateral scuffing of the paws Forelimbs: normal	Hindlimbs: normal or ipsilateral or bilateral plantigrade posture Forelimbs: normal
Peripheral nerves	Normal	Monoparesis, hemiparesis or tetraparesis. Movement is characterized by scuffing the paws; a stiff, short-strided gait; or inability to support weight	Postural reaction deficits and decreased extensor tone of the affected limbs
Skeletal muscle	Normal	Monoparesis, hemiparesis or tetraparesis. Movement is characterized by scuffing the paws; a stiff, short-strided gait; or inability to support weight	Postural reaction testing may be normal if the animal is supported, however, postural reaction deficits may occur in affected limbs

partial seizures. Therefore, if an animal presents with a seizure characterized by lateralized signs such as lifting one limb, turning to one side, or twitching over one side of the face, one should strongly consider secondary epilepsy.

Obtaining a good history
The following questions should be addressed:

- Is the animal vaccinated?
- Has there been any exposure to toxins? Strychnine, lead, mercury, metaldehyde, moulds, organophosphates, chlorinated hydrocarbons, ethylene glycol, amphetamines, caffeine, theobromine, cocaine, 5-fluorouracil, ivermectin and others may cause seizures
- Has the animal had seizures in the past? Is the animal currently taking anticonvulsants? How many seizures have occurred within the past year, 6 months or month? Generalized seizures occurring infrequently over years suggest idiopathic epilepsy or a static, structural lesion
- How old is the animal? The onset of seizures in dogs due to idiopathic epilepsy is between 6 months and 5 years of age (most commonly 9 months to 3 years). Idiopathic epilepsy is uncommon in cats
- What time of day did the seizure occur? Seizures following feeding may be associated with hepatic encephalopathy. Seizures occurring when a meal has been missed or soon before a meal may indicate hypoglycaemia

- Is the animal normal between seizures? Animals with idiopathic epilepsy appear normal between seizures. Animals with reactive epilepsy or secondary epilepsy may be normal between seizures or may be behaviourally abnormal, dull, circle, or show other signs of nervous system disease. These animals may also show signs of systemic disease.

Blood tests
It is recommended that a complete blood count, blood smear evaluation for inclusion bodies (seen with canine distemper virus infection) and nucleated red cells (seen with lead toxicity), urinalysis, and blood gas measurements be performed. Levels of serum electrolytes, blood glucose, alanine aminotransferase, blood urea nitrogen, serum ammonia, serum creatinine and cholesterol should be determined. Additional serum may be refrigerated for future determination of anticonvulsant, insulin or thyroid hormone concentrations, or for titres for infectious disease assays.

Seizures due to metabolic causes require specific therapy in addition to anticonvulsant medications. (see 'Abnormal mental status and metabolic encephalopathies' for the treatment of hypoglycaemia, hypocalcaemia and thiamine deficiency).

Status epilepticus and cluster seizures may result in hypoxia, acidosis and/or hyperthermia, which require specific treatment. Usually, seizures result in hyperglycaemia. Rarely, however, status epilepticus may result in hypoglycaemia and the patient may require supplementation with dextrose.

Segmental reflexes	Sensation	Cranial nerve function	Other
Normal or hyporeflexive sciatic nerve reflexes. Decreased anal sphincter tone. Depressed bulbocavernosus reflex	Decreased sensation of the perineal area, tail and skin over the limb innervated by the sciatic nerve	No abnormalities	Urinary incontinence with an easily expressible bladder. Faecal incontinence
Hyporeflexia in affected limbs. Decreased anal tone	Normal or decreased sensation of affected regions	Decreased sensation of the face, decreased jaw tone, masticatory muscle atrophy (CN V); decreased palpebral reflex (CN V and VII); medial strabismus, decreased globe retraction (CN VI); drooping lips, inability to blink the eyelids or move the ears (CN VII); nystagmus, head tilt and positional ventral strabismus (CN VIII); dysphagia, dysphonia, decreased gag reflex (CN IX and X); regurgitation, megaoesophagus (CN X); and decreased tongue motion and tongue muscle atrophy (CN XII) ipsilateral to the side of the lesion.	Urinary incontinence with an easily expressible bladder. Faecal incontinence. Quickly progressing and severe muscle atrophy. Exercise intolerance
Normoreflexia or hyporeflexia in affected limbs. Decreased anal tone	Normal or muscle may be painful on palpation.	Decreased jaw tone; ipsilateral or bilateral masticatory muscle atrophy; drooping lips; decreased ability to blink the eyelids or move the ears; dysphagia; dysphonia; decreased gag reflex; regurgitation; megaoesophagus; and decreased tongue motion with atrophy of the tongue muscle	Quickly progressing and severe muscle atrophy. Exercise intolerance. Limited joint motion

Figure 7.1: Clinical signs of neurological diseases.

Spinal cord disease results in no abnormalities of mental status or cranial nerve function. Deficits in gait, postural ability, reflexes and sensation occur at or caudal to the level of the lesion and ipsilateral to the side of the lesion. Bilateral deficits may occur if the lesion crosses the midline of the spinal cord.

Ataxia: incoordination; may be characterized by crossing over of the limbs, increased stride length, abduction or circumduction of a limb or limbs, walking on the dorsum of the paw, or the failure of an observer to be able to predict where a paw will land.

Paresis: partial loss of voluntary motor ability; may be characterized by an inability to support weight fully while walking or standing, scuffing of the paws when walking and tremoring when trying to stand.

Paralysis: complete loss of voluntary motor ability.

Spasticity: increased extensor tone of the limbs.

Abnormalities associated with hypothalamic involvement: diabetes insipidus, diabetes mellitus, hyperadrenocorticism and acromegaly; abnormalities in appetite, thirst, sleep, sexual behaviour, temperature regulation and electrolyte regulation.

Cheyne–Stoke's pattern of respiration: a repeating pattern of deep and shallow respiration followed by periods of apnoea.

Dysmetria: a form of ataxia, characterized by abnormal rate or range of a movement.

Horner's syndrome: miosis, ptosis, prolapsed third eyelid and enophthalmosis.

Schiff–Sherrington posture: characterized by increased extensor tone and normal postural ability of the forelimbs.

Bulbocavernosus reflex: squeezing the bulb of the penis or the vulva causes contraction of the anal sphincter in normal animals.

Administering anticonvulsant medication

If the seizure lasts less than 2 minutes and is not repeated, no medication is required.

Seizures over 2 minutes, seizure clusters or status epilepticus:

- Diazepam: 0.2–0.5 mg/kg i.v. or rectally may be repeated 2–3 times over 5–10 minutes.
- Phenobarbitone: a loading dose of 16 mg/kg i.v. is given divided into three or four doses over several hours. It may take up to 30 minutes before an effect is noted. (If the animal is currently on an adequate dose of phenobarbitone, there is little evidence that increasing the dose by another 16 mg/kg has any beneficial effect)
- Diazepam and phenobarbitone may be given concurrently.

If status epilepticus or seizure clustering continues, one of the following regimens may be used:

- Intravenous administration of 10–20 mg/kg thiopental (given as 2–4 mg/kg boluses to effect), endotracheal intubation and isoflurane anaesthesia
- Intravenous administration of 6 mg/kg propofol (given as 1–2 mg/kg boluses to effect), followed by a continuous rate infusion of 0.1–0.2 mg/kg/min propofol. (If hepatic disease is suspected from the history or blood work, the propofol regimen may be more appropriate than administering barbiturates.)
- Intravenous administration of 2–6 mg/kg pentobarbitone
- Continuous rate infusion of diazepam administered at a rate of 0.1–0.5 mg/kg/h in a 5% dextrose solution.

In all these second tier regimens, the patient is profoundly sedated or is anaesthetized. Endotracheal intubation and careful monitoring of respiratory and cardiovascular status may be required. The patient should be anaesthetized for 15–30 minutes with propofol or thiopentone. If seizures continue after recovery from anaesthesia, repeated anaesthesia for longer periods of time may be attempted. If seizures continue after discontinuing these regimens, potassium bromide (400 mg/kg) may be administered either rectally or via stomach tube.

Maintenance medication:
- Phenobarbitone (3–5 mg/kg orally every 12 hours). Serum concentration attains steady-state within 2 weeks

or
- Potassium bromide (30 mg/kg orally every 24 hours). Serum concentration attains steady state in 2–4 months.

Prognosis

Idiopathic epilepsy is rarely life threatening unless status epilepticus develops. However, blindness, weakness or changes in behaviour may continue for days to weeks following a seizure and may be made temporarily worse by anticonvulsant medications.

Animals with secondary epilepsy require further diagnostic testing including cerebrospinal fluid analysis and brain imaging. If secondary epilepsy is suspected, medication in addition to anticonvulsants may be required (e.g. mannitol, steroids, antifungals, antibacterials). Animals with reactive epilepsy require treatment of the underlying metabolic disease.

LOSS OF CONSCIOUSNESS AND COMA

Stupor is a state of depressed consciousness in which the animal is responsive only to strong, often noxious stimuli. Coma is a state of unconsciousness in which the animal is not aroused by even noxious stimuli. Both may result from: severe, bilateral and diffuse dysfunction of the cerebral hemispheres; destructive lesions of the brainstem; compression of the brainstem due to a mass or occipital lobe herniation; or metabolic encephalopathies.

Evaluation of the stuporous or comatose patient

Gait and postural ability are non-existent in stuporous or comatose animals. Segmental reflexes are normal or hyperreflexive.

Cerebral hemispheres/diencephalon

Cranial nerves: Diffuse bilateral disease of the cerebral hemispheres and diencephalon may cause blindness and bilaterally miotic pupils that are responsive to light. No abnormalities of physiological nystagmus are found.

Other: Cheyne–Stokes respiratory pattern may occur. Rhythmic walking movements may be elicited if the animal is supported.

Midbrain

Cranial nerves: The animal may or may not respond to visual testing. Unilateral or bilateral fixed midposition or dilated pupils and abnormal or absent physiological nystagmus may occur. Ipsilateral or bilateral ventrolateral strabismus may occur.

Other: Hyperventilation and/or a decerebrate posture may occur.

Pons/medulla

Signs of pons/medulla dysfunction in addition to midbrain dysfunction provide evidence of multifocal or diffuse brainstem disease. In addition to bilateral fixed midposition pupils, signs of cranial nerve V–XII dysfunction and apnoea may occur.

Causes and treatment of stupor or coma

Diffuse dysfunction of the cerebral hemispheres

Inflammatory diseases, lysosomal storage diseases, metabolic diseases, neoplasia with associated oedema and hydrocephalus can cause signs of diffuse, cerebral hemisphere/diencephalic dysfunction. Treatment is directed at the inciting cause and at decreasing intracranial pressure (see 'Head trauma').

Destructive brainstem disease versus herniation

Destructive disease: Neoplasia and encephalitis of the brainstem may result in an acute or progressive onset of brainstem dysfunction. Chemotherapy, antimicrobials/ antifungals or anti-inflammatories may be required.

Trauma and haemorrhage of the brainstem may result in acute onset of dysfunction. Brainstem haemorrhage is treated by supporting the patient and observing for evidence of improvement.

Herniation: Neoplasia, inflammation (e.g. canine distemper virus, granulomatous meningoencephalitis, feline infectious peritonitis, toxoplasmosis/neosporosis, mycotic diseases) or trauma of the cerebral hemispheres may result in increased intracranial pressure, unilateral or bilateral occipital lobe herniation and brainstem compression. Herniation is often preceded by hours to days of progressive cerebral hemisphere/diencephalon dysfunction including progressive depression of consciousness. Occipital lobe herniation is suspected from the development (over hours to days) of unilateral or bilateral non-responsive dilated or midposition pupils; progressive loss of physiological nystagmus; and alterations in respiratory patterns. Herniation of the cerebellum through the foramen magnum may result in apnoea. Increases in intracranial pressure causing herniation should be treated without delay by the methods discussed in the section 'Head trauma'.

Metabolic causes

Metabolic disease and toxins rarely result in deficits related to discrete lesions of the nervous system. Rather, bilaterally symmetrical deficits that suggest diffuse cerebrocortical dysfunction or diffuse brain disease are usual. Signs are progressive. Evidence of vision is present until stupor is profound or coma occurs. Pupils are responsive and usually of normal diameter but may be bilaterally miotic. Physiological nystagmus is generally present unless profound stupor or coma occurs. Metabolic causes for stupor or coma include: diabetic coma, heat stroke, hepatic encephalopathy, hypo- and hypernatraemia, hypoglycaemia, hypothyroid coma, hypoxia, renal encephalopathy and thiamine deficiency (see 'Abnormal mentation and metabolic encephalopathies'). Toxic causes include heavy metals, ethylene glycol, barbiturates, narcotics, ivermectin and tranquillizers. Intoxication is treated by gastric lavage, activated charcoal, specific antidotes and chelators and by supporting the patient.

A note on vascular causes

Stupor or coma may result from infarction/haemorrhage of the midbrain, or from infarction/haemorrhage in the cerebral hemispheres and diencephalon, resulting in increased intracranial pressure and occipital lobe herniation. Causes of cerebrovascular accidents in animals include metastatic neoplasia, coagulation disorders, cardiac disease, hypertension, parasitic emboli and feline ischaemic encephalopathy. Predisposing vascular disease, so common in humans, is rare in animals. As a consequence, infarction is not common. Infarction is treated by supporting the patient and decreasing intracranial pressure.

ABNORMAL MENTAL STATUS AND METABOLIC ENCEPHALOPATHIES

Metabolic encephalopathies result in bilaterally symmetrical signs of cerebrocortical dysfunction or in signs of diffuse brain disease. Abnormalities of mentation may progress to stupor and coma. History and blood workup are essential in determining that the signs are due to metabolic disease. However, cerebrospinal fluid analysis, titres for infectious disease and brain imaging are frequently necessary to rule out other causes of encephalopathy.

Electrolytes

Calcium

Hypocalcaemia (serum calcium <6.5 mg/dl; ionized calcium <0.6 mmol/l) may cause muscle twitching and spasms, disorientation, restlessness and seizures. Intravenous administration of 10% calcium gluconate (5–15 mg/kg) over 15 minutes, followed by calcium gluconate diluted in saline and given subcutaneously (5–15 mg/kg every 6–8 hours; Feldman, 1995) or 10 mg/kg/h i.v. by continuous rate infusion (CRI) often resolves clinical signs until the specific cause is identified. Hypoglycaemia and hypomagnesaemia may occur concurrently and supplementation may be necessary. Diazepam may be necessary to control seizures.

Hypercalcaemia (>12.0 mg/dl) may cause muscle weakness, seizures, depression, stupor or coma. Diuresis with 0.9% NaCl i.v. and frusemide may be performed until the cause is determined.

Sodium

Severe *hyponatraemia* (Na^+ <120 mEq/l) may cause disorientation, seizures, stupor or coma. Ideally, sodium is supplemented at the rate at which it was lost. Rapid correction of chronic hyponatraemia (>10 mmol/l/day) may cause weakness, hypermetria, ataxia and myoclonic jerking of the limbs 3–5 days after treatment (O'Brien *et al.*, 1994).

If *hypernatraemia* (Na^+ >170 mEq/l) occurs acutely, restlessness, irritability, seizures, stupor and coma may occur. If hypernatraemia is chronic, only depression and disorientation may be noted. Chronic hypernatraemia must be treated slowly (over 2–3 days) to avoid cerebral oedema.

Glucose

Hypoglycaemia (blood glucose <45 mg/dl) may cause weakness, muscle tremors, blindness, seizures, stupor or coma. Intravenous administration of 0.5 g/kg of 10–25% dextrose solution may be given until signs resolve. Intramuscular thiamine (25–50 mg) should be administered prior to giving dextrose, as thiamine is a co-enzyme necessary for glucose utilization by the brain. Anticonvulsants may be necessary to control seizures. When an insulin-secreting tumour is present, dextrose (by CRI), diazoxide (10 mg/kg every 12 hours) and prednisolone (0.5 mg/kg/day) are often necessary to maintain serum glucose concentrations.

Hyperglycaemia and hyperosmolality (>340 mOsm/l) may cause stupor and coma. Sodium chloride 0.45–0.9% i.v. and insulin may be given to correct hyperglycaemia over 24–36 hours in order to prevent cerebral oedema. Potassium supplementation should be provided.

Heat stroke

A body temperature of >41°C may result in blindness, ataxia, disorientation, stupor or coma. Cooling and hydrating the patient and correcting acidosis, hypernatraemia, hypokalaemia, hypophosphataemia and hypocalcaemia are recommended. If neurological dysfunction progresses, increased intracranial pressure may be present (see 'Head trauma' for treatment).

Hepatic encephalopathy

Disorientation, pacing, blindness and circling often develop with hepatic encephalopathy; seizures, stupor or coma occur less often. Treatment is directed at decreasing the intake and absorption of protein-derived toxins from the large intestine (Bunch, 1995). Warm-water cleansing enemas and lactulose enemas retained for 20 minutes (20 ml/kg of 3 parts lactulose to 7 parts water) may be given every 4–6 hours. Neomycin sulphate (22 mg/kg orally every 8 hours) and metronidazole (7.5 mg/kg orally every 8 hours) may be administered to decrease the bacterial load. Serum glucose and potassium concentrations should be monitored and deficits corrected. Hydration should be maintained and gastrointestinal bleeding must be controlled.

Seizures occasionally occur after surgery for portosystemic shunt ligation. These seizures are notoriously difficult to control with phenobarbital or diazepam. Potassium bromide or propofol may be more effective, although data are lacking.

Hypoadrenocorticism

Depression, lethargy, weakness and shock may occur. Depending on the severity of signs, intravenous 0.9% saline, dexamethasone sodium phosphate (0.5–2.0 mg/kg), dextrose and/or sodium bicarbonate may be necessary.

Hypoxia and ischaemia

Changes in mental status, blindness and ataxia may occur with PO_2 <55 mmHg. Treatment includes providing supplemental oxygen, treating the underlying cause of the hypoxia and providing mannitol to decrease cerebral oedema. Blindness and changes in mental status will often resolve over weeks but may be permanent.

Lead poisoning

Whole blood lead concentrations >40 µg/dl may result in dementia, seizures and running fits in addition to gastrointestinal signs. Chelation therapy with EDTA, D-penicillamine, or succimer (10 mg/kg orally every 8 hours for 10 days; Ramsey et al., 1996) are specific therapies for intoxication.

Thyroid hormone

Hypothyroidism may result in depression, disorientation, stupor or coma most commonly in the Dobermann Pinscher. Serum cholesterol concentrations of >1000 mg/dl may occur. Abnormalities are reversible with thyroid supplementation. Respiratory support, glucocorticoids and intravenous L-thyroxine may be necessary in cases of coma (Kelly, 1989).

Hyperthyroidism may cause restlessness, hyperexcitability, circling and seizures. Rarely, lethargy may occur. Treatment with methimazole resolves these signs.

Renal encephalopathy

Acute renal failure may result in seizures. Chronic renal failure more commonly causes mental dullness, weakness, muscle twitching and myoclonus. Treatment is aimed at monitoring blood pressure and maintaining hydration, acid–base status and electrolyte concentrations.

Thiamine deficiency

This is usually caused by a deficiency of dietary thiamine, through cooked food or a diet high in fish containing thiaminase. Clinical signs include signs of central vestibular disease, ataxia, ventroflexion of the head and neck, bilaterally dilated fixed pupils, and seizures, stupor and coma. Thiamine hydrochloride (25–50 mg i.v.) is used to treat signs and repeated intramuscularly daily until improvement is noted.

HEAD TRAUMA

An overall assessment of the patient must be performed, paying specific attention to ensuring a patent airway, providing respiratory support if necessary and maintaining cardiovascular function. Ideally, the initial assessment should be performed on a board or firm table where the neck and back can be stabilized and assessed for fractures or luxations. Manipulation for radiography of any suspicious areas should be done with care. The nasal cavity, ear canals and nasopharyngeal region should be examined for haemorrhage, which may imply a skull fracture with the possibility of entry of bacteria into the brain. The jugular vein should not be used to collect blood since, even temporary occlusion may increase intracranial pressure (ICP).

Neurological assessment

In general, trauma to the cerebral hemispheres causes less severe neurological dysfunction and a better prognosis than trauma to the brainstem. Trauma to the cerebellum alone is uncommon. The progression of clinical signs over time plays a large role in determining prognosis. Deterioration of mental status may indicate increasing ICP and the possibility of impending brain herniation. Immediate therapeutic intervention is necessary. Prolonged stupor or coma suggests severe brainstem disease and indicates a poor prognosis. In general, pupillary abnormalities which become normal over time are a good prognostic sign; pupils which change to mydriasis or to midposition and are unresponsive to light are poor prognostic signs indicating oedema, herniation and compression of the brainstem warranting more aggressive intervention. Progressive alterations in breathing patterns, increases in mean arterial blood pressure and bradycardia may indicate increases in ICP requiring immediate therapy.

Treatment

The objective of management is to prevent the brain from undergoing any further insult due to ischaemia, inflammatory mediators or the effects of increased ICP. The authors recommend the following treatments in the care of the closed head trauma patient (Bagley, 1995).

Elevate the body at a 30° angle above heart level

The patient may be placed on a solid board and the board elevated at a 30° angle. Make sure no blankets compress the jugular veins thus decreasing venous drainage.

Hyperventilation

Hyperventilation can rapidly decrease ICP. Recent studies, however, have revealed that its use may be contraindicated (Obrist *et al.* 1984; Muizelaar *et al.* 1991; Fortune *et al.* 1995; Skippe *et al.* 1997) After cranial trauma, oxygen extraction is maximal and blood flow is limiting (oligaemia). Assisted ventilation is recommended to preserve oxygenation, but $PaCO_2$ (as determined by blood gas analysis, or inferred from capnography) should be maintained within normal limits. If the patient is not stuporous and is stable, supplemental oxygen, in the form of nasal oxygenation or via an oxygen cage may be provided.

Maintain perfusion

Hypotension, hypoxia and hypertension must be avoided. Fluid therapy should be used to maintain mean arterial pressure between 70 and 110 mmHg. Hypotension due to peripheral vasodilation may be treated with 10 mg of phenylephrine placed in 250 ml of saline and titrated to effect. Hypertension due to excitement and pain may be addressed with sedation or analgesics. Rarely, a comatose animal may present with hypertension and bradycardia due to increased ICP; treatment should be aimed at decreasing ICP.

Frusemide and mannitol

Frusemide (1–4 mg/kg i.v.) may be given as a bolus prior to administering mannitol to prevent an initial rise in ICP associated with mannitol administration. Frusemide should be avoided in hypovolaemic patients. Mannitol can rapidly decrease ICP. Its effect is greatest 30–60 minutes after administration and its effects last 2–4 hours. A dose of 0.5–1 g/kg of a 25% solution over 20 minutes can be repeated every 3–8 hours with a maximum of three doses over a 24-hour period. Mannitol is contraindicated in shock, hypotension, dehydration, congestive heart failure, anuric renal failure and pulmonary oedema. Serum electrolytes and osmolality should be monitored.

Steroids

Although steroids are frequently used to treat head trauma, there is little evidence to support their efficacy. A dose of 30 mg/kg of methylprednisolone sodium succinate, followed by 15 mg/kg, 2 and 6 hours after the first dose, followed by a CRI of 2.5 mg/kg/h for the next 2 days has been recommended.

Craniotomy

Craniotomy produces a rapid decrease in ICP and may be performed when managing skull fractures with displacement of bone more than the thickness of the calvarium in the fractured area, to remove projectiles or to treat progressive increases in ICP refractory to medical management. In the future, the routine availability of ICP monitoring and computerized tomography may aid in determining when craniotomy is necessary.

Anaesthetic concerns

Drugs that do not increase ICP or cause large changes in blood pressure should be used in cases of head trauma. Premedication may be limited to use of an intravenous benzodiazepine immediately prior to induction. This minimizes the required dose of induction agents and their cardiovascular effects. Opioids do not increase ICP unless there is associated respiratory depression. Lignocaine (2 mg/kg i.v.) may be given for its antitussive effect immediately after induction. Isoflurane is the maintenance agent of choice as cerebral autoregulation of vascular tone is preserved if inspired concentration is < 1.5 x MAC. Where this is insufficient, supplemental agents such as fentanyl or propofol should be used. $ETCO_2$ monitoring (or blood gas analysis) coupled with IPPV is important to maintain arterial CO_2 levels within normal limits of 35–45 mmHg. Hyper- or hypoventilation must be avoided.

Sedation

Frequently, trauma-related pain or agitation may result in the patient flailing around the cage or constantly vocalizing. Both behaviours may increase ICP. Diazepam (0.2–0.5 mg/kg) or phenobarbitone (5 mg/kg) may be used to sedate the patient, and butorphanol (0.2–0.4 mg/kg) to reduce pain. In the rare instance, when neither of these results in a calm patient, small doses of acepromazine (0.01–0.02 mg/kg i.v.) may be given. In these instances, the possibility of seizure induction may increase and the patient should be carefully observed.

ACUTE VESTIBULAR OR CEREBELLAR SIGNS

Signs of vestibular system dysfunction which occur regardless of lesion location include:

- Loss of balance
- Ataxia characterized by regularly falling toward the

side of the lesion
- Abnormal posture characterized by: leaning; turning of the head, neck and body; and/or rolling toward the side of the lesion
- Head tilted toward the side of the lesion. A head tilt exists when an imagined horizontal line running through both ears is tilted from the horizontal plane
- Ventral strabismus of the eye on the side of the lesion. The strabismus may not be noted until the head is elevated or returned to the horizontal plane
- Abnormal nystagmus with the slow phase directed toward the side of the lesion.

Blindfolding the animal may accentuate the ataxia, lifting the animal off the ground may increase the head tilt and rolling, and placing the animal on its back may induce nystagmus.

A common mistake is attributing compulsive circling (associated with disease of the cerebral hemispheres and diencephalon) to disease of the vestibular system. With compulsive circling there is no ataxia, no loss of balance and no abnormal nystagmus.

Localizing signs of vestibular system dysfunction

Vestibular system dysfunction may result from disease of the inner ear, medulla or cerebellum. The location of the lesion may be determined by the presence of neurological deficits in addition to those listed above.

Inner ear

Disease of the inner ear alone results in only the signs listed above. Auditory dysfunction is rarely recognized. The direction of the nystagmus is usually horizontal or rotary and is unchanged when the position of the head is altered. If the middle ear is also affected, signs of cranial nerve VII dysfunction and a Horner's syndrome may result. No postural reaction deficits occur.

Medulla/cerebellum

Disease of the medulla may cause changes in mental status. Hemiparesis and postural reaction deficits and dysfunction of cranial nerves V–XII may occur ipsilateral to the side of the lesion. The direction of the nystagmus may be horizontal, rotary or vertical and may change when the position of the head is altered.

Disease of the cerebellum may cause dysmetria and menace deficits ipsilateral to the side of the lesion, and head and neck tremors.

Exceptions to rules of localization

Bilateral peripheral vestibular disease may result in a wide-based stance and swaying of the body. Often, no nystagmus or strabismus is noted. The animal is severely off balance and ataxic when blindfolded or when lifted off the ground.

Disease of the cerebellum and medulla occasionally result in head tilt, strabismus and slow phase of the nystagmus directed away from the side of the lesion (paradoxical vestibular syndrome). The postural reaction deficits are ipsilateral to the side of the lesion.

Causes and management of diseases of the vestibular system

Inner ear

Otitis interna/media: Images of the osseous bullae and/or deep otic examination may confirm middle ear disease. Treatment with cephalosporins, enrofloxacin, or trimethoprim–sulphadiazine ± bulla osteotomy are recommended.

Idiopathic labyrinthitis: Older dogs and cats of any age may be affected. CN VII dysfunction and Horner's syndrome do not occur. No abnormalities are found in blood, images of the bullae, deep otic examination, or thyroid testing. Antibiotics are recommended but may not be necessary. Spontaneous recovery is common.

Other causes: Polyneuropathy, tumours and trauma involving the inner ear may result in vestibular system dysfunction. Hypothyroidism may be associated with polyneuropathy, and occasionally vestibular signs resolve only after the institution of thyroid hormone supplementation. Aminoglycosides at high doses may result in deafness and signs of peripheral vestibular dysfunction. In general, these animals are treated with antibiotics until a definitive diagnosis is made.

Medulla/cerebellum
- Canine distemper virus, *Toxoplasma*, *Neospora*, *Cryptococcus neoformans*, granulomatous meningoencephalomyelitis, feline infectious peritonitis, parasitic migration and other meningoencephalidites may result in vestibular system dysfunction
- Neoplasia may be suspected on the basis of cerebrospinal fluid abnormalities and images of the brain
- Metronidazole intoxication at doses greater than 30 mg/kg frequently results in an acute onset of vestibular system dysfunction with vertical nystagmus and, occasionally, seizures. Supportive care, requiring a week or more of hospitalization, results in recovery, although months may be required before all signs resolve
- Thiamine deficiency may result in vestibular system dysfunction. Intramuscular thiamine hydrochloride (25–50 mg i.m., continued until signs improve) can resolve the signs
- Infarction of the medulla or cerebellum may be suspected on the basis of cerebrospinal fluid abnormalities and images of the brain.

HINDLIMB PARESIS AND PARALYSIS

Hindlimb paresis and paralysis may result from a lesion between the third thoracic spinal cord segment and the first sacral spinal cord segment, as well as from diseases of peripheral nerve, muscle and neuromuscular junction.

Causes and management of diseases of the spinal cord

Intervertebral disc disease

An acute onset of neurological dysfunction and/or pain on palpation over the affected area may occur. Intervertebral disc protrusion/herniation may be confirmed by myelography, computerized tomography or magnetic resonance imaging. Animals with pain and mild ataxia/paraparesis may be treated with strict cage confinement for 4 weeks and prednisone (0.5 mg/kg orally every 12 hours for 3 days; 0.5 mg/kg every 48 hours for three doses). Animals with moderate paraparesis or paraplegia may be treated with methylprednisolone sodium succinate within 8 hours of the onset of signs (30 mg/kg i.v.; then 15 mg/kg at 2 and 6 hours; then 2.5 mg/kg/h for 24–48 hours) and decompressive surgery performed within 24 hours of the onset of signs. Medical management without surgical intervention may result in a longer recovery time and recurrence of clinical signs. Animals with anaesthesia caudal to the site of the lesion have a poor prognosis for recovery.

Neoplasia

Neoplasia may result in a gradual or sudden onset of clinical signs. Imaging modalities confirm the presence and location of the mass. Cerebrospinal fluid rarely contains neoplastic cells; however, examination of spinal fluid may raise suspicion of inflammatory disease. Biopsy yields a definitive diagnosis. Cats with lymphosarcoma of the spinal cord frequently have multicentric disease, are frequently FeLV positive, and often have lymphoblastic leukaemia on bone marrow aspiration (Spodnick et al., 1992). Signs due to spinal cord compression may respond to steroids ± decompressive surgery. Cage rest is recommended for neoplasia that causes vertebral body lysis.

Discospondylitis

Fever, depression and pain over the affected area are common. Radiographs or bone scans may reveal lysis of the vertebral endplates; however, no abnormalities may be found early in the course of the disease. Culture of urine, blood or the affected disc may identify the causative organism. Treatment involves cage rest and antibiotics (cephalosporins, oxacillin, cloxacillin or tetracycline) for at least 6–8 weeks.

Distemper, feline infectious peritonitis, mycotic/bacterial/protozoal myelitis

Diagnosis is aided by signs of systemic disease, results of titres and cerebrospinal fluid analysis. For viral infections, steroids may be temporarily palliative. Toxoplasmosis/neosporosis may be treated with clindamycin and trimethoprim–sulphadiazine (see below).

Granulomatous meningoencephalomyelitis

Cerebrospinal fluid analysis may show increases in protein, mononuclear cells and non-degenerate neutrophils. Myelography may reveal an intradural/ extramedullary or intramedullary lesion. Definitive diagnosis requires biopsy. Prednisone (1 mg/kg every 12 hours for 5 days; then 1 mg/kg every 24 hours for 7 days; then 1 mg/kg every 48 hours) may result in improvement in neurological signs but recurrence is common. Radiation therapy may result in rapid improvement.

Trauma

Trauma, with or without vertebral body fracture or dislocation, may result in clinical signs. Plain radiography or myelography must be performed with extreme caution if vertebral instability is suspected. Treatment involves cage rest, methylprednisolone sodium succinate within 8 hours of the onset of signs (30 mg/kg i.v.; then 15 mg/kg at 2 and 6 hours; then 2.5 mg/kg/h for 24–48 hours), and surgical decompression and stabilization if marked spinal cord compression or vertebral column instability is present. An external splint applied from the scapulae to the base of the tail may be used to limit motion of the spinal column in cases of vertebral body fracture.

Fibrocartilaginous emboli

Signs in dogs commonly begin during a period of exercise; mild transient pain may be noted. Signs may progress over the first 12 hours and then stabilize. Hemiparesis/paralysis may occur. Myelography may reveal intramedullary swelling or may be normal. Methylprednisolone sodium succinate (30 mg/kg i.v.; then 15 mg/kg at 2 and 6 hours; then 2.5 mg/kg/h for 24–48 hours) may be given within 8 hours of the onset of signs. Supportive care should be provided. Severity of signs and prognosis vary with the extent of the cord infarct. Recovery may take months and may be imcomplete.

Diseases of peripheral nerve, muscle and neuromuscular junction

Toxoplasmosis/neosporosis

In puppies, flaccid paralysis progressing to increased extensor tone of the hindlimbs of such a degree that the joints no longer bend can occur. Evidence of systemic disease may be recognized. Increased antibody titres occur. Trimethoprim–sulphadiazine (15 mg/kg every 12 hours for 2 weeks) and clindamycin (10 mg/kg every 12 hours for 8 weeks) may result in improvement of clinical signs, however, once hind limb rigidity has developed, improvement will not occur with therapy.

Aortic thromboembolism

Animals are in pain, limbs are cool, pulses are weak or absent, and muscles are firm. Abdominal ultrasonography may identify a thrombus in the aorta. Analgesics, intravenous fluids, heparin, acepromazine and aspirin may be given. Thromboembolism has been associated with cardiomyopathy in cats, and with protein-losing nephropathy in dogs.

Others

Hypoadrenocorticism and diabetes mellitus may cause rear limb paresis in addition to signs of metabolic disease. Diabetic cats may have a plantigrade stance. Control of metabolic disease commonly results in resolution of neurological dysfunction. Early polyneuropathy and myasthenia gravis may each result in signs of rear limb paresis (see 'Episodic weakness').

TETRAPARESIS AND PARALYSIS

Tetraparesis and paralysis may result from peripheral nerve/muscle, cervical spinal cord and/or brain stem disease. Differentiating peripheral nerve and muscle disease from spinal cord and brainstem disease is essential to making the correct diagnosis (see Figure 7.1).

Peripheral nerve/muscle

Botulism

Signs of flaccid paralysis and hyporeflexia occur in dogs hours to days after ingesting pre-formed toxin. Cranial nerve deficits include decreased ability: to blink the eyelids; to lift the upper lip; to close the mouth; and to lap water or swallow. Change in bark, regurgitation, megaoesophagus, decreased perineal reflex, faecal and urinary incontinence, and respiratory paralysis may occur. Botulism is suspected from history, clinical signs and electrodiagnostic testing (decreased compound motor action potential following nerve stimulation). Toxin may be identified in food, serum, stomach contents or faeces early in the course of the disease. Supportive care is given, a gastrostomy tube is placed if needed, and the animal is monitored for aspiration pneumonia and respiratory paralysis. Signs may resolve with supportive care within 2–3 weeks.

Acute polyradiculoneuritis and polyneuritis

Affected dogs may have been recently vaccinated or have a history of exposure to racoons, or neither. Flaccid paralysis and hyporeflexia occur. Facial muscle paresis and a change in bark are common. Respiratory paralysis may occur. Interestingly, however, tail and neck motion, swallowing and faecal and urinary continence are often maintained. The animal may be hyperaesthetic to touch. Cerebrospinal fluid analysis may show an increase in protein; electromyography may show fibrillation potentials and positive sharp waves in the majority of muscles tested; nerve conduction velocity is slow and evoked potentials may be decreased in amplitude. Biopsy of nerve root or nerve may show inflammatory cell infiltrates, demyelination and axonal loss. Prednisone (1 mg/kg prednisone every 12 hours for 1–2 weeks; then 1 mg/kg prednisone every 24 hours for 1 month) may be given; however, there is controversy as to whether it has any effect on the progression of this disease. Supportive care to prevent and treat decubital ulcers and urinary tract infections and observation for respiratory muscle paresis should be performed. Recovery may take 6–8 weeks and may be incomplete. Signs may recur.

Tick paralysis

Affected dogs have a female tick attached. Flaccid paralysis and hyporeflexia occur. Nystagmus, change in voice, dysphagia, weakness of facial muscles and masticatory muscles, and respiratory paralysis may occur. Electrodiagnostic testing may show reduction in amplitude or absence of the compound motor action potential following nerve stimulation and a slow nerve conduction velocity. Removal of ticks results in resolution of clinical signs within 24–72 hours. This disease is reported in the US and a more severe form occurs in Australia.

Insulin-secreting tumours

Serum glucose concentration of <50 mg/dl may result in clinical signs. Flaccid paralysis, hyporeflexia, lethargy, bradycardia, muscle tremors, hypothermia, disorientation and seizures may occur. Electromyographic examination may show fibrillation potentials, positive sharp waves and complex repetitive discharges. Small quantities of food high in protein, fat and complex carbohydrates may be provided frequently. Diazoxide (10 mg/kg every 12 hours) and prednisone (0.5 mg/kg/day) may be given.

Cervical cord disease and/or brainstem caudal to the thalamus

Intervertebral disc disease, neoplasia, discospondylitis, myelitis, granulomatous meningoencephalitis, trauma and fibrocartilagenous emboli (see 'Hindlimb paresis and paralysis', above).

Atlantoaxial subluxation

Neck pain and signs attributable to disease of cervical spinal cord segments 1–5 may occur in young small breed dogs. Flexing the neck may result in pain, worsening of clinical signs and respiratory paralysis. Survey radiographs may show the subluxation of the first and second cervical vertebrae ± abnormalities of the dens. Cage rest, steroids ± a neck brace may result in improvement. Surgical stabilization may ultimately be required.

Caudal cervical spondylomyelopathy ('Wobblers')

Most common in young Great Danes and in middle aged Dobermann Pinschers. Signs of disease attributable to cervical spinal cord segment 6 to thoracic cord segment 2 are most common. Cord compression and instability is confirmed with myelography. Flexed, extended and traction views of the neck are useful. In the emergency situation, these animals may be treated in a manner similar to animals with intervertebral disc disease. Without surgery, many dogs will eventually show a progression of clinical signs.

Steroid-responsive meningitis

Signs of neck pain, fever, lethargy and neurological deficits attributable to disease of cervical spinal cord segments 1–5 may occur in young dogs. CSF analysis reveals marked increases in protein and in white blood cells, with non-degenerate neutrophils the most common cell type. Culture of the CSF is negative. Treatment with glucocorticoids (1 mg/kg prednisone every 12 hours for 3 days and then decreased over time to a dose necessary to control signs) is required for 2–4 weeks; relapse of clinical signs is common.

EPISODIC WEAKNESS/SYNCOPE

Episodic weakness and collapse may occur due to neuromuscular or brain disease, syncope, or metabolic disorders.

Neuromuscular disorders

Acquired myasthenia gravis

At least three clinical presentations may occur (Dewey *et al.*, 1997):

- Focal myasthenia gravis. Animals exhibit facial, pharyngeal and/or laryngeal muscle dysfunction without appendicular muscle involvement. Megaoesophagus, regurgitation and aspiration pneumonia may occur
- Generalized myasthenia gravis. Animals exhibit appendicular muscle weakness with a stiff, short-strided gait with or without signs of facial, pharyngeal and/or laryngeal muscle dysfunction. Strength may or may not return following periods of rest
- Acute fulminating myasthenia gravis. Signs include: a sudden, rapid progression of severe appendicular muscle weakness, resulting in recumbancy which is unabated by rest; frequent regurgitation associated with megaoesophagus; respiratory difficulty; and facial, pharyngeal and/or laryngeal muscle dysfunction.

Diagnosis: Blood acetylcholine receptor antibody concentrations may be elevated (>0.6 nM/l in dogs and >0.3 nM/l in cats).

Edrophonium (0.1–0.2 mg/kg i.v.) may result in dramatic improvement in gait for 1–2 minutes. Pretreatment with atropine (0.02 mg/kg i.v.) is recommended.

Compound action potentials recorded from the interosseous muscle may show a 10% or greater decremental response following repetitive stimulation (Hopkins, 1992).

Treatment: Oral pyridostigmine (0.2–2.0 mg/kg every 8–12 hours) is given; alternatively, to animals with significant dysphagia and regurgitation, intramuscular neostigmine is given (0.04 mg/kg every 6–8 hours). Animals should be kept warm and exercise restricted. Animals with dysphagia and megaesophagus should be fed from a height with the head and neck elevated for 10 minutes after eating. Aminoglycoside antibiotics should be avoided due to the possibility of neuromuscular blockade. Prednisone may result in a rapid worsening of clinical signs and its use is contraindicated in the presence of aspiration pneumonia. However, in the authors' experience, prednisone may improve pharyngeal dysfunction sooner than cholinesterase inhibitors alone. A starting dose of 0.5 mg/kg/day increased to 2 mg/kg/day over 1 week has been suggested when aspiration pneumonia is not present (Le Couteur, 1988).

Exertional rhabdomyolysis

Racing Greyhounds may present with scuffing of the nails of the hindlimbs, muscle pain, tachypnoea, collapse and hyperthermia within 72 hours of exercise. Increased creatine kinase, lactate dehydrogenase, aspartate aminotransferase, blood lactate and myoglobin may occur. Renal failure may also occur. Intravenous fluids to treat shock and to aid in the excretion of myoglobin, cold water baths, pain medication and intravenous bicarbonate may be given.

Polymyositis

Dogs and cats of any age may present with generalized weakness which worsens with exercise. The gait is stiff and short-strided and dysphagia, regurgitation, megaoesophagus, change in bark, painful appendicular muscles, fever and lethargy may occur. Increases in creatine kinase, aspartate aminotransferase, lactate dehydrogenase and antinuclear antibody may occur. Electromyography may reveal fibrillation potentials, positive sharp waves and bizarre high frequency discharges. Muscle biopsy reveals lymphoplasmacytic inflammation and muscle necrosis. Toxoplasmosis and neosporosis should be ruled out with titres and muscle biopsy. Prednisone may be given (1 mg/kg twice daily initially) and reduced to the lowest dose necessary to control signs. Pharyngeal and oesophageal muscle involvement may result in aspiration pneumonia.

Brain disease

Narcolepsy/cataplexy

Episodes last seconds to minutes and are marked by acute collapse, decreased muscle tone and rapid eye movement sleep. Episodes may be provoked by excitement, food, or physostigmine (0.025–0.1 mg/kg i.v.). Minimizing excitement and imipramine hydrochloride (0.5–1 mg/kg orally every 8 hours) may decrease the number of events.

Syncope

Cardiovascular disease

Episodic weakness, ataxia, lethargy, dyspnoea and syncope may occur. Evidence of a heart murmur, irregular heart rate or rhythm, bradycardia or tachycardia, weak or irregular pulses, polycythaemia, heartworm infection and electrocardiographic abnormalities between or during events suggest cardiovascular disease as the cause.

Respiratory disease

Hypoxia, particularly if chronic, may result in syncope.

Metabolic disorders

Hyperthyroidism

Episodic weakness, decreased ability to jump, muscle tremors and ventroflexion of the neck may occur in addition to other signs of hyperthyroidism (Joseph and Peterson, 1992). Post-insertional trains of positive sharp waves are reported on electromyographic examination. Stress should be decreased and methimazole begun (10–15 mg/day divided every 12 hours).

Hypoadrenocorticism

Episodic weakness, stiff, stilted hindlimb gait, muscle tremors, vomiting, anorexia, weight loss, dehydration, weak pulses and shock may occur. Intestinal parasites (whipworms in particular) may cause clinical signs mimicking those of an Addisonian crisis. Stress should be decreased; i.v. fluid support with 0.9% sodium chloride provided; and hypoglycaemia treated. Dexamethasone sodium phosphate (0.5–2.0 mg/kg i.v.) may be given until the diagnosis is confirmed.

Hyperkalaemia

Appendicular and neck muscle weakness, bradycardia, arrhythmias, weak pulses, electrocardiographic abnormalities and hyporeflexia may occur when serum potassium is >6.5 mEq/l. Weakness resolves with treatment of hyperkalaemia.

Hypokalaemic myopathy

Ventroflexion of the neck, a stiff, short-strided gait, episodic weakness, pain on muscle palpation and respiratory muscle paresis/paralysis may occur. A serum potassium <3.5 mEq/l, increased creatine kinase, azotaemia and metabolic acidosis may be found. Electromyographic examination may reveal fibrillation potentials and positive sharp waves. Mildly or moderately affected cats may be treated with oral potassium supplementation (5–8 mEq potassium every 12–24 hours). Intravenous potassium infusion (CRI <0.5 mEq/kg/h) may be given to those with severe weakness and respiratory depression. Occasionally, hypomagnesaemia may accompany hypokalaemia and exacerbate the weakness. Weakness resolves with treatment of hypokalaemia and, if present, hypomagnesaemia.

Others

Other diseases which may present with episodic weakness include mitochondrial myopathy of Clumber and Sussex Spaniels and Old English Sheepdogs; phosphofructokinase deficiency of English Springer Spaniels; panosteitis; hypertrophic osteodystrophy; polyarthritis; anaphylactic reactions; and the presence of a phaeochromocytoma. A good history is necessary to rule out epileptic activity as a cause for paroxysmal collapse.

REFERENCES AND FURTHER READING

Braund KG (1994) *Clinical Syndromes in Veterinary Neurology, 2nd edn.* Mosby, St Louis

Bunch SE (1995) Specific and symptomatic medical management of diseases of the liver. In: *Textbook of Veterinary Internal Medicine, 4th edn*, ed. SJ Ettinger and EC Feldman, pp. 1358–1371. WB Saunders, Phildelphia

de Lahunta A (1983) *Veterinary Neuroanatomy and Clinical Neurology, 2nd edn.* WB Saunders, Philadelphia

Dewey CW *et al.* (1997) Clinical forms of acquired myasthenia gravis in dogs: 25 cases (1988–1995). *Journal of Veterinary Internal Medicine* **11**, 50–57.Feldman EC (1995) Disorders of the parathyroid glands. In: *Textbook of Veterinary Internal Medicine, 4th edn*, ed. SJ Ettinger and EC Feldman, pp. 1462–1463. WB Saunders, Phildelphia

Fortune JB, Feustel PJ *et al.* (1995) Cerebral blood flow and blood volume in response to O_2 and CO_2 changes in normal humans. *Journal of Trauma* **39**, 463–471

Hopkins AL (1992) Canine myasthenia gravis. *Journal of Small Animal Practice* **33**, 477–484.

Joseph RJ and Peterson ME (1992) Review and comparison of neuromuscular and central nervous system manifestations of hyperthyroidism in cats and humans. *Progress in Veterinary Neurology* **3**, 114–119

Kelly MJ (1989) Canine myxoedema stupor and coma. In: *Current Veterinary Therapy X: Small Animal Practice*, ed. RW Kirk and JD Bonagura, pp. 998–1001

Le Couteur RA (1988) Disorders of peripheral nerves. In: *Handbook of Small Animal Practice*, ed. RV Morgan, pp. 299–318. Churchill Livingstone, New York.

Muizelaar JP, Marmarou A *et al.* (1991) Adverse effects of prolonged hyperventilation in patients with severe head injury: a randomized clinical trial. *Journal of Neurosurgery* **75**, 731–739

O'Brien DP *et al.* (1994) Myelinolysis after correction of hyponatraemia in two dogs. *Journal of Veterinary Internal Medicine* **8**, 40–48.

Oliver JE *et al.* (1997) *Handbook of Veterinary Neurologic Diagnosis.* WB Saunders, Philadelphia

Obrist WD, Langfitt TW *et al.* (1984) Cerebral blood flow and metabolism in comatose patients with acute head injury. Relationship to intracranial hypertension. *Journal of Neurosurgery* **61**, 241–53

Podell M *et al.* (1995) Seizure classification in dogs from a nonreferral-based population. *Journal of the American Veterinary Medical Association* **206**, 1721–1728.

Ramsey *et al.* (1996) Use of orally administered succimer (meso-2,3-dimercaptosuccinic acid) for treatment of lead poisoning in dogs. *Journal of the American Veterinary Medical Association* **208**, 371–375

Skippen P, Seear M *et al.* (1997) Effect of hyperventilation on regional cerebral blood flow in head-injured children. *Critical Care Medicine* **25**, 1402–1409

Spodnick GJ *et al.* (1992) Spinal lymphoma in cats: 21 cases (1976–1989). *Journal of the American Veterinary Medical Association* **200**, 373–376

Wheeler *et al.* (1994) *Small Animal Spinal Disorders: Diagnosis and Surgery*. Mosby-Wolfe, London

CHAPTER EIGHT

Ophthalmological Emergencies

Deborah C. Mandell

INTRODUCTION

Ocular emergencies can be intimidating and frustrating for veterinary surgeons. While most general practitioners do not have the equipment to perform thorough and detailed ophthalmic examinations or surgery (i.e. slit lamps, operating microscopes), the majority of ophthalmological emergencies can be treated successfully with the basic equipment available to every veterinary surgeon. This chapter discusses the diagnosis, treatment and prognosis of common ophthalmological emergencies. When a disease is not responding to treatment or where there are conflicting disease processes in the same eye, an ophthalmologist should always be consulted.

GLAUCOMA

Definition and causes

Glaucoma is an increase in intraocular pressure. The causes are listed in Figure 8.1. Owners should be warned that glaucoma is usually a bilateral disease even if animals present with unilateral signs. Long-term medical therapy should be started in both eyes after stabilization of the acute stage.

Clinical signs

Clinical signs include buphthalmos (Figure 8.2), scleral injection, dilated pupil, negative menace response, absent pupillary light reflex, corneal oedema, pain and

Primary
Primary open angle
Primary closed angle (goniodysgenesis)

Secondary
Uveitis*
Lens luxation*
Neoplasia*
Hyphaema
Cataracts — due to lens-induced uveitis or swelling of the lens

Figure 8.1: *Causes of glaucoma. *Most common causes of glaucoma in cats.*

possible decreased retinal vascularity. Commonly affected breeds include Cocker Spaniels, Poodles, Basset Hounds, Beagles and Samoyeds.

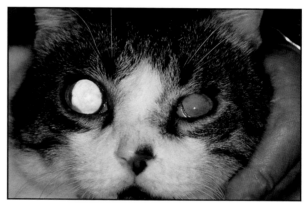

Figure 8.2: *Glaucoma in a cat (right eye). Notice the buphthalmos and dilated pupil. Uveitis is present in the left eye. The cat presented for a 2-day history of blindness.*

Diagnosis

The intraocular pressure (IOP) should be measured via a Shiotz or electronic tonometer. If using a Shiotz tonometer, it is important to keep the cornea parallel to the floor to obtain an accurate reading. Normal IOP is 15–25 mmHg. If the IOP is greater than 35 mmHg, emergency treatment should be initiated.

One of the differential diagnoses of a dilated pupil with acute blindness is sudden acquired retinal degeneration syndrome (SARDS), in which the ocular examination and IOP will be normal. SARDS is usually bilateral and can present with concurrent signs such as polyuria, polydipsia and polyphagia. The cause is unknown and there is no treatment.

Treatment

The treatment for glaucoma consists of lowering the IOP by medically drawing fluid out of the vitreous chamber, by increasing drainage and by decreasing aqueous production. Emergency treatment includes mannitol and pilocarpine. Mannitol, an osmotic diuretic that draws water from the vitreous into the vasculature, is given at a dose of 1 g/kg i.v. over 20–30 minutes. This can lower the IOP within 1 hour. The dose can be repeated in 4 hours if the IOP does not decrease below 30 mmHg. The main side effect of mannitol is dehydration from the osmotic diuresis, thus it should not be given to patients in which dehydration could result in serious adverse consequences, for example animals with renal insufficiency. Pilocarpine drops (2%) should be instilled every 15–60 minutes for 3–4 hours. Pilocarpine acts as a parasympathomimetic, constricting the pupil and thus opening the drainage angle. Side effects such as bradycardia are usually not seen.

Chronic medical therapy for glaucoma should be started. This can include a carbonic anhydrase inhibitor (CAI) which decreases the volume of aqueous fluid produced. Side effects of CAIs, including anorexia, nausea, vomiting and CNS sedation, occur less frequently with the newer CAIs such as dichlorphenamide. Timolol maleate (0.25–0.5% twice a day), a topical ß-blocker, can be used concurrently to further decrease the amount of aqueous production.

When glaucoma is secondary to another disease, the underlying disease such as lens luxation or uveitis must also be treated. Because long-term management is required, an ophthalmologist should be consulted. The IOP should be remeasured every 4–6 months, and owners should monitor for pain, buphthalmos and a dilated pupil.

Prognosis

If more than 24 hours have elapsed with an IOP of above 35 mmHg, the prognosis for vision becomes poor due to damage to the retina and optic nerve. Long-term prognosis is variable, depending on the length of time for which the medications control the IOP. Many cases eventually become refractory to medical management and need definitive treatment such as enucleation, cyclocryotherapy, laser treatment or intravitreous gentocin instillation.

PROPTOSIS

Definition and causes

Proptosis is forward displacement of the globe, which can occur secondary to trauma such as being hit by a car, bite wounds or any blunt trauma to the head (Figure 8.3). Brachycephalic breeds are predisposed because they have shallow orbits.

Clinical signs and management

Clinical signs and management depend on how far the eye has been proptosed and why it occurred. There are two options for therapy: enucleation or replacement with tarsorrhaphy. This decision is based on the severity of the proptosis. If the eye has ruptured all of the extraocular muscles are ruptured, and/or the extraocular muscles are necrotic or infected, the eye should be removed. If there is marked hyphaema or a dilated pupil, enucleation should also be considered. If the owner or veterinary surgeon is unsure whether the

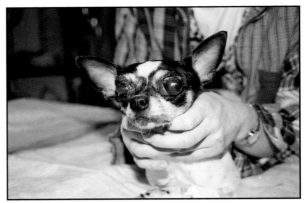

Figure 8.3: Traumatic bilateral proptosis secondary to a dog fight. One eye was enucleated and the other was replaced and a tarsorrhaphy was performed.

owner will be able to treat or monitor the eye, enucleation is usually the best option. Replacement can be attempted if the eye and extraocular muscles are relatively undamaged, few extraocular muscles have ruptured and the pupil is constricted.

Replacement with tarsorrhaphy

Although the eye should be replaced as soon as possible, if the animal has sustained significant head trauma, anaesthesia should be postponed until its condition is stable. Anaesthetic agents that increase IOP (e.g. ketamine) should be avoided. A topical sterile lubricant should be frequently applied to the globe to prevent desiccation.

Once the animal is anaesthetized, the surrounding area should be carefully clipped and aseptically scrubbed with chlorhexiderm or betadine. A stay suture with 2-0 or 3-0 nylon should be placed in the upper and lower eyelids close to the lid margin. A lateral canthotomy is usually needed to help replace the eye. Sterile lubricant is placed on the eye. While lifting out and up on the stay sutures, gentle pressure is placed on the eye to replace it. Once replaced, the stay sutures are crossed and held to prevent reproptosis. Tension relieving sutures are then placed as shown in Figure 8.4; 4-0 nylon can be used with pieces of a 3 or 5 French red rubber catheter or rubber band as stents. A horizontal mattress suture is used and all sutures should be preplaced before tying. The suture should go through a stent, enter 6–8 mm away from the upper lid margin, exit through the Meibomian glands and then enter through the lower Meibomian glands, exit 6–8 mm away from the lower lid margin and go through a stent. The needle then goes back in the reverse direction and the suture is tied at the dorsal aspect. This protects the cornea by everting the eyelids. The lateral canthotomy can then be sutured with 4-0 or 5-0 Vicryl. A small space should be left open medially to allow placement of medications.

Aftercare

Aftercare consists of topical antibiotics (tobramycin

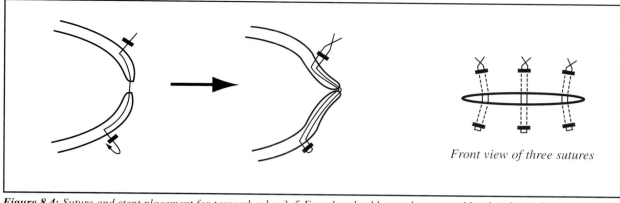

Front view of three sutures

Figure 8.4: *Suture and stent placement for tarsorrhaphy. 3–5 French red rubber catheter or rubber bands can be used as stents. The suture should go through a stent, enter 6–8 mm away from the upper lid margin, exit through the Meibomian glands, then enter the lower Meibomian glands, exit 6–8 mm away from the lower lid margin, then go through the stent. The needle then goes back in the reverse direction.*

0.3% four to six times a day) and topical atropine sulphate (1% twice a day). Oral broad-spectrum antibiotics should also be used. Frequent re-evaluations (every 2 days initially) should be performed to make sure that the client is able to administer medications, the sutures are not rubbing on the cornea, the animal is not febrile and that there is no discharge crusted over the eye. The sutures are removed in 14 days. Once the sutures are removed, the cornea should be stained to check for ulcers and treated appropriately. Topical corticosteroids can be used (prednisolone acetate 1% three times a day) if there is scarring with no corneal ulcer. When scarring is present along with a corneal ulcer, a topical non-steroidal anti-inflammatory drug like flurbiprofen (0.03% three times a day) should be used instead.

The eye should continue to be evaluated every 4–5 days for 2–3 weeks after suture removal to monitor for complications such as exposure keratitis. If the animal is lagophthalmic and has exposure keratitis, a partial permanent tarsorrhaphy may help. If the owners dislike the appearance of the eye with lateral strabismus, an ophthalmologist can correct it surgically.

Complications with replacement

Post-replacement complications include infection, dorsolateral strabismus due to rupture of the medial rectus muscle, blindness and ulcerative or exposure keratitis with a resultant corneal ulcer. Owners must be warned that enucleation may still be necessary.

Prognosis

Due to the stretching of the optic nerve, the prognosis for vision is poor but the prognosis for cosmetic repair is fair. The best way to success is to start treatment as soon as possible, and to follow with frequent evaluations to circumvent complications.

Enucleation

An ophthalmology or surgery text should be consulted for enucleation procedures.

UVEITIS

Definition

Uveitis is an inflammation of the iris, ciliary body and/or choroid. Many systemic disease processes manifest as uveitis in dogs and cats, and some examples are listed in Figure 8.5.

Dog
Trauma
Neoplasia (e.g. lymphosarcoma)
Sepsis
Toxoplasmosis
Fungal (blastomycosis, histoplasmosis, cryptococcidiosis)
Voyt–Koyanagi–Harada syndrome
Lens induced
Rickettsial diseases
Immune-mediated diseases

Cat
Trauma
Feline leukaemia virus
Feline immunodeficiency virus
Toxoplasmosis
Fungal
Lens induced
Feline infectious peritonitis

Figure 8.5: *Causes of uveitis.*

Clinical signs

Clinical signs include blepharospasm, a miotic pupil due to ciliary spasm, pain, a red, inflamed, dull or 'fluffy' iris, aqueous flare, hypopyon or hyphaema, decreased IOP and prolapsed nictitans.

Diagnosis

The diagnosis of anterior uveitis is based on clinical signs. Other differential diagnoses for patients presenting with a red painful eye include glaucoma and corneal ulcers. These diseases may not be mutually exclusive, for example uveitis can cause glaucoma, and trauma can cause both corneal ulcers and uveitis. Every eye should be stained with fluorescein, and IOP should be measured. Diagnostic tests should be geared towards identification of the suspected cause and can include any of the following: complete blood count, chemistry panel, urinalysis, fungal serology, rickettsial tick panel, toxoplasmosis titre and thoracic radiography. In a cat, feline leukaemia virus (FeLV)/feline immunodeficiency virus (FIV) and possibly feline infectious peritonitis (FIP) serology should also be performed. Vogt–Koyanagi–Harada (VKH) or uveodermatological syndrome is an immune-mediated disease associated with antibody production against melanocytes. It should be suspected in Japanese breeds of dog (e.g. Akita) presenting with uveitis (Figure 8.6).

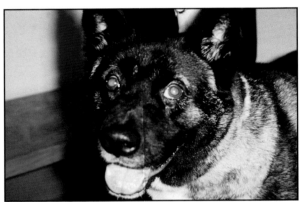

Figure 8.6: *A 3-year-old Akita with a 5-day history of blindness. There was severe uveitis and retinal detachment. This dog had Vogt–Koyanagi–Harada syndrome.*

Treatment

Topical atropine sulphate (1% two to three times a day to maintain a dilated pupil) should be used to prevent synechiae and to make the animal more comfortable. If secondary glaucoma is present, atropine is contraindicated, and adrenaline drops (1% three times a day) can be used to dilate the pupil and decrease aqueous production. Adrenaline is contraindicated in animals predisposed to arrhythmias. Topical corticosteroids (prednisolone acetate 1% three times a day) are necessary to decrease inflammation. In severe cases, systemic corticosteroids can be considered. VKH syndrome requires therapy with immunosuppressive doses of corticosteroids (prednisolone 1–2 mg/kg twice a day) and azathioprine. Any eye with uveitis should be rechecked in 4–5 days for progress.

Complications

The secondary complications include anterior or posterior synechia, glaucoma and cataracts. In cases involving either recurrent uveitis or multiple disease processes in the same eye, the animal should be referred to an ophthalmologist.

Prognosis

Many systemic disease processes have a fair to good short-term prognosis for control of uveitis but a poor long-term prognosis (e.g. FeLV/FIV infection). The prognosis is good, however, when the underlying cause can be controlled (i.e. sepsis, rickettsial or immune-mediated diseases). Traumatic uveitis should respond to treatment and resolve within 1 week.

CORNEAL ULCERS

Definition

Corneal ulcers are epithelial defects of the cornea, which are classified according to the layers that are affected. The most common causes of corneal ulcers are listed in Figure 8.7.

Trauma
Abrasions
Keratoconjunctivitis sicca
Foreign bodies
Infectious – bacterial, viral, fungal
Exposure keratitis
Topical irritants

Figure 8.7: *Causes of corneal ulcers.*

Clinical signs

Patients with corneal ulcers usually present with blepharospasm, ocular discharge and pain causing photophobia and possibly a miotic pupil. Miosis may also occur secondary to concurrent uveitis. Corneal oedema and/or vascularization may be found around the ulcer.

Monitoring

For all ulcers, regardless of the treatment, owners should monitor the eye carefully. Re-evaluation is warranted if: there is a discharge from the cornea; the animal keeps its eye closed; the eye appears red or pain recurs; the eye loses or changes shape; or the animal becomes lethargic or anorexic.

Basic management

Topical corticosteroids are always contraindicated if the corneal epithelium is not intact. If severe uveitis accompanies the ulcer, topical NSAIDs (e.g. flurbiprofen three times a day) or tapering doses of systemic corticosteroids can be used.

Superficial ulcers

Diagnosis

Superficial ulcers are diagnosed based on fluorescein stain retention. A Shirmer tear test should first be performed to rule out primary keratoconjunctivitis sicca (KCS) as the underlying cause. Normal tear production is 10–15 mm/min. A tear test result of <5 mm/min is indicative of KCS. The eye should be thoroughly examined for any foreign material.

Treatment

Treatment includes topical antibiotics (triple antibiotic solution is usually sufficient, four times a day) with or without atropine sulphate (1% twice a day) if a miotic pupil is present or the eye is painful. Cyclosporin (0.2–1%) should be started twice a day for 4 weeks if KCS is the initiating cause of the ulcer. If the ulcer was due to a topical irritant such as a shampoo or soap, irrigation with copious amounts of sterile eye wash or saline is performed. In cats, many corneal ulcers have a viral aetiology, and an antiviral medication (trifluridine or vidarabine four or five times a day) can be included. The eye should be restained after 4–5 days, at which time the ulcer should be healed. If not, an indolent or complicated ulcer should be suspected.

Prognosis

If there are no complications, the prognosis is excellent.

Indolent ulcers

Diagnosis

An indolent ulcer or boxer ulcer is a non-healing ulcer that occurs when the epithelium does not attach to the stroma. When the ulcer is stained with fluorescein, the stain extends further than the edges of the ulcer.

Treatment

A topical anaesthetic (proparacaine) is placed on the eye. A cotton swab (moistened with artificial tears or proparacaine) is used to debride the edges of the ulcer, creating a larger defect. Once the edges are debrided, a grid or punctate keratectomy is performed with a 20–25 gauge needle, avoiding going full thickness through the cornea (Figure 8.8). This aids healing and is thought to help the epithelium attach to the stroma. Topical antibiotics (tobramycin 0.3% four times a day) and atropine sulphate (1% twice a day) should then be started.

Prognosis

With treatment, the majority of indolent ulcers heal.

Deep corneal ulcer

Diagnosis

Deep corneal ulcers are also diagnosed based on fluorescein staining, although the defect may be appreciated on gross examination (Figure 8.9). Deep ulcers may not be as painful as superficial ulcers.

Treatment

For all deep ulcers, care must be taken to avoid excessive restraint of the patient, as this can lead to perforation. Therapy with topical antibiotics (tobramycin or

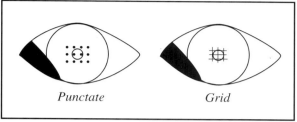

Figure 8.8: *Punctate and grid keratectomy. After topical anaesthetic and debridement with a cotton swab, a 25 gauge needle is used to make punctate or grid marks on, not through, the corneal epithelium.*

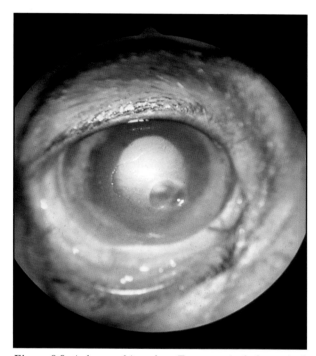

Figure 8.9: *A deep melting ulcer. Treatment includes topical antibiotics, atropine sulphate and an anticollagenase (serum or acetylcysteine). Perforation can occur with restraint or if the animal rubs or scratches the eye.*

gentocin 0.3% four to six times a day) and topical atropine sulphate (1% twice a day) should be started. A topical anticollagenase should also be added in patients with deep melting or infected ulcers (see Figure 8.9). Autologous serum can be used, in which α-macroglobulin acts as the anticollagenase. Acetylcysteine, diluted to a 5% solution with artificial tears, may also be used. Anticollagenases should be instilled every 15 minutes to 1 hour for the first day of treatment. If the animal is rubbing or scratching at the eye, an Elizabethan collar must be worn. A third eyelid or conjunctival flap should be considered in any patient with a deep ulcer.

Prognosis

With aggressive treatment the prognosis can be good. The eye should be monitored very carefully for the first 2–3 days, and then every 3 days for 2 weeks, to ensure that the ulcer continues to heal properly.

Descemetocoele

Diagnosis

When Desçemet's membrane protrudes through the ulcer, it looks clear or transparent (Figure 8.10) and does not retain fluorescein stain. In this case, the cornea is in imminent danger of perforation.

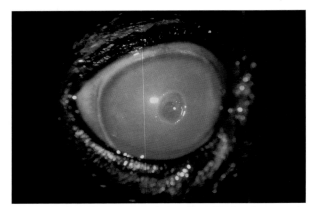

Figure 8.10: A descemetocoele in a Pug. Notice the central clear area, which will not retain fluorescein stain. The cornea should be sutured over the defect. A conjunctival or third eyelid flap will then be needed to protect the cornea.

Treatment

A descemetocoele is a true emergency. Topical antibiotics (tobramycin or gentocin 0.3% four to six times a day) should be started. If the animal is struggling or resents restraint, medications should wait until after surgical repair. The cornea can be sutured over the descemetocoele, inverting the membrane if possible, with 6-0 to 9-0 Vicryl in a simple interrupted or horizontal mattress pattern without penetrating full thickness through the cornea. Since the cornea is usually oedematous and weak, more support and protection can be achieved with a third eyelid or conjunctival flap. Atropine sulphate (1% twice a day) can then be added to the treatment.

Prognosis

The prognosis is variable depending on the extent of corneal disease and the cause of the ulcer. If the animal is lagophthalmic and predisposed to ulcers, the prognosis is guarded and further corrective surgery may be needed.

Iris prolapse

Diagnosis

The iris is visible protruding through the ulcer (Figure 8.11).

Treatment

Topical antibiotics (tobramycin or gentocin 0.3% four to six times a day) should be started. The iris must be removed from the ulcer. It can be freed from the edges of the cornea with an iris spatula or atraumatic forceps,

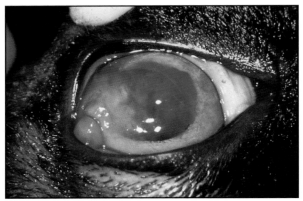

Figure 8.11: Iris prolapse. Notice the iris protruding through the edge of the ulcer. The exposed iris must be removed from the defect. The cornea can then be sutured closed with 6-0 to 9-0 Vicryl. A conjunctival or third eyelid flap is then performed after reinflation of the anterior chamber with saline or air.

and then the exposed iris can be excised with tenotomy scissors. The cornea is then sutured with 6-0 to 9-0 Vicryl in a simple interrupted or horizontal mattress pattern without penetrating full thickness through the cornea. Placing a needle at the limbus, sterile saline or air can be used to reinflate the anterior chamber. A third eyelid or conjunctival flap is then performed. An Elizabethan collar should be worn at all times and oral broad-spectrum antibiotics and topical atropine sulphate (1% twice a day) should be administered.

Prognosis

The prognosis is guarded. Frequent re-evaluations will determine whether the treatment is successful in sealing the cornea and preventing reperforation.

Corneal perforation

Diagnosis

The cornea can rupture and either seal with a fibrin clot or leak aqueous humor, which causes collapse of the anterior chamber. A large fibrin clot may be visible on top of the cornea. If there is a leak, the fluorescein stain will form rivulets at the site of perforation.

Treatment

Medical treatment with topical antibiotics and atropine sulphate, and an Elizabethan collar as described above, can be attempted when there is a fibrin seal and the anterior chamber is intact. The animal must be kept calm and ideally rested in a cage to help prevent the clot from dislodging and rupturing the eye. When there is a leak, the corneal edges should be debrided and sutured with 6-0 to 9-0 Vicryl in a simple interrupted or horizontal mattress pattern without penetrating full thickness through the cornea. The anterior chamber may require reinflation as described above. A third eyelid or conjunctival flap should then be performed and broad-spectrum oral antibiotics should be administered.

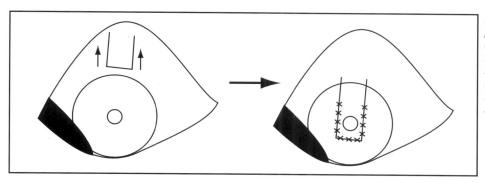

Figure 8.12: Pedicle flap placement. Starting 2 mm away from the dorsal limbus, the flap is extended using blunt dissection with tenotomy scissors. It can then be sutured on to the healthy cornea.

Prognosis

If uncomplicated, the prognosis is good.

Flaps

For a detailed discussion on flap surgery, an ophthalmology text should be consulted. Flaps provide support and protection to the damaged cornea. They provide fibroblasts to help seal the defect and a blood supply to deliver anticollagenases and antibiotics. Third eyelid flaps are technically an easy surgery, but they do not allow visualization of the cornea and monitoring of the ulcer. For this reason, most ophthalmologists prefer conjunctival flaps.

The two primary goals of conjunctival flaps are to make the flap as thin as possible and to have minimal tension on the flap. For pedicle flaps, the flap is started about 2 mm away from the dorsal limbus and extended using blunt dissection. As the flap is extended, care must be taken to keep it 'paper' thin. When the incisions are made perpendicular to the limbus, to mobilize the flap it is important to ensure that the flap is wide enough to cover the defect (Figure 8.12). Once the flap can cover the defect with minimal to no tension, it is sutured on to the healthy cornea surrounding the ulcer with 7-0 to 9-0 Vicryl in a simple interrupted pattern, going through about half the depth of the stroma (Figure 8.13). The part of the flap connecting it to the conjunctiva is not sutured. Topical antibiotics (tobramycin four to six times a day) and topical atropine sulphate (1% twice a day) should be used.

Monitoring

The owner must monitor for signs of discomfort, flap detachment, rupture of the eye or pain. The flap should be re-evaluated by the veterinary surgeon every 3–4 days. The sutures can be removed in 14 days, or the flap can simply be transected at its attachment to the conjunctiva. Topical corticosteroids with antibiotics (neomycin–polymyxin–dexamethasone) three or four times a day) can then be used to decrease scar formation. Re-evaluations should be performed at 1 and 2 weeks post-detachment.

CORNEAL LACERATIONS AND FOREIGN BODIES

Diagnosis

The history and clinical signs are similar to corneal ulcers. Corneal lacerations (Figure 8.14) usually have oedema around the edges and may be difficult to distinguish from corneal ulcers. Lacerations can cause a descemetocoele or iris prolapse and should be treated accordingly. All cases of corneal lacerations should be extensively evaluated for ocular foreign bodies. The area under and around the nictitans and under and at the margins of both eyelids should be carefully investigated, and a magnifying lens should be used to evaluate the cornea. A topical anaesthetic or general anaesthetic is usually necessary to perform a full evaluation and to prevent further damage.

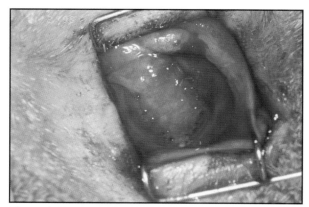

Figure 8.13: Post-conjunctival flap placement. The flap is very thin and there is no tension on it. This helps ensure that the flap will not break down or cause pain.

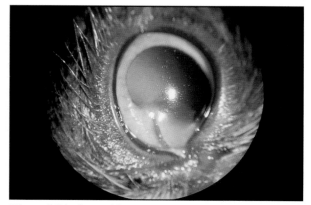

Figure 8.14: Corneal laceration in a cat. Notice the corneal oedema around the edges. All cases should be extensively evaluated for a foreign body. A twig caused the laceration in this cat.

Treatment

If a corneal foreign body is present, gentle irrigation with sterile eyewash or saline may dislodge it. Alternatively, it can be dislodged using a 25 gauge needle, taking care not to push it further into the stroma. If the foreign body is lodged deeply in the cornea, an incision is made next to it using a no. 11 scalpel blade. The foreign body can then be pushed upward with the needle and removed.

If the cornea is perforated or lacerated, it should be sutured with 6-0 to 9-0 Vicryl in a simple interrupted or horizontal pattern. Topical antibiotics (triple antibiotic solution or tobramycin 0.3% four times a day) and atropine sulphate (1% twice a day) should be used for 10–14 days. Broad-spectrum oral antibiotics should also be administered.

Monitoring

The eye should be monitored for signs of suture breakdown/dehiscence and infection (i.e. discharge, redness and pain), with re-evaluations every 3 days for the first 1–2 weeks until it is healed. A third eyelid or conjunctival flap may be necessary if the cornea appears weak or unhealthy.

Prognosis

If uncomplicated, the prognosis is excellent.

LENS LUXATION

Diagnosis

A lens luxation can be diagnosed based on the presence of an aphakic crescent (Figure 8.15), increased or decreased anterior chamber depth, abnormal iris movement, IOP and/or corneal oedema. The causes are listed in Figure 8.16. An anteriorly luxated lens can be an emergency due to the high possibility of secondary glaucoma. The IOP should therefore always be measured in these cases.

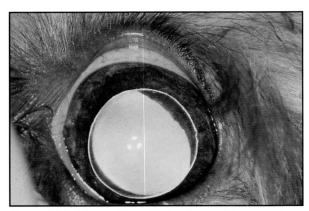

Figure 8.15: *A luxated lens. Notice the aphakic crescent. The ideal treatment is surgical lens extraction, to avoid secondary complications of glaucoma, uveitis, vitreous liquefaction and cataracts.*

Traumatic:	will see other evidence of trauma
Primary:	breeds predisposed include terriers
Secondary:	to glaucoma, neoplasia, uveitis

Figure 8.16: *Causes of lens luxations.*

Treatment

If IOP is increased, treatment with mannitol (1 g/kg over 20 minutes i.v.) is warranted. The ideal treatment is surgical lens extraction. An ophthalmology text or ophthalmologist should be consulted for lens extraction surgery. If surgery is not an option, the lens can be 'pushed' back into the vitreous using a short-acting mydriatic (tropicamide) followed by a miotic agent (pilocarpine) to keep it in the vitreous chamber. This is not ideal, since the presence of the lens will lead to secondary vitreous liquefaction and intraocular disease.

Prognosis

As lens luxations can lead to glaucoma, uveitis, vitreous liquefaction and cataracts, the prognosis is guarded unless the lens luxation is diagnosed and treated early.

HYPHAEMA

Definition and causes

Hyphaema is blood in the anterior chamber; the most common causes are listed in Figure 8.17.

Trauma
Infection ± uveitis
Neoplasia ± uveitis
Coagulopathy
Congenital

Figure 8.17: *Causes of hyphaema.*

Clinical signs

The clinical signs are dependent on the primary cause. Additional systemic signs of a coagulopathy, trauma or uveitis may also be present.

Diagnosis

Diagnosis is based on direct visualization of blood in the anterior chamber (Figure 8.18). When no other signs of trauma are found, the diagnostic plan should proceed as with uveitis, and a full coagulation panel (platelet count, prothrombin time, partial thromboplastin time, fibrin split products and buccal mucosal bleeding time) should also be submitted.

Treatment

Treatment consists of topical corticosteroids (prednisolone acetate 1%) or corticosteroid/antibiotic mixture (neomycin–polymyxin–dexamethasone every 6–8

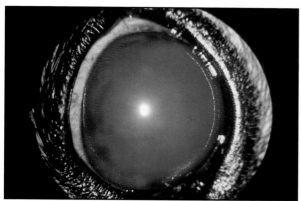

Figure 8.18: *Hyphaema. Trauma, coagulopathy and neoplasia are the most common causes. Once secondary glaucoma is ruled out, topical mydriatics and corticosteroids can be started.*

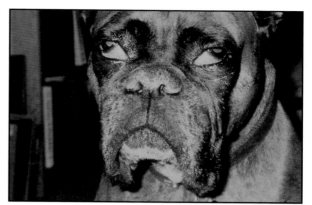

Figure 8.20: *Severe conjunctivitis in a 7-year-old Boxer. Note the ocular discharge. Other signs of seasonal atopy were present, including pododermatitis and pruritus.*

hours. There is controversy as to whether a mydriatic or miotic should be used in hyphaema. If there is no history of trauma, it can be difficult to rule out uveitis definitively, and then a mydriatic (atropine sulphate 1% twice a day) is most appropriate. Secondary glaucoma should be ruled out via tonometry before starting mydriatic therapy.

Prognosis

The prognosis is variable depending on the underlying cause. If bleeding can be controlled the prognosis is good. If the haemorrhage is due to uveitis, the prognosis depends on the primary diagnosis.

CONJUNCTIVITIS

Definition and causes

Conjunctivitis is inflammation and/or infection of the conjunctiva. The most common causes are listed in Figure 8.19.

Bacterial
Viral (herpes)
Chlamydia infection in cats
Corneal ulcers
Keratoconjunctivitis sicca
Allergy/atopy
Canine distemper
Chemical irritants

Figure 8.19: *Causes of conjunctivitis.*

Clinical signs

Clinical signs include blepharospasm, ocular discharge, chemosis and conjunctival hyperaemia (Figure 8.20).

Diagnosis

The diagnosis is based on clinical signs. In cats, infectious conjunctivitis is more common than in dogs, and conjunctival scrapings and bacterial cultures should be submitted. In dogs, allergic or non-infectious conjunctivitis is more common and other signs of allergies (e.g. alopecia, pruritus) might be present. Due to the fact that many ocular diseases can cause conjunctivitis, other diagnostic tests include a Shirmer tear test, fluorescein stain, tonometry and FeLV/FIV serology (cats).

Treatment

The treatment is based on the underlying cause. The eye(s) should be irrigated with sterile eyewash. In cats, topical antibiotic ointment (tetracycline or erythromycin three to four times a day) should be used. The antibiotic is then changed based on culture and sensitivity results. Topical antiviral ointment (vidarabine or trifluridine four to five times a day) should be considered in cats with recurrent herpes conjunctivitis. In dogs, once bacterial conjunctivitis is ruled out (via cytology), topical corticosteroids with or without antibiotics (prednisolone acetate 1% three times a day, neomycin–polymyxin–dexamethasone four times a day) can be used.

Prognosis

Many cases of allergic and viral conjunctivitis are recurrent. Owners should be warned of this because many get frustrated when the disease returns. An ophthalmologist should be consulted in recurrent or nonresponsive cases.

FURTHER READING

Bachrach Jr A (1992) Ocular emergencies. In: *Veterinary Emergency and Critical Care Medicine,* ed. RJ Murtaugh *et al.,* pp. 273–287. Mosby

Gionfriddo JR (1995) Identifying and treating conjunctivitis in dogs and cats. *Veterinary Medicine* **90,** 242–253

Gionfriddo JR (1995) Recognizing and managing acute and chronic cases of glaucoma. *Veterinary Medicine* **90,** 265–275

Gionfriddo JR (1995) The causes, diagnosis, and treatment of uveitis. *Veterinary Medicine* **90,** 278–284

Morgan RV (1989) Vogt–Koyanagi–Harada syndrome in humans and dogs. *Compendium on Continuing Education* **11,** 1211–1218

Peiffer RL Jr and Petersen-Jones SM (1997) *Small Animal Ophthalmology: A Problem-Oriented Approach.* WB Saunders, London

Severin GA (1989) *Veterinary Ophthalmology Notes*. Colorado State University, Fort Collins, CO

Slatter D (1990) *Fundamentals of Veterinary Ophthalmology*. WB Saunders, Philadelphia

Whitley RD, Whitley EM and McLaughlin SA (1993) Diagnosing and treating disorders of the feline conjunctiva and cornea. *Veterinary Medicine* **88**, 1138–1149

Whitley RD, Hamilton HL and Weigand CM (1993) Glaucoma and disorders of the uvea, lens and retina in cats. *Veterinary Medicine* **88**, 1164–1173

Wilkie DA (1993) Therapeutics in practice. Management of keratoconjunctivitis sicca in dogs. *Compendium on Continuing Education* **15**, 58–63.

CHAPTER NINE

Acute Abdominal and Gastrointestinal Emergencies

David Holt and Dorothy Brown

Animals with an acute abdominal crisis present several challenges. The veterinarian must perform a rapid thorough physical examination and begin resuscitation to stabilize the animal's condition, then accurately diagnose the cause of the problem and decide whether surgery is indicated. The animal must be as stable as possible before anaesthesia. During surgery, the clinician must do a complete abdominal exploratory and avoid focusing on an obvious lesion. Emergency gastrointestinal surgery requires critical evaluation of bowel viability and exacting technical skill for best results. Adept postoperative management, including careful monitoring and an index of suspicion for potential complications, is vital.

INITIAL EXAMINATION AND RESUSCITATION

Animals frequently present to veterinarians for a sudden onset of vomiting with or without diarrhoea. In many situations the condition is a low-grade acute gastroenteritis associated with a change in diet or dietary indiscretion, will be self-limiting and can be treated conservatively. Some animals, however, may have life-threatening disease. Each case must be carefully evaluated to determine which are true emergencies requiring extensive initial resuscitation and aggressive diagnostic investigation. The rapid initial examination and resuscitation of animals with vomiting and diarrhoea should focus on the degree of dehydration, hypovolaemia and electrolyte abnormalities and the possibility of shock or sepsis. The subsequent patient evaluation should focus on whether the vomiting and diarrhoea might be caused by an immediately life-threatening disease or toxicity and should determine the best means to evaluate, diagnose and treat the underlying cause.

Vomiting and diarrhoea have a variety of aetiologies, many of which are not related to the gastrointestinal tract (Figures 9.1 and 9.2). The signalment is often helpful as a starting point in the diagnostic evaluation. Older female dogs may be more likely to have pancreatitis, pyometra or diabetic ketoacidosis. Young puppies may have viral gastroenteritis, severe parasitism or a swallowed foreign body. Older male dogs may have abdominal pain secondary to prostatitis. Geriatric cats may have renal failure, diabetic ketoacidosis or hyperthyroidism, while string foreign bodies are common in younger cats.

The owner should be thoroughly questioned about the vaccination status, worming history and pre-existing medical conditions, the possibility of foreign body ingestion and possible access to toxins (lead, other heavy metals, ethylene glycol) or medications the owner may not consider dangerous (aspirin, acetaminophen, ibuprofen). When taking a history, it is important to ask questions that distinguish between vomiting and regurgitation. Vomiting is characterized by retching and repeated contractions of the abdominal muscles. Regurgitation is more passive, with owners often reporting that the animal 'just opens its mouth and the food falls out'; this tends to indicate oesophageal rather than gastric or small intestinal disease. However, animals that are initially vomiting can begin to regurgitate because of oesophagitis caused by the vomited material. Finally, the veterinarian should perform a 'systems review', asking the owner questions about other clinical signs that might indicate an underlying disease process. For example, polydypsia and polyuria might indicate renal disease, diabetes mellitus, pyometra or hepatic disease.

A rapid examination is performed, concentrating on the degree of dehydration or hypovolaemia and the cardiovascular, respiratory, renal and central nervous systems. In less severely affected animals, dehydration (lack of interstitial fluid volume) is estimated from skin turgor and capillary refill time. If the animal is dehydrated, fluid deficits are corrected in the first 2–4 hours, with additional fluid administered to account for ongoing losses and maintenance requirements. For example, a 10 kg dog which is 5% dehydrated and vomiting 50 ml every 2 hours requires 500 ml to correct dehydration. When fluid for ongoing losses and maintenance (1–2 ml/kg/h) are added, the fluid rate is 170 ml/h (dehydration = 125 ml/h for 4 hours, plus 25 ml/h for ongoing loss, plus 20 ml/h for maintenance).

Animals with acute abdominal crises often have hypovolaemia (decreased intravascular volume) in addition to dehydration. Pale mucous membranes, a rapid heart rate and weak thready pulses indicate the

Physical obstruction
Foreign bodies
Pyloric hypertrophy
Mural thickening (granulomas, neoplasms, strictures)
Extraluminal compression (masses, adhesions)
Intussusception
Delayed gastric emptying
Ileus
Constipation

Inflammation/irritation of the gastrointestinal tract or other abdominal organs
Pharyngitis
Gastritis (e.g. acute/chronic, atrophic, hypertrophic, eosinophilic)
Inflammatory bowel disease (small and large intestine)
Gastrointestinal neoplasia
Gastroduodenal ulcers
Lymphangiectasia
Gastrinoma
Adverse reactions to food (infections, intolerances, allergies)
Hepatobiliary (neoplasia, bile duct obstruction, cholelithiasis, portosystemic shunts)
Pancreatitis and pancreatic neoplasia
Nephritis
Peritonitis
Pyometra, metritis
Organ ischaemia (avulsion, infarction, torsion)

Endogenous toxins (local and systemic)
Uraemia
Sepsis and endotoxaemia
Diabetic ketoacidosis
Hypoxia
Electrolyte disturbances (hypokalaemia, hypercalcaemia, others)

Exogenous toxins (local and systemic)
Apomorphine
NSAIDs
Chemotherapeutic agents
Digoxin
Insecticides
Copper sulphate
Heavy metals (lead, others)
Ethylene glycol
Mycotoxins
Household plants
Others

Infectious or parasitic agents
Bacterial infections (e.g. *Salmonella*, *Campylobacter*)
Viral infections (e.g. parvovirus, panleucopenia, infectious canine hepatitis)
Fungal infections (e.g. histoplasmosis)
Parasites (e.g. ascarids, heartworm (cats), salmon poisoning)
Neurological disorders
Dysautonomia
Myenteric ganglionitis
CNS tumours
Meningitis
Encephalitis
Hydrocephalus
Vestibular disturbances
Visceral epilepsy

Figure 9.1: Commonly recognized causes of vomiting. Adapted from King and Donaldson (1994).

Self-limiting
Idiopathic
Dietary indiscretion
Parasites
Viral enteritis — coronavirus
Bacterial enteritis
Drugs and toxins

Life-threatening
Severe dietary indiscretion or parasitism
Viral enteritis — parvoviruses, distemper
Bacterial enteritis
Intestinal obstruction
Haemorrhagic gastroenteritis
Systemic diseases
    Acute pancreatitis
    Acute renal failure
    Acute liver disease
    Hypoadrenocorticism
    Ketoacidotic diabetes mellitus

Figure 9.2: *Differential diagnoses of acute diarrhoea. Adapted from Matz (1996).*

potential for hypovolaemic shock. Large amounts of fluid are lost in vomitus and diarrhoea. Additional fluid is sequestered in inflamed non-motile intestines. When the gastrointestinal tract has ruptured, the inflammation caused by chemicals (gastric acid, bile, pancreatic enzymes) and bacteria causes vasodilation, increased peritoneal vessel permeability, and subsequent loss of intravascular fluid and protein into the peritoneal cavity. Fluid losses are often accompanied by dangerous electrolyte and acid–base abnormalities. The presence of injected brick red mucous membranes may indicate the 'hyperdynamic' phase of sepsis, which is associated with peripheral vasodilation caused by the release of endotoxin and cytokines. In more advanced sepsis, this clinical sign is not apparent; animals have severe vasoconstriction, pale mucous membranes and may be hyper- or hypothermic. Animals may also be septic from aspiration pneumonia.

Treatment should begin immediately in unstable shock patients. In animals with no previous history of heart disease, no respiratory abnormalities and no murmur evident on initial examination, a shock bolus of up to 50–100 ml/kg of balanced electrolyte solution may be administered intravenously in the first 60 minutes. Two large bore intravenous catheters are inserted and prior to fluid therapy, blood is obtained for an initial database, including packed cell volume (PCV), total protein (TP) and dipstick estimation of blood glucose and blood urea nitrogen. Ideally, urine is obtained before aggressive fluid therapy is begun. Evidence of isosthenuria (urine specific gravity 1.007–1.015) in the presence of dehydration indicates poor renal function. Azotaemia (pre-renal, renal or post-renal) can be confirmed by dipstick. A blood smear should be made to provide an indication of the white blood cell and platelet count.

The PCV and TP are usually increased in non-anaemic animals that are dehydrated, but should be interpreted in the light of clinical findings. For example, an animal with a 'normal' initial PCV may actually be quite anaemic following rehydration. Extremely high PCVs (60–80%) are seen with canine haemorrhagic gastroenteritis (HGE). Animals with acute haemorrhage may have a normal PCV and TP initially. During an acute haemorrhagic crisis, the PCV may be maintained in the normal range by splenic contraction, but the TP is often low, indicating the severity of blood loss. As intravenous fluids are given, both the PCV and TP drop to dramatically low values. Blood transfusion is required in animals in which the PCV rapidly drops below 25%. In these cases, blood (10–20 ml/kg) is administered at a rate of 10 ml/kg/h. In severely anaemic hypovolaemic animals, this rate can be doubled if necessary. Colloids (plasma, hetastarch, dextran) should be considered in cases with low total protein levels (less than 4 mg/dl).

High blood glucose could indicate diabetes but occurs very commonly with stress in cats. The urinalysis can provide an inexpensive and valuable tool in these cases; ketones in the urine help confirm diabetic ketoacidosis. Glucose supplementation should be considered in animals with blood glucose concentrations less that 60 mg/dl. Dextrose (0.25–0.5 g/kg of 25–50% solution) can be administered slowly, intravenously as a bolus and the intravenous fluids are supplemented to achieve a glucose concentration between 2.5 and 5%.

Serum electrolytes should be measured and blood gas analysis should be performed. Since severe electrolyte and acid–base disturbances can occur with vomiting and diarrhoea, these provide valuable information and help determine the appropriate fluid for resuscitation. Animals vomiting gastric contents secondary to a pyloric obstruction will lose sodium, potassium and chloride and have a metabolic alkalosis. For these animals, 0.9% sodium chloride supplemented with potassium is the ideal replacement fluid. Hyperkalaemia associated with hyponatraemia should increase suspicion of Addison's disease. Animals vomiting secondary to small intestinal obstruction will lose not only sodium, potassium and chloride, but also bicarbonate, and their acid–base status can be more variable.

A thorough physical examination is performed after the initial resuscitation is begun and a complete history is obtained. The animal's mouth should be carefully examined for the presence of a linear foreign body or evidence of ulcers that might indicate toxin ingestion or underlying systemic disease. The chest should be auscultated for evidence of arrhythmias or crackles and wheezes caused by aspiration pneumonia. Abdominal palpation is an important part of assessing the gastrointestinal system. In many instances, a foreign body or intussusception can be readily palpated, making a diagnosis straightforward. The abdomen is palpated with the animal's forelimbs held off the ground or examination table to allow the abdominal contents to slide caudal to the last ribs. A rectal examination is performed to assess the urogenital tract and the character of the faeces, and a sample is obtained for faecal floatation. The peripheral lymph nodes are carefully palpated and the skin carefully checked for any masses, which may be histamine releasing mast cell tumours.

The cardiovascular status should be re-evaluated at this time. The mucous membrane colour, capillary refill time and skin turgor should all be improved after the initial fluid bolus. The heart rate should have decreased and the pulse quality should have improved. If the animal still appears to be dehydrated or in shock, the following questions should be considered: (i) was the initial fluid bolus adequate or is the animal losing additional fluid that was not accounted for, perhaps into the bowel lumen or peritoneal cavity?; (ii) could the animal's poor response be associated with sepsis?

Initial therapy for potentially septic animals should include further aggressive intravenous crystalloid and colloid therapy and broad spectrum bactericidal antibiotics (see Chapter 20).

In stable patients who respond well to initial fluid resuscitation and have no obvious abnormalities on physical examination, the extended database or plain abdominal radiographs, conservative treatment is indicated. The animal can be monitored either in the hospital or at home with the owner. Food and water should be withheld for 12–24 hours. Small amounts of water should be offered initially, followed by small amounts of easily digestible food, such as boiled chicken and rice.

Some animals respond to initial fluid resuscitation but still have signs of systemic illness, such as fever and abdominal pain, without an obvious cause apparent on the initial extended database or plain abdominal radiographs. These animals should be hospitalized and their fluid and electrolyte balance closely monitored. Food and water are withheld. Intravenous fluid therapy is continued, with fluid rates taking into account potential losses from diarrhoea and vomiting, and glucose and electrolytes, particularly potassium, are supplemented as needed. Ongoing systemic illness or recurrent vomiting should prompt a more extensive diagnostic investigation. Animals with signs of systemic illness should be carefully monitored. The physical examination should be repeated and if symptoms change, diagnostic tests should be repeated. For example, abdominal radiography should be repeated if the animal develops abdominal pain, to evaluate for evidence of pancreatitis, gastrointestinal obstruction or peritonitis. Clinical parameters, such as capillary refill time, mucous membrane colour, heart rate, pulse quality and temperature and laboratory parameters, including blood pressure, serial PCV/TP/glucose, electrolytes and urine output, are monitored.

In some cases, severe acute diarrhoea can occur without vomiting. Diarrhoea occurs because of increased faecal water content. This, in turn, results from malabsorption (osmotic diarrhoea), excessive fluid secretion (secretory or exudative diarrhoea) or altered intestinal motility. Life-threatening diarrhoea is associated with severe dietary indiscretion, severe parasitism (especially in younger dogs), bacterial (*Salmonella*, *Campylobacter*) or viral (parvovirus) enteritis, haemorrhagic gastroenteritis and several systemic diseases including diabetes, renal failure, pancreatitis and hypoadrenocorticism. The initial resuscitation, physical examination and diagnostic investigation are similar to that described for the vomiting animal.

SYMPTOMATIC MANAGEMENT OF VOMITING AND DIARRHOEA

Antiemetics are often required in animals with persistent vomiting. Metoclopramide acts centrally to inhibit the chemoreceptor trigger zone. In the gut, it increases the co-ordination of upper gastrointestinal motility, decreasing gastric emptying time and intestinal transit time. For these reasons it may be contraindicated if there is any suspicion of intestinal obstruction. Metoclopramide can be administered at a dose of 0.2–0.5 mg/kg s.c. or ideally, added to the intravenous fluids at a dose of 1–2 mg/kg/24 h. Prochlorperazine (0.1–0.5 mg/kg i.m. or i.v. every 6–8 h) and chlorpromazine (0.25–0.5 mg/kg i.m. every 6–8 h) are phenothiazine derivatives that suppress the vomiting centre. They should be used with extreme caution in animals with hypovolaemia, possible shock or poor perfusion, as they are α-adrenergic antagonists and can cause profound hypotension.

Antibiotics should not be universally administered to animals with vomiting and/or diarrhoea. Animals with loss of integrity of the gut mucosa (for example, with haemorrhagic vomiting or diarrhoea), high fevers (>39°C), signs of sepsis or evidence of pneumonia or pyometra should receive broad spectrum bactericidal antibiotics intravenously. Ampicillin (22 mg/kg i.v. every 8 hours) or cefazolin (22 mg/kg i.v. every 8 hours) can be supplemented with enrofloxacin (2.5–5 mg/kg i.m./i.v. every 12 hours). Alternatively, an aminoglycoside (amikacin 15 mg/kg i.v. every 24 hours or gentamicin 6 mg/kg i.v. every 24 hours) can be used once the animal is rehydrated and the initial database shows no evidence of renal disease.

Gastric acid inhibitors are indicated in animals with haematemesis or melaena; cimetidine (10 mg/kg i.v. every 6–8 hours) or ranitidine (2 mg/kg i.v. every 8 hours) can be given.

Anthelmintics are often indicated as part of symptomatic treatment of diarrhoea, as some animals can have severe parasite burdens yet still have negative faecal floatation results. Pyrantel pamoate (20 mg/kg) is effective against *Toxocara* and *Ancylostoma* species. Fenbendazole (50 mg/kg orally daily for 3 days) is effective against *Toxocara*, *Ancylostoma* and *Trichuris* species. *Giardia* infection is treated with metronidazole (dogs: 50 mg/kg orally once daily or divided into two daily doses; cats: 30 mg/kg divided into two daily doses). Coccidiosis is treated with sulphamethoxine (55 mg/kg orally initially, followed by 25 mg/kg once daily for 2 weeks). *Salmonella* infection is treated with enrofloxacin (5 mg/kg orally every 12 hours for 10 days) and *Campylobacter* infection is treated with enrofloxacin or erythromycin (10 mg/kg orally every 8 hours for 7 days).

Opioids such as loperamide (0.1 mg/kg orally every 8 hours) are used to decrease intestinal motility and intestinal secretion in dogs with acute diarrhoea in which a bacterial aetiology is not suspected. Their use in cats is controversial. Side-effects such as constipation, bloat and sedation can occur, particularly at inappropriate doses. Opioids should be discontinued if the diarrhoea has not resolved in 48 hours. Bismuth subsalicylate (1 ml/kg orally every 6–8 hours) is often a useful treatment for acute, non-specific diarrhoea. The compound is thought to have anti-endotoxic and weak anti-bacterial properties. The salicylate compound is rapidly absorbed and salicylate toxicity may occur with overdoses, particularly in cats.

PATIENT EVALUATION AND DIAGNOSTIC INVESTIGATION

Results from a complete blood count and serum biochemical analysis including amylase and lipase, although not always immediately available, often indicate potential underlying metabolic diseases or inflammatory conditions. The majority of dogs with parvoviral enteritis have severe leucopenia. Animals with haemorrhagic gastroenteritis often have marked haemoconcentration.

If diarrhoea is present in an unvaccinated animal, faecal samples should be tested for parvovirus with a commercial ELISA kit. Faecal floatation and zinc sulphide sedimentation are used to test for helminths, coccidia and *Giardia*. In animals with severe diarrhoea that are negative for Parvovirus and faecal parasites, additional faeces should be Gram stained and cultured to rule out bacterial infections such as *Campylobacter* and *Salmonella*. Canine haemorrhagic gastroenteritis (HGE) has been associated with a heavy growth of *Clostridium perfringens* on faecal cultures.

Additional diagnostic tests, such as radiography, are performed based on the results of physical examination. Plain abdominal radiographs are indicated in animals with abdominal pain or persistent vomiting. Plain cervical and thoracic radiographs should be made to evaluate the oesophagus for foreign bodies in animals presenting with regurgitation. The radiographs should be critically evaluated for evidence of gastrointestinal obstruction, foreign bodies, pancreatitis and the pres-

ence of free air or fluid in the peritoneal cavity. Radiographic signs of obstruction include the presence of gas- or fluid-distended small bowel loops (Figure 9.3). Severe intestinal gas distension can be associated with a mesenteric volvulus. Decreased radiographic contrast in the right cranial abdomen, displacement of the stomach to the left, widening of the angle between the pyloric antrum and the duodenum, displacement of the duodenum to the right and static gas in the duodenum are all radiographic signs associated with pancreatitis (Figure 9.4). Evidence of free gas in the abdominal cavity without prior abdominocentesis or surgery indicates intestinal perforation or the presence of gas-forming organisms in the abdominal cavity and is an indication for immediate laparotomy. The free gas often accumulates caudal to the diaphragm, outlining the crura of the diaphragm clearly (Figure 9.3). Loss of abdominal detail due to fluid should prompt abdominal paracentesis and peritoneal fluid analysis.

Contrast radiographs should be made if gastric or intestinal obstruction is suspected but not definitive on plain abdominal radiographs. Five to ten ml/kg body weight of a 25% liquid barium suspension is given. Iodine-based contrast agents (Iohexol 2–5 ml/kg orally) should be used if intestinal perforation is suspected, as

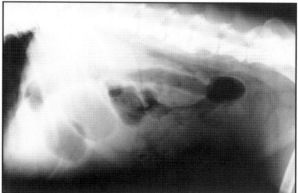

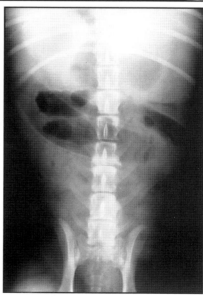

Figure 9.3: Lateral and dorsoventral abdominal radiographs of a dog with a small intestinal obstruction. Note the gas distension of several parts of the small intestine. The gas-filled descending duodenum is clearly visible on the lateral radiograph.

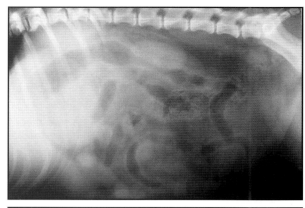

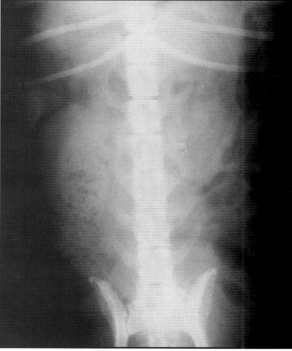

Figure 9.4: Lateral and dorsoventral abdominal radiographs of a dog with pancreatitis. Radiographic signs suggestive of pancreatitis include: increased soft tissue opacity and decreased abdominal detail in the right cranial abdomen; a static, gas-filled descending duodenum; displacement of the pyloric antrum to the left; and displacement of the duodenum to the right, producing a widened angle between the stomach and the duodenum.
Courtesy of Dr H M Saunders, University of Pennsylvania School of Veterinary Medicine.

barium worsens peritonitis if it leaks from the gastrointestinal tract.

Abdominal paracentesis is performed if peritoneal fluid is detected on physical examination or there is loss of detail on plain abdominal radiographs. The ventral abdomen is clipped and prepared as for aseptic surgery. A four-quadrant tap is performed with a 20 to 22 gauge needle. Retrieved fluid should be examined microscopically for evidence of degenerative neutrophils and the presence of intracellular bacteria. In many cases, peritoneal fluid is present but cannot be recovered by paracentesis, presumably because the needle becomes plugged with omentum. In this situation,

ultrasound guidance can assist in fluid aspiration; alternatively, diagnostic peritoneal lavage is indicated. The bladder is expressed and the ventral abdomen is prepared aseptically. An over-the-needle catheter or dialysis catheter is introduced into the abdomen 2 cm caudal to the umbilicus and 20 ml/kg of warm balanced electrolyte solution is rapidly infused through the dialysis catheter. The fluid is distributed by abdominal massage and then collected. Only a few millilitres of fluid may be retrieved. In normal animals, lavage fluid leucocyte counts before surgery are usually less than 1000 cells/mm^3. After uncomplicated intra-abdominal surgery, lavage fluid neutrophil numbers generally increase to 10,000 cells/mm^3 or less. Toxic degenerative neutrophils with intracellular bacteria indicate septic peritonitis and are an indication for immediate exploratory laparotomy. Creatinine and bilirubin levels may also be measured on the peritoneal exudate or lavage fluid. Values for bilirubin, creatinine and amylase that exceed corresponding serum levels indicate biliary leakage, urinary tract leakage or pancreatitis, respectively. The use of peritoneal fluid glucose levels and acid–base measurements to diagnose septic peritonitis is currently under investigation. Contraindications for peritoneal lavage include dyspnoea, diaphragmatic hernia and severe organomegaly.

Abdominal ultrasound can be used to evaluate the abdominal organs, especially when free peritoneal fluid makes radiographic interpretation difficult. Particular attention should be paid to the pancreas in animals with abdominal pain. The spleen and liver should be carefully evaluated for possible neoplasms or ruptured haematomas in cases of haemoperitoneum and for evidence of splenic torsion or thrombosis. The biliary tree, urogenital tract (especially the prostate or uterus) and mesenteric lymph nodes are carefully evaluated.

In animals with respiratory difficulty, thoracic radiographs will help confirm suspected aspiration pneumonia secondary to vomiting. Arterial blood gas analysis will indicate the severity of hypoxia, and a transtracheal wash will provide important information on the type and antibiotic sensitivities of bacteria associated with the pneumonia. Further evaluation of the vomiting animal could include ACTH stimulation tests for hypoadrenocorticism, endoscopy and gastrointestinal biopsies.

Complete stabilization of the animal with an acute abdominal crisis may not be possible until the underlying cause is treated. In many cases this requires abdominal surgery. Indications for exploratory abdominal surgery include:

• Free gas visible in the peritoneal cavity of an animal that has not had recent (within 1 month) abdominal surgery
• Gastric dilatation/volvulus
• Gastrointestinal obstruction (including intussusception) or linear foreign body

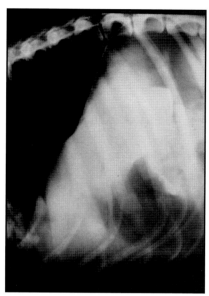

Figure 9.5: *Lateral radiograph of a dog with gastric perforation, illustrating free gas in the peritoneal cavity. Note the diaphragm outlined clearly by the lungs cranially and the free peritoneal gas caudally.*

- Intracellular bacteria and toxic neutrophils on peritoneal tap or lavage
- Bilirubin or creatinine levels in the peritoneal lavage fluid greater than those of serum
- Animals with abdominal haemorrhage that do not stabilize after initial resuscitation
- Splenic torsion/mesenteric volvulus
- Pyometra/prostatic abscessation
- Penetrating abdominal injury (gunshot, impalement).

If surgery is required, anaesthetic agents with minimal depressant effects on the cardiovascular and respiratory systems are used (see Chapter 18). If bacterial contamination of the peritoneal cavity is suspected or anticipated, broad-spectrum bactericidal antibiotics are administered (ampicillin, 20 mg/kg i.v. every 8 hours and gentamycin 6 mg/kg i.v. every 24 hours). A large incision is made, extending from the xiphoid to caudal to the umbilicus. A complete exploratory laparotomy is performed and all organ systems examined sequentially. Definitive treatment depends on the organ system affected and the nature of the disease.

OESOPHAGUS

Oesophageal foreign bodies should be suspected in any animal presenting with a history of regurgitation. Foreign bodies tend to lodge at points of narrowing in the oesophagus: the thoracic inlet, the heart base and cranial to the gastro-oesophageal sphincter. Bones, fish hooks and needles are common in dogs and cats. Bones usually lodge at the heart base or between the heart base and diaphragm. Sharp objects may lodge anywhere. The animal may continue to attempt to eat but regurgitates soon after. Many hypersalivate. Radiopaque foreign bodies and bones are visualized on plain radiographs (Figure 9.6). Non-radiopaque foreign bodies require a positive contrast oesophagram for visualization. Although barium may be used, if oesophageal perforation is suspected an iodinated contrast agent is required. Removal of foreign bodies should be immediate. Local changes occur in the oesophagus at the point(s) of contact with a foreign body. Spasm of the oesophageal muscles and mucosal necrosis can occur. Necrosis may extend through the entire oesophageal wall, with perforation, escape of intraluminal contents and subsequent mediastinitis, pleuritis and sepsis.

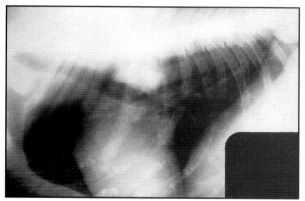

Figure 9.6: *Lateral thoracic radiograph of a dog illustrating a thoracic oesophageal body present over the heart base.*
Courtesy of Dr Colin Harvey, University of Pennsylvania School of Veterinary Medicine.

The foreign body should always be removed by the simplest means possible. The mouth and tongue should be carefully examined for a thread in animals with a hook or needle lodged in the oesophagus. Rigid proctoscopes or flexible fibreoptic endoscopes and long blunt-ended forceps can be used to remove most foreign bodies. Under anaesthesia, the animal is placed in left lateral recumbency so that the oesophagus is over the aorta. The oesophagus is suctioned and the foreign body grasped. Some instruments allow insufflation of air, dilating the oesophagus around the foreign body. Gentle twisting (1/4 turn) will sometimes disengage the foreign object and allow removal. Some are too large to grasp and can be gently pushed into the stomach. Once in the stomach, bones will generally be digested and do not have to be removed. Sharp objects require proper planning for removal to prevent additional damage. After removal, the oesophageal wall is re-examined. Clean lacerations that do not extend through the full thickness of the oesophageal wall (as judged by gently pushing the tip of a forceps or endoscope against the laceration) can be left to heal by epithelialization.

Full-thickness tears or areas of necrotic oesophageal wall require immediate surgical management.

Surgical removal of foreign bodies is necessary when endoscopic removal fails or in cases with associated oesophageal perforation. The cervical oesophagus is accessed via a ventral midline incision in the neck. The ventral sternohyoideus and sternothyroideus muscles are separated on the midline and the oesophagus is located on the left of the trachea. For foreign bodies lodged at or cranial to the heart base, a right 3rd or 4th intercostal thoracotomy provides the best exposure of the oesophagus. For foreign bodies lodged caudal to the heart base, a left 8th intercostal thoracotomy is used. Foreign bodies in the distal oesophagus can sometimes be retrieved by manipulation through a gastrotomy incision. The foreign body is located by palpation. Fish hooks can be difficult to feel in the thoracic oesophagus and occasionally an assistant must locate the hook using an endoscope per os while the thorax is open. A longitudinal oesophagotomy is performed. The oesophageal wall opposite the incision is checked for perforation and the incision is closed with a single layer of interrupted, appositional sutures. The authors prefer 3/0 or 4/0 monofilament suture material. The oesophagus lacks a serosal covering, necessitating careful apposition of the oesophageal layers to prevent dehiscence. Factors inherent in oesophageal surgery which may predispose to dehiscence are impairment of its intramural blood supply, tension and motion at the anastomosis site, lack of omentum, general debilitation of the patient and movement of food and saliva across the oesophageal anastomosis. All tissues must be handled extremely gently. The areas are lavaged thoroughly. Omental, diaphragmatic and pericardial grafts have been used to reinforce the anastomosis. Adequate nutrition is vital to wound healing and the ability to fight infection. In the nutritionally compromised patient, consideration should be given to the insertion of a gastrostomy tube (for feeding) via a flank laparotomy at the time of oesophageal surgery.

After uncomplicated endoscopic foreign body removal, animals are held off food for at least 24 hours, then fed a small amount of soft food or a slurry. The major complication is mediastinitis, due to oesophageal perforation and is manifested by fever, reluctance to eat and widening of the mediastinum on a dorsoventral thoracic radiograph. The diagnosis is confirmed by repeat oesophagoscopy or a contrast oesophagram using a water-soluble iodinated contrast agent. Surgical repair of the perforation and thoracic drainage via chest tubes are indicated.

Oesophageal perforation may occur as a sequel to chronic foreign body obstruction, ingestion of a sharp foreign body or foreign body removal, direct cervical or thoracic trauma, penetrating bite wounds or oesophagoscopy. Clinical signs of obstruction may or may not be present. Pleuritis, mediastinitis, abscessation, broncho-oesophageal fistulation or cervical cellulitis may occur. Perforation should be suspected in patients with a history of oesophageal obstruction and depression, fever, elevated white blood cell count, cough, dyspnoea, or a cervical soft tissue swelling. Diagnosis is by oesophagoscopy or contrast radiography using soluble iodine based agents. Treatment is initially aimed at stabilizing the potentially septic patient with volume support and intravenous broad-spectrum bactericidal antibiotics. Leakage of the cervical oesophagus is treated by establishing drainage, controlling the infection and repairing the oesophagus. Thoracic oesophageal perforation requires exploratory thoracotomy, removal of infected debris and repair of the damaged area. The chest cavity is thoroughly lavaged and drained via chest tubes.

Megaoesophagus is a general term for the clinical sign of oesophageal dilation. Megaoesophagus has been classified as congenital idiopathic, adult onset idiopathic and secondary acquired. Idiopathic megaoesophagus is inherited in the Wire-Haired Fox Terrier and the Miniature Schnauzer. German Shepherd Dogs, Great Danes, Irish Setters and Siamese cats are also predisposed. No clear sex predilection is evident. The cause and site of the neuromuscular lesion are unknown. Clinical signs include regurgitation, poor body condition and signs of pneumonia. Regurgitation may occur immediately after eating or may be delayed. Megaoesophagus must be differentiated from other causes of regurgitation, vomiting and aspiration pneumonia. In young dogs, vascular ring anomalies are frequent causes of oesophageal dilation. Oesophageal diverticula also occur occasionally. Survey radiographs may establish the diagnosis, although mild oesophageal dilation may not be visible on plain films. The radiographs should also be examined carefully for evidence of aspiration pneumonia. Contrast fluoroscopy provides a definitive diagnosis. Once the diagnosis of megaoesophagus is made, possible underlying causes should be investigated, as the diagnosis of idiopathic megaoesophagus is only made by exclusion. Secondary megaoesophagus has been associated with many different diseases. Any abnormality of the oesophageal muscles (myositis, myopathy) or the neurological pathways controlling oesophageal motility could result in megaoesophagus. Additionally, toxins such as lead, autoimmune and endocrine conditions, foreign bodies, infections and neoplasia have been associated with megaoesophagus.

Treatment involves feeding affected animals small frequent meals from a height and maintaining them in a vertical position for some time after feeding. Individual animals may respond better to different food consistencies. In severe cases in which the animal is very debilitated, a gastrotomy feeding tube may be surgically or endoscopically placed, to provide nutritional support to the animal. In secondary megaoesophagus, the primary cause should be treated, if possible. The prognosis depends on the cause of the megaoesophagus and the age of onset of the clinical signs. In general, congenital megaoesophagus has a better prognosis than adult onset megaoesophagus, although reports document recovery from both conditions.

Oesophageal strictures are almost always acquired lesions resulting from oesophageal foreign bodies, trauma, oesophageal surgery and, most commonly, reflux oesophagitis. The last is believed to occur secondary to reflux of gastric contents which produces epithelial erosion, then ulceration, resulting in stricture formation. Alkalis (i.e. pancreatic secretions) and bile are more damaging to the oesophagus than gastric acid. The deeper the ulceration, the more severe the stricture. The reflux almost always occurs with the animal under general anaesthesia in dorsal recumbency. At this time protective reflexes such as swallowing and secondary peristalsis are abolished by anaesthesia. Strictures are seen within 1–8 weeks.

Clinically, affected animals show a gradually increasing difficulty with solid food, progressing to an inability to retain anything but liquid food. There may be weight loss in long standing cases and the potential for aspiration pneumonia always exists. Some animals may be depressed, febrile or salivate excessively. The diagnosis is made by barium contrast fluoroscopy and oesophagoscopy.

The most successful means of treatment is conservative: balloon dilation of the stricture followed by prednisolone to minimize stricture reformation. An angiographic guide wire is passed beyond the stricture under fluoroscopic guidance. A polyethylene balloon dilating catheter with the balloon deflated is passed over the guidewire. Balloon size is based on normal oesophageal lumen size and the diameter of the stricture. The balloon is slowly filled and the stricture (seen as an 'hourglass' indentation in the balloon) is observed under fluoroscopy. Upon completion of the dilation, the oesophageal mucosa should be examined endoscopically for signs of damage. It is important to prevent repeat scarring after stricture dilation. Prednisolone is given at 1 mg/kg initially then in a gradually diminishing dose over 4 weeks to prevent new collagen formation.

Vascular ring anomalies cause regurgitation in puppies, beginning shortly after weaning. Persistent right fourth aortic arch (PRAA) is the most common anomaly. Normally, the embryological branchial arch system develops so that the left fourth arch becomes the dorsal aorta located to the left of both the trachea and oesophagus. In animals with a functional right fourth arch and a normal left ductus arteriosus (6th branchial arch), the oesophagus is trapped between the heart base, pulmonary artery, and the abnormally positioned right aortic arch. German Shepherds, Irish Setters, Weimaraners and Siamese and Persian cats are predisposed. Regurgitation occurs immediately on weaning and beginning solid food intake. Physical condition and prognosis worsen when correction is delayed. The diagnosis is made by a barium oesophagram. Typically, the oesophagus is grossly enlarged cranial to the heart base and narrows considerably at the heart base. Treatment involves ligation and division of the left ligamentum arteriosum via a left 4th intercostal space thoracotomy. Prognosis ranges from good to poor depending on the severity of oesophageal dilation and presence of aspiration pneumonia. Postoperatively, animals are fed from an elevated platform to utilize gravity in the passage of food into the stomach.

STOMACH

Gastric dilatation/volvulus (GDV) is a range of syndromes varying from severe gastric distension without volvulus, to volvulus without distension. Massive distension of the stomach with swallowed food or air results in obstruction of the portal vein and caudal vena cava. Decreased venous return from these vessels results in severely decreased cardiac output and poor tissue perfusion. Ischaemia affects the heart, resulting in arrhythmias, and the stomach, causing necrosis in severe cases. Many GDV dogs have disseminated intravascular coagulation (DIC) and are endotoxaemic.

Resuscitation with shock doses of crystalloids (or initially hypertonic saline/dextran: 5 ml/kg slowly i.v.) prior to anaesthesia and surgery is vital. Additional therapies, such as corticosteroids, flunixin meglumine and desferrioxamine have not been proven to have clinical benefits. Once fluid resuscitation is underway, the stomach is decompressed by carefully passing an orogastric tube or, if this is not possible, gastric trocharization. Radiographs, including a right lateral view, are made to differentiate dilatation from volvulus. On a right lateral view, the pylorus will appear gas filled and dorsal to the rest of the stomach in most dogs with a volvulus (Figure 9.7).

The GDV patient should be anaesthetized with great care (see Chapter 18). At surgery, the stomach is decompressed, derotated, and replaced in a normal position. In most dogs, the pylorus rotates from its normal position on the right side of the abdomen, passing between the fundus of the stomach and the ventral body wall to end up either on the left side of the abdomen (180° volvulus), dorsal to the rest of the stomach (270° volvulus) or towards the right side of the abdomen (360° volvulus). The surgeon, standing on the right side of the dog, locates the duodenum and traces it to the pylorus. The pylorus is then gently pulled back into a normal position with one hand, while the other hand gently pushes the remainder of the stomach dorsally to facilitate derotation. The spleen is exteriorized and examined for viability, venous or arterial thrombosis, and short gastric vessel rupture. A splenectomy is performed, if necessary. The remainder of the abdomen is explored and then the stomach is re-examined for necrosis, particularly along the greater curvature. As a guide, areas of the stomach which are discoloured dark

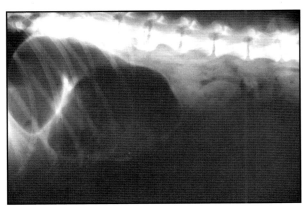

Figure 9.7: Right lateral radiograph of a dog with gastric dilatation/volvulus (GDV), showing the gas filled pylorus dorsal to the stomach. In a right lateral view, the pylorus in a normal dog should be on the down side and hence filled with fluid and not visible. In a dog with a GDV, the pylorus is displaced to the left side and so is often filled with gas and clearly visible on a right lateral view.

purple or grey/green, feel paper thin or do not bleed when incised, must be removed. If there is doubt concerning the viability of an area it should be removed, using either a stapling device or manual resection and suturing. A permanent gastropexy is performed to attach the antrum to the body wall. The authors use a tube gastropexy to allow for postoperative gastric decompression, but at least seven other 'pexy' techniques are described. The abdomen is copiously lavaged and closed.

Postoperatively, GDV patients require intensive care and monitoring. The rate of intravenous fluid administration is based on an assessment of perfusion. Tissue perfusion is estimated from clinical examination, blood pressure and urine output measurements and laboratory parameters. Cardiac arrhythmias often develop in the first 24–48 hours after surgery. They are not necessarily associated with a poor prognosis as previously thought. Antiarrhythmic therapy is given if the arrhythmias are associated with poor cardiac output (subjectively assessed from mucous membrane colour, heart rate and arterial blood pressure) or severe electrical disturbance (frequent 'R on T' phenomena). An infusion of lignocaine is started (50–80 µg/kg/min) and a bolus of 1–2 mg/kg is administered to convert the arrhythmia to sinus rhythm.

Most gastric foreign bodies are not true surgical emergencies. However, needles should be removed as soon as possible to prevent migration or perforation. In most cases, this is readily accomplished using a flexible endoscope.

Occasionally, severe gastric ulceration and bleeding can be successfully treated surgically. Gastric ulceration and haemorrhage is associated with gastric neoplasia, mast cell tumours, gastrinomas, and exogenous corticosteroids. Severe haemorrhage also occurs frequently after non-steroidal anti-inflammatory medication. Surgery is considered for those cases with massive bleeding in which medical therapy fails. The animal is

stabilized with transfusions of packed red blood cells and plasma. Rapid endoscopy is useful to differentiate focal from diffuse gastric haemorrhage. The peritoneal cavity is explored, a large gastrotomy incision made and the stomach mucosa examined. Focal bleeding ulcers are resected.

SMALL INTESTINE

Foreign bodies are the most common small intestinal condition requiring emergency surgery. The clinical signs, degree of dehydration and electrolyte and acid–base imbalance vary with the location, duration and severity of the obstruction. Many foreign bodies can be detected on abdominal palpation. Plain and sometimes contrast radiographs are useful in making a diagnosis of obstruction. The classic sign of mechanical obstruction is the presence of multiple loops of gas-dilated small intestine of various diameters. Contrast radiography is sometimes needed to confirm the diagnosis. Most proximal small intestinal obstructions will be evident within 6 hours of administration of the barium suspension, but more distal small intestinal obstructions may require a 24-hour study for effective diagnosis. Prophylactic antibiotics are given before surgery if peritoneal contamination is anticipated. Surgery involves a thorough, sequential examination of the entire gastrointestinal tract. The affected area is packed off from the remainder of the peritoneal cavity with moistened laparotomy sponges. When the bowel is healthy, the foreign body is removed through an incision made in the antimesenteric border immediately distal to the foreign body. This ensures that the suture line is placed in healthy bowel. The enterotomy is closed with single interrupted appositional sutures; 3/0 polydioxanone (PDS) is used in medium and large dogs and 4/0 PDS in small dogs and cats. In cases where the bowel is of questionable viability, a generous area of small intestine is resected and an end-to-end anastomosis is performed. The area can be 'reinforced' by omental wrapping or serosal patching.

Linear foreign bodies pose some specific challenges. The clinician must examine the tongue carefully. The authors have seen several cases in which the string cut through the lingual frenulum, which subsequently healed. At laparotomy, the plicated area of bowel should be isolated from the peritoneal cavity before cutting the 'anchor' under the tongue; mesenteric areas of the plicated bowel can be perforated but may be prevented from leaking until the tension on the string is released and the plications relax. The entire length of string is removed, necessitating multiple enterotomies. Large sections of the intestine may have multiple mesenteric perforations, necessitating resection and anastomosis.

Intussusceptions are common in youngeranimals. Although a cause is often not apparent, all affected animals should be treated for intestinal parasites. At surgery, gentle traction on the intussusceptum and pressure on the intussuscipiens aids reduction. Resection and anastomosis are required in cases in which the lesion cannot be reduced or if the involved bowel is necrotic. This often means apposing bowel segments with different lumen diameters, as the majority of intussusceptions involve the ileocolic junction. This can be managed by an incision on the antimesenteric surface of the smaller bowel loop or oversewing of the larger bowel loop.

Small intestinal neoplasms are rarely true emergencies; however, when they cause obstruction, haemorrhage or intestinal rupture, immediate surgical intervention is warranted. Thoracic radiographs should be made before surgery to check for metastatic disease if neoplasia is suspected. Similarly, the abdominal contents, especially the liver and regional lymph nodes, should be carefully examined during the exploratory laparotomy. Intestinal neoplasms are removed by resection and anastomosis, with generous margins. Enlarged lymph nodes are removed or biopsied.

Mesenteric torsion is rare in dogs. The root of the mesentery twists, completely occluding the mesenteric veins and partially to completely occluding the mesenteric arteries. The intestinal mucosa is rapidly compromised, allowing bacteria and endotoxins to translocate into the peritoneal cavity and systemic circulation. Animals present with a peracute abdominal crisis and cardiovascular collapse. Within hours, the abdomen becomes markedly distended by gas-filled intestinal loops, which are obvious on survey abdominal radiographs. Treatment includes rapid fluid resuscitation and immediate surgery to reduce the twisted mesenteric root. Unless recognition and treatment of the condition is immediate, the prognosis for recovery is grave.

LARGE INTESTINE

Isolated large intestinal disease associated with an acute abdominal crisis is uncommon. More often, the large intestinal disease is associated with concurrent small intestinal disease, such as viral gastroenteritis, severe parasitism or viral infections. Surgical emergencies of the colon are uncommon, but include obstruction, perforation and haemorrhage. Perforation of the colon is a true emergency because of the high colonic bacterial content. Untreated, colonic perforations are rapidly fatal. Perforation occurs secondary to trauma (e.g. gunshot), rupture of colonic neoplasms or, rarely, from foreign bodies. Perforation has also been associated with corticosteroid administration in animals with intervertebral disc prolapse. The diagnosis is initially one of peritonitis, based on the clinical signs of shock, abdominal distension and pain, and a peritoneal tap or lavage showing severe peritonitis, with degenerating neutrophils and intracellular bacteria. Emergency fluid

resuscitation, antibiotics, and laparotomy are indicated. At surgery, the peritoneal cavity is explored, the affected area of bowel packed off with moistened laparotomy sponges and the peritoneal cavity lavaged to remove gross debris and contamination. The affected area of colon is packed off and either debrided and sutured or resected. Treatment for peritonitis is discussed later in this chapter.

Severe colonic obstruction occurs secondary to intussusception or neoplasia. Surgical treatment involves reducing the intussusception. In situations where this is not possible, the affected area of bowel is resected and the ends anastomosed. This often involves resection of the ileum and anastomosing a jejunal segment of small diameter to a colonic segment of large diameter. To equalize the lumen sizes, part of the colonic segment is oversewn with a single interrupted Lembert suture pattern to slightly invert the colonic mucosa, and the antimesenteric border of the jejunum is incised to widen its lumen. The ends are anastomosed with a single layer of single interrupted appositional sutures (Figure 9.8). The authors prefer 3/0 synthetic absorbable monofilament suture for dogs and 4/0 for cats. Colonic neoplasms are removed by resecting and anastomosing the affected area. The sample is submitted for histopathology, with particular emphasis placed on the margins of the resection. The local lymph nodes are carefully inspected and biopsied to rule out possible metastatic disease.

Rectal perforation occasionally occurs secondary to trauma or foreign bodies. The rectum should be carefully evaluated by digital and proctoscopic examination in any animal with a gunshot wound in the pelvic area. A dorsal approach (an inverted U-shaped incision from one ischial tuberosity to the other, passing dorsal to the anus) is used for exposure of caudal rectal lesions and a ventral approach using a pelvic symphysiotomy or pubic flap is used for more cranial lesions. The affected area is debrided and sutured or resected and the rectal end anastomosed. The abdomen is explored and lavaged if there is any suspicion of contamination of

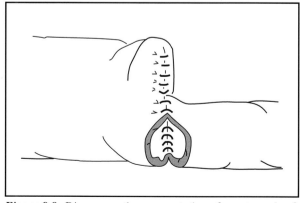

Figure 9.8: *Diagrammatic representation of anastomosis of the small intestine to the large intestine. The large intestine has been oversewn so that its lumen approximates the size of the small intestine. The front is still to be sutured.*

the peritoneal cavity. If the perforation is secondary to a gunshot or arrow injury, the entire tract of the penetrating wound is explored, debrided and lavaged.

Rectal prolapse occurs most frequently in young parasitized animals. It can also occur secondary to other conditions which cause tenesmus, such as perineal hernia, prostatic disease and colitis. It is important to differentiate simple rectal prolapse from small or large intestinal intussusception with prolapse. With rectal prolapse, a blunt lubricated probe will not pass into a 'lumen' because the prolapsed tissue converges with the mucocutaneous junction of the anus. The viability of the prolapsed tissue should be assessed carefully. In simple cases with viable rectum, the prolapse is reduced digitally with the animal under general anaesthesia. A purse string suture is placed, avoiding the anal sacs and ducts and tied loosely to allow the passage of soft faeces. An epidural anaesthetic (2% lignocaine, 1 ml/5 kg) reduces immediate postoperative straining. In cases in which manual reduction is difficult or has failed and in which the tissue is viable, a colopexy is performed using a caudal midline approach to the abdomen. The prolapse is reduced by gentle traction on the colon, and the colon is sutured to the transverse abdominus muscle to maintain reduction. Rectal amputation is required in prolapse cases with necrotic rectal tissue. The animal is placed on a well padded rectal stand, with the area around the prolapse clipped and prepared for aseptic surgery. Two stay sutures may be placed through all layers of the prolapse, one dorsally and one ventrally, cranial to the level of proposed resection. The dorsal half of the prolapsed rectum is incised 180° and the outer and inner layers of the prolapse identified and anastomosed with single interrupted 3/0 monofilament absorbable sutures, spaced 2–3 mm apart. The ventral half is then incised and sutured in a similar manner. The anastomosis is carefully checked, the stay sutures are removed and the anastomosis is replaced in the pelvic canal.

PANCREAS

Acute pancreatitis is a common condition associated with an acute abdominal crisis in the dog. Pancreatic enzymes, usually stored within the gland as inactive zymogen granules, are activated and begin to damage the pancreas and surrounding tissue. The severity of pancreatitis varies substantially. Mild episodes are associated with oedematous pancreatitis, while more severe pancreatic inflammation results in haemorrhage and necrosis, with activation of many systemic inflammatory cascades, leading to a 'septic' or 'systemic inflammatory response' state. Potential causes of pancreatitis include diet change, hyperlipidaemia, some drugs (frusemide, azathioprine, L-asparaginase and tetracyclines), hypotension during general anaesthesia and pancreatic ischaemia or trauma secondary to surgical manipulations.

Clinical signs of pancreatitis are unfortunately non-specific and include depression, anorexia, abdominal pain, vomiting and diarrhoea. Signs vary widely and may not initially reflect the potential severity of the disease. Animals may be mildly to severely dehydrated on presentation, with mild or severe abdominal discomfort. In some cases a cranial abdominal mass (the enlarged pancreas) is palpated; in others, an effusion is suspected on abdominal palpation. Animals are often obese and may have a history of similar episodes in the past. They may have recently ingested a large or fatty meal.

Definitive diagnosis of pancreatitis is difficult. The plain radiographic signs of pancreatitis have been described above. Ultrasound is increasingly used to evaluate the abdomen in cases in which pancreatitis is suspected. The inflamed pancreas has a non-homogenous appearance, with variable hypoechoic areas in the parenchyma. Large hypoechoic areas can represent developing pseudocysts or abscesses. Computed tomography is the modality used most frequently to image the pancreas in humans.

On haematology evaluation, neutrophilia or severe neutropenia may be present. Severe hyperlipidaemia may be present in the serum of some animals with pancreatitis; grossly, the serum appears milky. It is important to remember that hyperlipidaemia prevents accurate determination of serum biochemical values. Serum alkaline phosphatase and alanine transaminase values are often elevated, because of cholestasis and hepatic damage caused by ischaemia or toxins from the inflamed pancreas in the portal blood. Azotaemia may be present, often secondary to dehydration, but sometimes associated with acute renal failure. Serum amylase and lipase activities may be increased, but these enzymes are also produced by extra pancreatic tissue and their elevations may be transient. Decreased clearance of amylase and lipase occur secondary to renal failure or poor renal perfusion. Serum trypsin-like immunoreactivity (TLI) tends to increase early and then decrease sooner than other enzymes. If an effusion is apparent on radiographs or ultrasound scans, samples should be obtained by paracentesis. Samples are submitted for amylase and lipase determinations and examined for cytological evidence of peritonitis.

The cornerstones of pancreatitis treatment are maintaining fluid and electrolyte balance and withholding food. Fluids should be administered intravenously. Ideally, a central venous line should be placed in the jugular vein, allowing for fluid administration, blood sampling, monitoring of central venous pressure and administering total parenteral nutrition, if required. Fluid choice and electrolyte supplementation should be guided by serial monitoring of electrolytes and acid-base status. Parenteral antibiotics (enrofloxacin, trimethoprim sulphadiazine) are given to animals that are febrile or have toxic changes on their haemogram. Plasma is increasingly being administered to animals with pancreatitis. It provides colloid osmotic pressure support and acute phase proteins such as α-macroglobulin, which bind circulating activated proteases released from the inflamed pancreas. The bound proteases/macroglobulin complexes are then cleared from the plasma by the reticuloendothelial system. Experimentally, once the α-macroglobulin binding capacity is exceeded, free circulating proteases activate the inflammatory, coagulation and fibrinolytic cascades, and rapid death ensues. Other colloid solutions (Dextran 70, Hetastarch) are administered to provide oncotic support and improve pancreatic microcirculation. Controversial treatments for pancreatitis include gastric suctioning via a nasogastric tube, anti-secretory therapy (atropine, somatostatin or its analogues), enteral feeding, free radical scavengers and peritoneal lavage.

Emergency surgery of the pancreas is usually limited to abscess drainage or removal. Abscesses are diagnosed by ultrasonographic evaluation of the pancreas. They appear as large hypoechoic areas within the inflamed pancreas and are an indication for surgical exploration. The surgeon should be thoroughly familiar with the anatomy of the pancreas, its blood supply and the pancreatic and common bile ducts to avoid damaging vessels supplying the duodenum and stomach, the pancreatic papillae or the common bile duct. If the abscess is thick-walled and well delineated, it may be treated by closed-suction drainage. A balloon catheter (such as a Foley) is placed through the body wall and into the abscess cavity. The abscess cavity is thoroughly drained and flushed repeatedly at surgery. The abscess is then drained for 5–10 days, postoperatively. Alternatively, the affected area of the pancreas is removed. This is often a difficult, technically exacting surgery. The abdomen is generously lavaged with warm, balanced electrolyte solution. Open peritoneal drainage is preferred in cases with severe peritonitis associated with the pancreatitis (see Peritonitis, below).

UTERUS

Pyometra describes a pus-filled uterus and is a disease of the dioestrus phase of the ovarian cycle. During this phase, the corpus luteum is actively secreting progesterone, which increases the secretions of the uterine glands, inhibits myometrial contraction and maintains closure of the cervix. Short-term progestational compounds (megoestrol acetate) can also lead to pyometra if given when endogenous oestrogen concentrations are high. Long acting progestational compounds (medroxyprogesterone) administered to intact animals can cause an environment sufficient for the formation of pyometra regardless of the phase of oestrus.

Pyometra should be considered in any ill dioestral bitch or queen and occurs within 4–8 weeks of the last oestrus. The type and severity of the clinical signs depend on the patency of the cervix and the duration of the illness. Vaginal discharge may not be present if the cervix is closed. An enlarged uterus may be found on abdominal palpation, but care must be taken to avoid rupturing a distended uterus. Laboratory findings are not pathognomonic for pyometra, but total leucocyte count is often greater than 15,000 cells/mm^3 and a degenerative left shift is common. On survey abdominal radiographs, homologous tubular structures of fluid density may be seen in the caudal abdomen. Ultrasonography is useful for determining the presence of fluid in a uterus that leaves no visible uterine silhouette on survey radiographs. Although 30% of dogs with pyometra have urinary tract infection, cystocentesis is not performed prior to treatment for fear of lacerating the friable uterus and causing contamination of the peritoneal cavity.

The usual treatment for pyometra is ovariohysterectomy. Corrective therapy for fluid deficits, acidosis and sepsis is started before surgery and is continued, as needed, during and after surgery. The standard triple clamp technique at the cranial cervix with individual ligation of the uterine arteries is the recommended method for handling the uterine body. The uterus is isolated from the abdomen with laparotomy sponges before it is severed to prevent abdominal contamination. The small amount of exposed uterine stump is lavaged to remove residual purulent material. If the cervix is greatly distended a Parker–Kerr oversew may be necessary. If the uterus has ruptured or is torn during surgery, the abdomen is copiously lavaged and therapy for peritonitis and sepsis is initiated. *Escherichia coli* is the predominant organism cultured so appropriate antibiotic therapy can be initiated.

Medical therapy for pyometra (prostaglandin F$_2$) is reserved for valuable breeding animals with an open cervix. Systemically ill animals are not candidates for this therapy because clinical improvement is not observed for at least 48 hours after the initiation of treatment. Recurrence of pyometra is very common in dogs; therefore, breeding at the next oestrus after treatment is recommended.

Uterine torsion is uncommon in dogs and cats. One or both uterine horns can twist around the long axis or around the opposite horn, or the entire uterine body can rotate. Clinical signs are non-specific and usually include acute abdominal pain, straining as if in labour or repeated attempts to defaecate. The caudal aspect of the rotated uterus may be felt on vaginal examination. Survey radiographs often reveal a large air- or fluid-filled tubular structure. The treatment of choice is ovariohysterectomy. If the uterus is gravid, viable fetuses may be present in the normal horn and can be delivered via Caesarean section.

TESTES

Torsion of the spermatic cord is rare and is usually

associated with a retained testis in the abdominal cavity. It rarely involves an inguinal cryptorchid testis. The condition is most common in young animals, 5–10 months of age. Clinical signs of abdominal discomfort are not specific. A firm mass can usually be palpated in the abdomen and the mass is evident on survey abdominal radiographs. The presence of these signs in a cryptorchid animal should arouse suspicion. In untreated cases, the testis undergoes fibrosis or necrosis. Following destruction of the testis, spontaneous recovery occurs, but it is preferable to do an exploratory laparotomy and remove the affected testis.

In the case of an intra-abdominal testis, an incision is made lateral to the penis and the abdomen is opened through the linea alba. If the testis is not found near the internal ring of the inguinal canal, a search must be made for either the vas deferens near the neck of the urinary bladder or the spermatic vessels, which join the aorta and vena cava near the kidney. A standard three-clamp technique for removal of the affected testicle is recommended.

PERITONITIS

The peritoneum is a serous membrane lining the abdominal cavity and reflecting around the abdominal organs. In the normal animal, a small amount of fluid separates the parietal and visceral peritoneal layers and decreases friction between the abdominal contents. Fluid (or contamination) disperses rapidly throughout the peritoneal cavity. Fluid in the peritoneal space drains by diaphragmatic lymphatics to sternal and mediastinal lymph nodes and the thoracic duct.

Peritonitis is defined as any inflammatory process involving the peritoneum. In most cases, peritonitis occurs as a sequela of another disease process and can be aseptic or septic. Aseptic peritonitis may be secondary to foreign bodies (surgical sponges), ruptured neoplasms or chemical agents such as pancreatic enzymes, bile (which can contain bacteria), urine and stomach or proximal duodenal contents, in which bacterial concentrations are low. Primary peritonitis occurs most commonly in cats with Coronavirus infection (feline infectious peritonitis; FIP).

Septic peritonitis results from bowel perforation distal to the duodenum, penetrating wounds, surgical contamination or extension of a urogenital infection (ruptured pyometra or prostatic abscess). The peritoneum is exposed to large numbers of usually Gram-negative organisms as well as chemical bowel contents. Endotoxin is liberated and produced as bacteria grow in the peritoneal exudate.

Chemical injury results in inflammation of the peritoneum. Vasodilation and increased vascular permeability initially results in loss of isotonic fluid into the peritoneal cavity. As vascular permeability increases, albumin is lost into the peritoneal space. Given the large peritoneal surface area, fluid and protein loss can be massive. Diaphragmatic lymphatics, which normally return peritoneal fluid to the systemic circulation, become overloaded and plugged with fibrin. Concurrent vomiting and diarrhoea exacerbate fluid loss. Fluid loss decreases circulating blood volume and results in decreased cardiac output and poor tissue perfusion, which in turn results in cellular hypoxia and anaerobic cellular metabolism. Cellular energy depletion causes loss of cell membrane integrity, cell death and eventually organ failure.

Different aetiological agents cause some variation in the pathophysiology of chemical peritonitis. For example, uroperitoneum rapidly causes a life-threatening hyperkalaemia. This should be initially treated by a slow intravenous injection of calcium gluconate (a functional antagonist of potassium) at a dose of 0.5 ml/kg. Although it does not lower serum potassium, it returns membrane excitability to normal for approximately 20–30 minutes. Regular insulin (1 IU/kg) and glucose (1–2 g/IU of insulin) can also be administered intravenously. Animals are often also severely acidotic. Sodium bicarbonate can be administered (1–2 mEq/kg i.v.) to correct acidosis. This can, however, paradoxically lower ionized calcium and worsen the effects of hyperkalaemia. Bile, although usually sterile, can cause permeability changes in the intestinal wall, allowing transmural bacterial migration. Gastric and pancreatic secretions are more irritating than bile and produce a rapid and severe peritonitis.

In septic peritonitis, bacteria are initially rapidly opsonized by white blood cells or absorbed by diaphragmatic lymphatics. Haemoglobin and mucus enhance the virulence of intraperitoneal organisms. Bacterial synergism, wherein the virulence of total bacterial load is greater than the sum of the individual organisms, occurs. Bacterial destruction liberates endotoxins, exotoxins and proteases. Endotoxin and cell membrane damage can both activate the arachidonic acid pathways, generating prostaglandins and leucotrienes. The complement, clotting and fibrinolytic systems are also activated. Macrophages are stimulated to release tumour necrosis factor, stimulating the release of other inflammatory cytokines. Ongoing absorption of bacteria and toxins and generation of inflammatory mediators results in sepsis or the systemic inflammatory response syndrome.

Systemically, the animal responds to these profound changes by trying to maintain perfusion to the heart and brain. Hypotension stimulates the carotid baroreceptors; subsequent inhibition of vagal tone and sympathetic stimulation increase heart rate and cause peripheral vasoconstriction. Vasoconstriction is augmented by angiotensin II, produced after hypotension-induced stimulation of the renin–angiotensin–aldosterone system. Angiotensin II stimulates aldosterone release from the adrenal cortex, resulting in sodium and water retention by the kidneys.

Peritonitis is often difficult to diagnose. The clinical signs are largely non-specific. Depression and diffuse abdominal pain are often present, to a degree greater than that usually seen following abdominal surgery or trauma. Most animals splint their abdominal wall at the slightest touch. Vomiting is also a prominent sign of peritonitis. Peritoneal inflammation often causes a paralytic ileus and intestinal dilatation, in addition to the effusion. In septic peritonitis, fever and leucocytosis are not consistent findings. Animals with peritonitis may have a leucocytosis with a left shift or a neutropenia. In uroperitoneum, elevations in BUN, serum creatinine and potassium are detected. SAP, SGPT and total bilirubin levels are elevated in cases of bile peritonitis. Abdominal radiographs may show free gas or a lack of intestinal detail and a ground glass appearance from free fluid in the abdominal cavity. Recovery and examination of peritoneal exudate is extremely valuable in the diagnosis of peritonitis. A four-quadrant tap is performed and if this does not yield fluid, peritoneal lavage should be considered. Toxic degenerative neutrophils with intracellular bacteria indicate septic peritonitis. Creatinine, potasssium and bilirubin levels may also be measured on the peritoneal exudate.

Aggressive patient stabilization is required prior to anaesthesia and surgery. Intravenous fluids are administered at shock doses. Capillary refill time, heart rate, arterial blood pressure, urine output and central venous pressure are monitored to assess the response to therapy. Plasma or synthetic colloids are often required because of the massive loss of albumin into the peritoneal cavity. The choice of fluid type and electrolyte supplementation is based on the results of sequential electrolyte and blood gas measurements.

Broad-spectrum, bactericidal antibiotics are administered intravenously as soon as the diagnosis of peritonitis is made. Antibiotics effective against Gram-positive and -negative, aerobic and anaerobic bacteria are recommended. A combination of a penicillin or cephalosporin with an aminoglycoside antibiotic can be used in animals without pre-existing renal disease. Cefazolin (20 mg/kg i.v. four times daily) should be used in preference to cephalothin, which does not reach adequate tissue levels in dogs. Gentamycin should be administered once daily at 6 mg/kg, as the single high dose is more effective and less nephrotoxic. Metronidazole (10 mg/kg orally or i.v. every 8 hours) may be added for additional anaerobic coverage. Penicillins, cephalosporins and aminoglycosides all reach intraperitoneal levels equivalent to their serum levels.

Corticosteroid administration in septic shock is controversial. Doses recommended are 15–30 mg/kg for methyl prednisolone sodium succinate and 4–6 mg/kg for dexamethasone. Theoretically, corticosteroids increase myocardial function, block formation of several pro-inflammatory mediators, stabilize lysosomal membranes and prevent complement activation. However, in some human clinical studies, corticosteroid administration either failed to improve or worsened clinical outcome. In experimental studies demonstrating benefit, steroid administration was often before or immediately after bacterial challenge, a situation rarely encountered in clinical practice. Once all of the proinflammatory cascades of sepsis are activated, steroids are likely to have limited beneficial effects. Because of risks of immunosuppression and gastric ulceration, corticosteroids are now rarely used for management of septic shock.

Non-steroidal anti-inflammatory drugs (NSAIDs) are also controversial in the treatment of septic shock. Again, in experimental septic shock models demonstrating therapeutic benefit, the NSAID (aspirin, indomethacin, phenylbutazone, flunixin meglumine) was administered prior to the onset of shock. Potential side effects of NSAIDs include gastrointestinal haemorrhage (especially if administered in conjunction with corticosteroids), nephrotoxicosis and blood dyscrasias. Potential benefits include improved cardiac index, increased blood pressure, decreased microvascular damage and permeability and improved survival. The suggested dose of ibuprofen is 1 mg/kg i.v.; the suggested dose of flunixin is 1–2 mg/kg i.v. NSAIDs should not be administered to cats and are rarely used for management of canine septic shock in the author's institution.

One of the most important aspects of treating peritonitis is prompt removal of the inciting cause. While the animal should be stabilized before anaesthesia and surgery, the underlying source must be addressed to resolve the peritonitis. Exploratory laparotomy is mandatory to treat the source of the peritonitis, remove peritoneal contamination and exudate and provide a route for enteral nutrition. A large ventral midline incision is used for exposure. A complete exploratory laparotomy is performed. The source of the peritonitis is identified and isolated from the remainder of the abdomen using moistened laparotomy sponges. In animals with generalized peritoneal contamination, the authors prefer to lavage the peritoneal cavity with a large volume of warm sterile saline before proceeding with definitive treatment. The fluid is immediately aspirated from the peritoneal cavity.

Definitive treatment of peritonitis often involves resection and anastomosis of damaged bowel. Omental wrapping or serosal patching are recommended to reinforce anastomoses in the face of peritonitis. Serosal patching is a technique in which loops of healthy bowel are loosely sutured to the bowel adjacent to the anastomosis (Figure 9.9). The serosal surfaces of the healthy bowel are then in contact with the anastomosis site allowing a reinforcing fibrin seal to form.

Few animals with peritonitis will eat voluntarily and many vomit during the postoperative period, so methods for nutritional support should be considered during surgery. Placement of a gastrostomy or jejunostomy

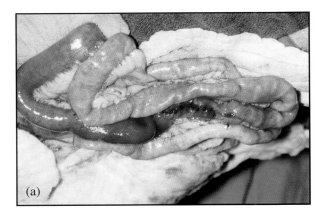

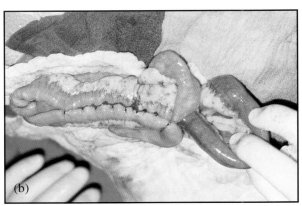

Figure 9.9: *Serosal patching. (a) Two healthy loops of small intestine are brought alongside the loop of bowel to be patched. Sutures are placed between the mesenteric side of the normal and affected intestine loops. (b) The antimesenteric surfaces of the two healthy loops of intestine are apposed with single interrupted sutures, covering the affected area with bowel. Please note: this procedure should only be performed to reinforce healthy bowel. Patching does not remove the need for accurate assessment of bowel viability and resection of unhealthy bowel.*

tube should be considered unless it interferes with the repair of leaking intestine. Enteral nutrition also improves enterocyte function, which may help minimize bacterial translocation from the intestines.

The peritoneal cavity should be thoroughly lavaged with a large volume of warm sterile balanced electrolyte solution to remove bacteria and debris. The volume of fluid required varies from 500 ml in a cat to several litres in a large dog. All lavage fluid must be aspirated. Lavage with inadequate aspiration merely spreads bacteria throughout the peritoneal cavity and sequesters them from phagocytosis.

The addition of antiseptics to the lavage fluid is controversial. Several human studies have concluded that there is no benefit to adding povidone–iodine to lavage fluid. Experimental studies have shown that 2 ml/kg of povidone–iodine (10% solution, 1% available iodine) instilled into the peritoneal cavity of dogs with peritonitis is lethal. Intraperitoneal povidone–iodine also decreases the neutrophil percentage and increases bacterial numbers in the peritoneal cavity in rats with experimental peritonitis.

The addition of antibiotics to peritoneal lavage fluid is also debated. Most studies indicate that this treatment is not beneficial in patients receiving the appropriate antibiotics parenterally. However, a recent human study indicated that the addition of tetracycline to the lavage solution completely inhibited bacterial growth in the residual peritoneal fluid.

Contamination often remains within the peritoneal cavity even after extensive debridement and lavage. The veterinarian must decide which cases require postoperative peritoneal drainage. Local peritoneal drainage is important in cases in which the inflammation is confined to a specific area of the peritoneal cavity. Drainage tubes, with or without suction, can be used in such cases; examples include prostatic and pancreatic abscesses. Ideally, drain exit points should be covered with a sterile dressing. Drainage tubes are ineffective for draining the entire peritoneal cavity, as they are rapidly sealed by fibrin and omentum. The presence of drains, which are effectively foreign bodies, resulted in increased bacterial translocation and histological inflammation in an experimental peritonitis model. Drainage of the entire peritoneal cavity is best accomplished by incompletely closing the abdominal incision. The falciform ligament is removed and the linea is sutured with a continuous monofilament suture leaving a gap of 2–4 cm between the wound edges (Figure 9.10). The wound is bandaged using a sterile dressing of petroleum jelly-impregnated gauze covered by sterile towels. This primary dressing is covered with an absorbent layer of combine material, then adhesive tape. The dressing usually requires changing every 6 hours, initially, as fluid from the peritoneum soaks through. Bandage changes are performed under sterile

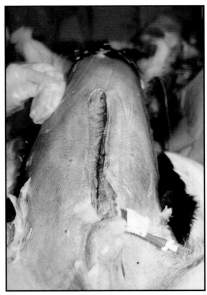

Figure 9.10: *Open peritoneal drainage. The linea alba is sutured approximately 3 cm apart with non-absorbable material. This open incision is then covered with a sterile bandage that will require changing every 6–12 hours.*

conditions with the animal sedated. Fibrous adhesions, which may entrap peritoneal exudate, are gently freed. There are no exact criteria to help the clinician judge either which cases of peritonitis require open abdominal drainage or when to close the open incision. In general, the incision is closed when drainage has decreased and the peritoneum appears grossly healthy at bandage changes. Closure should be performed as a complete laparotomy and the peritoneal cavity examined for any evidence of residual infection.

HAEMOPERITONEUM

Severe haemoperitoneum occurs most commonly due to bleeding from vascular splenic or hepatic neoplasms and from trauma injuring the spleen, liver, kidneys and great abdominal vessels. Successful management involves rapid aggressive blood volume expansion and early definitive haemorrhage control by surgical exploration. Animals presenting with haemoperitoneum have pale mucous membranes and, often, a slow capillary refill time. The heart rate is often elevated and the pulses are weak or even not palpable. The abdomen is moderately to severely distended. Rapid volume expansion is imperative. Two large-bore intravenous catheters are placed and blood is drawn for a minimum database. Intravenous fluids are started at 60–90 ml/kg in the first hour; however, if haemorrhage is not self-limiting, blood transfusion and surgical intervention will be necessary. The abdomen should be tapped. Blood from an abdominal tap in an animal with haemoperitoneum should not clot unless the spleen is inadvertently penetrated. The PCV of the abdominal blood is compared to the peripheral PCV. Often, the peripheral PCV is 10–15 points lower than that of the blood in the abdomen. If paracentesis is negative, diagnostic peritoneal lavage is performed and the lavage catheter is left in place and aspirated every 15 minutes. An increasing PCV in the returning lavage fluid indicates active haemorrhage. External pressure may be applied by wrapping a temporary, well padded bandage around the abdomen. The external tape layer of the bandage is applied tightly to generate counter pressure.

The owner should be questioned thoroughly about the possibility of trauma. If trauma was not a likely cause of the haemorrhage, neoplasia should be considered. Thoracic radiographs should be made to evaluate the lungs for possible metastases. The cardiac silhouette should also be critically evaluated for evidence of tamponade, as animals with splenic or hepatic haemangiosarcoma can have concurrent right atrial neoplasia. Evidence of pulmonary or cardiac neoplasia in animals with severe haemoperitoneum is an indication that euthanasia should be considered.

The animal is carefully monitored for the response to initial resuscitation. Mucous membrane colour, capillary refill time, heart rate, blood pressure and the PCV and TP are all evaluated every 10–15 minutes. Blood transfusions are necessary when the PCV falls rapidly below 25%. In some instances, veterinarians are reluctant to transfuse an animal with ongoing haemorrhage, reasoning that the blood they are administering is going 'straight into the abdomen.' However, transfusions are necessary in this situation to provide red cells for tissue oxygen delivery and to make the animal as stable as possible during anaesthesia and surgery. In the severely anaemic shocked animal, the blood should be administered as rapidly as possible, using a pressure bag. Autotransfusion is a lifesaving alternative when other blood products are not available. Blood from the abdomen should only be used in cases in which intra-abdominal neoplasia is not suspected. In addition, a sample of the retrieved blood should be smeared, stained and examined to rule out the possibility of contamination from a ruptured loop of intestine. Blood is retrieved from the abdomen using a large-bore, fenestrated catheter and administered through a line containing the standard 170 µm filter.

Some animals with traumatic or neoplastic abdominal haemorrhage will stabilize with initial resuscitation. However, if clinical indicators of perfusion remain poor, the PCV continues to fall or if the animal deteriorates after initially improving, emergency surgery is indicated. Anaesthetic agents with minimal cardiovascular depression are used, the surgery room and instruments are prepared, then the abdominal bandage is removed and the entire ventral abdomen and thorax is prepared rapidly for surgery. A large ventral midline laparotomy is performed. A hand can be placed along the left abdominal wall, cranial to the left kidney, to occlude the aorta on the dorsal midline while the blood is suctioned from the abdomen. If neoplastic disease is the suspected cause of the haemorrhage, the spleen should be exteriorized and examined immediately. Ongoing splenic haemorrhage can be controlled by rapidly isolating and ligating the splenic artery and vein. The remaining splenic vessels are then ligated and the spleen is removed. In traumatic haemoperitoneum, large laparotomy pads or skin towels are used to pack the abdomen into quadrants to facilitate identification of the bleeding site(s). The abdominal incision can be extended into a paracostal approach by cutting just caudal to the last rib or to a sternotomy if additional exposure of the liver is necessary. Severe haemorrhage from the liver often requires lobectomy of the affected lobe(s). Tears of large vessels, such as the vena cava, can initially be controlled with direct pressure, but must be clamped and sutured, subsequently.

POSTOPERATIVE MANAGEMENT OF THE ACUTE ABDOMEN

During the postoperative period, tissue perfusion is

maintained by ensuring adequate hydration. Fluid can be sequestered in or lost from the peritoneal cavity (especially in severe peritonitis treated with open peritoneal drainage) and in inflamed distended non-motile bowel loops. Fluid can also be lost through ongoing vomiting and diarrhoea. Consequently, fluid rates much higher than maintenance are often required. Indicators of tissue perfusion, including capillary refill time, skin turgor, blood pressure and urine output, are monitored. Electrolyte and acid-base balance are monitored. Plasma protein losses can also be substantial, leading to decreased plasma oncotic pressure. Supplementation of fluids with plasma or synthetic colloids may be necessary. Enteral nutrition is considered early in the postoperative period to improve enterocyte function and increase liver production of plasma proteins. Feeding through a gastrostomy tube may be contraindicated by persistent vomiting or pancreatitis. The clinician should anticipate and monitor for possible complications (see Chapter 19).

LIVER FAILURE

Liver failure is an uncommon cause of acute gastrointestinal crises in dogs and cats. Although the presentation may be one of acute crisis, the disease may be chronic with a recent acute decompensation of liver function. There are many potential causes of acute liver failure; aetiological agents include chemicals, drugs, viruses and other infectious agents and neoplasms. The most commonly reported causes include drug toxicities (adverse reactions to trimethoprim/sulphonamides and benzodiazepines), hepatic lymphosarcoma, leptospirosis and feline hepatic lipidosis. Animals may present with a history that includes lethargy, abnormal mentation, polydypsia, polyuria, vomiting and diarrhoea. On physical examination, the mucous membranes may be icteric; petechial haemorrhages, hepatomegaly and ascites may or may not be present. Venepunctures may result in excessive bleeding due to lack of clotting factor synthesis. Serum biochemical analysis should reveal low blood urea nitrogen (BUN), albumin and cholesterol concentrations and may reveal elevated bilirubin, alanine amino transferase (ALT) and alkaline phosphatase (ALP) values. Coagulation times are usually prolonged and blood ammonia concentrations may be elevated. Definitive diagnosis of the cause of liver failure requires hepatic biopsy. This must often be postponed until the animal is more stable and fresh frozen plasma is available to normalize blood clotting. Liver biopsy is performed either at exploratory laparotomy or by using a biopsy needle percutaneously.

The goals of stabilization of the animal with acute liver failure include normalizing fluid and electrolyte balance, improving colloid osmotic pressure and blood clotting ability and decreasing the concentration of ammonia and other encephalopathic substances in the blood. Animals with acute liver failure have low colloid osmotic pressures due to failure to produce albumin. Fluid resuscitation with crystalloid solutions further lowers the colloid osmotic pressure and may worsen ascites and decrease blood coagulation by diluting clotting factors in the blood. Ideally, animals with acute hepatic failure should receive fresh frozen plasma as the fluid of choice for initial volume resuscitation, since it provides volume, albumin for oncotic support and coagulation factors; however, it is often not available in sufficient quantity. Synthetic colloids can worsen coagulation and should be used with caution. If a transfusion of red blood cells is required, fresh, rather than stored, packed cells are used, as they have a lower ammonia content. Food is initially withheld to minimize intestinal ammonia production. Lactulose (0.5 mg/kg every 2–4 h) is given, by enema in vomiting animals or by mouth, once vomiting is controlled. Lactulose promotes an osmotic diarrhoea, decreasing ammonia absorption. Flumazenil, (0.01–0.02 mg/kg i.v.) a centrally-acting benzodiazepine blocking agent, may be administered to improve neurological signs in profoundly stuporous animals.

REFERENCES

King LG and Donaldson MT (1994). Acute vomiting. *Veterinary Clinics of North America* **24**, 1191.

Matz ME (1996) Acute diarrhoea — rational approach to drug therapy. *Proceedings of the Fifth International Veterinary Emergency and Critical Care Symposium*, p. 192.

CHAPTER TEN

Haematological Emergencies

Susan G. Hackner

ANAEMIA

Anaemia is defined as a decrease in the red blood cell mass, occurring due to decreased production, increased destruction (haemolysis) or loss (haemorrhage) of red blood cells. The consequences of anaemia are tissue hypoxia and, ultimately, death. Successful management depends on a systematic diagnostic approach and timely effective intervention.

Approach in the emergency situation

Anaemic patients are usually presented for progressive weakness, which may culminate in collapse. The duration of clinical signs ranges from peracute to chronic. The patient in an anaemic crisis requires rapid intervention (Figure 10.1), with an initial goal of stabilization of life-threatening emergencies. The primary survey of the emergency patient is an initial rapid assessment of vital organ systems to determine if a life-threatening situation exists. Pallor is the hallmark sign of anaemia, and should be differentiated from pallor associated with hypoperfusion by determination of perfusion parameters and the packed cell volume (PCV). Patients in an anaemic crisis are moribund or extremely depressed, with marked pallor, tachypnoea, tachycardia and bounding pulses. If the anaemia is due to severe blood loss, signs of hypoperfusion will predominate.

Venous access is achieved by placement of a large bore peripheral catheter, ideally the largest bore catheter possible, in case aggressive fluid therapy is warranted. In large dogs with evidence of hypoperfusion, two catheters may be required. Blood is collected from the catheter for a minimum data base (MDB) including a PCV and total protein (TP). Blood samples should be collected prior to initiating therapy, to avoid treatment-induced changes in laboratory parameters. In addition to the MDB, samples should include a blood smear, an in-saline agglutination test, blood typing, serum and EDTA- and citrated-plasma samples for later laboratory testing.

Following the collection of blood samples, therapy should be initiated to stabilize the patient. In severe anaemia, blood transfusion is usually required. The decision to transfuse should be based on the patient's clinical signs rather than on the PCV. Animals with

1. Primary survey

2. Establish vascular access

3. Collect pretreatment samples:
   - Minimum data base (PCV/TP)
   - Blood smear
   - EDTA plasma (for later CBC, reticulocyte count, platelet count, blood typing, immune testing)
   - Serum (for later chemistry profile and/or serological testing)
   - In-saline agglutination test, if haemolysis suspected
   - Citrated plasma, if bleeding suspected (for later coagulation testing)

4. Initiate therapy to stabilize the patient:
   - Support of airway and/or breathing, if indicated
   - Fluid therapy to maintain adequate perfusion
   - Control of haemorrhage, if present
   - Blood transfusion, if indicated

5. Secondary survey:
   - Complete history
   - Thorough physical examination

6. Diagnostic work-up (see text)

7. Specific therapy (see text)

Figure 10.1: *Emergency approach to the anaemic patient.*

chronic anaemia may tolerate remarkably low PCVs with few clinical signs. Conversely, patients acutely affected by moderate anaemia may be extremely decompensated if concurrent hypoperfusion or hypoxaemia exacerbates tissue hypoxia.

Selection of blood components should be based on the PCV and TP. If only the PCV is low, packed red blood cells should be transfused. If both the PCV and TP are low, whole blood transfusion is indicated. If only packed cells are available, synthetic colloid solutions can be used instead of plasma to provide colloidal support during resuscitation. All cats must be blood typed prior to transfusion to avoid potentially fatal transfusion reactions. As a general guide, whole blood is transfused at a dose of 20 ml/kg. A transfusion rate of

5 ml/kg/h is recommended in patients that are not in shock. In the hypovolaemic patient, this rate can be substantially increased depending on individual needs. Slower transfusion rates (1–2 ml/kg/h) are recommended in patients with significant cardiac disease, hypertension or hyperviscosity disorders. Blood transfusion is generally sufficient for the initial stabilization of the anaemic patient, unless ongoing haemorrhage is present. All patients should be closely monitored for changes in PCV and perfusion parameters following resuscitation.

Following initial stabilization, the secondary survey includes a complete history and thorough physical examination. A diagnostic plan is formulated to determine the cause of the anaemia. Following PCV/TP assessment, laboratory testing should begin with blood smear examination, a complete blood count (CBC) and a reticulocyte count.

Clinical and laboratory assessment

History and physical examination

The signalment of the animal may be informative. Young animals are more likely to have a congenital disease or blood loss due to parasites, whereas older animals are at greater risk of malignancies. The history should include a detailed enquiry into vaccines, medications, diet, travel and past illnesses. Vaccination and drug therapy may predispose to immune-mediated disease, marrow suppression or thrombopathia. Dietary indiscretion (onions, zinc) may result in haemolysis. Travel to certain locations might alert the clinician to the possibility of tick-borne disease or red cell parasites. Previous bleeding episodes should arouse suspicion of haemorrhage, and the owner should be questioned about melaena, haematuria or epistaxis. Since many anaemic cats have viral disease, detailed questions should be asked regarding serological testing and exposure to other cats.

Animals with acute onset of haemolysis or bleeding will develop clinical signs at a higher PCV than animals with gradual onset of anaemia due to decreased erythropoiesis. Physical examination should include a thorough search for any evidence of haemorrhage: evaluation of the body cavities, examination of the skin, mucous membranes and joints, as well as rectal and fundic examinations. The clinician should also actively seek evidence of neoplasia, infectious disease or immune-mediated disease (arthritis, uveitis, glomerulonephritis or cutaneous lesions). Icterus may be due to haemolysis or to hepatic or biliary disease. Splenomegaly may be due to haemolysis, neoplasia, infectious disease or extramedullary haematopoiesis. Fever may result from infectious disease, neoplasia or acute haemolysis.

PCV and TP

A decreased PCV confirms anaemia. Typically, a decreased TP suggests blood loss, whereas a normal TP suggests haemolysis or decreased red cell production. With acute blood loss (for example following trauma), the PCV may be normal or increased due to splenic contraction and because fluid shifts have not yet occurred. In these patients a decreased TP is an important clue to active haemorrhage. The plasma should be examined for evidence of haemolysis or icterus.

Blood smear examination

Blood smear examination is probably the single most useful tool in evaluating anaemia. It permits evaluation of the regenerative response and frequently indicates the cause of the anaemia (Figure 10.2). If the anaemia is judged to be non-regenerative, erythrocyte morphology may indicate an aetiology (e.g. iron deficiency). If haemolysis is suspected, erythrocytes may show toxic damage (Heinz bodies, eccentrocytes), immune-mediated destruction (spherocytes), physical damage (schizocytes) or parasites.

If the patient is bleeding, smear examination is vital to rapidly assess platelet numbers and morphology. In addition, evaluation of leucocytes is informative with regard to white cell numbers and proportions and may indicate the presence of a left shift, morphological/neoplastic changes or parasites. Approximately 18–51 leucocytes per x10 objective field indicates a normal count.

Complete blood count

The CBC determines absolute cell numbers and red cell parameters. Cell types are distinguished based on a size threshold. In cats, there is often considerable overlap between erythrocyte and platelet volumes, and automated cell counters cannot resolve the cells into two distinct populations, resulting in inaccuracy of automated platelet counts.

Reticulocyte count

A reticulocyte count should be performed in all anaemic patients, providing accurate quantitation of the regenerative response. Reticulocyte counts are performed by staining blood with a vital stain that allows visualization of ribosomes. Usually, a few drops of blood are mixed with an equal volume of 0.5% new methylene blue in physiological saline, 1000 red blood cells are counted and the percentage of reticulocytes is recorded.

Reticulocyte counting is simple in the dog, as there is essentially only one type of reticulocyte. The cat, however, has two types of reticulocytes: aggregate reticulocytes, in which the organelles are coalesced into aggregates; and punctate reticulocytes, in which the organelles are present as small particles. Aggregate forms are released from the marrow and, after approximately 12 hours, develop into punctate forms that persist in the circulation for 10–12 days. Aggregate forms therefore indicate active regeneration, whereas punctate forms indicate recent, cumulative regeneration.

Abnormality	Interpretation
Polychromasia	Regeneration
Macrocytosis	Regeneration; dyserythropoiesis; FeLV infection; breed-associated (Poodles)
Microcytosis	Iron deficiency; copper deficiency; portosystemic shunt; breed-associated (Akitas)
Hypochromia	Iron deficiency; copper deficiency
Nucleated red blood cells	Regeneration; lead toxicity; splenic disease; haemangiosarcoma; corticosteroid therapy; systemic stress (cats)
Spherocytosis	Immune-mediated haemolytic anaemia; other haemolytic anaemias
Schizocytosis	Microangiopathy (haemangiosarcoma; disseminated intravascular coagulation; dirofilariasis; myelofibrosis; glomerulonephritis)
Heinz bodies	Oxidative red cell injury; may be normal in cats
Eccentrocytosis	Onion toxicity
Codocytosis	Iron deficiency; hepatic disease; post-splenectomy
Parasitic inclusions	Babesiosis, haemobartonellosis, distemper inclusion bodies

Figure 10.2: Common erythrocyte abnormalities observed on blood smear examination.

Since punctate forms are not recognizable on routine staining, the degree of regeneration may be underestimated in cats. If both forms are counted and not distinguished, active regeneration may be overestimated.

The degree of reticulocytosis must be interpreted relative to the degree of anaemia, by calculation of the absolute reticulocyte count (numbers/µl of blood) or a corrected reticulocyte count (%). In dogs, an absolute reticulocyte count >60,000 per µl is evidence of regeneration. In cats, >50,000 aggregate reticulocytes/µl is considered regenerative. The corrected reticulocyte count is calculated by the formula: corrected reticulocyte % = (observed reticulocyte count) x (PCV of the patient/mean normal PCV). Mean normal PCV is 45% for the dog and 37% for the cat. A corrected reticulocyte count above 1% indicates active erythropoiesis.

Saline agglutination test

Evaluation for autoagglutination is performed by mixing a drop of blood with an equal or greater volume of saline on a glass slide. Microscopic evaluation of a fresh wet mount will allow detection of microagglutination and differentiation from rouleau formation. Autoagglutination, if present, should persist following a procedure of washing the cells three times in saline. Convincing agglutination is evidence of immune-mediated haemolytic anaemia, but is present in only a small percentage of cases.

Diagnostic approach

The essential first step of diagnosis in the anaemic patient is to determine the mechanism of the anaemia: decreased erythropoiesis, haemolysis or haemorrhage (Figure 10.3).

Regenerative versus non-regenerative

First, it is important to determine whether the anaemia is regenerative or non-regenerative by performing a reticulocyte count or, in the emergency setting, examination of a blood smear. On a routinely stained smear, reticulocytes (the only reliable indicator of regeneration) are seen as larger, more basophilic erythrocytes, resulting in anisocytosis and polychromasia (Figure 10.4). Nucleated red blood cells are not a reliable indicator of erythroid hyperplasia, as they may be present in numerous conditions in spite of a quiescent marrow (e.g. lead toxicity, splenic disease and haemangiosarcoma).

In general, regeneration indicates either haemolysis or haemorrhage, and the absence of regeneration suggests decreased erythropoiesis. There are three important exceptions: (1) acute haemorrhage or haemolysis of less than 2–4 days' duration, as there has been insufficient time for bone marrow response; (2) concomitant disease that precludes an appropriate bone marrow response, e.g. renal failure; and (3) immune-mediated haemolytic anaemia where the immune response is targeted to the red cell precursors (Figure 10.5). Therefore, if the anaemia is regenerative, the next step is to determine if it is due to haemolysis or haemorrhage. If the anaemia is non-regenerative, decreased erythropoiesis should not be assumed.

Haemolysis versus haemorrhage

Several clinical clues are available to differentiate haemolysis from haemorrhage (Figure 10.6). Blood loss is not always obvious, so a careful search must be made for evidence of haemorrhage. In some patients, haemorrhage and haemolysis occur simultaneously.

Haemolysis

Antibody mediated:
    Immune-mediated haemolytic anaemia
    Neonatal isoerythrolysis
    Transfusion reaction

Toxic:
    Zinc toxicity
    Oxidative injury (onions, paracetamol (acetaminophen),
    propylthiouracil, methylene blue, DL-methionine, lead,
    cephalosporins, fenbendazole, dapsone, gold salts,
    phenacetin, modified live virus vaccine)

Infectious:
    Erythroparasites
        Babesiosis (*Babesia canis, B. gibsoni*)
        Haemobartonellosis (*Haemobartonella canis, H. felis*)
        Cytauxoonosis (*Cytauxoon felis*)
        Ehrlichiosis (*Ehrlichia canis*)
    Viral
        Feline leukaemia virus
        Feline immunodeficiency virus

Microangiopathic:
    Disseminated intravascular coagulation
    Splenic torsion
    Haemangiosarcoma
    Vena caval syndrome

Congenital:
    Pyruvate kinase deficiency (Basenji, Beagle, West Highland
    White Terrier, Abyssinian cats)
    Phosphofructokinase deficiency (English Springer Spaniel,
    American Cocker Spaniel)
    Congenital porphyria
    NADH methaemoglobin reductase deficiency
    Vitamin B$_{12}$ deficiency (Giant Schnauzer)

Miscellaneous:
    Hypophosphataemia
    Copper toxicosis
    Snake bites

Haemorrhage

Trauma/surgery
    Bleeding disorders
    Ectoparasites
    Gastrointestinal (endoparasites, ulceration, neoplasm)
    Neoplasia (haemangiosarcoma, others)

Decreased erythropoiesis

Extra-marrow disease:
    Anaemia of chronic disease/inflammation
    Renal failure
    Endocrine disease (hypoadrenocorticism, hypothyroidism)
    Feline leukaemia virus

Intra-marrow disease:
    Myeloaplasia
    Drug-associated (chemotherapy, oestrogen, phenylbutazone,
    griseofulvin, trimethoprim-sulphadiazine, thiacetarsamide,
    quinidine, chloramphenicol)
    Infectious (feline leukaemia virus, canine ehrlichiosis,
    parvovirus)
    Idiopathic aplastic anaemia
    Haematopoietic malignancy
    Myelodysplasia
    Myelofibrosis

Nutritional:
    Iron deficiency
    Inadequate protein intake

Figure 10.3: *Causes of anaemia.*

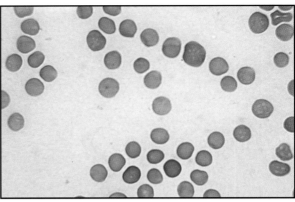

Figure 10.4: *Regenerative anaemia in a dog with immune-mediated thrombocytopenia, showing anisocytosis and polychromasia (Diff-Quik®).*

The serum protein concentration is generally normal with haemolysis and decreased with haemorrhage. There are, however, exceptions: patients with concomitant haemolysis and protein loss (e.g. protein-losing nephropathy) or those with pre-existing hyperglobulinaemia. Haemoglobinaemia and haemoglobinuria indicate haemolysis. Splenomegaly and icterus usually suggest haemolysis, but are not consistent or specific findings.

Having determined the mechanism for the anaemia, a comprehensive list of differential diagnoses can be constructed, and further diagnostic testing allows determination of the specific cause (see Figure 10.3).

Haemorrhagic anaemia

Acute haemorrhage is treated by arresting the bleeding and restoring the circulating blood volume. Internal sources of significant blood loss include: the pleural cavity, the peritoneal cavity, the retroperitoneal space, the fasciomuscular planes and the gastrointestinal tract. Large volumes of blood can accumulate in the intestines for several days before melaena becomes evident. When haemorrhage is identified without evidence of trauma, it is important to determine whether the bleeding is due to local factors or a systemic bleeding disorder, based on the history or the presence of multiple sites of bleeding. Where doubt exists, haemostasis should be tested.

Patients with chronic blood loss generally do not become emergencies until they are severely anaemic due to depletion of iron stores. Since younger animals have smaller stores, they become anaemic more readily than adults, usually from endo- and ectoparasitism. The anaemia is variably regenerative and is usually microcytic and hypochromic. Thrombocytosis may be present. Chronic blood loss is usually from the gastrointestinal tract. Even when parasites are identified in the adult, additional testing is indicated to eliminate the possibility of an additional cause of haemorrhage (e.g. neoplasia, ulceration).

Haemolytic anaemia

Haemolytic anaemia is common in dogs, often occurring acutely. Most haemolysis is extravascular, with

Regenerative	Non-regenerative
Haemolysis Haemorrhage	Decreased erythropoiesis Peracute haemolysis/haemorrhage Haemolysis/haemorrhage with concurrent disease precluding regeneration Immune-mediated destruction of erythrocyte precursors

Figure 10.5: *Regenerative versus non-regenerative anaemia.*

Clinical feature	Haemorrhage	Haemolysis
Evidence of bleeding	Common	Rare
Serum protein	Low to normal	Normal to high*
Haemoglobinaemia/uria	No	Common
Icterus	No*	Common
Splenomegaly	No*	Common

Figure 10.6: *Clinical features to assist in differentiating haemorrhage from haemolysis. *Exceptions can occur in the presence of concurrent or associated disease.*

erythrocyte destruction occurring in the spleen and liver. Splenomegaly is frequently present. Intravascular haemolysis is less common and results in haemoglobinaemia and haemoglobinuria, which may cause acute nephrosis. With either process, the rate of erythrocyte destruction may exceed the rate of hepatic clearance, resulting in hyperbilirubinaemia and icterus.

The evaluation of patients with haemolytic anaemia should always include a blood smear examination and a saline agglutination test. In cats, viral serology should also be included. Morphological abnormalities highly suggestive of a particular cause are frequently detectable, for example spherocytes, Heinz bodies, erythroparasites and schizocytes (see Figure 10.2). There are numerous causes of haemolytic anaemia (see Figure 10.3), which can be divided into six major categories: (1) immune mediated, (2) toxic, (3) infectious, (4) microangiopathic, (5) congenital and (6) miscellaneous. The most common are briefly discussed here.

Immune-mediated haemolytic anaemia (IMHA)

IMHA is the most common cause of haemolysis in dogs. Haemolysis is usually extravascular, but may be intravascular. IMHA may be primary (idiopathic) or secondary to drug administration (e.g. sulphonamides), live-virus vaccination, neoplasia (especially lymphosarcoma and haemangiosarcoma), tick-borne disease (babesiosis, ehrlichiosis), dirofilariasis and bacterial infection (leptospirosis, others). It may be accompanied by other immune-mediated processes such as immune-mediated thrombocytopenia or systemic lupus erythematosus (SLE).

The onset of signs is usually acute. Splenomegaly is common, as is icterus and fever. The anaemia is usually regenerative, and neutrophilia occurs frequently. Up to 33% of cases may have reticulocytopenia, which may indicate recent haemolysis or the destruction of red cell precursors in the bone marrow. Thrombocytopenia may be present due to antibody-mediated destruction or as a result of consumption (thrombosis or disseminated intravascular coagulation (DIC)).

Diagnosis of IMHA requires elimination of other causes of haemolysis and demonstration of immune-mediated erythrocyte injury. Spherocytosis is the most reliable feature of IMHA (Figure 10.7). Autoagglutination is the next most convincing evidence, but is not always present. A positive direct Coombs' test supports the diagnosis, but a negative test does not rule out IMHA. When spherocytosis is not convincing and autoagglutination and Coombs testing are negative, a saline fragility test may help to document erythrocyte injury.

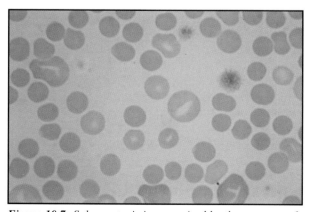

Figure 10.7: *Spherocytosis is recognized by the presence of many small round erythrocytes that lack central pallor. The finding of large numbers of these cells is highly suggestive of immune-mediated haemolytic anaemia.*
Courtesy of Dr Patricia McManus, University of Pennsylvania.

If the anaemia is non-regenerative, recognition of spherocytes is an important clue to the presence of IMHA. In this case, a longer period of time should be anticipated for a response to therapy. Bone marrow examination is indicated, usually revealing a distinct maturation block at one stage of erythroid development, with an absence or paucity of later stages. Erythrophagocytosis may be evident. Immune-mediated pure red cell aplasia might exist, due to destruction of stem cells. Diagnosis of IMHA in these cases can be difficult, and response to therapy provides important diagnostic information.

Once a diagnosis of IMHA is made, a thorough search for underlying causes or systemic immune-mediated disease should begin. In addition to a CBC, chemistries and urinalysis, indicated diagnostic tests include radiology/ultrasound, an antinuclear antibody test (ANA) and serology for tick-borne diseases and occult dirofilariasis.

IMHA is uncommon in the cat. Since recognition of spherocytes is difficult in the cat, the saline fragility test can be used to detect erythrocyte injury. Haemobartonellosis is frequently associated with IMHA. A direct association between FeLV and IMHA is equivocal, but cats with IMHA should be evaluated for viral disease.

Treatment of IMHA includes the elimination of any underlying cause, adequate immunosuppression and appropriate supportive care. Glucocorticoids are the backbone of immunosuppressive therapy, either prednisolone (1–2 mg/kg bid orally or s.c. for animals <10 kg and 15 mg/m^2 bid for animals >10 kg) or dexamethasone (0.1–0.3 mg/kg i.v. bid). The use of gastrointestinal protectants (H$_2$-receptor antagonists and/or sucralfate) is recommended. When tick-borne disease is possible in the dog, or haemobartonellosis in the cat, doxycycline should be administered (10 mg/kg sid orally).

Most patients with IMHA respond to glucocorticoid therapy within 7 days. Response to therapy is evaluated based on the haematocrit, which depends on the balance between cell destruction and bone marrow regeneration. The need for more potent immunosuppressive agents remains unclear, as their efficacy has yet to be firmly established in small animals. Cyclophosphamide is most commonly advocated for the acutely unresponsive patient (200 mg/m^2 total dose i.v. or orally once or divided over 3–4 consecutive days). Rapid responses to human intravenous immunoglobulin (0.5–1.5 g/kg as a single infusion) have been described in the dog, but require further investigation.

The guidelines for blood transfusion are no different from other forms of anaemia. There is no basis for the statement that transfusion is contraindicated in this disease. Intravenous fluid therapy is indicated in severely affected patients to prevent blood stasis and associated hypercoagulability (thromboembolism and DIC) and to ensure adequate diuresis in patients with intravascular haemolysis. The use of heparin remains controversial.

Corticosteroids are continued at the initial dosage until the haematocrit begins to increase, usually a minimum of 2–3 weeks. Then they are gradually tapered over the following months. The addition of other immunosuppressive agents may provide a synergistic effect. Options include danazol (5 mg/kg bid) or azathioprine (2.2 mg/kg sid). If the haematocrit decreases with tapering of the corticosteroid, more potent immunosuppressive agents can be used, such as cyclophosphamide (200 mg/m^2 divided over 3–4 consecutive days weekly) or cyclosporine (10 mg/kg daily).

The prognosis for animals with IMHA is variable. A poorer prognosis is associated with intravascular haemolysis, severe hyperbilirubinaemia and some underlying diseases (e.g. neoplasia). Thromboembolic complications, particularly pulmonary thromboembolism, are common. A small proportion of cases may have protracted disease that precludes discontinuation of corticosteroids. The prognosis is more guarded in cats because of the likelihood of viral disease.

Zinc toxicity

Zinc poisoning should be considered in any patient with acute haemolytic anaemia without autoagglutination or morphological abnormalities on the blood smear. Ingestion of pennies, zinc nuts or bolts or topical protectants can result in toxic concentrations of zinc, causing severe intravascular haemolysis, gastrointestinal irritation and even acute renal failure. A tentative diagnosis can be made based on a history of exposure, and foreign objects in the gastrointestinal tract can often be demonstrated radiographically. Since the mere presence of metal-dense foreign bodies does not confirm zinc toxicity, diagnosis requires the presence of convincing clinical signs or an elevated blood zinc concentration. Due to the high mortality associated with zinc toxicity, these cases are serious emergencies and treatment should not be delayed pending the results of zinc concentrations.

Treatment of zinc toxicity begins with patient stabilization, followed by the removal of the object via

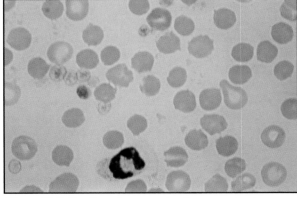

Figure 10.8: Small erythrocytes that have sustained intravascular membrane damage may occasionally be mistaken for spherocytes, for example in this case of zinc intoxication.

Courtesy of Dr Patricia McManus, University of Pennsylvania.

endoscopy or laparotomy. Appropriate fluid therapy is given based on renal function, and packed red blood cells should be transfused if necessary. Treatment with H$_2$-receptor antagonists (cimetidine, famotidine) is recommended to decrease 'leaching' of zinc from the source prior to removal. Chelation therapy with calcium ethylenediamine tetra-acetic acid (CaEDTA) should be initiated (25 mg/kg diluted in 5% dextrose, s.c. qid). Since CaEDTA can be nephrotoxic, careful attention should be paid to dosing and adequate fluid therapy. The duration of chelator therapy remains unclear, as zinc concentrations may take 2–21 days to decline following removal of the object. Where feasible, the decision should be based on normalization of the serum zinc concentration. The prognosis for complete recovery is good with timely and aggressive intervention.

Oxidative injury

Oxidative injury may cause denaturation of haemoglobin resulting in Heinz body formation, or oxidation of haem iron resulting in methaemoglobinaemia. Heinz bodies result in altered erythrocyte deformability and shortened red cell survival. Heinz bodies usually appear within 24 hours of exposure and result in haemolysis after several days.

The most common cause of Heinz bodies in the dog is the ingestion of onions (raw, cooked or dehydrated). Haemolysis generally occurs approximately 5 days after ingestion. Heinz bodies in the dog are usually small, occur in multiples and are readily identified with reticulocyte staining. When large they may be seen as clear 'blebs' protruding from the cell surface. Eccentrocytes — erythrocytes with a clear non-haemoglobinized zone on one side — frequently accompany Heinz bodies in the dog (Figure 10.9).

Feline haemoglobin is highly sensitive to oxidative denaturation, and Heinz body formation is common in the cat (up to 96% of erythrocytes in normal cats). Heinz bodies accompany numerous feline primary diseases, including lymphosarcoma, hyperthyroidism and diabetes mellitus. Commercial cat foods containing propylene glycol are associated with susceptibility to oxidant injury, but do not generally cause clinical anaemia. A variety of other agents may induce Heinz body formation and severe anaemia in cats (see Figure 10.3). Diagnosis of overt Heinz body anaemia requires relatively large Heinz bodies in many erythrocytes, with convincing evidence of haemolysis. Heinz bodies in the cat are usually single, may project from the membrane and are best visualized with one of the reticulocyte stains.

Treatment of Heinz body anaemia involves removal of the offending toxin, blood transfusion where indicated and supportive care.

Erythroparasites

Haemobartonella felis can cause acute anaemia, especially in cats with an underlying infection such as feline leukaemia virus (FeLV) or feline immunodeficiency

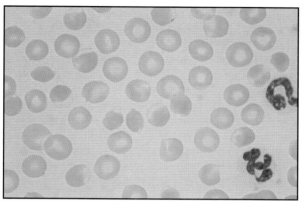

Figure 10.9: *Eccentrocytes and Heinz bodies in a dog, caused by the ingestion of onions.*
Courtesy of Dr Patricia McManus, University of Pennsylvania.

virus (FIV). Diagnosis requires identification of ring or rod forms of the organism on erythrocytes on blood smear examination (Figure 10.10). Ring forms consist of a fine basophilic ring with a hollow centre. Rod forms are observed on the periphery of the cell. Identification may require examination of a fresh blood smear on several consecutive days. Since the organisms are epicellular, they can be easily dislodged from the cells or washed off the cells in EDTA. Prolonged alcohol fixation decreases the displacement of organisms during staining. Treatment consists of tetracycline (60 mg/kg orally tid) for 2–3 weeks. Corticosteroid therapy has been advocated, since an immune-mediated process is likely. Supportive care and specific therapy for concurrent disease are intuitive.

Haemobartonella canis is rare, usually only occurring in splenectomized, severely debilitated or immunosuppressed dogs. Organisms are readily seen as chains across the surface of the red cell. Spherocytosis is common, indicating an immune-mediated pathophysiology. Treatment should consist of tetracyclines, using the same regimen as for the cat. Corticosteroids can be added to the regimen if the response to antibiotics alone is inadequate.

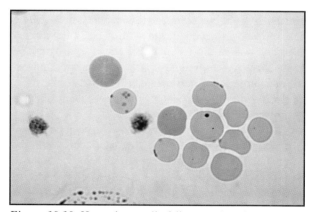

Figure 10.10: Haemobartonella felis *organisms in a cat (Diff-Quik®). Note the difference between the peripherally located* Haemobartonella *organisms and the larger, refractile, centrally located Howell–Jolly body in one cell.*

The tick-transmitted protozoans *Babesia canis* and *Babesia gibsoni* cause haemolytic anaemia in dogs. The clinical manifestations range from acute disease with severe intravascular haemolysis to subacute or chronic disease with mild or moderate anaemia. Immune-mediated haemolysis appears to occur frequently, and concurrent infection with *Ehrlichia canis* is common. The diagnosis requires identification of intra-erythrocytic pyriform bodies on blood smear examination (Figure 10.11). Since parasitized erythrocytes tend to 'sludge' in the capillaries, yield is best using an ear-stick blood smear. When babesiosis is suspected, but organisms cannot be found, serological testing is indicated. A direct Coombs' test and serological testing for ehrlichiosis should also be performed. Treatment includes appropriate supportive therapy and antiparasitic drugs such as diminazene aceturate and imidocarb diproprionate. Tetracyclines have limited efficacy.

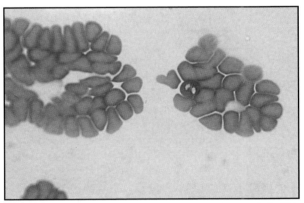

Figure 10.11: Babesia canis *piroplasms in a dog (Diff-Quik®).*

Congenital disorders

Inherited enzyme deficiencies are rare, but may mimic IMHA. Phosphofructokinase (PFK) deficiency has been described in English Springer and American Cocker Spaniels. Mild to moderate chronic anaemia occurs, with superimposed episodes of intravascular haemolysis precipitated by vigorous exercise or panting, due to the sensitivity of these erythrocytes to alkalaemia. These dogs present at a young age with acute intravascular haemolysis, a strong regenerative response and spontaneous recovery. If immunosuppressive therapy is initiated, recovery may be erroneously ascribed to the drug. Diagnosis of PFK deficiency is made using enzyme assay by specific laboratories.

Pyruvate kinase (PK) deficiency has been described in Basenjis and Beagles. It is characterized by chronic severe haemolysis and moderate to severe anaemia usually first recognized at 3–6 months of age. The haematocrit slowly declines over the following 1–3 years. It is typically highly regenerative, but terminal myelofibrosis may develop. Diagnosis is presumptive based on elimination of other causes, and confirmed by enzyme assay by specialized laboratories.

Microangiopathy

Microangiopathic haemolytic anaemia is caused by mechanical fragmentation of erythrocytes. Causes include splenic torsion, haemangiosarcoma, DIC and caval syndrome associated with heartworm disease. Erythrocyte fragmentation is recognized by finding schizocytes (sheared erythrocytes) on blood smear examination. Ordinarily, anaemia is subclinical, but in severe cases overt anaemia develops (splenic torsion and caval syndrome).

Decreased erythropoiesis

Decreased erythropoiesis can be caused by extra-marrow or intra-marrow disease (Figure 10.3). Extra-marrow anaemia is the result of systemic diseases that selectively depress erythropoiesis. The anaemia is generally mild (haematocrit range 25–35% in dogs and 20–25% in cats). Because anaemia develops slowly, clinical signs of the underlying disease usually predominate. Intra-marrow disease, such as myeloaplasia (aplastic anaemia), myelodysplasia, myeloproliferative disorders and myelofibrosis, results from injury to the stem cells and/or microenvironment. Depending on the course of disease, variable cytopenias are observed. Acute disease is characterized by granulocytopenia and thrombocytopenia, with mild to non-existent anaemia. Chronic marrow disease is characterized by moderate to severe anaemia, with variable degrees of leucopenia and thrombocytopenia.

Evaluation of patients with non-regenerative anaemia includes questioning the owner regarding drug exposure, a CBC to determine other blood cell counts, evaluation for systemic disease, serological testing for FeLV and FIV in the cat and for ehrlichiosis in the dog, and bone marrow examination. The bone marrow aspirate is evaluated for evidence of neoplasia or dysplasia and for estimation of cellularity. A core bone marrow biopsy is required to determine the degree of cellularity or fibrosis.

Treatment for non-regenerative anaemia depends on the cause, but may include blood transfusion and/or the administration of colony stimulating factors.

BLEEDING DISORDERS

Bleeding disorders may be classified as primary (platelet or vascular disorders) or secondary (coagulation factor disorders). They may be inherited or acquired.

Approach in the emergency situation

Bleeding disorders should always be considered life threatening. Animals suffering a haemorrhagic crisis usually show typical signs of hypovolaemic shock. Establishing a diagnosis and instituting rational therapy can represent a major challenge.

Blood samples should be collected prior to initiating therapy, including a minimum data base (MDB), a blood smear, and EDTA- and citrated-plasma samples for later laboratory testing. The MDB usually reveals a decreased PCV and TP. In acute haemorrhage, the PCV may be normal or elevated due to compensatory splenic contraction, but the TP may be low reflecting blood loss. A blood smear should be examined, with emphasis on platelet numbers and morphology and the presence of schizocytes. Depending on the findings in the individual patient, further testing may include a CBC, chemistry profile, immune testing and screening coagulation tests.

Stabilization of the bleeding patient requires (1) control of haemorrhage and (2) blood volume replacement. The most life-threatening problem in these animals is shock, so initial therapy should involve aggressive fluid replacement (crystalloid ± synthetic colloids) until blood is available. There is no justification to withhold the fluid therapy in the anaemic patient. Fluid therapy will not alter the absolute red cell mass, and hypoperfusion will only exacerbate tissue hypoxia.

Animals should be kept quiet and unstressed, subcutaneous injections should be avoided and venepunctures performed only when required for platelet enumeration. Sites should be held off with manual pressure for 5 minutes. An intravenous catheter can usually be safely placed and used to collect all other blood samples (including regular PCV monitoring; see Chapter 21). Patients should be closely monitored for evidence of ongoing haemorrhage, including evaluation of perfusion, respiratory rate and effort, mucous membrane colour, neurological status and PCV/TP.

Once the patient has been stabilized, three initial questions must be answered:

- Is the bleeding due to local factors or does the animal have a generalized haemostatic abnormality?
- If a systemic disorder does exist, what is the nature of the haemostatic defect?
- Is the defect congenital or acquired?

This is generally achieved based on the history, physical examination and screening laboratory tests.

Pathophysiology

The haemostatic system can divided into three major parts: primary haemostasis, secondary haemostasis and fibrinolysis.

Primary haemostasis

Primary haemostasis involves interactions between the vessel wall and the platelets, terminating in the formation of a primary haemostatic plug a temporary seal over the injured vessel. At the site of vascular injury, platelets adhere to the subendothelial collagen, mediated by von Willebrand's factor (vWF) and membrane glycoproteins. Following adherence, the platelets undergo conformational changes and release bioactive substances that stimulate platelet aggregation. Aggregated platelets constitute the primary haemostatic plug and expose platelet phospholipid (platelet factor 3) that plays an important role in secondary haemostasis. Defects in primary haemostasis may be due to vascular or platelet disorders. Vasculopathies may lead to excessive fragility or abnormal interaction with platelets. Platelet disorders may be quantitative (thrombocytopenia) or qualitative (thrombopathia).

Secondary haemostasis

Secondary haemostasis involves the formation of fibrin by the coagulation factors, in and around the primary haemostatic plug. All coagulation factors are produced in the liver, with the exception of factor VIII. Vitamin K is required for the formation of factors II, VII, IX and X, as well as protein C. Classically, two pathways for activation of the coagulation cascade are recognized: an intrinsic and an extrinsic pathway. The intrinsic pathway is surface activated and operates strictly with components present in the blood, whereas the extrinsic pathway requires a tissue factor for activation. These two pathways converge in a final common pathway of fibrin formation. Defects of secondary haemostasis may include quantitative or qualitative coagulation factor disorders.

Fibrinolysis

The fibrinolytic system consists of plasminogen and all substances that convert it to its active form, plasmin. Plasmin is responsible for dissolution of the fibrin clot, resulting in the production of various fragments. Fibrin split products (FSPs) (or fibrin degradation products) have anticoagulant activity by interfering with platelet function and inhibiting thrombin, and are ultimately removed from the circulation by the liver (half-life approximately 9–12 hours). Excessive fibrinolysis and generation of FSPs may occur in conditions such as DIC and hepatic disease, and may contribute to a bleeding tendency.

Clinical and laboratory assessment

Following initial stabilization, the first step is to determine whether the bleeding is due to a systemic bleeding disorder. Then bleeding disorders are categorized as defects of primary or secondary haemostasis. The history and physical examination often provide important clues about the type of coagulation problem, but definitive classification requires laboratory testing.

History

A detailed history is vital. Severe inherited disorders are generally apparent within the first 6 months of life. Milder forms may not be diagnosed until surgery, trauma or concurrent disease precipitate excessive bleeding. Certain inherited disorders are breed-related, for example von Willebrand's disease in the Dobermann. It is important to ascertain whether previous bleeding episodes have occurred in the patient or in family members. The history should include detailed enquiries about previous illnesses and medications. Live-virus vaccines and certain drugs may cause thrombocytopenia 3–10 days post-treatment. Specific enquiries about the environment and patient behaviour may reveal the potential of exposure to toxins or trauma. Some animals with bleeding disorders are presented for apparently unrelated disease; for example, shifting leg lameness may result from recurrent haemarthrosis, and acute blindness may be due to hyphaema.

Physical examination

Evaluation of the distribution, extent and nature of current haemorrhage requires careful examination of all body systems including the skin, mucous membranes, eyes and joints, as well as the urine and faeces. The nature of the haemorrhage helps to characterize the haemostatic defect (Figure 10.12). Defects of primary haemostasis are characterized by petechiation/ecchymosis and spontaneous bleeding from mucosal surfaces, including epistaxis, gingival bleeding, haematuria, melaena and ocular haemorrhage. Platelet and vascular abnormalities generally cannot be distinguished on physical examination alone. Defects of secondary haemostasis are usually characterized by single/multiple bruises and bleeding into subcutaneous tissue, body cavities, muscles or joints. Some acquired abnormalities, such as DIC, defy this classification because multiple haemostatic defects are present. Likewise von Willebrand's disease (vWD) usually has the characteristics of a primary haemostatic defect, but in its most severe form it may mimic a secondary haemostatic disorder.

Screening coagulation tests

Laboratory tests are essential to confirm and characterize the haemostatic defect (Figures 10.13 and 10.14). These tests should be performed and interpreted carefully, together with the clinical findings. Blood samples should be collected via atraumatic venepuncture prior to the initiation of therapy. The common screening tests are discussed below (for normal values see Figure 10.15).

Platelet enumeration/estimation: Quantitative platelet disorders are detected by performing platelet counts in animals with suspected bleeding disorders. Examination of a blood smear allows rapid estimation of platelet numbers (approximately 11–25 platelets per high-power field (hpf) is normal). Platelet clumping at the feathered edge of the smear may result in artefactually

Disorders of primary haemostasis	Disorders of secondary haemostasis
Petechiae common	Petechiae rare
Haematomas rare	Haematomas common
Bleeding often involves mucous membranes	Bleeding into muscles and joints common
Bleeding usually at multiple sites	Bleeding frequently localized
Prolonged and repeated bleeding from cuts (rebleed)	Bleeding may be delayed in onset

Figure 10.12: Clinical features helpful in differentiating between primary and secondary haemostatic abnormalities.

Process	Screening test	Component/factors evaluated
Primary haemostasis	Platelet enumeration Platelet estimation* Bleeding time (BT)*	Platelet numbers Platelet numbers and function, vascular integrity
Secondary haemostasis	Activated clotting time (ACT)* Partial thromboplastin time (PTT) Prothrombin time (PT) Thrombin time (TT)	Intrinsic and common pathways: factors XII, XI, IX, VIII, X, V, II and fibrinogen, platelet numbers As with ACT, but more sensitive Extrinsic and common pathways: factors III, VII, X, V, II and fibrinogen Terminal common pathway: fibrinogen quantity and quality
Fibrinolysis	Fibrin split products (FSPs)*	Products of fibrinolysis

*Figure 10.13: Screening tests for the evaluation of haemostasis. *In-office tests.*

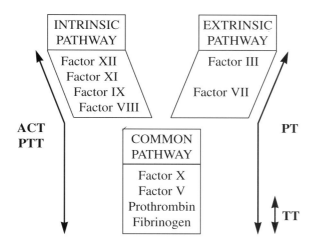

Figure 10.14: *Factors evaluated with the screening coagulation tests. ACT: activated clotting time, PTT: partial thromboplastin time, PT: prothrombin time, TT: thrombin time.*

low estimates. Large platelets (macroplatelets or 'shift' platelets) generally indicate megakaryocytic hyperplasia (a regenerative response). In addition, the blood smear should be examined for schizocytes (fragmented erythrocytes), which suggest microangiopathic haemolysis.

Samples for platelet counting should be collected in EDTA and analysed within 12 hours of collection, either manually (by haemocytometer) or by an automated cell counter. Both techniques are reliable for canine blood. In cats there is considerable overlap between erythrocyte and platelet volumes, resulting in erroneous results from automated cell counters. Feline platelets should therefore be enumerated manually.

Bleeding time: The bleeding time is the duration of haemorrhage resulting from infliction of a small standardized injury involving microscopic vessels. The buccal mucosal bleeding time (BMBT) is considered the most reliable and reproducible method. Cats usually require light sedation. The patient is restrained in lateral recumbency and a strip of gauze is tied around the maxilla to fold up the upper lip, tightly enough to cause

moderate mucosal engorgement. A two-blade, spring-loaded device is used to make two 1 mm deep incisions in the mucosa of the upper lip. The incisions should be made at a site devoid of visible vessels and inclined so that the blood flows toward the mouth. Shed blood is carefully blotted with filter paper, taking extreme care not to disturb the incision sites. The time from incision to cessation of bleeding is measured. The cuticle bleeding time — the duration of bleeding after the tip of the dermis of the nail has been severed by a guillotine-type nail clipper — is far less reliable and reproducible.

The bleeding time reflects *in vivo* primary haemostasis. It may be prolonged by thrombocytopenia, thrombocytopathies or vascular anomalies and is indicated in patients with a suspected primary haemostatic defect when the platelet count is adequate. This test is unnecessary if the patient is thrombocytopenic.

Activated clotting time (ACT): The ACT is a simple screening test for the intrinsic and common pathways. Blood (2 ml) is drawn into a prewarmed (37°C) commercial tube containing diatomaceous earth, which serves as a chemical activator of factor XII. The first few drops of blood are discarded because of the possible presence of tissue factor. The sample is mixed by inversion and then placed into a 37°C heat block or water bath for 50 seconds. It is then inverted every 10 seconds, observed for clot formation and replaced. The ACT is the time interval to first clot formation, which is prolonged by severe abnormalities of the intrinsic and/or common pathways. It is a relatively insensitive, but easily performed and valuable screening test. Severe thrombocytopenia ($<10{,}000/\mu l$) causes mild prolongation of the ACT (10–20 seconds). Similarly, hypofibrinogenaemia and some thrombopathias may result in ACT prolongation.

Partial thromboplastin time (PTT): The PTT tests the intrinsic and common pathways. Usually, at least one factor must be less than 30% of the normal value before prolongation occurs. This test is more sensitive than the ACT and is not affected by primary haemostatic

Variable	Dog	Cat
Platelet count ($\times 10^3/\mu l$)	150–500	200–600
Buccal mucosal bleeding time (minutes)	1.7–4.2	1.4–2.4
Cuticle bleeding time (minutes)	2–8	2–8
Activated clotting time (seconds)	60–110	50–75
Prothrombin time (seconds)*	7–10	9–12
Partial thromboplastin time (seconds)*	9–12	15–21
Fibrin split products (µg/ml)	<10	<10

Figure 10.15: *Normal values for screening coagulation tests. *'Normal' values are dependent on laboratory and technique.*

disorders. Samples for coagulation testing should be collected into plastic or siliconized glass tubes and anticoagulated with 3.8% citrate at a ratio of 1:9 with the blood sample. If samples cannot be analysed within 12 hours, the plasma should be separated and frozen. Factor deficiencies may be differentiated from the effects of an anticoagulant, such as heparin, by repeating the PTT following dilution of the abnormal plasma 1:1 with normal plasma. Correction of the test indicates a factor deficiency, whereas failure to correct suggests the presence of an anticoagulant.

Prothrombin time (PT): The PT is the principal test of the extrinsic pathway. Because of the short half-life of factor VII, this test is very sensitive to vitamin K deficiency or antagonism. It is less sensitive to heparin than is the PTT. Sample collection and handling is as for the PTT.

Thrombin time (TT): The TT determines the reactivity of fibrinogen to exogenous thrombin. It assesses the conversion of fibrinogen to fibrin (the common pathway) and bypasses all other steps. It may be prolonged by hypofibrinogenaemia (<100 mg/dl) or dysfibrinogenaemia or by substances that inhibit thrombin, such as heparin or FSPs. Sample collection and handling is as for the PT and PTT.

Fibrin split products/fibrin degradation products: FSPs, the end products of fibrinolysis, are commonly quantified with a commercial kit. Elevated concentrations of FSPs implies increased fibrinolysis, commonly due to DIC. Hepatic disease may also result in enhanced fibrinolysis and reduced clearance of FSPs. False elevations occur when fibrinogen is not clotted by thrombin and remains in solution, for example in patients on heparin therapy or those with dysfibrinogenaemia.

Disorders of primary haemostasis
The causes and diagnostics for primary haemostatic disorders are listed in Figures 10.16 and 10.17.

Thrombocytopenia
Thrombocytopenia is the most common primary haemostatic defect and may be due to decreased platelet production, destruction, consumption or sequestration. Clinical evidence of bleeding does not occur until platelet counts are lower than approximately 40,000/µl, unless another concomitant bleeding disorder exists. Many animals tolerate lower counts without evidence of haemorrhage.

The secondary haemostatic mechanisms should be evaluated in all thrombocytopenic animals to exclude DIC or other combined defects, which are consistent with consumption or sequestration. If these are normal, a bone marrow aspirate or biopsy is indicated to evaluate platelet production. Megakaryocytic hypoplasia

---

Quantitative platelet disorders (thrombocytopenia)

Decreased production:
Drug-induced (oestrogen, chloramphenicol, cytotoxics)
Immune-mediated megakaryocytic hypoplasia
Viral (FeLV)
Chronic rickettsial disease
Oestrogen-secreting neoplasm
Myelophthisis (myeloproliferative disease)
Myelofibrosis
Cyclic thrombocytopenia (*Ehrlichia platys*)
Radiation
Idiopathic bone marrow aplasia

Increased destruction:
Immune-mediated (IMTP)
    Primary
        Idiopathic
        Evan's syndrome (IMHA and IMTP)
        Systemic lupus erythematosus
    Secondary
        Drugs
        Live-virus vaccination
        Tick-borne disease
        Neoplasia
        Bacterial infection
Non-immune
    Drug-induced
    Ehrlichiosis
    Rocky Mountain spotted fever
    Dirofilariasis

Consumption/sequestration:
Disseminated intravascular coagulation
Microangiopathies
Sepsis
Vasculitis
Splenic torsion, hypersplenism
Hepatic disease
Heparin-induced
Profound acute haemorrhage
Haemolytic uraemic syndrome

Qualitative platelet disorders (thrombopathia)

Inherited:
Von Willebrand's disease (numerous dog breeds)
Canine thrombopathia (Basset Hound)
Canine thromboasthenic thrombopathia (Otterhound)

Acquired:
Drug-induced (e.g. NSAIDs, synthetic colloid solutions, antibiotics, heparin)
Uraemia
Hepatic disease
Pancreatitis
Myeloproliferative disorders
Dysproteinaemia (e.g. myeloma)

Vascular disorders

Inherited:
Ehrlers–Danlos syndrome

Acquired:
Vasculitis
Hyperadrenocorticism

Figure 10.16: *Causes of disorders of primary haemostasis.*

---

may result from numerous conditions. In the absence of a compatible drug history or evidence of myelophthisis on bone marrow examination, further testing should include investigation of potential neoplastic, infectious or immune-mediated aetiologies. Oestrogen-secreting tumours, chronic rickettsial disease (*Ehrlichia canis*)

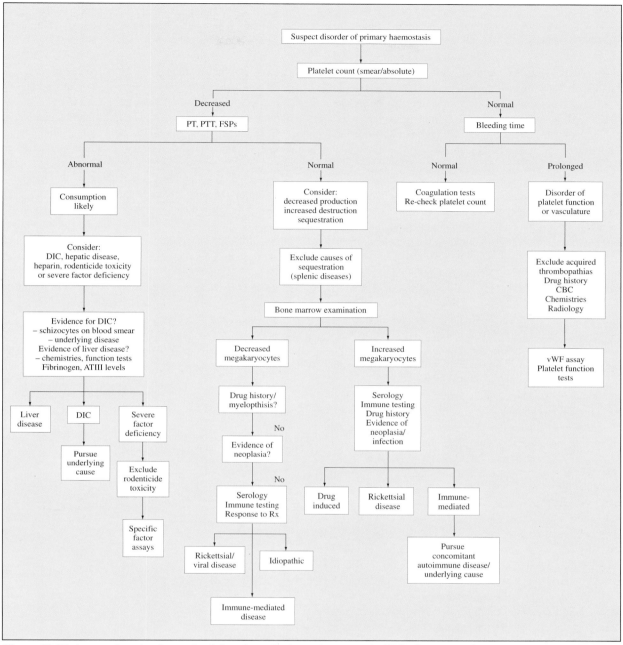

Figure 10.17: *Approach to the diagnosis of disorders of primary haemostasis. DIC: disseminated intravascular coagulation, ATIII: antithrombin III, vWf: von Willebrand Factor.*

and viral infections such as FeLV and FIV should be considered where appropriate. Immune-mediated megakaryocytic hypoplasia can present a diagnostic dilemma, which is usually resolved by exclusion of other differentials and evaluation of the response to immunosuppressive therapy.

Normal or increased numbers of megakaryocytes in thrombocytopenic patients indicate increased platelet destruction, consumption or sequestration. Some common causes of platelet consumption and sequestration include DIC, sepsis, vasculitis and splenic torsion, which can usually be excluded based on clinical findings. Immune-mediated thrombocytopenia (IMTP) is a

common cause of thrombocytopenia in the dog (see Figure 10.4). Diagnosis of IMTP is based on exclusion of other causes of thrombocytopenia. Tick-borne diseases may be diagnosed by examination of an earstick blood smear (*E. canis morulae* or *Babesia canis* trophozoites) or serologically (ehrlichiosis, Rocky Mountain Spotted Fever). A negative titre, however, does not exclude tick-borne disease and should be repeated in 10–14 days. IMTP may be idiopathic, may be associated with other autoimmune processes such as IMHA or SLE, or may develop secondary to drug administration (notably sulphonamides), live-virus vaccination, neoplasia (especially lymphoid) and infection. Suspicion of IMTP should prompt a thorough search for underlying disease. In addition to a CBC, chemistries and urinalysis, diagnostic testing should include radiology/ultrasound, a direct Coombs' test, an antinuclear antibody (ANA) test and serology for tick-borne diseases and occult dirofilariasis.

Management of IMTP includes treatment of any underlying cause, adequate immunosuppression and appropriate supportive care. Glucocorticoids are the backbone of immunosuppressive therapy: either prednisolone (1–2 mg/kg bid for animals <10 kg and 15 mg/m^2 bid for animals >10 kg) or dexamethasone (0.1–0.2 mg/kg i.v. bid). The use of gastrointestinal protectants (H$_2$-antagonists and/or sucralfate) is recommended. When tick-borne disease is possible, doxycycline should be administered (10 mg/kg sid orally or i.v.). Response to glucocorticoid therapy generally requires 2–7 days. Vincristine (0.01–0.025 mg/kg i.v.) has been advocated in dogs with IMTP and megakaryocytic hyperplasia, to cause a more rapid increase in platelet numbers, but its efficacy is not well documented. In dogs, danazol (5 mg/kg orally bid) may be used as an adjunctive immunosuppressive agent. Anecdotal reports of rapid responses to human intravenous immunoglobulin have been described in the dog, but remain to be adequately investigated.

Thrombocytopenic patients can deteriorate rapidly due to massive haemorrhage (most commonly in the gastrointestinal tract) or due to haemorrhage into a vital organ (e.g. lungs or brain). Patients should be hospitalized until platelet counts are above 50,000/µl and bleeding has ceased. Thereafter, platelet counts should be regularly monitored. When these are within reference range, prednisolone dose is decreased by approximately 25%. The dose is then decreased gradually over 2–4 months, with close monitoring of platelet counts.

Relapses of thrombocytopenia with decrease of the prednisone dose are unpredictable and not uncommon. Periodic monitoring of the platelet count is therefore essential. If relapse occurs, the prednisolone dose should be increased temporarily and danazol (5 mg/kg orally bid), azathioprine (2.2 mg/kg/day orally) or cyclophosphamide (200 mg/m^2 weekly, divided over 3–4 days) added to the treatment regimen. Experience with cyclosporine in dogs with IMTP is limited. Splenectomy is generally reserved for patients that have splenomegaly and exhibit refractory IMTP. Prior to splenectomy, it is crucial to ascertain (via bone marrow examination) that the spleen is not a significant source of extramedullary haematopoiesis.

Thrombopathia

Vascular disorders are a relatively uncommon cause of bleeding. In patients with primary haemostatic disorders and normal platelet numbers, a platelet function defect is likely. A prolonged bleeding time in a patient with adequate platelet numbers generally confirms thrombopathia. The drug history should be carefully appraised, as drugs often cause thrombopathia. Numerous diseases can precipitate platelet dysfunction, including uraemia, hepatic disease, pancreatitis, myeloproliferative disorders and myeloma. If no obvious cause of thrombopathia can be found, a hereditary disorder is suspected. Von Willebrand's Factor can be assayed. Other thrombopathias require specific platelet function testing, performed by specialized laboratories.

Control of haemorrhage in a dog with vWD includes administration of von Willebrand's Factor (vWF) in plasma products and desmopressin acetate (DDAVP). Cryoprecipitate is the ideal plasma product, as it contains relatively large quantities of vWF, but alternatively fresh frozen plasma may be used. DDAVP (1 µg/kg s.c.) may have a positive clinical effect, but a limited duration of action. It can be administered during a bleeding crisis or 20–30 minutes prior to an anticipated trauma such as surgery. Efficacy can be determined by repeating the BMBT 30–60 minutes after administration.

Disorders of secondary haemostasis

Defects of secondary haemostasis may be hereditary or acquired (Figures 10.18 and 10.19). The hereditary coagulopathies are deficiencies of specific coagulation factors, usually noted in purebred dogs. Specific factor assays are performed by specialized laboratories.

Inherited
Deficient factor:
  I: Hypo/dysfibrinogenaemia (St Bernard, Borzoi)
  II: Hypoprothrombinaemia (Boxer)
  VII: Hypoproconvertinaemia (Beagle, Malamute)
  VIII: Haemophilia A (numerous dog breeds, mongrels, cats)
  IX: Haemophilia B (numerous dog breeds, British Shorthair cats)
  X: Stuart Prower trait (Cocker Spaniel)
  XI: Plasma thromboplastin antecedent deficiency (Springer Spaniel, Great Pyrenees)
  XII: Hageman factor deficiency (numerous dog breeds, cats)
Acquired
Vitamin K deficiency/antagonism
Hepatic disease
DIC
Circulating anticoagulants (e.g. heparin)

Figure 10.18: Causes of disorders of secondary haemostasis.

Acquired disorders include vitamin K deficiency or antagonism, hepatic disease, DIC and the presence of anticoagulants (e.g. heparin). These conditions tend to affect multiple factors in both the intrinsic and extrinsic pathways. Factor VII has the shortest half-life (4–6 hours) so prolongation of the PT may precede PTT prolongation in early vitamin K deficiency or early acute hepatic failure. Conversely, the PTT alone may be prolonged with chronic hepatic disease, DIC or heparin therapy.

Anticoagulant rodenticide toxicity

The most common cause of vitamin K deficiency or ingestion of anticoagulant rodenticides. Synthesis of

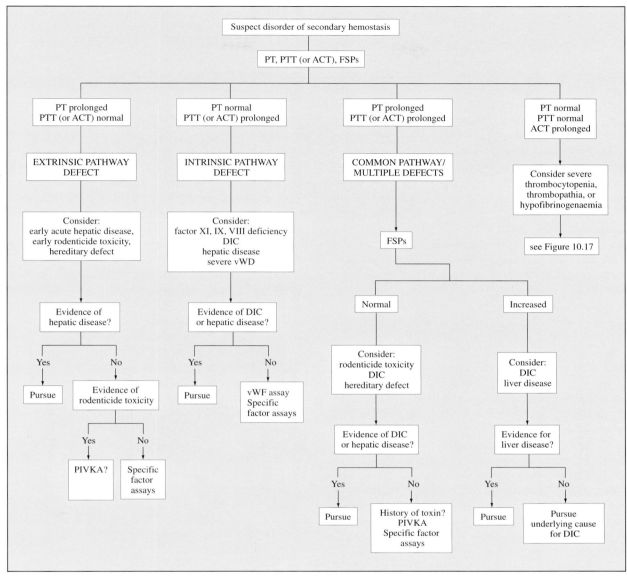

Figure 10.19: *Approach to the diagnosis of disorders of secondary haemostasis. DIC: disseminated intravascular coagulation, vWF: von Willebrand Factor, vWD: von Willebrand's disease, PIVKA: test for Proteins Induced by Vitamin K Absence/Antagonism.*

vitamin K-dependent factors occurs in the liver. Vitamin K is an essential cofactor for carboxylation of these proteins, rendering them functional. During this reaction, vitamin K is converted to an epoxide metabolite, which is recycled back to vitamin K. Anticoagulant rodenticides interfere with this recycling, resulting in rapid depletion of vitamin K.

Clinical signs of a secondary haemostatic disorder generally occur 2–3 days post-ingestion. Prolongation of the PT occurs first, but by the time haemorrhage is evident, the PT, PTT and ACT are usually all prolonged. FSPs and fibrinogen concentration are normal. The platelet count is usually normal, but may be decreased by consumption during bleeding. Toxicological testing for warfarin or for proteins induced by vitamin K antagonism (PIVKA) is not usually helpful in the emergency situation, but may serve to confirm an uncertain diagnosis.

Vitamin K_1 is essential to management. Improved coagulation, however, requires the synthesis of new factors which commonly takes up to 12 hours. Emergency needs for clotting factors can be met only via transfusion of plasma (9 ml/kg). Fresh whole blood (20 ml/kg) or packed red blood cells with fresh frozen plasma are indicated when anaemia is present. Because the half-life of transfused clotting factors is relatively short, plasma transfusion should be repeated after approximately 6 hours. Parenteral administration of vitamin K_1 (5 mg/kg bid) is recommended for initial therapy, ideally subcutaneously using a small gauge needle. The intravenous route should be avoided, due to the potential for anaphylaxis. The intramuscular route is discouraged as it may result in haematoma formation. After 24 hours, if the patient is not vomiting, vitamin K_1 is administered orally (0.25–2.5 mg/kg daily in warfarin exposure, 2.5–5.0 mg/kg for long-acting rodenticides).

Vitamin K_1 has no effect on toxin elimination. Therapy must be maintained until the toxin has been metabolized, with varying durations depending on the type of rodenticide. If the anticoagulant is known to be warfarin, 1 week of therapy is usually sufficient. If the anticoagulant is unknown or a second-generation rodenticide, oral vitamin K_1 should be continued for at least 3–4 weeks. The PT must be evaluated 48–72 hours after cessation of therapy. If it is prolonged, therapy should be reinstituted for an additional 2 weeks and the PT again re-evaluated after discontinuation.

Hepatic disease

Severe hepatocellular damage results in variable factor deficiencies and/or abnormalities in vitamin K metabolism. Reduced synthesis of inhibitors of fibrinolysis and reduced clearance of plasminogen activators leads to excessive fibrinolysis. In addition, both quantitative and qualitative platelet disorders may occur. FSPs may be elevated and antithrombin III and fibrinogen concentrations may be reduced. Differentiation from DIC is sometimes impossible based on coagulation testing alone, and may depend on clinical findings, serum chemistries and liver function testing. Bleeding in patients with hepatic failure often occurs into the gastrointestinal tract, resulting in a protein meal that may precipitate hepatic encephalopathy. Bleeding tendencies must be corrected before pursuing a hepatic biopsy. Transfusion of fresh frozen plasma can temporarily offset factor deficiencies. Vitamin K_1 may be beneficial in some patients with hepatic disease; efficacy should be ascertained by repeating coagulation tests at least 12 hours after initiating therapy.

Disseminated intravascular coagulation

DIC refers to intravascular activation of haemostasis with resultant microcirculatory thrombosis. Exaggerated consumption of platelets and clotting factors results in defective haemostasis and a bleeding tendency. Fibrinolysis of microthrombi generates FSPs, further exacerbating the bleeding disorder. Consumption of the natural anticoagulants can precipitate a thrombotic tendency.

DIC occurs secondary to a wide variety of underlying diseases including sepsis, severe infections (viral, bacterial and protozoal), neoplasia, shock, heat stroke, haemolysis, pancreatitis, severe hepatic disease, trauma and tissue necrosis. Three basic 'trigger' mechanisms have been proposed: (1) activation of the extrinsic coagulation pathway by tissue factor released during cell injury; (2) contact activation of the intrinsic coagulation pathway via endothelial damage and exposure of the subendothelial matrix; and (3) direct activation of coagulation factors by certain enzymes (for example, trypsin in pancreatitis). Numerous factors can act as 'enhancers' of DIC. Acidosis and hypoxia increase endothelial damage and inhibit antithrombin III.

Vascular stasis decreases the removal of activated coagulation factors and exacerbates local acidosis and hypoxia. The functional capacity of the mononuclear phagocytic system and the liver may be overwhelmed, hindering the removal of endotoxins, FSPs, enzymes and antigen–antibody complexes.

The clinical manifestations of DIC vary depending on the inciting cause, the ability to replace depleted factors and platelets, the concentrations of natural anticoagulants and the efficacy of clearance of activated factors and FSPs. DIC may be subclinical, mild or severe, and acute or chronic. It may manifest as multiple organ failure due to microvascular thrombosis or as bleeding due to consumption of coagulation factors and platelets. Microthrombosis leads to ischaemia, which may manifest as renal failure, respiratory insufficiency, hepatic failure, neurological signs or gastrointestinal disorders. Bleeding tendencies may manifest as prolonged bleeding from venepuncture sites, petechiae, ecchymoses, epistaxis, gastrointestinal haemorrhage and/or haematoma formation.

The diagnosis of acute fulminant DIC is usually easy, while chronic or subclinical DIC may prove more difficult. The laboratory findings are extremely variable. Thrombocytopenia is almost invariably present, but relative changes may be undetected unless a recent count is available for comparison. The PT and more often the PTT may be prolonged, but both may be normal if compensatory factor production is adequate. Significant elevations of FSPs are highly suggestive of DIC, but are a non-specific finding. Schizocytes on the blood smear are significant, but may occur with other conditions. Antithrombin III levels are decreased in 85% of dogs with DIC. Fibrinogen concentrations are usually low, but may be normal or increased as fibrinogen is an acute phase reactant. Diagnosis of DIC therefore requires careful consideration of both the clinical and the laboratory findings, with no single finding being pathognomonic.

The treatment of DIC is fourfold: (1) correction of the underlying cause; (2) fluid therapy; (3) prevention of secondary complications; and (4) control of the haemostatic defects. Correction of the underlying cause must be the primary focus because until it is removed, haemostatic activation will continue. In many cases, removal of the inciting cause is impossible or infeasible. Fluid therapy is essential to remove activated clotting and fibrinolytic factors from the microcirculation and to maintain adequate tissue perfusion, thereby alleviating vascular stasis, tissue hypoxia and acidosis. The prevention or control of secondary complications includes: correction of acid–base and electrolyte disorders, oxygen therapy where indicated, maintenance of adequate perfusion to prevent renal and gastrointestinal ischaemia and the prevention of secondary sepsis.

Control of the haemostatic defects of DIC can be attempted via blood product transfusion and heparinization. Plasma administration provides antithrombin III and replaces depleted coagulation factors. If the patient is actively bleeding, fresh whole blood can replace red blood cells, coagulation factors and platelets. The adage that the administration of blood products to a patient in DIC 'adds fuel to the fire' has not proven to be true. In fact, experimental studies have shown that the administration of antithrombin III (ATIII) is an effective therapy. The use of heparin in the treatment of DIC is controversial as studies are lacking. The primary mechanism of action of heparin is by potentiation of ATIII activity, thus inhibiting the activity of thrombin and other factors. Therefore, heparin is not effective unless adequate concentrations of ATIII are present. The optimal dose of heparin is unclear. In mild cases of DIC, mini- or low-dose heparin (5–10 or 75–200 IU/kg s.c. tid) is generally recommended. In moderate to severe cases, intermediate or high doses (300–500 or 750–1000 IU/kg s.c. tid) may be necessary.

Monitoring of patients on heparin therapy is difficult. Ideally, the PTT should not exceed 1.5–2 times the pretreatment value. The PTT indicates the risk of haemorrhage and not the adequacy of anticoagulation. Therefore, the PTT may be normal in an adequately heparinized patient. It may be impossible to ascertain whether increased PT/PTT is due to heparinization or to changes in the basal coagulation status. Abrupt cessation of heparin therapy is contraindicated because of the risk of rebound thrombotic complications. Heparin should be weaned over several days.

HYPERCOAGULATION AND THROMBOSIS

Thrombosis is the deposition of a fibrin-platelet mass (thrombus) within the vasculature, resulting in tissue ischaemia. Fragmentation of the thrombus produces emboli in the bloodstream that obstruct remote sites. Hypercoagulability is an unusual predisposition to thromboembolism.

Pathophysiology

Thrombosis depends on three major risk factors: changes in the vessel wall (vascular injury), impairment of blood flow (stasis) and alterations in blood constituents (hypercoagulability). Vascular injury leads to the exposure of subendothelial vessel wall components, resulting in platelet adhesion and activation of the coagulation system. Factors resulting in vascular injury include trauma, catheterization, inflammation, neoplastic invasion, parasitic damage and plaque deposition (atherosclerosis, amyloidosis). Vascular stasis retards the removal of activated coagulation factors and causes local hypoxia and vascular injury. Stasis can result from hypovolaemia, shock, cardiac insufficiency, blood vessel compression, immobility and hyperviscosity. True hypercoagulability refers to a change in the coagulation system, which can result from: platelet hyperaggregability, excessive activation or decreased removal of coagulation factors, deficiencies of natural anticoagulants or defective fibrinolysis.

Hyperaggregability of platelets increases thrombotic risk. Platelet aggregation is controlled by the interaction between platelets and the vascular endothelium. Platelets produce and release various proaggregating substances, while the endothelium releases several inhibitors of platelet aggregation. Disturbance in this balance can lead to thrombosis. There is no correlation between thrombocytosis and hypercoagulation.

The coagulation system is finely regulated by three principal mechanisms: antithrombin III, protein C and the fibrinolytic system. These mechanisms operate to prevent thrombus formation in normal circumstances and to limit and localize the formation of the haemostatic plug. If one or more of these mechanisms fail, coagulation is favoured.

Antithrombin III (ATIII) is synthesized primarily in the liver. It accounts for approximately 80% of the total anticoagulant effect of plasma. ATIII binds to and neutralizes thrombin and factors IXa, Xa, XIa and XIIa. The rate of neutralization is markedly increased by heparin. ATIII deficiency may result from decreased production, loss or consumption. Decreased hepatic production of ATIII occurs with liver disease, but thrombosis generally does not result because coexisting factor deficiencies favour haemorrhage. A similar situation occurs with protein-losing enteropathies. In contrast, protein-losing nephropathies permit selective loss of smaller plasma proteins such as ATIII, creating an imbalance that favours hypercoagulability. Disseminated intravascular coagulation (DIC) is associated with increased ATIII consumption.

Protein C is a natural anticoagulant that inactivates factors Va and VIIIa, suppressing thrombin production.

The fibrinolytic system is complex and poorly understood, but the presence of persistent thrombi implies defective fibrinolysis. The fibrinolytic system consists of plasminogen and the activators that convert plasminogen to plasmin. Plasmin causes dissolution of the fibrin clot. There are two physiological plasminogen activators — tissue-type plasminogen activator (t-PA) and urokinase — and numerous inhibitors of these activators. Hypofibrinolysis and resultant thrombosis can occur due to decreases in plasminogen or plasminogen activators, or due to increases in inhibitors.

Causes

Hypercoagulable states are acquired disorders, secondary to several systemic diseases; the pathophysiology is multifactorial and complex. Frequently, a hypercoagulable state will not result in thrombosis unless it is combined with changes in vascular integrity or blood flow. Numerous conditions have been associated with thromboembolism in dogs (Figure 10.20). In the critical patient, multiple factors promote thrombosis, including hypoperfusion, dehydration, immobility, venous catheterization, tissue injury and inflammatory cytokines.

> Renal disease (nephrotic syndrome,
> glomerulonephritis, acute renal failure)
>
> Cardiac disease (vegetative endocarditis,
> heartworm disease, cardiomyopathy)
>
> Neoplasia (carcinomas and sarcomas)
>
> Acute pancreatic necrosis
>
> Immune-mediated haemolytic anaemia
>
> Hypercortisolism (hyperadrenocorticism, chronic
> corticosteroid therapy)
>
> Atherosclerosis (hypothyroidism)
>
> Diabetes mellitus
>
> Sepsis

Figure 10.20: Conditions associated with thromboembolism in dogs.

Clinical signs

The clinical signs of thrombosis/embolism depend on the function of the ischaemic organ, the acuteness of vasculature obstruction and the ability of collateral circulation to maintain adequate perfusion. Clinical signs vary from mild subclinical effects to severe life-threatening complications such as acute dyspnoea in the case of pulmonary thromboembolism (PTE). Embolization of the central nervous system can cause a variety of neurological signs or death. Renal thromboembolism may cause abdominal pain, haematuria and/or vomiting. Visceral arterial thrombosis causes acute abdominal pain, vomiting, diarrhoea and/or haematochezia. Emboli related to cardiac disease in cats frequently lodge in the aortic bifurcation. Signs are peracute and the affected limb is painful, cool, paretic, pale and pulseless. Aortic thromboembolism in dogs varies from peracute to chronic (months), and chronic cases may show only lameness or paresis.

Diagnosis

The diagnosis of thromboembolism should include:

- Confirmation of the presence of a thrombus/embolus
- Laboratory evaluation of coagulation
- Identification of an underlying systemic disorder.

Thromboembolism should be included in the differential diagnoses for dyspnoea, abdominal effusion, intestinal compromise, acute abdomen, haematuria, hindlimb lameness/paresis/paralysis and acute neurological signs. Diagnosis depends on the exclusion of other causes and confirmation of the presence of a thrombus by ultrasonography, contrast angiography or nuclear imaging.

Laboratory detection of hypercoagulability is difficult as routine screening tests are designed to evaluate bleeding disorders, not thrombotic tendencies. There is little evidence for a relationship between thrombocytosis, shortened bleeding times, shortened PT and PTT and a thrombotic tendency. Increased concentrations of FSPs indirectly imply thrombus formation, but are also influenced by other factors, such as fibrinolytic activity and hepatic clearance. Routine screening coagulation tests, therefore, may be normal. ATIII and fibrinogen concentrations are more useful, but less widely available. ATIII concentration is well correlated to thrombotic risk when ATIII deficiency is the primary mechanism for thrombosis. Thrombotic tendency is moderate when ATIII levels are between 50% and 75% and high when levels are below 50%. Only a few hypercoagulable states, however, are associated with an ATIII deficiency. Similarly, significant elevations of fibrinogen are believed to be associated with hypercoagulation, but not all hypercoagulable states are associated with hyperfibrinogenaemia.

Treatment and prevention

Treatment and prevention of thromboembolism include reduction of vascular stasis by maintenance of adequate perfusion, minimization of vascular injury by the appropriate use and handling of venous catheters and direct pharmacological manipulation of the haemostatic system. Pharmacological agents that inhibit haemostasis are categorized as antiplatelet drugs, anticoagulants and fibrinolysins. In general, antiplatelet drugs and anticoagulants do not lyse existing thrombi, but they can help to inhibit their growth and prevent recurrences.

Antiplatelet drugs

Antiplatelet drugs inhibit platelet adhesion and aggregation, preventing formation of the primary platelet plug. Antiplatelet drugs are most useful for prevention of arterial thrombosis (e.g. heartworm disease, glomerulonephritis).

Aspirin (acetylsalicylic acid): Aspirin is the only widely used antiplatelet drug in small animals. It acts by acetylation of cyclo-oxygenase, thus preventing the formation of prostaglandins, thromboxanes and prostacyclin. The effect on the platelets is irreversible because platelets are unable to produce additional cyclo-oxygenase. The effect on endothelial production of prostacyclin is reversible, however. Effective antiplatelet therapy with aspirin depends on using a low dose that would affect the platelets irreversibly, but allow the endothelial cells to recover. In dogs, aspirin (0.5 mg/kg orally bid) has been shown to be effective in decreasing platelet aggregation, while sparing anti-aggregators such as prostacyclin. In cats, a lower aspirin dose (25 mg/kg orally twice weekly) effectively inhibits platelet aggregation, but the effect on prostacyclin is unknown.

Anticoagulants

Anticoagulants inhibit the coagulation system by

enhancing natural anticoagulants or by decreasing factor production. Anticoagulants are most useful in preventing venous thrombosis.

Heparin: The primary mechanism of action of heparin is the potentiation of ATIII activity. ATIII deficiency may result in resistance to heparin. While heparin therapy alone will decrease ATIII levels, it will generally not lower levels enough to result in resistance. Low levels are more commonly related to the disease process, e.g. nephrotic syndrome or DIC. In these situations, fresh plasma should be given prior to heparin. Guidelines for the administration and monitoring of heparin are discussed above. The major complication of heparin administration is haemorrhage. If uncontrollable haemorrhage occurs, treatment with protamine sulphate should be instituted. If administered within minutes of a heparin dose, a full neutralizing dose should be given: 1 mg of protamine sulphate per 100 units heparin, via slow intravenous infusion (over 10 minutes). If 1 hour has elapsed since the last heparin dose, 50% of the dose of protamine should be given. If 2 hours have elapsed, 25% of the dose should be given.

Warfarin: Warfarin is a vitamin K antagonist, making the carboxylation of vitamin K-dependent factors II, VII, IX, X and protein C impossible. The anticoagulant effect of warfarin is not immediate. Factor VII and protein C have the shortest half-lives, and during the first 24–48 hours after initiating therapy only these factors are significantly affected. Decreased activity of factor VII leads to anticoagulation and prolongation of the PT. Inhibition of protein C, however, is prothrombotic, which may lead to thrombosis, especially during the first 24–48 hours, before the other factors are inhibited. Heparin therapy should overlap warfarin for the first 2–4 days. Following initiation of warfarin (starting dose 0.05–0.1 mg/kg sid in dogs and cats), the PT should be monitored and the dose adjusted to maintain it at 1.3–1.5 times pretreatment values. The major complication of warfarin therapy is haemorrhage. In the event of uncontrollable haemorrhage, therapy should be discontinued and plasma or fresh blood administered. Vitamin K is seldom indicated, as the onset of effect is delayed and the patient is refractory to further warfarin therapy for up to 2 weeks.

Fibrinolysins

Fibrinolysins (streptokinase, urokinase and tissue-type plasminogen activator) are effective to some degree in almost all instances of thrombosis. Their efficacy depends on numerous factors including the age of the thrombus, fibrin content, plasminogen content and whether the thrombus is arterial or venous. Recent thrombi and arterial thrombi lyse more readily. The major concern during fibrinolysin use is the possible induction of systemic haemorrhage. This life-threatening complication is not uncommon when agents are used in high doses intravenously. Systemic lysis is less common when small doses are administered directly at the site of the thrombus, but this is often not feasible in veterinary medicine. The introduction of newer, fibrin-specific agents may allow intravenous administration with reduced risk. Contraindications for fibrinolysin therapy include: active internal bleeding, hypertension, recent (within 10 days) surgery, organ biopsy and severe gastrointestinal bleeding.

FURTHER READING

Catalfamo JL and Dodds WJ (1988) Hereditary and acquired thrombopathias. *Veterinary Clinics of North America (Small Animal)* **18**, 185–193

Fogh JM and Fogh IT (1988) Inherited coagulation disorders. *Veterinary Clinics of North America (Small Animal)* **18**, 231–243

Giger U (1992) The feline AB blood group system and incompatability reactions. In: *Kirk's Current Veterinary Therapy XI*, eds. RW Kirk and JD Bonagura, pp. 470–474. WB Saunders, Philadelphia

Giger U (1998) Emergency management of anaemia and the transfusion trigger. *Proceedings of the Sixth International Veterinary Emergency and Critical Care Symposium*, 202–204

Giger U (1998) Emergency management of the bleeding patient: plasma and platelet transfusions, vitamin K and DDAVP. *Proceedings of the Sixth International Veterinary Emergency and Critical Care Symposium*, 205–206

Hackner SG (1998) Intravenous immunoglobulins: hope or hype in acute immune-mediated disease. *Proceedings of the Sixth International Veterinary Emergency and Critical Care Symposium*, 211–214

Jain NC (1993) Erythrocyte physiology and changes in disease. In: *Essentials of Veterinary Haematology*, ed. NC Jain, pp. 133–158. Lea and Febiger, Philadelphia

Johnson JS *et al.* (1988) Canine vonWillebrand's disease: a heterogenous group of bleeding disorders. *Veterinary Clinics of North America (Small Animal)* **18**, 195–229

Harvey JW (1995) Methemoglobinaemia and Heinz-body haemolytic anemia. In: *Kirk's Current Veterinary Therapy XII*, ed. JD Bonagura, pp. 437–442. WB Saunders, Philadelphia

Jordan HL *et al.* (1993) Thrombocytopenia in cats: a retrospective study of 41 cases. *Journal of Veterinary Internal Medicine* **7**, 261–265

Lewis DC and Meyers KM (1996) Canine idiopathic thrombocytopenic purpura. *Journal of Veterinary Internal Medicine* **10**, 207–218

Rackear DG (1988) Drugs that alter the haemostatic mechanism. *Veterinary Clinics of North America (Small Animal)* **18**, 67–77

Stewart AF and Feldman BF (1993) Immune-mediated haemolytic anemia. Part II: clinical entity, diagnosis and treatment theory. *Compendium on Continuing Education for the Practicing Veterinarian* **15**, 1479–1491

Stone MS and Cotter SM (1992) Practical guidelines for transfusion therapy. In: *Kirk's Current Veterinary Therapy XI*, ed. RW Kirk and JD Bonagura, pp. 475–479. WB Saunders, Philadelphia

Troy GC (1988) An overview of haemostasis. *Veterinary Clinics of North America (Small Animal)* **18**, 5–20

Weiser MG (1995) Erythrocyte responses and disorders. In: *Textbook of Veterinary Internal Medicine IV*, ed. S. Ettinger, pp. 1864–1891. WB Saunders, Philadelphia

Weiser G (1995) Haematologic technology for diagnosing anemias. In: *Kirk's Current Veterinary Therapy XII*, ed. JD Bonagura, pp. 437–442. WB Saunders, Philadelphia

CHAPTER ELEVEN

Reproductive and Paediatric Emergencies

Gary C.W. England

INTRODUCTION

In contrast to several large animal species, there are many reproductive disorders that produce acute onset and potentially fatal clinical disease in dogs and cats. These conditions can be considered to occur in the non-pregnant female and the pregnant and post-parturient female, as well as the male. Many of these conditions can be diagnosed and treated relatively easily. Information about the management, diagnosis and treatment of neonatal disease is, however, scant, and for many breeding establishments perinatal losses are a disgraceful 20%. This is despite the fact that most neonatal care simply requires an understanding of the normal physiological requirements of these species. The aim of this chapter is to review the diagnosis and treatment of reproductive tract emergencies as well as the care and management of the neonatal dog and cat.

REPRODUCTIVE EMERGENCIES IN THE NON-PREGNANT FEMALE

Pyometra

Aetiopathology

Pyometra is a disease of the luteal phase, with most bitches and queens showing clinical signs between 5 and 80 days after the end of oestrus. In the queen, a luteal phase only follows ovulation, which is most commonly induced by coitus. Whilst corpora lutea are always present within the ovaries of bitches and queens with pyometra, progesterone concentrations are similar to those in healthy bitches at the same stage of the luteal phase, and the functioning capacity of the corpora lutea has been shown to be normal. In the spontaneous disease, it appears that anogenital bacteria enter the uterus during oestrus and are able to proliferate during metoestrus. A further factor that must be considered in the aetiology of pyometra is the use of exogenous progestogens (for the control of oestrus) and oestrogens (for the treatment of unwanted mating). Progestogens have a stimulatory effect upon the uterus whilst oestrogens enhance the effects of progesterone.

Clinical signs

Animals are initially lethargic and inappetent with vomiting, polydipsia and polyuria. Later there may be a vulval discharge, which in some cases is associated with improvement in the general health. In other cases, the animal remains unwell and there is no discharge of pus. These cases if undiagnosed generally end fatally, often within 14–21 days from the onset of clinical signs; the cervix remains closed throughout. Death may be due to toxaemia alone or it may be associated with peritonitis due to rupture of the uterus. Occasionally the cervix relaxes and there is an outpouring of pus just before death. In other cases there may be intermittent opening of the cervix, with relative good health following the discharge of pus, and malaise during the intervening periods. Such cases generally become toxaemic within 6–8 weeks. Some cases of open-cervix pyometra may persist for years with a more or less continuous vulval discharge.

Rectal temperature may be normal in cases of open-cervix pyometra, whilst there is commonly pyrexia in cases of closed-cervix pyometra. In toxaemic patients the temperature may be subnormal.

The character of the vulval discharge may vary considerably; often it is a light chocolate-brown colour and has a characteristic odour. In other cases it is yellow in colour, often blood tinged and varying from watery to a creamy consistency. The vulva is generally enlarged and there may be discoloration or scalding of the perivulval tissues and perineum.

An increased thirst is common and is due to reduced water permeability in the distal convoluted tubule of the kidney. Renal dysfunction is probably caused by the formation of immune complexes.

Diagnostic features

Most cases can be diagnosed on the basis of the clinical signs. In addition, ultrasonography (Figure 11.1) and radiography are valuable diagnostic tools for the detection of an enlarged or fluid-filled uterus. The total number of leucocytes is frequently increased in cases of pyometra, although the degree is lower in cases of open-cervix compared with closed-cervix pyometra.

Therapeutic considerations

Renal dysfunction is common and many patients have

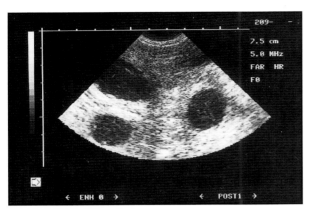

Figure 11.1: Ultrasound image of a bitch with pyometra showing three sections of the uterus filled with echogenic fluid (5.0 MHz transducer, scale in cm).

polydipsia and polyuria. There may also be vomiting such that fluid, electrolyte and acid–base balance are frequently disturbed. Intravenous fluid therapy is therefore mandatory; urine output should be maintained at approximately 1–2 ml/kg/h. Balanced electrolytes, for example Hartmann's solution, should be used to restore volume and allow any acid–base and electrolyte imbalance to be corrected. The rate of fluid administration should be according to individual requirements, but in hypovolaemic animals it may be necessary to give up to 90 ml/kg/h. The lactate precursor in Hartmann's solution should be sufficient to correct the metabolic acidosis; however, if blood pH decreases below 7.2, bicarbonate may need to be administered. Hypokalaemia may also be present and appropriate addition of potassium to the intravenous fluids may be required in these cases. It is often worthwhile monitoring the blood pressure of these patients at presentation and during stabilization and anaesthesia. This can be performed using indirect external methods or by percutaneous direct measurement. Mean blood pressure should be maintained above 60–80 mmHg.

Animals with septic shock, including some cases of pyometra, are hypoglycaemic as a result of depleted glycogen stores. If this is detected, dextrose may be added to the intravenous crystalloid fluid. Frequently, dextrose is administered as a 2.5–5.0% solution.

The common bacteria cultured in cases of pyometra are *Escherichia coli*, as well as *Staphylococcus* spp. and *Streptococcus* spp. For these reasons, broad-spectrum bactericidal antimicrobial agents may be administered intravenously, particularly those with actions against both Gram-positive and Gram-negative organisms. Suggested agents include cephalosporins, clavulanic acid-potentiated amoxycillin and trimethoprim-potentiated sulphonamides.

A number of complications may occur in patients with pyometra; secondary hepatic disease may follow sepsis or endotoxaemia, or poor hepatic perfusion associated with hypovolaemia. This is quickly reversible in most cases following removal of the uterus and restoration of fluid and electrolyte balance. A non-regenerative normochromic anaemia may also develop subsequent to bone marrow suppression, blood loss at surgery and aggressive fluid replacement. Blood transfusion is rarely indicated, unless the packed cell volume (PCV) decreases below 20%.

Treatment
Ovariohysterectomy is the treatment of choice for pyometra. Animals that are presented early in the course of the disease are usually a low surgical risk and high success rates should be expected.

The aim of the surgeon is, whenever possible, to stabilize the patient prior to surgery and then quickly to remove the uterus without causing it to rupture. Postoperative management involves continuation of fluid and antimicrobial therapy and general nursing care.

If the condition is not life threatening and the animal has a high breeding value, the question of restoration of fertility may be considered. Attempts have been made to drain the uterine fluid using a catheter placed via the cervix; however, this technique is difficult to perform and therefore surgically introduced drains have been advocated by some workers. These are inserted transcervically via a hysterotomy and are used to flush the uterus after surgery. Reasonable success rates have been reported using this method, although such treatment does not induce lysis of the corpora lutea, which are responsible for stimulating the condition.

In those cases where it is essential to retain reproductive function, or where surgery is not possible because of intercurrent disease, medical therapy may be considered. There have been several reports of successful medical management using oestrogens (presumably to induce cervical relaxation), as well as drugs to induce uterine contraction, including ergometrine, quinine and etamiphylline. However, since pyometra is a disease of the luteal phase and ovariectomy has been shown to produce resolution of the clinical signs, there has been considerable interest in the use of prostaglandins to cause lysis of the corpora lutea as well as for their uterine spasmogenic action. Recently, prostaglandins have been successfully used in the treatment of cases of open-cervix pyometra, even in those cases in which progesterone concentrations were low. A protocol of 0.25 mg/kg prostaglandin $F_{2\alpha}$ administered daily by subcutaneous injection has been recommended, although the twice daily administration of 0.125 mg/kg may result in fewer adverse effects, including restlessness, pacing, hypersalivation, tachypnoea, vomiting, diarrhoea, pyrexia and abdominal pain. These may be severe and can persist for up to 60 minutes. More recent studies have used lower dosages (20 µg/kg) three times daily for up to 10 days with good success. Hospitalization and careful observation of the patient are necessary during such treatment. Prostaglandin therapy should be combined with appropriate broad-spectrum antimicrobial agents and intravenous fluid administration. Whilst prostaglandins have been used in cases of closed-cervix pyometra, this is not recommended because of the risk of uterine rupture. Following prostaglandin treatment, up to 80% of bitches have subsequently become pregnant and whelped. More recently, there has been interest in the use of progesterone receptor antagonists. One such agent, RU46534 (aglepristone), was shown to be useful for the treatment of pyometra in bitches, producing no adverse effects and a good return to fertility. Further investigations with this agent appear warranted.

Vaginal hyperplasia

Aetiopathology
Vaginal hyperplasia (commonly termed prolapse) reflects an accentuated response of the caudal vaginal floor to normal circulating oestrogen concentrations. Usually, the vaginal mucosa cranial to the external urethral orifice is involved, becoming oedematous and thickened. This rapidly increases in size and a large smooth pink mass protrudes from the vulva. Occasionally, the circumference of the vagina may be involved. In a very small proportion of cases, dysuria may occur due to obstruction by the bulk of the tissue. The condition has not been reported in the queen.

Clinical signs
The features of the condition are easy to identify, since the hyperplastic tissue is evident protruding through the vulval lips. There is often excessive licking, and self-trauma of the site is a common sequel. If self-trauma is severe the tissue may become necrotic.

Diagnostic features
Clinical examination and speculum examination will confirm the nature of the problem.

Therapeutic considerations
In most bitches, the hyperplastic tissue decreases in size at the end of oestrus when oestrogen concentrations decrease and progesterone concentrations increase. The tissue usually completely disappears and is absent even upon careful speculum examination. The greatest problem is often that of reassuring the owner that the mass will regress. The tissue may need to be surgically removed if self-trauma has been severe.

Treatment
Conservative management with local cleansing and lubrication is usually sufficient. Self-trauma should be prevented by the application of an Elizabethan collar. It is possible to speed the termination of oestrus by the administration of progestogens such as proligestone or megoestrol acetate. Ovariohysterectomy during the subsequent anoestrus will prevent recurrence. Artificial insemination may be necessary in bitches that are required for breeding, or sub-mucosal resection of the tissue may be performed during early oestrus before mating. Sub-mucosal resection may also be required in cases where there has been self-trauma. This surgery involves performing an episiotomy, placing a urinary catheter into the urethra and resecting the hyperplastic tissue. There is often considerable blood loss at the time of surgery. A minority of surgically treated cases will recur and those that are not required for breeding should be neutered. The use of surgery in breeding animals has been questioned, since a familial tendency has been reported in certain breeds.

REPRODUCTIVE EMERGENCIES IN THE PREGNANT FEMALE

Hypocalcaemia

Aetiopathology
Eclampsia or puerperal tetany occurs most commonly during early lactation or late pregnancy in small to medium sized bitches and in multiparous queens with a large litter 2–4 weeks post-partum. The aetiology of hypocalcaemia is probably related to calcium loss in the milk combined with poor dietary availability. In some animals, reduced appetite after parturition contributes to the problem.

Clinical signs
Hypocalcaemia causes loss of cell membrane-bound calcium and subsequent changes in membrane potential. Early clinical signs are restlessness, panting, increased salivation and a stiff gait, which progress to muscle fasciculations and pyrexia. If untreated, tetany and death result.

Diagnostic features
The condition is most readily diagnosed by the clinical signs and history of late pregnancy or recent parturition. Measurement of plasma calcium concentration is diagnostic; most animals are severely hypocalcaemic with values less than 1.6 mmol/l.

Therapeutic considerations
The principal aim in the short term is to restore plasma calcium concentrations to normal. Factors that increase the protein-bound fraction of plasma calcium may contribute to the development of clinical signs; such causes include hypoglycaemia and systemic alkalosis.

Treatment
The slow intravenous administration of a 10% calcium gluconate solution to effect (5–15 mg Ca/kg) produces a rapid response; the required dose is in the region of 10 mg/kg. Cardiac rate and rhythm should be monitored during administration preferably using an electrocardiogram. If bradycardia or premature ventricular

complexes are observed, administration should temporarily cease. The response to treatment is usually dramatic; however, the effect is only maintained for between 1 and 12 hours and therefore short-term maintenance therapy is required. In clinical practice this is achieved by giving further supplementation subcutaneously and orally to prevent recurrence. Prevention of hypocalcaemia may be achieved by oral calcium supplementation in the last few days of pregnancy and during lactation. Excessive oral calcium administration reduces intestinal absorption of calcium and inhibits the secretion of parathyroid hormone, and although this is clinically significant in several species, this does not appear to be the case in the bitch or queen.

In some bitches there is a poor response to treatment and this may be related to either a contributing or primary hypoglycaemia (see below).

Hypoglycaemia

Aetiopathology
It is very rare for a bitch or queen to become hypoglycaemic during pregnancy. Normally, progesterone acts as a potent peripheral insulin antagonist and results in hyperglycaemia (see below). Indeed, dioestrus or pregnancy diabetes are well recognized, as is the difficulty in stabilizing known diabetics during dioestrus or pregnancy. However, there are reports in bitches of an apparently primary hypoglycaemia of unknown aetiology occurring during pregnancy. In some cases it is thought that hypoglycaemia worsens the clinical signs noted with hypocalcaemia. The condition has not been reported in the queen.

Clinical signs
Bitches with pregnancy hypoglycaemia are weak and may become comatose. The clinical features may be mistaken for those of hypocalcaemia, although tetany is not a usual clinical finding.

Diagnostic features
Diagnosis is based on the measurement of plasma glucose concentration. Such investigation may be stimulated by a lack of effect of intravenous calcium administration (in the initial belief that the bitch was hypocalcaemic).

Therapeutic considerations
The aim of treatment is to restore plasma glucose concentrations and provide frequent intake of glucose until the onset of parturition. The condition disappears following parturition and some authors have suggested that a Caesarean operation may be required in severe cases.

Treatment
Rapid resolution of the clinical signs is achieved following the intravenous administration of glucose to effect. Subsequently, increased frequency of feeding can be used to prevent recurrence until the onset of parturition.

Hyperglycaemia
Increased plasma progesterone concentration has a direct antagonistic effect upon insulin and also stimulates the secretion of growth hormone. Progesterone reduces insulin binding and glucose transportation within tissues. Growth hormone also has an antagonistic effect upon insulin, mediated by a decrease in the number of insulin receptors and inhibition of glucose transport.

Development of a diabetic state may therefore occur in the bitch during pregnancy; the condition is rare in the queen.

The clinical signs, diagnostic features, therapeutic considerations and treatment of hyperglycaemia associated with diabetes mellitus are discussed in Chapter 12.

Prolonged gestation

Aetiopathology
Prolonged gestation does not normally occur in the queen unless there has been unnoticed uterine inertia or dystocia. However, a common concern of many bitch owners is that parturition is 'overdue' when pregnancy length exceeds 65 or 66 days. In these cases there is a misunderstanding of the normal reproductive physiology, since whilst the 'endocrinological' length of pregnancy is 65 days, there is a large variation in the 'apparent' length of pregnancy. The latter, which is the interval from the day of mating to the day of parturition, can vary from 58 to 72 days in normal bitches of all breeds. Other causes for prolonged gestation include the bitch that has had unnoticed primary uterine inertia or dystocia, or the non-pregnant bitch that is mistakenly thought to be pregnant.

Clinical signs
Bitches that are within their physiological pregnancy length and those that are non-pregnant do not have abnormal clinical signs. Those bitches and queens that have had primary uterine inertia may have previously had a small volume vulval discharge and may have exhibited uterine and possibly abdominal contractions which were unnoticed by the owner. Subsequently, there is placental separation and the onset of a green-coloured vulval discharge. Dams then become systemically ill as the fetuses die and decompose; a large volume vulval discharge may be present. Initially, rectal temperature may be normal, but this may subsequently increase and terminally it may become subnormal.

Diagnostic features
Several methods may be used to predict the time of expected parturition in the bitch and may therefore be useful to determine whether this has been exceeded. If

the bitch has been monitored during oestrus (using measurement of plasma progesterone concentration to detect the optimal mating time), the time from ovulation to parturition is tightly regulated (63 ± 1 days). Similarly, the use of vaginal cytology during oestrus may be useful since the onset of the metoestrus vaginal smear is related to parturition (58 ± 4 days), although not as precisely as the time of ovulation. A third useful assessment is to instruct the owner to record the rectal temperature twice daily during the last one-third of pregnancy, since a decline in rectal temperature precedes partition by approximately 12–36 hours. In the queen, prediction of the time of expected parturition can be achieved by counting the number of days from mating. In many bitches, however, none of these procedures has been undertaken and in many queens mating is frequently unnoticed. It is important, therefore, to perform a full clinical examination to ensure that the dam is clinically well and that she is pregnant. Measurement of plasma progesterone concentration can then be used to assess whether parturition is imminent. Progesterone concentrations decrease approximately 24–36 hours before parturition in both species (Figure 11.2). Demonstration of high plasma progesterone concentration therefore indicates that parturition is not imminent, whilst a low progesterone concentration indicates that parturition is imminent or should already have occurred. Intermediate values are difficult to interpret. Plasma progesterone can be easily measured in the practice laboratory by the use of ELISA kits.

From the above, it can be seen that bitches that are still within their normal physiological pregnancy length will have high plasma progesterone concentrations, whilst bitches and queens that have had primary uterine inertia will have low plasma progesterone concentrations. Non-pregnant bitches may have high or low plasma progesterone concentrations, since the luteal phase of pregnancy and non-pregnancy is remarkably similar. Non-pregnant queens will have low plasma progesterone concentrations unless the queen has returned to oestrus and subsequently ovulated.

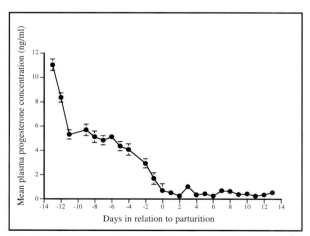

Figure 11.2: *Changes in mean plasma progesterone concentration (± SEM) in 10 periparturient bitches.*

Treatment

No treatment is required for the bitch that has a normal long apparent pregnancy length or the bitch or queen that is non-pregnant. For the dam that has suffered primary uterine inertia, the best option is to perform a Caesarean operation to remove the retained fetuses, which are likely to be dead. This should be performed as described below, although the requirements for fluid therapy may differ if the bitch is endotoxaemic or septicaemic.

Dystocia

Aetiopathology

There are many causes of dystocia in the bitch and queen and it is not possible to describe these fully within this review. It is sufficient to classify dystocia as either non-obstructive (primary uterine inertia) or obstructive (dystocia secondary to maternal or fetal causes). Primary uterine inertia occurs most commonly in dams with a small litter, very large litter, or in obese females or those at their first parturition. Obstructive dystocia may be related to breed, previous injury of the dam or a multiple of fetal causes. Secondary uterine inertia may develop after the correction of an obstructive dystocia.

Clinical signs

In non-obstructive dystocia, there may be few clinical signs (see prolonged gestation above); however, the observant owner may notice that first stage parturition has commenced but that this has not progressed.

In cases of obstructive dystocia, the female has entered second stage parturition and continues to strain unproductively. This may occur during the birth of any of the fetuses depending upon the cause.

Diagnostic features

Females with non-obstructive dystocia have relaxation of the perineal musculature, dilation of the cervix (this can only be assessed upon endoscopic examination and not digital palpation) and already have had a decline in plasma progesterone (and in bitches a subsequent decline in rectal temperature). If placental separation occurs, a green-coloured vulval discharge will be evident. Early in the course of the condition the fetuses will be alive, and fetal movement may be palpated and fetal movement and heart beats may be detected ultrasonographically. Fetal death can be recognized immediately using ultrasonography by an absence of fetal movement and by a non-moving echogenic appearance to the heart. Fetal death can be detected radiographically by a change in the fetal posture, by the accumulation of gas within the fetus and/or uterus and by overlapping of the bones of the skull, although these changes may take several days before they are evident.

Similar diagnostic methods may be used when there is obstructive dystocia, where fetuses can be identified lodged within the birth canal as a result of fetal or maternal abnormalities.

Therapeutic considerations

Females with primary uterine inertia will respond to the administration of exogenous oxytocin. However, the aetiology of the condition is not entirely clear and such therapy should be considered in light of the clinical condition of the dam, as well as the likely number of fetuses to be delivered. For example, it may be preferable to undertake a Caesarean operation in a bitch that has a large number of puppies and is debilitated, rather than to administer oxytocin repeatedly, resulting in an extended parturition with the possibility of dead fetuses.

In females with obstructive dystocia, the primary aim is to remove the obstruction. This can be achieved using retropulsion, realignment and traction techniques if the obstruction is the result of an abnormality of fetal presentation, position or posture. Care should be taken to ensure that parturition continues normally after such correction, since there is a risk of the development of secondary uterine inertia. However, in many cases, the dystocia is the result of a fetal or maternal abnormality that cannot be corrected to allow normal delivery, and in such circumstances it is necessary to resort to a Caesarean operation. In such cases it should be remembered that: (a) the dam may be 'normal' or she may be debilitated and require careful anaesthetic management, (b) there is often no time for pre-anaesthetic preparation and (c) the dam may have recently been fed. The general aims of the procedure are to ensure adequate oxygenation (by intubation and provision of inspired oxygen), to maintain blood volume and prevent hypotension (by the administration of intravenous fluid therapy) and to minimize maternal and fetal depression during surgery and after delivery (by reducing the dose of anaesthetic agents used). A number of factors are important when considering the most appropriate fluid for intravenous administration, for example there may be increased alveolar ventilation (an effect of progesterone) causing respiratory alkalosis, although the enlarged abdomen may produce a decreased tidal volume causing respiratory acidosis, there may be loss of acid because of vomiting and there may be loss of blood as a result of the surgery. The best choice agent is probably lactated Ringer's solution administered at a rate of 10–20 ml/kg/h.

It is not possible to discuss all of the anaesthetic options for Caesarean operation in this text; however, there are a few points worth considering. For premedication, atropine is best not given routinely, since it blocks the normal bradycardic response of the fetus to hypoxia and it relaxes the lower oesophageal sphincter, making aspiration more likely. Phenothiazine tranquillizers are very useful agents, since they smooth anaesthetic induction and reduce the subsequent dose of induction and maintenance agents; they are, however, rapidly transported across the placenta. Alpha$_2$-adrenoceptor agonists such as medetomidine and xylazine are contraindicated because of their severe cardiorespiratory depressant effects. Similarly, the respiratory depressant effect of opioids make them unpopular. Metoclopramide may be administered intravenously prior to induction to reduce the risk of vomiting during the procedure. For the induction of anaesthesia, dissociative agents such as ketamine are best avoided because they produce profound depression of the fetuses. The ultrashort-acting barbiturates and propofol appear to be most useful, since they are either rapidly redistributed or metabolized and therefore have limited effect upon the fetuses after delivery.

For maintenance of anaesthesia, the volatile agents are preferable, especially those with low partition coefficients such as isoflurane. This agent has a rapid uptake and elimination by the animal and it may have a better cardiovascular margin of safety than the more soluble agents such as halothane.

Whilst nitrous oxide may be used to reduce the dose of other anaesthetic agents, it is rapidly transferred across the placenta and, although it has minimal effects upon the fetus *in utero*, it may result in a significant diffusion hypoxia after delivery. In certain cases, inhalational agents are used for anaesthetic induction and in this case nitrous oxide is useful for speeding the induction of anaesthesia via the second gas effect.

Treatment

In females with primary uterine inertia, or secondary uterine inertia after the correction of an obstruction, the intramuscular administration of oxytocin (0.25–1.0 IU/kg) may be all that is required to ensure continuation of parturition. In some cases, the effectiveness of uterine contractions can be improved by the administration of 50–150 mg/kg 10% calcium borogluconate. When there is a large litter, oxytocin administration may need to be repeated approximately every 30 minutes.

In debilitated dams or those with an obstructive dystocia that cannot be resolved, a Caesarean operation should be performed after stabilization and consideration of the anaesthetic requirements discussed above. Operative speed is important since surgical delay is associated with increased fetal depression and asphyxia. Following a conventional Caesarean operation, the uterus should rapidly begin to contract. If this is not the case, oxytocin should be administered to promote uterine involution. This may be required especially if halothane anaesthesia has been used, since this agent is known to delay uterine involution. The administration of oxytocin should, however, not be taken lightly since it may produce peripheral vasodilation and hypotension.

REPRODUCTIVE EMERGENCIES IN THE POST-PARTURIENT FEMALE

Metritis

Aetiopathology

There are a number of causes of acute metritis in the

bitch and queen, some of which are discussed in greater detail below. The common causes include prolonged parturition, poor uterine involution, retained placentae, retained fetuses and obstetrical intervention. The condition is principally a bacterial infection of the uterus, usually with bacteria that are normally considered commensal organisms.

Clinical signs

There is most frequently a purulent or serosanguineous vulval discharge. The dam is often lethargic and anorexic and there may initially be pyrexia, although if untreated the rectal temperature may become sub-normal. The dam is often weak and may be dehydrated and may continue to strain.

Diagnostic features

Often the uterus is palpably enlarged, but enlargement can be detected radiographically and by the use of ultrasound. The latter technique usually demonstrates echogenic material present within the uterine lumen, and thickening of the uterine wall.

Therapeutic considerations

Stabilization of the patient by the administration of appropriate fluid therapy is essential, as is the administration of suitable broad-spectrum antimicrobial agents such as ampicillin or trimethoprim-potentiated sulphonamides. There is no underlying endocrine component of this condition unlike pyometra, and the primary aim is to establish drainage of the uterus.

Treatment

Trans-cervical lavage of the uterus with physiological saline is extremely useful to encourage drainage of the infected material. This can be difficult without endoscopic guidance, although in these cases, the cervix usually remains open. Drainage can also be stimulated by the administration of ecbolic agents such as oxytocin and prostaglandin. Local application of antimicrobial agents into the uterus is valuable, however, because of the problems of administration of most agents are given systemically. In severe cases ovariohysterectomy may be necessary.

Haemorrhage

Aetiopathology

Haemorrhage is an uncommon post-partum condition in the bitch and queen that may occur as a result of physical injuries to the uterus or vaginal wall, or as a result of placental necrosis.

Clinical signs

Blood loss is common at the time of parturition, although this is normally limited to the time of delivery of each fetus. A small volume of haemorrhagic fluid may be passed after the termination of parturition in the normal female, but this rapidly decreases in volume and changes in colour due to the release of the pigment uteroverdin from the marginal haematoma. Persistence of a haemorrhagic discharge is abnormal. The dam may initially be unsettled, but later may be depressed and have pale mucous membranes.

Diagnostic features

Inspection of the vaginal wall either digitally or using a speculum or endoscope may demonstrate the site of a physical injury. Uterine bleeding may be detected by the presence of haemorrhagic fluid exiting via the cervix, or by transabdominal ultrasound imaging of the uterus. It is not normally necessary to measure the PCV of the fluid.

Therapeutic considerations

The principle consideration is to prevent further blood loss and to maintain blood volume as discussed in uterine prolapse (see below).

Treatment

Cases of vaginal trauma can be treated either by direct pressure or the application of a vaginal tampon, or occasionally by clamping of the bleeding tissue using artery forceps followed by subsequent ligation. For uterine bleeding in the first instance, it is appropriate to attempt to speed uterine involution by the administration of oxytocin (0.25–1.0 IU/kg) or ergometrine (0.2–0.5 mg/kg). If there is no response, a laparotomy and ovariohysterectomy may be indicated, although a coagulopathy should always be suspected and assessments of clotting function should be performed prior to surgery.

Retained fetuses or placentae

Aetiopathology

Retained placentae are very uncommon in bitches and queens, despite the concern expressed by many breeders. Most commonly the condition is mistaken, since placentae are not always expelled after each fetus and several are delivered some time later during parturition. Retained fetuses should be investigated as described in primary and secondary uterine inertia (see above).

The aetiology of placental retention is unknown, but it appears to be more common in toy breeds of dog.

Clinical signs

In cases of true placental retention in the bitch, there is usually persistence of a green-coloured vulval discharge, and the bitch may be restless and not allow the puppies to suck. If the condition is not treated, the discharge will become malodorous and the bitch may become depressed, septicaemic and toxaemic. In general, queens have similar clinical signs, although in some there are no signs of vulval discharge until several weeks after parturition.

Diagnostic features

Diagnosis of the condition soon after parturition can be very difficult without ultrasonographic or endoscopic examination. Transabdominal palpation is often misleading because the involuting uterus may have sections which are dilated, and adjacent regions that are smaller in diameter.

Therapeutic considerations

In many cases there are no placentae retained and the problem is simply the concern of the owner. In true cases the bitch or queen may become septicaemic and toxaemic. In such instances, removal of the infected material is imperative; however, stabilization of the patient with appropriate fluid and antimicrobial therapy is essential. The principles as described in pyometra (see above) should be followed.

Treatment

In the early stages, repeated administration of oxytocin may be sufficient to cause expulsion of the retained placentae. This results in resolution of the clinical signs, although the dam should be treated with broad-spectrum antimicrobial agents such as ampicillin or trimethoprim-potentiated sulphonamides to prevent the development of a secondary metritis.

In the later stages of the condition, the number of uterine oxytocin receptors have decreased and the administration of exogenous oxytocin has little or no clinical effect. In these instances repeated low-dose prostaglandin treatment may be contemplated (as described for pyometra – see above); however, it may be difficult to dislodge the placenta, and hysterotomy may be indicated. In animals not required for breeding, ovariohysterectomy is the treatment of choice.

Uterine prolapse

Aetiopathology

Prolapse of one or both uterine horns is rare in the bitch and queen and is only associated with pregnancy. The condition occurs following parturition or abortion. It may occur in females of all ages and, although the aetiology is uncertain, it is claimed to be due to over-relaxation and stretching of the pelvic musculature, uterine atony, trauma of the uterus and prolonged tenesmus during dystocia. Following prolapse, there is commonly rupture of the uterine vessels and the vessels in the broad ligament resulting in haemoperitoneum and hypovolaemic shock.

Clinical signs

The history is that of a dam that has recently undergone parturition or has aborted, and either one or both uterine horns can be identified at the vulva. Frequently, the patient continues to have abdominal contractions. The prolapsed uterus may be traumatized, in which case there is considerable haemorrhage.

Diagnostic features

The condition can be diagnosed by the history and presenting clinical signs. In the bitch, uterine prolapse can be easily differentiated from vaginal hyperplasia since the latter occurs during oestrus and has an insidious onset.

Therapeutic considerations

The principal consideration is the loss of blood volume. This can be restored by the use of plasma expanders and crystalloids administered intravenously. In most cases crystalloids should be administered at a rate of 2.5 times the anticipated volume that has been lost. Blood transfusion may be considered when the PCV decreases to 20%, or in patients in whom arterial pressure cannot be maintained by infusion of balanced electrolyte solutions. In cases of severe haemorrhage, autotransfusion may be considered by collecting blood aseptically from the peritoneal cavity.

Treatment

Prompt laparotomy with traction of the prolapsed uterus is necessary to allow inspection of the uterine vessels. In cases that are presented early, replacement and pexy of the uterus may be attempted; however, in most cases there is marked pathology of the uterine vasculature, and ovariohysterectomy is the treatment of choice.

Hypocalcaemia

See above.

Septic mastitis

Aetiopathology

In many cases mastitis is a minor clinical disease. However, acute septic mastitis can occur following the introduction of bacteria during the process of suckling. The condition may occur in a single gland, or occasionally may involve all glands. The common bacteria involved are *E. coli* and *Staphylococcus* spp.

Clinical signs

The affected gland is normally hot, swollen and painful and there may be discoloration of the skin surrounding the teat. The dam is normally pyrexic and lethargic.

Diagnostic features

Examination of strippings from the affected gland or glands often demonstrates a haemorrhagic discoloration of the milk. Microscopic examination may be useful to demonstrate the presence of bacteria, and culture may be undertaken to identify the sensitivity of the organism to antimicrobial agents.

Therapeutic considerations

Topical instillation of antimicrobial agents into the teat canal is not possible and systemic antimicrobials should be used with care, since the aim is to have high milk concentrations, which will be ingested by the neonates. However, in the case of a severe septic mastitis the dam is so unwell that it is often necessary to remove the litter and institute artificial feeding.

Treatment

Stripping of the affected glands and the use of hot compresses is important to encourage drainage of the infected material. The administration of appropriate antimicrobial agents is essential; however, in many cases it is not possible to wait for the results of culture and sensitivity, and therefore broad-spectrum agents are often chosen. Ampicillin is the agent of choice, although chloramphenicol has also been recommended. Agents that are weak bases tend to achieve high concentrations, since milk is slightly more acidic than plasma. Occasionally, severely affected glands become necrotic and surgical drainage is necessary.

REPRODUCTIVE EMERGENCIES IN THE MALE

Paraphimosis

Aetiopathology

Paraphimosis is a failure of the glans penis to be retracted fully into the prepuce. This may be the result of a small preputial orifice, inversion of the preputial skin and hair, a short prepuce or neurogenic factors affecting the preputial muscles. In the tom, the condition has only been reported associated with an abnormality of the preputial orifice. Paraphimosis may become an emergency because there is swelling of the penis, interference with the circulation within the penis and ultimately ischaemic necrosis. Secondary urethral obstruction may result.

Clinical signs

Initially, clinical signs are extrusion of the penis, associated with pain and continuous licking. Self-trauma may progress to mutilation. After several hours, the penis becomes cold and the male may pay less attention to the area.

Diagnostic features

The condition can be diagnosed by inspection, and differentiated from other conditions, since normally the penis is engorged.

Treatment

The application of ice packs and lubricants may be sufficient to allow replacement of the penis, which is the primary goal. In some cases the male will not allow any manipulation, and sedation is required; this can be helpful since it reduces systemic blood pressure and causes detumescence of the penis. Surgical enlargement of the urethral orifice may be necessary to allow replacement

of the penis, and in some cases amputation of the necrotic organ is required.

Torsion of the spermatic cord (testicular torsion)

Aetiopathology

Rotation of one of the testes around the vertical axis causes occlusion of the pampiniform plexus, followed by swelling and necrosis of the testicle. The aetiology is unknown although it may be related to rupture of the scrotal ligament. Torsion is more common in enlarged neoplastic intra-abdominal testes. The condition has not been reported in the tom.

Clinical signs

Torsion results in severe pain, unilateral swelling of the scrotum and thickening of the spermatic cord (Figure 11.3). Frequently, dogs are unwilling to walk and continually self traumatize the scrotum. Clinical signs are diagnostic when the condition occurs in a scrotal testis, but may be confusing when the torsion relates to an abdominal testis. In these cases there may be lethargy, inappetence, abdominal pain and vomiting. Later in the course of the condition, the animal may develop ascites and become shocked. A firm mass may be palpated within the caudal abdomen.

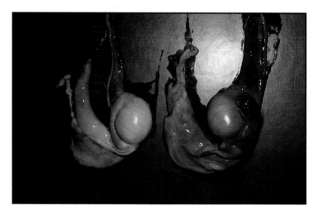

Figure 11.3: *Normal testicle and testicle with torsion of the spermatic cord demonstrating severe haemorrhage and oedema.*

Diagnostic features

Diagnosis can be made upon the clinical signs for scrotal testes; however, ultrasonography and/or exploratory surgery may be necessary in dogs with torsion of intra-abdominal testes.

Therapeutic considerations

Dogs with this condition require treatment for shock using fluid therapy and possibly the administration of corticosteroids.

Treatment

Prompt surgical removal of the affected testis is essential.

Acute bacterial prostatitis

Aetiopathology

Adult dogs may develop prostatitis following ascending infection of bacteria, commonly *E. coli*, *Staphylococcus* spp. and *Streptococcus* spp. Prostatitis does not occur in the tom. In dogs, certain conditions increase the likelihood of contamination of the prostate gland, including benign prostatic hyperplasia and squamous metaplasia. It is likely that diseases which increase the number of bacteria within the prostatic urethra including cystitis, urethral calculi and neoplasia also increase the chance of prostatitis developing.

Clinical signs

The clinical signs often include systemic illness, with pyrexia, vomiting and caudal abdominal pain. There may be a purulent or haemorrhagic discharge at the prepuce. Urethral obstruction or colonic compression can occur if the prostate becomes large enough.

Diagnostic features

Dogs are commonly neutrophilic and the gland is painful and has an irregular contour upon palpation. Urine culture, urethral washings and fine needle aspiration may help with the diagnosis. An often overlooked technique is to collect a semen sample and cytologically examine the third fraction of the ejaculate.

Therapeutic considerations

The blood–prostatic fluid barrier is thought to be lost when there is severe inflammation, and therefore many antimicrobial agents can be used for the treatment of prostatitis. Inadequately treated lesions may become chronic and pockets of purulent exudate may form (prostatic abscessation), producing signs of recurrent cystitis or destruction. Treatment of these cases is difficult.

Reduction of the size of the gland may be helpful in speeding the resolution of the disease.

Treatment

Prompt antimicrobial treatment should preferably be undertaken on the basis of culture and identification of sensitivity; potentiated sulphonamides and enrofloxacin are particularly useful if treatment is required before this can be established. Penicillins and cephalosporins have limited penetration into prostatic fluid. Treatment should be continued until no bacteria are found within the prostatic fluid; this may require 3 weeks of therapy or more, but is necessary to prevent the development of chronic disease. If chronic infection and abscessation are diagnosed, surgical investigation and drainage is required.

Recovery in many cases can be enhanced by reducing prostatic size, either by castration or the administration of exogenous progestogens or oestrogens. Exogenous steroids produce only a temporary response, and it should be remembered that prolonged oestrogen therapy may produce prostatic metaplasia which predisposes to prostatitis.

EMERGENCIES IN THE NEONATE

Resuscitation of neonates

Neonates may require to be resuscitated following a Caesarean operation, or following a normal delivery. In both cases, the primary cause of mortality is hypoxia. This can be reduced by the rapid removal of fetuses from the amniotic sac. The nostrils and oropharynx should be cleared of fluid using a plastic pipette or cotton swabs. Fluid can also be removed by supporting the head and neck and swinging the neonate slowly downwards in a large arc. Care must be paid to ensure that a whiplash or concussive injury does not occur. The neonate should be vigorously dried, since this stimulates respiratory drive. Gentle compression of the chest usually results in the establishment of respiratory effort. If this is not the case and the heart is beating, respiratory stimulation should be continued by rubbing the thorax. In certain cases the administration of respiratory stimulant agents such as doxopram hydrochloride (1–2 drops sublingually), may be efficacious, as may the administration of oxygen. If respiration does not commence, then artificial respiration should be performed by endotracheal intubation using a 20 gauge plastic catheter, or by blowing gently into the nose and mouth. These should both be performed carefully to induce only slight lung expansion without over-inflation. If the heart is not beating, external cardiac massage combined with artificial respiration may be attempted.

Once regular respiratory efforts are maintained, the neonate may be placed into a prewarmed box or incubator until it is active, when it should be returned to the dam and encouraged to suck.

Sucking normally occurs immediately after birth and at intervals of 2–3 hours for the first few days. The umbilicus should be cut approximately 3 cm from the fetal abdomen; excessive bleeding can be prevented by the application of a ligature or haemostatic clip.

Nursing care of neonates

Once born, the puppies and kittens should be carefully examined and their body weight should be recorded. Normal neonates increase in body weight by 5–10% per day; a failure to achieve this rate may indicate ill-health. Examination should ensure that the umbilicus is clean and there should be no evidence of herniation. Respiration should be regular and without excessive noise; the normal respiratory rate is 15–40 breaths per minute. There should be no discharge from the eyes or ears. The neonate should be examined for the presence of congenital diseases. The normal rectal temperature is 32–34°C in the first week after birth.

The environmental temperature is critical; hypothermia is a major cause of neonatal mortality.

Recommended temperatures (25–30°C) are only necessary for the first few days; these are often unbearable for the dam and can be safely reduced (22°C) as long as draughts are avoided.

One method to reduce heat exposure of the dam is to heat only half of the box. Underfloor heating is the ideal; however, warm hot water bottles or circulating water blankets provide a good alternative. Heat lamps that are suspended above the nest should be used with caution, since the environment may become too hot.

Neonatal puppies and kittens are unable to stand at birth. They should, however, be quite mobile by using their limbs to crawl. Neonates should be assessed for their general strength and the weakest should be carefully observed, since these often do not feed adequately and may fail to thrive. Standing may be seen from 10 days after birth, and most neonates should be able to walk at 3 weeks of age.

Puppies and kittens are born with their eyes closed; separation of the upper and lower lids and opening of the eyes occurs approximately 10–14 days after birth. The cornea at this stage may appear slightly cloudy, although this will disappear over the first 4 weeks. In the first few weeks of life, the dam will provide all the care for her offspring provided that the environment is clean and dry. Many types of bedding material may be used including shredded paper, newspaper and blankets or newspaper and synthetic rugs. Materials should be washable or easily disposed of. The dam normally licks the perineal region of each neonate for the first 2–3 weeks after birth to stimulate urination and defaecation. Puppies and kittens defecate and urinate voluntarily at 3 weeks of age and at this time soiling of the bedding increases; regular changing of the bedding is therefore necessary.

When considering pharmacological therapy for neonates, it should be remembered that drug distribution differs considerably from that of adults because of differences in body composition (lower body fat stores and plasma albumin concentrations, higher percentage of total body water and a poorly developed blood–brain barrier). For these reasons, drug dosages may need to be reduced by up to 50% and the frequency of administration may need to be reduced.

Fading puppies and kittens

Perinatal losses are generally thought to be higher in dogs and cats than other species; approximately 15% are reported to be dead at birth and a further 8% to have died shortly afterwards. Examination of dead puppies shows that asphyxia is the most common cause. This probably relates to the fact that oxygenation is threatened at birth because: (a) there is reduced blood flow to the uterus during contractions, (b) the umbilicus is stretched (it is very short anyway) and (c) the placenta separates some time prior to delivery. Immediately after birth there are therefore marked physiological changes for the neonate; the arterial oxygen concentrations decrease and the arterial carbon dioxide concentrations increase. Neonates are therefore born with a moderate to severe acidosis. Recovery of normal blood values should occur over a period of 3–6 hours. This is mediated by normal respiration and can therefore be inhibited by poor respiratory function (i.e. carbon dioxide is not reduced if breathing is poor). It is clear that suitable supervision at the time of parturition can reduce the loss rates considerably; indeed, in high quality breeding establishments the total losses are in the order of 5%.

However, in addition to perinatal losses caused by asphyxia many puppies and kittens are lost without an apparent cause being found. These neonatal losses are often said to be attributed to fading puppy/kitten syndrome. The first signs of this can often be detected within a few hours of life and it is possible that these neonates are not fully viable at birth. Occasionally, a primary infectious agent, such as parvovirus, is identified; however, in most cases bacteriological and viral investigations are unrewarding. In general, most of these losses occur because of congenital abnormalities, nutritional disease (including inadequate feeding), abnormally low birth weight, trauma during or immediately after birth, neonatal isoerythrolysis (kittens) and various infectious disease. There are no consistent reports of successful treatment of fading puppies and kittens, probably because many are in *extremis* at the time of presentation. Often, whatever the cause, there appears to be an early failure to suck and subsequent establishment of a fatal cycle of dehydration and further failure to feed. Early supplementary feeding may improve the survival rates, as may the administration of antimicrobial agents in cases of neonatal sepsis. However, many cases are not related to a primary bacterial infection and such treatment alone is often unrewarding. Intensive therapy, including the administration of intravenous fluids and antimicrobial agents, and intravenous nutrition may be valuable; however, the prognosis for most cases is extremely guarded. Prevention is aimed at: the early recognition of weak neonates, or dams that have inadequate milk or poor mothering behaviour; and instituting rapid and aggressive supplementary feeding. Accurate post-mortem examination is essential to establish the causative factors so that these can be eliminated prior to the next breeding.

Artificial nutrition of neonates

Maternal illness, death of the dam, poor nursing, inadequate lactation and a large litter are all factors that contribute to malnutrition of the neonate. In these cases, partial hand-rearing (with rotation of the offspring between the dam and artificial feeding), complete hand-rearing or a foster dam (a bitch in pseudopregnancy or a bitch/queen who has lost her litter) are required.

When contemplating artificial feeding, a well formulated milk replacer is essential and, whilst home-prepared replacers using cows' milk have been advocated, it is the author's opinion that a commercially available replacer should be used. It has been suggested that some neonates should be reared entirely artificially rather than alternating the whole litter. However, all neonates should remain with the dam to ensure a normal social development.

It is essential that all neonates receive colostrum from the dam during the first few hours after birth to ensure an adequate uptake of maternal immunoglobulins. Should the dam have died, it may still be possible to milk some colostrum from the mammary glands as long as it is not contaminated with high concentrations of drugs or toxins. Orogastric intubation is relatively simple and may be useful in the first few days of life for the rapid feeding of especially sick neonates. A soft polythene tube (2 mm diameter) measured from the mouth to a level with the 9th rib is optimal.

Artificial feeding is time consuming and demanding, particularly if the litter is being reared without the dam. Milk substitutes may be administered using syringe feeders, eye droppers, sucking devices or stomach tube. In most cases it may be easiest to feed from a small syringe (2 ml) for the first 2–5 days. After this time, a small bottle with a nipple may be used; this encourages normal sucking but takes the greatest time. When these devices are used the aperture should be large enough to prevent wind sucking but small enough to prevent excessive volumes being administered, since this may result in aspiration.

Normally neonates feed every 2–4 hours for the first 5 days of life. It is best to mimic this with artificial feeding. The interval can be reduced to every 4 hours after day 5. The milk replacer should be warmed to body temperature (39°C) before feeding and then fed to the manufacturer's instructions, depending upon body weight. After each feeding, the perineal area of the neonate should be stimulated with a moist towel, to mimic the licking action of the dam and stimulate urination and defecation.

CONCLUSION

It is clear that there are many reproductive disorders which produce acute onset and potentially fatal clinical disease in dogs and cats. Similarly, there are many management factors responsible for perinatal mortality in puppies and kittens. There have been substantial advances in our knowledge of reproductive and neonatal physiology and pharmacology over the past 15 years, and with prompt recognition many of these conditions can be quickly and effectively treated without subsequent loss of reproductive performance.

FURTHER READING

England GCW (1998) *Allen's Fertility and Obstetrics in the Dog.* Blackwell Science, Oxford

Gilbert RO, Nothling JO and Oettle EE (1989) A retrospective study of 40 cases of canine pyometra-metritis treated with prostaglandin F-2alpha and broad spectrum antibacterial drugs. *Journal of Reproduction and Fertility Supplement* **39**, 225–229

Gourley IM (1975) Treatment of canine pyometra without ovariohysterectomy. In: *Current Techniques in Small Animal Surgery*, ed. MJ Bojrab. Lea and Febiger, Philadelphia

Hoskins JD (1990) *Veterinary Pediatrics: Dogs and Cats from Birth to Six Months.* WB Saunders, Philadelphia

Jackson PGG (1995) *Handbook of Veterinary Obstetrics.* WB Saunders, London

CHAPTER TWELVE

Endocrine and Metabolic Emergencies

Tim Hackett

ENDOCRINE EMERGENCIES

Diabetic ketoacidosis

Diabetic ketoacidosis (DKA) is one of the most common small animal endocrine emergencies. DKA may be discovered when a previously undiagnosed patient is found to be an insulin-dependent diabetic after presenting in a ketoacidotic crisis. Alternatively, a known diabetic animal with poorly regulated disease may become ketoacidotic because of inadequate insulin therapy. In this case, problems with insulin therapy may involve the use of outdated or mishandled insulin products, incorrect administration or insulin resistance.

Pathophysiology and diagnosis

Diabetes mellitus causes accumulation of glucose in plasma, as a result of impaired glucose uptake, utilization and storage. When the renal threshold of glucose is exceeded, the resulting glucosuria causes an osmotic diuresis and primary polyuria. With progression of the disease, the secondary polydipsia is insufficient to maintain fluid balance, and dehydration results. Insulin deficiency leads to a relative lack of calories in insulin-dependent tissues, which stimulates fat mobilization as an alternate energy source. Increasing levels of glucagon activate hormone-sensitive lipase, which mediates the transport of long-chain free fatty acids (FFAs). When excess glucagon is present, FFAs are oxidized in the liver to produce the ketone bodies ß-hydroxybutyrate, acetone and acetoacetate. In the presence of insulin and glucose substrate, ketone bodies can be metabolized to carbon dioxide and water, which together can form bicarbonate. In the absence of insulin, ketone production exceeds its metabolism, resulting in ketonuria and metabolic acidosis.

It is worth noting that the colorimetric urine dipsticks used to check for ketonuria detect only acetoacetate. In highly reduced states such as severe hypovolaemia and hypoperfusion, ß-hydroxybutyrate predominates. For this reason, severely ketotic patients may show only trace levels of ketones using a dipstick. Addition of 1-2 drops of hydrogen peroxide to the urine sample will oxidize the ß-hydroxybutyrate to acetoacetate. After retesting, the strip should show a strong positive reaction for ketones. Similarly, patients showing an excellent response to fluid therapy may test more strongly positive for ketones on subsequent urine tests, as acetoacetate begins to predominate over ß-hydroxybutyrate with rehydration and improved perfusion.

Management

Emergency treatment of DKA is aimed at correcting severe dehydration, electrolyte abnormalities and metabolic acidosis, in addition to providing insulin. A central intravenous large bore (16-18 gauge) catheter should be placed, in anticipation of a large fluid requirement and to facilitate the collection of multiple blood samples over time. Drawing small blood samples through the catheter instead of using needles for every sample can minimize patient discomfort and iatrogenic blood loss. Blood glucose should be measured no less than every 2 hours. Intravenous fluid resuscitation is initiated with 0.9% NaCl. Potassium supplementation will be required once the acidosis and poor perfusion are corrected, as most DKA patients have a total body potassium deficit, even though they may initially have hyperkalaemia at presentation.

Hyperglycaemia and ketoacidosis should be addressed with regular insulin. Regular insulin will result in the most rapid ketone metabolism and by virtue of its short duration of action provides the most accurate control of blood glucose in critical patients. There are several protocols for administration of regular insulin in DKA (Figure 12.1). Because of the severe dehydration, subcutaneous administration is contraindicated. Either low dose intramuscular injections of regular insulin, or constant rate infusion using an infusion pump can be used. The goal is not to normalize blood glucose, but to metabolize ketones and to bring the plasma glucose concentrations below the renal threshold for glucose loss. Maintenance of blood glucose within the 6-17 mmol/l range is an acceptable degree of control for most DKA patients. When the blood glucose levels drop with insulin therapy, glucose may need to be added to the intravenous fluids, as adequate dextrose is required for metabolism of ketone bodies by insulin.

As insulin corrects the hyperglycaemia, potassium and phosphorus are driven into the cells. Potassium and phosphorus should be monitored and if necessary added to the maintenance fluids as therapy continues.

Fluid replacement

1. Place a central, large bore (16—18 gauge) intravenous catheter
2. Obtain baseline blood samples for CBC, diagnostic profile, electrolytes, blood glucose. Obtain a urinalysis
3. Begin resuscitation with 0.9% NaCl, shock bolus up to 90 ml/kg if required
4. When pulse quality is improved and patient is not showing clinical signs of shock, assess serum electrolytes to determine optimal maintenance fluid plan:
   - If blood glucose <11 mmol/l, add 5% dextrose
   - If normokalaemic or hypokalaemic add 20-80 mEq/l potassium chloride (Figure 12.6)
   - If hypophosphataemic or showing evidence of haemolysis add potassium phosphate to fluids so that the patient receives 0.03-0.12 mmol phosphorus/kg/h

Insulin therapy

If an infusion pump is available, use a continuous infusion of intravenous regular insulin. If accurate infusion methods are not available use an hourly intramuscular regular insulin protocol.

Continuous intravenous regular insulin infusion:
- Dogs – give 2.2 IU/kg/day regular insulin by continuous infusion
- Cats – give 1.1 IU/kg/day regular insulin by continuous infusion
- Insulin can be mixed with maintenance fluids but at least 50 ml of fluid should be allowed to run through all plastic tubing first, to allow insulin to bind to the tubing
- Blood glucose should be rechecked every 1-2 hours and fluid therapy and dextrose concentrations adjusted to maintain blood glucose between 6 and 17 mmol/l
- Potassium and phosphorus should be rechecked at least every 6 hours
- Continue therapy until the patient is rehydrated, no longer ketonuric and eating

Hourly intramuscular regular insulin:
- After a loading dose of 0.2 IU/kg, the patient should receive 0.1 IU/kg every hour
- Blood glucose should be rechecked every 1-2 hours and fluid therapy and dextrose concentrations adjusted to maintain blood glucose between 6 and 17 mmol/l
- Potassium and phosphorus should be rechecked at least every 6 hours
- When the patient is well hydrated, regular insulin can be given every 6 hours by subcutaneous injection until ketonuria has resolved

Figure 12.1: Emergency treatment of diabetic ketoacidosis.

Hypokalaemia can result in weakness, while severe hypophosphataemia (<0.5 mmol/l) causes weakness, haemolysis and even thrombocytopenia. If phosphorus cannot be measured, anaemic patients or those with haemolysed plasma can be assumed to be hypophosphataemic unless azotaemia is also present. Phosphorus should be supplemented using potassium phosphate (0.03-0.12 mmol/kg/h). The potassium contained in the phosphorus infusion should be taken into consideration as part of the overall potassium supplementation. If hypokalaemia is refractory to supplementation, serum magnesium should be measured and magnesium should be supplemented (1 mEq/kg/24 h) if the levels are low.

As therapy progresses and the patient becomes rehydrated, insulin therapy can be continued with subcutaneous regular insulin every 6 hours. Close attention to patient condition and frequent rechecks of blood glucose and urine ketones should continue while providing insulin and substrate. When the ketones have disappeared from the urine and the patient is eating, a main-

tenance insulin regimen can be started.

If the pet was on insulin for previously diagnosed diabetes mellitus, the owners should be asked about their daily insulin routine. Outdated, mishandled and inappropriately administered medications are some common causes of treatment failures. If the problem persists with proper administration of an adequate dose of fresh insulin, then insulin resistance should be investigated. Systemic infections and hyperadrenocorticism are the most common causes of insulin resistance (Figure 12.2) and often require appropriate therapy before diabetes can be properly regulated.

Hypoadrenocorticoid crisis

Adrenocortical insufficiency can cause profound shock and is usually associated with gastrointestinal signs and bradycardia. Hypoadrenocorticism or Addison's disease is usually caused by immune destruction of the adrenal cortex and is primarily a disease of young to middle-aged female dogs. There is often a waxing and waning history of ill-defined gastrointestinal problems

Infections
Bacterial pyoderma
Pneumonia
Pyelonephritis/lower urinary tract infection

Concurrent endocrine diseases
Hyperadrenocorticism
Hypothyroidism (dogs)
Hyperthyroidism (cats)
Acromegaly
Glucagonoma (dogs)
Phaeochromocytoma

Renal insufficiency
Pancreatitis
Obesity
Dioestrus (intact bitch)

Figure 12.2: *Common causes of insulin resistance.*

including vomiting, diarrhoea, lethargy and weight loss. Animals may respond dramatically to fluid replacement and/or corticosteroid administration, and repeated episodes may occur before more thorough diagnostics reveal the aetiology. Animals presenting in a hypoadrenocorticoid crisis classically display all the signs of hypovolaemic shock (weak pulses, cool extremities, depression and weakness) with the exception of heart rate. Bradycardia in the setting of shock should alert the clinician to the possibility of hyperkalaemia and adrenocortical insufficiency.

Pathophysiology

Primary hypoadrenocorticism presents with both mineralocorticoid and glucocorticoid deficiency. Atypical or secondary hypoadrenocorticism involves only glucocorticoid deficiency. Clinical manifestations of glucocorticoid deficiency include vomiting, diarrhoea, weight loss, lethargy and weakness. Without aldosterone, renal sodium and chloride loss occurs, resulting in loss of the renal medullary concentrating gradient, inability to retain water and eventually hypovolaemia, acidosis and hypotension. Clinically, these animals become polyuric with a secondary polydipsia. Aldosterone deficiency also results in decreased potassium excretion. As serum potassium levels rise, cardiac function is impaired as conduction is slowed (see Chapter 4). The result is decreased heart rate in the face of hypovolaemia and impaired cardiac output.

Glucocorticoid deficiency by itself may be more difficult to identify. Glucocorticoids are important hormones in the body's battle with daily stress. Cortisol is an important counter-regulatory hormone to insulin. Patients deficient in cortisol are often hypoglycaemic. Cortisol is also important for cellular integrity, especially within the gastrointestinal tract. Many of the non-specific gastrointestinal signs associated with hypoadrenocorticism are related to glucocorticoid deficiency. A normal blood count is another interesting finding in these patients. Normal cortisol release during times of stress causes lymphopenia, eosinopenia and neutrophilia. Instead, a normal leucogram in a stressed, shocked animal should alert the clinician to possible glucocorticoid deficiency and secondary (atypical) hypoadrenocorticism.

It may be difficult to distinguish hypoadrenocorticism from acute renal failure. Because of the loss of sodium the renal medulla loses its ability to concentrate urine, resulting in hyposthenuria in the face of dehydration. Azotaemia and hyperphosphataemia may be evident in both conditions. Hyperkalaemia, profound hyponatraemia, an episodic history and lack of a stress leucogram all raise hyperadrenocorticism higher on the list of differential diagnoses.

Management

Therapy for a hypoadrenocorticoid crisis consists of expansion of fluid volume, glucocorticoid and mineralocorticoid replacement, correction of electrolyte abnormalities and treatment of gastrointestinal haemorrhage. Emergency treatment should begin with intravenous fluid therapy with shock doses of 0.9% NaCl (up to 90 ml/kg over 1 hour in the dog); this precedes glucocorticoid therapy. Care must be taken, however, not to cause excessively rapid changes in serum sodium, which could lead to cerebral injury. Mortality associated with hypoadrenocorticism is usually due to hypovolaemic shock and complications associated with hypotension.

Steroid supplementation is the next priority and the choice of steroid is important to prevent problems with definitive diagnosis. An adrenocorticotropic hormone (ACTH) stimulation test should be performed as part of the admission database. Since the test involves drawing blood samples for serum cortisol levels at baseline and then 1 hour after aqueous ACTH (0.5 IU/kg i.v.), the steroid chosen for replacement should not cross react with the cortisol assay. Dexamethasone sodium phosphate (0.5-2.0 mg/kg) is the ideal choice. It is an inexpensive, fast acting steroid which, unlike prednisone sodium succinate, does not interfere with the cortisol assay.

If the patient has life-threatening hyperkalaemic bradycardia, serum potassium can be corrected rapidly by administration of either intravenous sodium bicarbonate (1-2 mEq/kg) or a combination of intravenous regular insulin (0.25-0.5 IU/kg) followed by 2 g dextrose for each unit of insulin. Intravenous administration of 0.5-1.5 ml/kg of 10% calcium gluconate often results in normalization of the ECG, although it does not change the plasma potassium concentration. As fluid resuscitation continues, further dilution of potassium occurs and it should be monitored and supplemented if necessary.

The remainder of the emergency care is supportive.

Close attention to the treatment of gastrointestinal haemorrhage is warranted, as gastroenteritis can be severe. Blood loss and damage to the gut mucosal barrier can result in significant anaemia, hypoproteinaemia and bacterial sepsis. Gastrointestinal protectants are required and, if necessary, blood transfusions. Parenteral antibiotics may be required to treat septicaemia due to enteric bacteria.

Following diagnosis and resolution of the hypoadrenocortical crisis and associated complications, long-term replacement therapy with physiological doses of corticosteroids and mineralocorticoid supplements can begin.

Life-threatening complications of hyperadrenocorticism

Hyperadrenocorticism is a progressive disease with multiple aetiologies. Excess endogenous corticosteroids may be the result of a pituitary adenoma or a primary adrenal tumour, while iatrogenic hyperadrenocorticism is a potential consequence of high dose or long term administration of corticosteroids. The disease is often insidious in onset and may not be associated with an acute, emergency presentation. However, chronically elevated steroid levels may result in serious complications, such as pulmonary thromboembolism, acute pancreatitis, pyelonephritis, systemic hypertension, diabetes mellitus and neurological complications associated with a growing pituitary tumour. Complications of therapy are also possible and are related to iatrogenic cortisol deficit and signs of hypoadrenocorticism.

Pulmonary thromboembolism

One of the most serious complications is pulmonary thromboembolism (PTE). Glucocorticoids alter the balance of coagulation and anticoagulation factors and excess steroids (either endogenous or iatrogenic) can predispose patients to thrombosis. Other risk factors for PTE are often present, including obesity, hypertension, glomerular disease and elevated haematocrit, and the risk is increased if central venous catheterization has been performed. The clinical signs of PTE include acute severe dyspnoea, fever and sometimes sudden death. Arterial blood gas analysis reveals low arterial PO_2, which may dramatically improve with supplemental oxygen. In response to acute hypoxia, alveolar hyperventilation leads to a concurrent decrease in PCO_2. Clinicopathological findings are typical of hyperadrenocorticism, but thrombocytopenia supports the diagnosis of PTE. Radiographic findings are variable, either normal or demonstrating any of the following abnormalities: diffuse interstitial pattern, alveolar pattern, pleural effusion and/or pulmonary arterial distension. Therapy is supportive and includes supplemental oxygen and the use of anticoagulants. The chance of repeated thromboembolism is very high and the prognosis is guarded.

Acute pancreatitis

Anorexia, vomiting and abdominal pain may indicate acute pancreatitis, which must be carefully differentiated from iatrogenic hypoadrenocorticism. Pancreatitis in the hyperadrenocorticoid patient may be the result of pancreatic ductule hyperplasia, lipaemia, hypercholesterolaemia and inspissated pancreatic secretions, in addition to polyphagia and a tendency to eat garbage or high fat food. Patients suspected of having iatrogenic adrenocortical insufficiency should respond quickly to fluid and glucocorticoid supplementation. If the vomiting animal with abdominal pain has not been previously treated for hyperadrenocorticism, pancreatitis should be considered (see Chapter 9).

Renal complications and hypertension

Elevated glucocorticoid levels can impact upon the kidney in several ways. Glucocorticoids inhibit white blood cell recruitment, resulting in a lowered resistance to infection. Cystitis, urolithiasis and pyelonephritis are all potential complications. Glomerulonephritis is a potential complication of chronic inflammatory disease or infection anywhere in the body, when antigen-antibody complexes cause damage to the glomerular membrane. Systemic hypertension may occur in dogs with hyperadrenocorticism due to elevation of plasma renin by cortisol. The cascade of events starts with renin release, leading to angiotensin activation and vasoconstriction. Hypertension can lead to acute blindness due to intraocular haemorrhage or retinal detachment, neurological signs due to intracranial haemorrhage, glomerulosclerosis and thromboembolism.

Diabetes mellitus

Overt diabetes mellitus occurs in 10-15% of dogs with hyperadrenocorticism and up to 60% of dogs have elevated fasting glucose concentrations due to the anti-insulin effects of cortisol. Initially, compensation occurs by increased insulin secretion, but chronic stimulation can eventually lead to ß-cell exhaustion and clinical diabetes mellitus. Concurrent treatment of hyperadrenocorticism and diabetes mellitus can be complicated and requires careful dosing of both insulin and o,p´-DDD. If possible, the diabetes mellitus should be well controlled before induction therapy with o,p´-DDD. It may be necessary to reduce the dose of insulin during the induction phase, as cortisol-induced insulin resistance will be lost and hypoglycaemia may develop.

Iatrogenic hypoadrenocorticism

A hypoadrenocortical crisis is a potential emergency arising during the treatment of hyperadrenocorticism with the adrenocorticolytic drug o,p´-DDD. Common signs include weakness, ataxia, anorexia, diarrhoea and vomiting. Since o,p´-DDD primarily destroys the zona reticularis and the zona fasciculata, most dogs have glucocorticoid deficiency alone, although occasional animals also have mineralocorticoid deficiency. One study (Kinzer and Peterson, 1991) showed that 25% of 200 dogs treated with o,p´-DDD for pituitary dependent hyperadrenocorticism developed one or more adverse reactions to therapy. Recognizing the non-specific gastrointestinal symptoms and characteristic electrolyte changes of hypoadrenocorticism, the clinician can quickly diagnose and treat this potentially serious complication. Treatment includes fluid and steroid replacement, along with a mineralocorticoid supplement if electrolyte abnormalities are present. It may be necessary to lower the maintenance dose of o,p´-DDD by 25-50% after resolution of clinical hypoadrenocorticism.

METABOLIC EMERGENCIES

Hypoglycaemia

Serum glucose concentrations below 3.5 mmol/l are considered hypoglycaemic. Laboratory error is a common cause that should be considered. If a delay is expected before blood glucose analysis, collection tubes containing sodium fluoride must be used to inhibit glycolysis. Alternatively, the sample can be promptly centrifuged, separating the serum and the red blood cells, and the serum refrigerated or frozen for later analysis. Polycythaemia may also cause artefactual hypoglycaemia due to accelerated glycolysis.

Since the brain requires adequate glucose for energy, does not store glycogen and is unable to utilize other sources of energy, most symptoms of hypoglycaemia are related to central nervous system dysfunction. Clinical signs of hypoglycaemia include behavioural changes, weakness, ataxia, stupor, blindness, seizures and coma. Signs do not occur at specific blood glucose values, but instead are related to the duration and rate of decline in blood glucose concentration. Animals with prolonged hypoglycaemia, such as those with functional pancreatic ß-cell tumours, may appear neurologically normal yet have dramatically low blood glucose concentrations.

A complete diagnostic plan requires a basic understanding of glucose kinetics. Blood glucose concentration represents a balance between production, storage and consumption. Insulin is released from pancreatic ß-cells in response to a postprandial rise in glucose, amino acids and gastrointestinal hormones. Insulin increases hepatic glycogen and triglyceride synthesis and inhibits glycogenolysis and gluconeogenesis, with a net effect of enhanced glucose storage. Approximately half of the body's glucose is stored within the liver as glycogen. The remainder is stored as glycogen in muscle and other tissues, or used as energy by the brain. During exercise, stress, illness and prolonged fasting, glucose counter-regulatory hormones start to work. Glucagon and adrenaline rapidly antagonize the effects of insulin, increasing blood glucose by inhibiting glucose utilization and increasing glycogenolysis and gluconeogenesis. These hormones also directly inhibit insulin secretion. Other, longer-acting inhibitors of insulin include growth hormone and cortisol. In order for glycogenolysis and gluconeogenesis to occur, adequate stores and glucose substrates need to be available. Gluconeogenic substrates include amino acids, glycerol and lactate.

Hypoglycaemia therefore develops as a result of decreased production of glucose, increased utilization, or a combination of the two. Decreased production may result from inadequate stores or an excess of circulating insulin, while systemic inflammatory diseases such as septic shock can lead to hypoglycaemia through increased glucose utilization and impaired gluconeogenesis. There are numerous causes of hypoglycaemia (Figure 12.3), each of which may be considered or eliminated based on signalment, physical examination and medical history.

Insulin-secreting tumours

Tumour-associated hypoglycaemia may be due to the secretion of insulin or insulin-like factors, decreased hepatic glycolysis or gluconeogenesis and accelerated glucose utilization by the tumour. Insulin hypersecretion from a functional ß-cell tumour is one of the most common causes of tumour-associated hypoglycaemia.

Insulin-secreting ß-cell tumours (insulinomas) are uncommon in dogs and rare in cats. Usually affecting older dogs with a mean age of 9 years, they have been seen in dogs as young as 3 years of age. Clinical signs are associated with the central nervous system manifestations of hypoglycaemia, usually occur long after eating and may be associated with exercise. 'Whipple's triad' is a clinical syndrome that suggests an insulin-secreting tumour, including: (1) neurological signs consistent with hypoglycaemia; (2) hypoglycaemia while these signs are occurring; and (3) resolution of signs with glucose replacement.

Pancreatic islet cell tumours are often very small and difficult to image. The tumour rarely metastasizes to the lungs but will spread to the liver and other sites within the abdomen. Serum insulin concentrations should be measured and interpreted in relation to a concurrent serum glucose concentration. Definitive diagnosis requires exploratory surgery and histopathological analysis of an islet cell tumour. Biopsies of the liver and local lymph nodes at the time of surgery are indicated to stage the disease and for prognosis. Clinical signs will return if functional residual tumour remains after surgery.

Medical management of non-surgical or metastatic insulinoma includes feeding multiple small meals throughout the day. Meals should preferably be high in complex carbohydrates and low in simple sugars. Prednisolone (0.25-3 mg/kg bid) can be used to control clinical signs by inducing insulin resistance. Diazoxide, a benzothiadiazide diuretic (5-30 mg/kg bid), has also been used to inhibit insulin secretion and increase

Increased circulating insulin Functional pancreatic ß-cell tumour
Hypoadrenocorticism
Neoplasia Lymphosarcoma Hepatocellular carcinoma Haemangiosarcoma Hepatoma Leiomyosarcoma/leiomyoma
Hepatic insufficiency
Sepsis/systemic inflammatory response syndrome
Neonatal hypoglycaemia
Hunting dog hypoglycaemia
Juvenile (toy breed) hypoglycaemia
Iatrogenic Insulin overdose o,p´-DDD therapy Oral hypoglycaemic agents
Laboratory error Polycythaemia Sample allowed to sit too long

Figure 12.3: Commom causes of hypoglycaemia.

gluconeogenesis and glycogenolysis through the release of adrenaline. If given with food, gastrointestinal side effects of diazoxide can be minimized.

Sepsis and the systemic inflammatory response syndrome

Hypoglycaemia is often associated with sepsis and septic shock, due to impaired gluconeogenesis and increased peripheral utilization of glucose. Serial blood glucose monitoring becomes very important in patients at risk of sepsis and if necessary glucose (2.5-5%) should be added to the maintenance crystalloid fluids to maintain normal blood glucose levels. This support should continue while treating the primary disease, in addition to other supportive therapy for sepsis (see Chapter 3).

Juvenile and neonatal hypoglycaemia

Starvation alone, a common cause of hypoglycaemia in man, usually does not cause hypoglycaemia in adult dogs. Neonatal hypoglycaemia is usually a combined problem of inadequate glycogen reserves and poorly developed hepatic function. Very young animals can

become hypoglycaemic as a result of poor glucose regulation, decreased food intake and slow hepatic gluconeogenesis.

Transient juvenile hypoglycaemia affects miniature and toy breeds of dog between 6 weeks and 6 months of age. Probably related to the large brain to liver ratio and the immature gluconeogenic and glycogenolytic systems, puppies usually grow out of this condition by the time they reach 6 months. In the meantime frequent feedings, parasite control and environmental strategies to minimize cold stress may be all that is required to prevent hypoglycaemia.

Hypoglycaemic neonates showing neurological signs should be given 1-2 ml/kg of 25% dextrose. The 25% dextrose solution should ideally be given intravenously. Alternatively, an intraosseous catheter placed in the medullary cavity of a long bone (femur, humerus, or tibia) can provide rapid vascular access to even the smallest patient. Using an 18-gauge bone marrow needle or a spinal needle with stylet, the medullary cavity is entered as if placing an intramedullary pin. Fluids, colloids, blood products, drugs and dextrose can all be given via the intraosseous route.

Hepatic failure

Hepatic dysfunction and portosystemic vascular anomalies can lead to decreased glucose through diminished gluconeogenesis and glycogenolysis. Liver function must be very severely abnormal before hypoglycaemia is a clinical problem. For this reason other signs of liver dysfunction, such as hypoalbuminaemia, coagulopathy or icterus, may predominate. Central nervous system signs often manifest soon after eating and are more often the result of hepatic encephalopathy rather than hypoglycaemia.

Hypoadrenocorticism

Because cortisol is a counter-regulatory hormone important in maintaining blood glucose in times of stress, hypoadrenocorticism is a potential cause of hypoglycaemia. Atypical hypoadrenocorticism (glucocorticoid deficiency alone) may not be accompanied by the typical electrolyte changes associated with decreased mineralocorticoid levels. However, with decreased cortisol, hypoglycaemia may occur in times of stress. Provocative adrenal function testing using the ACTH stimulation test should be performed to establish the diagnosis. Treatment includes hormone replacement with physiological levels of corticosteroid.

Others

A complete drug history may identify other possible causes of hypoglycaemia. Insulin overdosage, ingestion of oral hypoglycaemic drugs and the adrenocorticolytic drug o,p´-DDD can all cause hypoglycaemia. A review of administration protocols, drug concentrations and progression of the primary disease can aid the clinician in finding the best course of treatment.

Other miscellaneous causes of hypoglycaemia include glycogen storage diseases, hunting dog hypoglycaemia and hypopituitarism. Glycogen storage diseases are inherited defects in the glycogenolytic pathway. Because of glycogen deposition in the liver, kidneys and myocardium, the liver of these patients is often enlarged and the patient may be stunted or have abnormal growth. Hunting dog hypoglycaemia is seen in lean, active hunting dogs after lengthy exercise. These dogs often recover rapidly but may be quite weak. In dogs that are prone to this problem, signs can be minimized by frequent feedings of small meals. Physiological doses of prednisolone (2.5-5 mg orally) several hours before exercise may also prove beneficial.

Management of the hypoglycaemic patient

Regardless of cause, symptomatic treatment for patients with neurological manifestations of hypoglycaemia should take place immediately. Dextrose administration should be instituted immediately after collection of baseline blood samples. Dextrose is administered as a bolus (0.5 g/kg of 25% dextrose i.v. or orally), followed by addition of dextrose to the intravenous fluids, to make a solution of 2.5-10% dextrose. Blood glucose should be closely monitored (minimum every 2 hours) to determine the percent glucose required in the fluids. Infusions that contain more than 5% glucose should always be administered through a central vein because of their hypertonicity. Neurological signs usually resolve with rapid glucose replacement, but may persist if the hypoglycaemia was extreme or prolonged. Serum should be collected for biochemical and endocrine testing and for determination of serum insulin levels. High insulin levels in the face of hypoglycaemia are inappropriate and suggestive of a functional ß-cell tumour of the pancreas.

Disorders of calcium

Total serum calcium consists of ionized and protein-bound fractions. The ionized fraction is the physiologically active moiety and is carefully regulated within a very narrow range under normal circumstances. Changes in plasma protein concentration can therefore alter total serum calcium without affecting biological activity. Abnormal albumin and protein levels should be considered when interpreting total serum calcium concentrations. In dogs, total serum calcium can be corrected for hypoproteinaemia by the following equation:

Corrected calcium = measured Ca (mmol/l)
(mmol/l) $- \dfrac{\text{Albumin (g/l)}}{40} + 0.875$

Where available, ionized calcium measurement provides a more precise assessment of biologically active calcium.

Hypercalcaemia

Serum calcium concentrations above 3 mmol/l are abnormal in adult dogs and cats although mild increases may be seen in puppies. Hypercalcaemia in older animals is most often indicative of malignancy. A variety of tumours produce parathyroid-like substances that alter calcium homeostasis to increase serum calcium levels (Figure 12.4). Other causes of hypercalcaemia include hyperproteinaemia from dehydration, acute renal failure, vitamin D and calcium toxicoses, granulomatous disorders, non-neoplastic disorders of bone, hypoadrenocorticism, true hyperparathyroidism and chronic disuse osteoporosis. In most animals with hypercalcaemia, ionized calcium is 55-60% of total calcium. Patients in renal failure are an exception as the ionized calcium is often below that expected based on the total calcium.

Immediate diagnostics should involve repeat calcium measurement to rule out laboratory error. Assessment of electrolytes, blood urea nitrogen and creatinine may help identify non-neoplastic causes of hypercalcaemia. Elevated immunoreactive parathormone levels in association with hyperphosphataemia may suggest ectopic hormone production.

Hypercalcaemia is a medical emergency because of its effects on the kidney. Increased calcium levels damage ADH receptors, leading to decreased sodium and chloride transport into the medullary interstitium (nephrogenic diabetes insipidus) and eventually to calcium mineralization of renal tubular cells. Renal concentrating ability is impaired and animals display primary polyuria with secondary polydipsia. Total serum calcium levels >3.75 mmol/l, accompanied by renal insufficiency or abnormal mentation, constitute a hypercalcaemic crisis that requires immediate treatment.

Treatment for hypercalcaemia begins with rapid volume expansion. Isotonic saline (0.9% NaCl) is the fluid of choice. In addition to being an excellent fluid for rehydration, the sodium chloride causes a natriuresis that increases calcium excretion in the urine. Fluid therapy alone may be enough to correct mild to moderate hypercalcaemia. After the patient is rehydrated, frusemide, a potent loop diuretic, can be given (2-4

| **Hypercalcaemia associated with osteoclastic tumour activity** |
| Lymphoma |
| Multiple myeloma |
| Mammary gland adenocarcinoma |

| **Hypercalcaemia associated with parathyroid hormone-related peptide (PTH-rp)** |
| Lymphoma |
| Anal sac adenocarcinoma |

Figure 12.4: Common tumours associated with hypercalcaemia.

mg/kg i.v.) to potentiate calciuria. Aggressive saline diuresis with or without frusemide is usually enough to bring calcium levels down.

Glucocorticoids are another adjuvant treatment for hypercalcaemia. Glucocorticoids decrease bone resorption, decrease intestinal calcium absorption and enhance renal excretion of calcium. Glucocorticoids are also important in treating lymphosarcoma, the most common malignancy associated with hypercalcaemia. Since glucocorticoids can cause rapid tumour lysis, they can impair a later diagnosis of lymphosarcoma. In hypercalcaemic patients, every effort must be made to identify or rule out lymphosarcoma before administering steroids. Thoracic and abdominal radiography, palpation and aspiration of lymph nodes, and lymph node and bone marrow biopsy should be performed before instituting glucocorticoid therapy.

Hypocalcaemia

Hypocalcaemia is defined as a total calcium concentration below 2 mmol/l. Clinical signs are associated with increased neuromuscular excitability. Early signs include twitching of the ears and face that may be most notable in the whiskers. With more severe or acute changes in calcium levels, generalized muscle tremors and seizures are seen. The increased muscular activity results in an increase in body temperature (hyperthermia). Hypocalcaemia can also affect cardiac conduction, manifested as a prolonged Q-T segment.

Hypoalbuminaemia is the most common cause of low total calcium, but the biologically active ionized fraction is unaffected. Renal failure is another common cause of hypocalcaemia, due to progressively increasing serum phosphorus concentrations and decreased calcitriol synthesis. Eclampsia (lactation tetany) also results in clinical hypocalcaemia. Eclampsia is usually seen 1-3 weeks postpartum, usually during the period of peak lactation when calcium is diverted into milk production. If intake of a calcium deficient diet occurs and the litter size and calcium loss is too great, severe depletion can occur. Primary hypoparathyroidism has been reported in the dog, and iatrogenic hypoparathyroidism occurs following the removal of a functional parathyroid adenoma or within 5 days after bilateral thyroidectomy. Miscellaneous causes of hypocalcaemia include ethylene glycol intoxication, pancreatitis, intestinal malabsorption and massive transfusions with citrated whole blood.

Regardless of cause, patients showing clinical signs of hypocalcaemia should receive immediate parenteral calcium supplementation. Calcium gluconate (10%) is given (0.5-1.5 ml/kg i.v.) slowly over 15-30 minutes, preferably with continuous electrocardiographic monitoring. If an ECG is unavailable, the heart should be ausculted and pulses palpated simultaneously. If arrhythmias, pulse deficits or severe bradycardia occur, the calcium infusion should be stopped.

Calcium chloride (10%) is also available and should be administered in a similar cautious manner (1.5-3.0 ml per animal). Following resolution of clinical signs of hypocalcaemia, the cause should be addressed and the need for continuous supplementation assessed. Calcium gluconate (10%) can be given subcutaneously but should be diluted with 0.9% sodium chloride before injection. Calcium chloride should not be given subcutaneously. In patients that require ongoing parenteral supplementation, calcium gluconate can be given at 10 mg/kg/h CRI (1 ml 10% calcium gluconate = 100 mg). Long-term management of hypocalcaemia involves oral calcium salts (100-500 mg/kg divided tid) or vitamin D supplementation. Oral calcium is better suited for short-term problems such as eclampsia, while vitamin D supplements are ideal for long-term disorders such as chronic renal failure. Calcium and vitamin D analogues should only be given together with caution as the combination is likely to result in hypercalcaemia.

Disorders of sodium

Sodium is the most important osmotically active solute in the extracellular fluid and as such is vital to the maintenance of extracellular fluid volume. Sodium balance is regulated by osmoreceptors in the hypothalamus, which regulate thirst and the release of antidiuretic hormone (ADH). The kidney, controlled by the effects of ADH and aldosterone, is the organ responsible for balancing the excretion of salt and water.

Hypernatraemia

Hypernatraemia is defined as a serum sodium concentration greater than 155 mEq/l. Clinical signs are related to cerebral dehydration as fluid moves out of the brain cells toward the higher osmolality of the serum. Hypernatraemia is most commonly due to loss of fluid with a low sodium concentration, but occasionally occurs due to gain of fluid with a high sodium concentration (Figure 12.5). When pure water is lost, the extracellular fluid becomes hypertonic in relation to the intracellular fluid. Since water moves freely from the intracellular compartment to the extracellular compartment, all compartments share in this dehydration.

Because hypovolaemia is the most immediate concern, volume replacement should be initiated immediately. Isotonic saline (0.9% NaCl) is used to replace the deficit and restore volume. Giving sodium-containing fluids may not seem logical. However, with prolonged hypernatraemia, the brain lessens cellular fluid loss by generating intracellular substances called idiogenic osmoles. These osmoles cause cerebral oedema if plasma sodium levels are corrected too rapidly. In hypernatraemia, 0.9% NaCl (containing 154 mEq/l of Na^+) often has a lower sodium concentration than that of the patient, resulting in gradual dilution of sodium as the intravascular volume is replaced. Residual free water

Water restriction
Salt poisoning
Hyperthermia Environmental Fever
Gastrointestinal fluid loss Vomiting Diarrhoea
Renal loss of free water Nephrogenic diabetes insipidus Post-obstruction diuresis Polyuric renal failure
Endocrine Hyperadrenocorticism Diabetes mellitus — glucosuria
Neurological Central diabetes insipidus
Third space fluid loss Gastrointestinal obstruction Peritonitis
Burns
Iatrogenic Diuretic administration Hypertonic saline Sodium bicarbonate Sodium phosphate enema

Figure 12.5: *Common causes of hypernatraemia.*

deficits should then be replaced slowly, correcting the plasma sodium concentration gradually over 48-72 hours.

Only after hypovolaemia is corrected should the remaining free water deficit be addressed. Ideally, hypernatraemia should trigger thirst, stimulating the animal to drink, thereby naturally ingesting the appropriate amount of water. If the patient is hydrated, unable to drink and still hypernatraemic, the free water deficit can be calculated using the following formula:

$$\text{Water deficit (litres)} = \text{Current bodyweight (kg)} \times \left(\frac{\text{Plasma [Na}^+] \text{ (patient)}}{\text{Plasma [Na}^+] \text{ (normal)}} \right) - 1$$

The free water deficit can be replaced by giving 0.45% NaCl or 5% dextrose intravenously. Glucose rapidly enters the cells and is metabolized, leaving only free water.

Hyponatraemia

Hyponatraemia is defined as a serum sodium concentration less than 137 mEq/l. Since sodium is the most abundant extracellular cation, hyponatraemia reflects whole body hypo-osmolality. Clinical signs are related to hypo-osmolality and are generally only present when there have been rapid changes in serum osmolality. The blood-brain barrier is not permeable to sodium. With systemic hypo-osmolality, water can move into the central nervous system along a concentration gradient. The resulting influx of water can lead to cerebral oedema and diffuse cranial signs including lethargy, nausea and coma. This is only usually seen with water intoxication. Chronic hypo-osmolar conditions allow the brain time to adjust by losing osmotically active osmoles.

Pure water retention and/or loss of solute can cause hyponatraemia. Examples of solute loss include protracted vomiting and diarrhoea. Treatment should be directed at electrolyte replacement, the fluid of choice being 0.9% NaCl. Rapid correction with hypertonic saline fluids (3-7.5%) may lead to central pontine myelinolysis, although this point is now the subject of debate. Severe acute hyponatraemia is rare in small animal patients. Mild and chronic hyponatraemia is usually asymptomatic, requiring only treatment of the primary disease and gradual electrolyte replacement.

Disorders of potassium

Potassium is the most abundant intracellular cation, with approximately 95% of the total body potassium found within cells. Serum levels therefore do not reflect tissue concentrations. Normal potassium balance is maintained through renal elimination, enhanced by aldosterone. Potassium is important in maintaining cellular membrane potential; disruption of the normal potassium gradient can affect excitable tissues such as the heart, nerves and muscle.

Hyperkalaemia

Hyperkalaemia is caused by failure to eliminate potassium from the body via the renal tubules, by liberation of intracellular potassium from damaged cells or by translocation of potassium out of the cells during extreme acidosis. Specific problems associated with hyperkalaemia include hypoadrenocorticism, acute oliguric/anuric renal failure, ruptured urinary bladder and uroperitoneum and urethral obstruction. Massive cell damage with release of intracellular potassium can be seen with snakebite, heatstroke, trauma, thromboembolism and tumour lysis syndrome.

The most serious consequence of increased serum potassium is cardiac conduction abnormalities. As serum potassium levels climb, changes are seen in the ECG. The first change is an increase in the amplitude of the T wave, decreased amplitude of the R wave and a prolonged P-R interval. With higher levels, atrial standstill and absence of a P wave are noted. Bradycardia and widening of the QRS complex are eventually seen. Without treatment, cardiac arrest will occur due to ventricular fibrillation or asystole.

Treatment of hyperkalaemia may be required before an aetiology is established. Rapid restoration of potassium balance can be accomplished with either intravenous sodium bicarbonate (1-2 mEq/kg) or a combination of intravenous regular insulin (0.25-0.5 IU/kg) followed by 2 g of dextrose for each unit of insulin. Intravenous fluid therapy is usually necessary and the crystalloid fluid of choice is 0.9% NaCl. The myocardium can be protected from the arrhythmogenic effects of hyperkalaemia with 10% calcium gluconate (0.5-1.5 ml/kg) by slow intravenous infusion.

Following the intracellular movement of potassium, fluid therapy with potassium-free fluids should commence, but correction of the underlying disease is necessary to prevent recurrence. Urinary obstruction must be cleared or the urine removed via cystocentesis. If a ruptured bladder is present, placement of an abdominal drain and urinary catheter will divert urine and potassium out of the body until the patient can be stabilized and prepared for reparative surgery. If possible, anuric renal failure should be converted to oliguric or polyuric renal failure with intravenous fluid diuresis and diuretics if necessary (see Chapter 6). The prognosis for refractory anuric renal failure is grave. If urine flow is not established within a few hours of initiating treatment, peritoneal or haemodialysis are the only treatment options.

Hypokalaemia

Hypokalaemia (serum potassium below 4.0 mEq/l) is a common finding in critically ill patients. It is not usually clinically important until levels fall below 3.5 mEq/l. Hypokalaemia is caused by gastrointestinal (vomiting, diarrhoea) or renal potassium loss, or by translocation of extracellular potassium into cells. Anorexia and diets deficient in potassium can also contribute to hypokalaemia. Renal potassium loss is associated with chronic renal failure, tubular acidosis, intravenous fluid diuresis and post-obstruction diuresis. Drugs, including mineralocorticoids, penicillins and amphotericin B, have also been associated with renal potassium loss. Rapid shifts between the intracellular and extracellular compartment can cause changes in circulating potassium levels. Potassium is driven into the cells by insulin and glucose administration. Alkalosis, including that caused by sodium bicarbonate administration, can result in intracellular movement of potassium in exchange for hydrogen ions. Upper gastrointestinal obstruction can result in significant potassium loss through vomiting and an intracellular shift due to hypochloraemic metabolic alkalosis.

Signs of hypokalaemia are non-specific and include weakness, lethargy, ileus and anorexia. Muscle weakness can occasionally become so severe that respiratory paralysis can lead to death. Signs may be referable to the primary disease such as polyuria, polydipsia, vomiting or diarrhoea. In cats with renal disease, or those fed potassium-deficient diets, hypokalaemia can result in ventroflexion of the neck and a stilted forelimb gait.

Potassium can be supplemented orally or added to intravenous fluids. If the patient is stable and not vomiting, oral potassium supplementation is desirable because it is safe and avoids the dilutional effects of intravenous fluids and further loss of potassium from diuresis. If oral supplementation is not possible, the amount of potassium to add to maintenance fluids should be based on measured serum potassium (Figure 12.6). When replacing estimated fluid losses or giving shock boluses of fluids, it is important not to use fluids that have been supplemented with extra potassium. Because of risks of hyperkalaemia and cardiotoxicity, potassium doses of 0.5 mEq/kg/h should not usually be exceeded. Normally, 14-20 mEq/l of potassium in maintenance fluid is sufficient to maintain normal potassium levels, but patients with pre-existing deficits may require much more.

Magnesium is essential in the normal sodium-potassium exchange. Hypomagnesaemia, another common finding in the critically ill, can therefore lead to refractory hypokalaemia. If hypokalaemia fails to resolve following aggressive replacement therapy, hypomagnesaemia should be considered. Because serum magnesium represents less than 1% of total body magnesium, there is no easy way to document overall magnesium deficiency. Magnesium replacement (0.75-1 mEq/kg/24 h) may result in rapid resolution of the hypokalaemia.

Acidosis

Acidosis may be primarily a metabolic disorder (characterized by a decrease in HCO_3^-) or a respiratory disorder (with an elevated PCO_2). Metabolic acidosis can be caused by loss of HCO_3^- containing fluids, addition of fixed (non-volatile) acids, or production of fixed acids within the body. Fixed acid production occurs during cellular metabolism: when perfusion is poor, fixed acids accumulate. In addition, anaerobic metabolism during tissue hypoxia leads to production of lactic acid. Bicarbonate, the body's major buffering system, is regulated by the kidney. Renal hypoperfusion can affect HCO_3^- balance and the excretion of fixed acids. Diarrhoea contains higher concentrations of HCO_3^- than plasma and is another important cause of metabolic acidosis.

Metabolic acidosis is a common finding with circulatory shock and should be considered in any severely ill patient. Left uncorrected, acidosis can lead to life-threatening cardiac dysfunction. Acidosis sensitizes the

Serum potassium (mEq/l)	mEq/l potassium chloride added to fluids
3.6-5.0	20
3.1-3.5	30
2.6-3.0	40
2.1-2.5	60
<2.0	80

Figure 12.6: *Potassium replacement.*

myocardium to ventricular arrhythmias and impairs cardiac contractility.

The anion gap can be used to evaluate patients with metabolic acidosis, specifically to determine whether the problem is an accumulation of hydrogen ions or a loss of bicarbonate. To achieve electrical neutrality, the concentration of positively charged cations must balance that of the negatively charged anions. The only measured cations are sodium and potassium, while the measured anions are chloride and bicarbonate. The following formula helps visualize this relationship:

$$[K^+ + Na^+] + UC = [Cl^- + HCO_3^-] + UA$$

where UC represents unmeasured cations and UA is unmeasured anions.

$$\text{Anion gap} = [Na^+ + K^+] - [Cl^- + HCO_3^-]$$

The normal anion gap is 10-27 in cats and 8-25 in dogs. Causes of high anion gap metabolic acidosis include ethylene glycol intoxication, salicylate intoxication, diabetic ketoacidosis, lactic acidosis and some forms of renal failure. Normal anion gap metabolic acidosis is associated with hypoadrenocorticism, renal tubular acidosis and protein losing enteropathies.

Therapy for metabolic acidosis should begin with treatment of the primary problem. Resolution of hypoperfusion and enhanced tissue circulation is often sufficient and crystalloid fluid resuscitation with a balanced electrolyte replacement solution is the mainstay of shock therapy. As volume is restored, if the acidosis persists, an alkalinizing fluid such as 0.9% NaCl with sodium bicarbonate (24 mEq/l) can be considered. Lactated Ringer's solution contains lactate, a bicarbonate precursor requiring hepatic metabolism. Other available fluids contain acetate and gluconate, which are converted to bicarbonate in peripheral tissues. The end point of therapy for acidosis is the restoration of oxygen delivery to the tissues. If a patient is anaemic, whole blood, packed red cells or a free haemoglobin replacement product may be required. If the patient is hypoxic, supplemental oxygen should be administered.

Bicarbonate therapy should be guided by measured blood gas values and is usually only necessary when the pH is less than 7.1. Respiratory acidosis, caused by elevations in PCO_2, should never be treated with bicarbonate. If a severe metabolic acidosis is not responding to volume expansion, the total bicarbonate deficit is calculated using the following formula:

Bicarbonate deficit = Body weight (kg) x base excess x 0.3

Approximately one third to a half of the calculated deficit is administered slowly intravenously and then blood gases should be re-evaluated to determine whether further bicarbonate replacement is required.

If blood gases are unavailable, empirical doses of sodium bicarbonate are 1, 3 and 5 mEq/kg i.v. for mild, moderate and severe metabolic acidosis respectively. Overcorrecting a metabolic acidosis is undesirable. The resulting iatrogenic alkalosis causes an increased affinity by haemoglobin for oxygen, making it more difficult for oxygen to leave the red blood cell and find its way to the peripheral tissues where it is so urgently needed.

Alkalosis

Alkalosis can either be metabolic (increase in plasma bicarbonate), or respiratory (decrease in carbon dioxide). Elevated blood pH results in impaired cellular function and a left shift of the oxygen/haemoglobin dissociation curve, resulting in impaired oxygen delivery to the tissues. Metabolic alkalosis is caused by loss of hydrogen and chloride ions from the upper gastrointestinal tract and/or kidneys. Loss of hydrogen ions is associated with an increase in HCO_3^- concentration. Hypochloraemic metabolic acidosis due to pyloric or high duodenal obstruction is the most common reason for metabolic alkalosis in the dog and cat. Hypovolaemia worsens alkalosis, as the kidneys are forced to reabsorb sodium and HCO_3^- instead of chloride. Loop and thiazide diuretic administration can also result in renal chloride loss and hypochloraemic metabolic alkalosis. Respiratory alkalosis is due to alveolar hyperventilation, which is most commonly caused by severe hypoxaemia.

Treatment for alkalosis should be directed at the primary disease. Treating the cause of vomiting, discontinuing diuretic therapy and treating respiratory disease will help the body's buffer systems correct the acid base disorder. Hypovolaemia and hypokalaemia should be avoided but treated with intravenous fluids if they do occur. Hypochloraemic metabolic alkalosis is best treated with 0.9% NaCl, supplemented with potassium chloride.

Hypoproteinaemia

Hypoproteinaemia may be due to decreased production or increased loss of albumin or globulin. Decreased production of albumin is seen with liver disease and starvation, while increased loss can be seen with protein-losing renal or gastrointestinal disease. Gastrointestinal protein loss is unique in that it usually causes panhypoproteinaemia, whereas liver failure and renal disease usually only result in low albumin with normal globulins. Haemorrhage with crystalloid fluid replacement also causes hypoproteinaemia with a concomitant anaemia. Critically ill animals with exudates from extensive skin wounds (burns, bites), peritoneal or pleural effusions, may also rapidly develop clinically significant and severe hypoproteinaemia. Hypoproteinaemia is therefore a serious complication of several diseases, which has been associated with poor outcome. One study (Michel, 1993) found that admission serum albumin level could predict clinical outcome and identify a population of critically ill animals that could benefit from nutritional support.

Renal protein loss occurs secondary to glomerular diseases such as amyloidosis and glomerulonephritis, resulting in loss of small proteins such as albumin and antithrombin III. The normal glomerulus is a charge and size selective barrier preventing plasma protein entry into the urine. Very small proteins like immunoglobulin light chains (Bence-Jones proteins) and myoglobin can find their way through a normal glomerulus. Mucoproteins and secretory immunoglobulins may also find their way into urine, so that a small amount of protein may be found in normal animals, especially when urine is concentrated.

The urine protein:creatinine ratio is not affected by urine volume or concentration, so it is a useful means of quantifying an abnormal urine protein content (normal <0.5). A ratio greater than 1.0 is consistent with urine protein loss while a ratio greater than 5 is typical of patients with significant glomerular disease. If there is an inflammatory urine sediment (large numbers of cells or casts) urine protein content and even the protein:creatinine ratio should be interpreted cautiously. Abnormally high urine protein loss may be further investigated with a renal biopsy. Glomerulonephritis is a potentially correctable cause of renal protein loss and may require a thorough antigen hunt to find any sites of chronic inflammation, infection or immune stimulation.

Clinical signs associated with hypoproteinaemia depend in large part on the underlying disease. Animals with gastrointestinal malabsorption and maldigestion may have severe weight loss, diarrhoea and vomiting. Patients with renal protein loss may show signs of uraemia and nephrotic syndrome including nausea, anorexia, dehydration and hypercholesterolaemia. With advanced hepatic insufficiency, signs may relate to hepatic encephalopathy, hypoglycaemia and defects in coagulation. In addition to hypoalbuminaemia, laboratory abnormalities associated with advanced liver insufficiency include: decreased blood urea nitrogen; decreased cholesterol; hypoglycaemia; increased bilirubin; elevated pre- and postprandial bile acids; and abnormal coagulation testing.

Gastrointestinal disease should be suspected in patients with hypoproteinaemia, adequate liver function and no proteinuria or other obvious source of protein loss. With diffuse gastrointestinal disease, plasma proteins are lost in the intestinal lumen. In addition, protein, peptide and amino acid substrates may not be adequately absorbed due to intestinal disease. With the increased loss of serum proteins and inadequate substrates for hepatic protein synthesis, panhypoproteinaemia occurs. Faecal examination for parasites, bacterial overgrowth, the presence of un-split fats and a serum biochemical profile should precede more invasive diagnostics. Intestinal biopsies can be problematic as surgical healing may be impaired. Endoscopic evaluation of the intestinal tract with pinch biopsies of the stomach and small bowel can provide diagnostic material with minimal risk of breakdown and peritonitis.

Normal levels of serum albumin are required to maintain an oncotic pressure gradient within blood vessels. If the serum albumin level drops much below 1.5 g/dl, fluid leaves the vessels causing interstitial oedema, ascites and pleural effusion, presenting clinically as pitting oedema of the brisket and distal extremities. Analysis of pleural or peritoneal fluid reveals low cellularity and protein concentration less than 3 g/dl. Treatment must be directed at the primary problem while supportive care is instituted to prevent further loss of fluid and protein.

Emergency treatment involves the replacement of lost albumin with colloidal fluids. If the patient is anaemic and hypoproteinaemic, a whole blood transfusion is indicated. If the packed cell volume is normal, plasma or a synthetic colloid should be administered. Plasma contains albumin and many clotting factors that may also be deficient in a patient with protein losing disease. Since the dose of plasma is 6-10 mg/kg, the disadvantage is its relative cost and difficulty keeping enough in stock to treat a severe albumin deficit. Numerous synthetic colloid solutions, for example hydroxyethyl starch and dextrans, are available to provide oncotic support while the primary disease is treated (see Chapter 2).

REFERENCES AND FURTHER READING

Batt RM and Hall EJ (1989) Chronic enteropathies in the dog. *Journal of Small Animal Practice* **30**, 3-12

Bruskiewicz KA *et al.* (1997) Diabetic ketosis and ketoacidosis in cats: 42 cases (1980-1995). *Journal of the American Veterinary Medical Association* **211**, 188-192

Concannon KT (1993) Colloid oncotic pressure and the clinical use of colloidal solutions. *Journal of Veterinary Emergency and Critical Care* **3**, 49-62

Dhupa N and Proulx J (1998) Hypocalcaemia and hypomagnesemia. *Veterinary Clinics of North America: Small Animal Practice* **28**, 587-608

DiBartola SP (1992) Disorders of sodium and water: hypernatremia and hyponatremia. In: *Fluid Therapy in Small Animal Practice*, ed. DeBartola SP, pp. 57-88. WB Saunders, Philadelphia

Forrester D and Moreland KJ (1989) Hypophosphatemia – causes and clinical consequences. *Journal of Veterinary Internal Medicine* **3**, 149-159

Greco DS (1997a) Endocrine emergencies. Part I. Endocrine pancreatic disorders. *Compendium of Continuing Education for the Practicing Veterinarian* **19**, 15-23

Greco DS (1997b) Endocrine emergencies Part II. Adrenal, thyroid and parathyroid disorders. *Compendium of Continuing Education for the Practicing Veterinarian* **19**, 27-39

Haskins SC (1992) Management of septic shock. *Journal of the American Veterinary Medical Association* **200**, 1915-1924

Kintzer PP and Peterson ME (1991) Mitotane (o,p′-DDD) treatment of 200 dogs with pituitary-dependent hyperadrenocorticism. *Journal of Veterinary Internal Medicine* **5**, 182-190

Kintzer PP and Peterson ME (1997) Treatment and long term follow-up of 205 dogs with hypoadrenocorticism. *Journal on Veterinary Internal Medicine* **11**, 43-49

Kruger JM (1994) Canine and feline hypercalcemic nephropathy. Part 1. Causes and consequences. *Compendium of Continuing Education for the Practicing Veterinarian* **16**, 1299-1310

Langlais-Burgess L *et al.* (1995) Concurrent hypoadrenocorticism and hypoalbuminaemia in dogs: a retrospective study. *Journal of the American Animal Hospital Association* **31**, 307-311

Lifton SJ *et al.* (1996) Glucocorticoid deficient hypoadrenocorticism in dogs: 18 cases (1986-1995). *Journal of the American Veterinary Medical Association* **209**, 2076-2081

Loeb RG *et al.* (1988) Insulin/dextrose therapy of hyperkalaemia: a comparison of two doses. *Veterinary Surgery* **18**, 251

Macintire DK (1993) Treatment of diabetic ketoacidosis in dogs by continuous low-dose intravenous infusion of insulin. *Journal of the American Veterinary Medical Association* **202**, 1266-1272

Macintire DK (1995) Emergency therapy of diabetic crises: insulin overdose, diabetic ketoacidosis and hyperosmolar coma. *Veterinary Clinics of North America: Small Animal Practice* **25**, 639-650

Macintire DK (1997) Disorders of potassium, phosphorus and magnesium in critical illness. *Compendium on Continuing Education for the Practicing Veterinarian* **19,** 41-49

Martin LG (1998) Hypercalcemia and hypermagnesemia. *Veterinary Clinics of North America: Small Animal Practice* **28**, 565-586

Melian C and Peterson ME (1996) Diagnosis and treatment of naturally occurring hypoadrenocorticism in 42 dogs. *Journal of Small Animal Practice* **37**, 268-275

Michel KS (1993) Prognostic value of clinical nutritional assessment in canine patients. *Journal of Veterinary Emergency and Critical Care* **3**, 96-104

Moreau R and Squires RA (1992) Hypercalcemia. *Compendium on Continuing Education for the Practicing Veterinarian* **14**, 1077-1087

Nichols R (1994) Concurrent illness and complications associated with canine hyperadrenocorticism. *Seminars in Veterinary Medicine and Surgery* **9**, 132-136

Ortega TM *et al.* (1996) Systemic arterial blood pressure and urine protein/creatinine ratio in dogs with hyperadrenocorticism. *Journal of the American Veterinary Medical Association* **209**, 1724-1729

Peterson ME and Kintzer PP (1997) Medical treatment of pituitary-dependent hyperadrenocorticism. Mitotane. *Veterinary Clinics of North America: Small Animal Practice* **27**, 255-272

Peterson ME *et al.* (1996) Pretreatment clinical and laboratory findings in dogs with hypoadrenocorticism: 225 cases (1979—1993). *Journal of the American Veterinary Medical Association* **208**, 85-91

Rosol TJ *et al.* (1995) Pathophysiology of calcium metabolism. *Veterinary Clinical Pathology* **24**, 49-63

Sadek D and Schaer M (1996) Atypical Addison's disease in the dog: a retrospective survey of 14 cases. *Journal of the American Animal Hospital Association* **32,** 159-163

Steiner JM and Bruyette DS (1996) Canine insulinoma. *Compendium on Continuing Education for the Practicing Veterinarian* **18,** 13-24

Walters PC and Drobatz KJ (1992) Hypoglycaemia. *Compendium on Continuing Education for the Practicing Veterinarian* **14**, 1150-1159

Wheeler SL (1988) Emergency management of the diabetic patient. *Seminars in Veterinary Medicine and Surgery* **3**, 265-273

Whitley NT *et al.* (1997) Insulin overdose in dogs and cats: 28 cases (1986—1993). *Journal of the American Veterinary Medical Association* **211**, 326-330

CHAPTER THIRTEEN

Acute Management of Orthopaedic and External Soft Tissue Injuries

Matthew Pead and Sorrel Langley-Hobbs

INTRODUCTION

Many animals with orthopaedic injuries or wounds will also have injuries to vital organ systems. Fractures and wounds are often obvious and may be spectacular but must initially be assigned a low priority in emergency treatment, as they are rarely life threatening. Concurrent injuries, especially those involving the thoracic and abdominal cavities, commonly occur during the trauma. The thoracic problems most frequently encountered include pulmonary contusions (46–66%), pneumothorax (12–50%) and rib fractures (10–25%) (Spackman *et al.*, 1984; Tamas *et al.*, 1985; Houlton and Dyce, 1992; Griffon *et al.*, 1994) (Figure 13.1). If the animal is in shock, this should be addressed prior to any investigations or even a full physical examination. Shock can result from internal injury or from the wound or fracture alone. Fluid loss in burns, or osseofascial haemorrhage in fractures, can be sufficient to lead to irreversible shock and death. The initial investigative plan for a trauma case should include: conscious thoracic and abdominal radiographs; an electrocardiogram; and evaluation of blood packed cell volume and total protein. If abnormalities are detected, further investigations may be deemed appropriate.

While potentially life-threatening problems are a priority, temporary and emergency management of wounds and fractures should not be ignored. Such treatment should be directed towards prevention of any additional injury or deterioration at the site of trauma, minimizing contamination and improving patient comfort. Emergency management of wounds and fractures should control any systemic implications of the traumatized tissues and prepare them for the start of definitive treatment.

WOUNDS

Wounds are tissue injuries caused by chemical, thermal or physical trauma. In most cases the skin is damaged and there will be a variable involvement of underlying tissues. Particular consideration should be given to the major structures adjacent to the site (Figure 13.2).

Wound types

Wounds related to physical trauma
These wounds result from the breakdown of tissue by physical force and are the most common type seen in

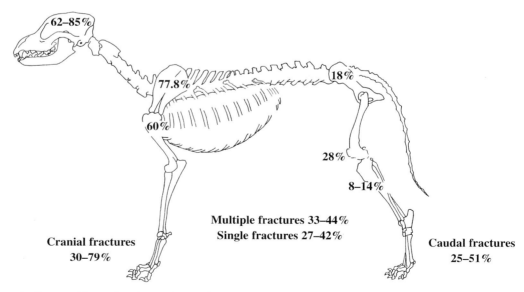

Figure 13.1: *Schematic diagram illustrating the incidence of thoracic injuries associated with fractures in specific areas.*

Area	Examples	Considerations
Head	Cranial fractures	Impacted cranial fractures or jaw fractures need removal of fragments or repair. Risk of meningitis
	Brain damage — swelling, oedema and haemorrhage	Continual monitoring of neurological status required to detect deterioration that may require surgical decompression
Neck	Tracheal rupture	Pneumomediastinum and subcutaneous emphysema
	Recurrent laryngeal nerve damage	Assess laryngeal function by observation under a light plane of anaesthesia
	Cervical spinal cord injury	Assess neurological function, evidence of fracture/dislocation of cervical vertebrae
	Carotid artery severance	Emergency haemostasis
	Oesophageal injuries	Exploration for foreign body, consider gastrostomy tube
Thorax	Fractured ribs, pneumothorax, pulmonary contusions	Often treat conservatively. Large wounds must be covered to allow lung expansion. Air may need drainage if severe or a tension pneumothorax. Supplement oxygen. Flail chest — bandage and delay treatment
	Ruptured diaphragm	Usually delay repair until systemically stable, unless there is respiratory distress
Appendicular	Bone, ligament, tendon, nerve, artery and vein	Check integrity of tendons, nerves (including spinal cord) and vasculature, prior to surgical intervention and anaesthesia
Abdomen	Damage to any abdominal viscera. Abdominal wall or diaphragm rupture with herniation	Monitor for damage by regular physical examination, auscultation, ultrasound and abdominocentesis. Biochemical and cytological analysis of blood and peritoneal fluid

Figure 13.2: Consideration of wounds affecting specific areas.

veterinary practice. Punctures, lacerations, shearing or degloving of the skin and the impact of projectiles, may all cause wounds. They may be complicated by the presence of a foreign body. Recognition of the type of wound can give an early indication of the treatment required (Figures 13.3 and 13.4). In general, the physical breakdown of the skin layer allows damage and exposure of the deeper tissues and so the immediate concern is to control haemorrhage and minimize contamination. All wounds should be covered immediately with a sterile dressing to prevent further contamination from the patient and the hospital environment, as nosocomial infection can be more serious and difficult to eliminate than infection resulting from the original injury.

Burns

Burns cause cell death and the subsequent breakdown of tissue integrity. Although common in the human population, they are relatively rare in veterinary practice. In thermal and electrical burns, the build-up of thermal energy cannot be dissipated before the cells are disrupted. In chemical and radiation burns, cellular

integrity is directly disrupted by toxic substances or ionizing radiation. In all types of burns, destruction of tissue may continue after removal of the source of the injury. There can be a life-threatening loss of fluid in burn injuries, and emergency treatment is based on the removal of the source of the injury and assessment of the severity of the burn to determine the need for fluid therapy. Partial thickness burns involve the epidermis and a variable degree of the dermis. Full-thickness burns involve the entire skin layer. Partial-thickness burns eventually progress to a separation between the viable and non-viable tissue, but this can take up to 10 days to happen naturally. Full-thickness burns progress to a brown or black eschar, which may become hard to the touch (see Figure 13.3b).

In general, any deep partial- or full-thickness burn involving more than 15–20% of the animal's surface will involve major complications requiring emergency systemic supportive therapy (Swaim, 1980; Pavletic, 1993). Burns are vulnerable to infection, and the same care must be taken to prevent contamination as would be exercised for an open wound.

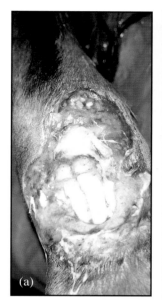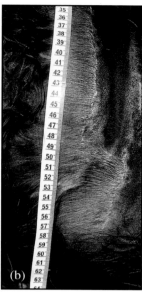

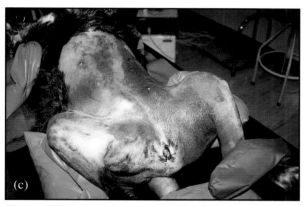

Figure 13.3: Different wound types. (a) A large wound over the carpus, with extensive skin loss and exposure of the deep tissues (bone and joint). There are elements of abrasion, avulsion, laceration and crushing. (b) An extensive burn caused when the animal was trapped against the exhaust pipes of a car. The pale clipped normal skin contrasts with the blackened eschar delineated by a line of exudation. (c) Abrasion and crushing have produced extensive bruising in this dog with a pelvic fracture.

Treatment of wounds

Although it is advisable to progress to definitive treatment of wounds as soon as possible, other more serious complications of trauma may take priority. Treatment of wounds can be divided into emergency procedures (which can and should be done as soon as possible) and the initiation of definitive treatment. In many cases it is possible to combine these procedures without compromising the animal overall. It should not be forgotten that wounds themselves might pose a considerable systemic threat to the patient, especially in terms of fluid loss. All animals with wounds should be evaluated for analgesic therapy.

As successful treatment of wounds ultimately involves care over a considerable period of time, owners should be made aware as soon as is practical of the implications of treatment in terms of their time and finance. Continued effective communication is important throughout the period of treatment.

Emergency treatment

Emergency treatment of wounds often takes place at the time of initial presentation, while systemic involvement in trauma is being assessed and treated. Analgesia should be considered as soon as possible. The animal should be muzzled or restrained to prevent it further traumatizing or contaminating the wound and to ensure that veterinary staff can treat the animal effectively without being bitten.

Haemostasis: Bleeding should be addressed first. Direct pressure can be achieved using a wad of sterile gauze swabs or a bandage, and will be sufficient in most cases to stop minor bleeding. The addition of adrenaline 1:1000 (1 ml to 4–5 ml of sterile saline) to the swabs may facilitate haemostasis. Use of adrenaline is contraindicated at extremities, where prolonged vasoconstriction may lead to ischaemia and necrosis, and in the presence of cardiac arrhythmias. Wounds also can be packed with haemostatic agents such as calcium alginate fibre. With more profuse arterial haemorrhage, it may be necessary to use 'pressure point' haemostasis. At sites where major arteries run superficially, such as the brachial and femoral arteries in the axilla and femoral triangle, respectively, digital pressure is applied over the pressure points proximal to the area of haemorrhage. Head, nose and oral cavity arterial bleeding can be controlled by applying direct digital pressure to the deep area ventral and directly adjacent to the angle of the mandible where the common carotid arteries give rise to the maxillary artery tributaries. Superficial pressure will occlude the jugular, linguofacial or maxillary veins and further venous bleeding can occur, so it is important to apply pressure accurately.

Pressure cuffs and tourniquets: Blood pressure cuffs may be placed proximal to appendicular wounds and inflated 20–30 cm H2O higher than measured arterial pressure. These should not be left in place for more than 6 hours, or irreversible neurovascular compromise will occur. Tourniquets of narrow bands of elastic material such as Penrose drains will place significant pressure on neurovascular structures and may cause permanent deficits. They are not recommended unless the limb is to be amputated or they are applied distal to the tarsus or carpus, where major motor nerves are not present. However they can still only safely be used for 3–5 minutes, although bands 5–10 cm wide can be used for up to 30 minutes. Ligation, surgical stapling and electrosurgery may then be used for definitive haemostasis. Profuse haemorrhage will require clamping and ligation of major vessels; lesser haemorrhage can usually be controlled by the application of a pressure bandage (Feliciano, 1992).

Wound type	Description	Treatment considerations
Abrasion	Superficial wound involving destruction of varying depths of skin by friction or shearing forces. Usually bleeds minimally	When associated with a fracture, normal skin barrier is incompetent — treat fracture as grade I open
Avulsion	Characterized by tearing of tissues from attachments and creation of skin flaps. Limb avulsion injuries with extensive skin loss are called 'degloving'	Blood supply to skin may be compromised leading to skin necrosis 2–5 days after injury. Repeat examinations and consider secondary debridement
Chemical burns	Direct exposure to noxious chemicals	Copious lavage to remove chemical. Ensure animal cannot lick area and ingest harmful substances
Contusion	Blunt trauma may cause blood to pool in the subcutaneous tissue	Application of cold and analgesics. Beware of compartment syndrome
Crushing injuries	Combination of other injuries with extensive damage and contusion to the skin and deeper tissues	Assess neurological and vascular supply prior to treatment
Gunshots	These are contaminated. The heat generated in firing a bullet does not render it sterile (Wolf *et al.*, 1978). Open fractures may be present	Remove metal if encountered but not usually necessary to remove all fragments unless intra-articular or impinging on major structures such as nerves and arteries
Laceration	Created by tearing, which damages the skin and underlying tissues and may be superficial or deep and have irregular edges	Debridement and primary closure may be used if treatment is early
Penetrating or puncture wound	Related to the impact of a missile or sharp object such as a knife or tooth. Tissue damage is directly proportional to the velocity of the impact	Excise a 2–3 mm wide full thickness rim of skin around the puncture site. Check vital signs as may be significant internal haemorrhage. Penetrating abdominal wounds require exploratory laparotomy
Penetrating foreign bodies	Foreign bodies such as sticks and glass can fragment causing widespread contamination	May need extensive exploration to remove all fragments (90% of glass shards show on radiographs (Tandberg, 1982)). Protruding foreign bodies should be left in place for transport but can be cut 2–3 cm from the body wall to minimize further internal damage by preventing the protruding shaft acting as a fulcrum
Thermal burns	Check for reddened, crusted or blackened skin. Check for injuries around the head and neck, which may compromise respiration	Beware of systemic complications of the burn. Attend to analgesia and cooling the area

Figure 13.4: *Recognition and treatment of specific wounds.*

Initial control of contamination: A 'golden period' of 6 hours exists in which a contaminated wound may be cleaned and primarily closed or covered without development of infection (Johnson, 1974). The procedure for cleaning wounds is summarized in Figure 13.5. Sterile apparel, especially gloves and instruments, should be used to minimize further contamination. A large volume of lavage fluid is used to remove contaminants, debris and bacteria and to rehydrate the tissues, and a minimum of 500 ml is recommended. The pressure at which the fluid is applied should be sufficient to dislodge contaminants. Applying fluid under too high a pressure and inserting the needle deep into the wound will force material deeper and open up uncontaminated tissue planes. Fluid applied through a 20–50 ml syringe with a 19 gauge needle will produce satisfactory pressure of 7–9 psi and will significantly decrease the number of bacteria and thus the incidence of infection. The ideal

Haemostasis

Cover wound with sterile dressing whilst preparing for lavage

Wear sterile gloves (and hat, mask, gown)

Apply gel or sterile saline-soaked swabs to the wound

Clip away hair, working from wound outwards if possible

Flush wound with sterile saline, remove all contaminants from chemical burns

Take a bacterial swab for culture

Apply a sterile dressing and bandage

Figure 13.5: Summary of emergency wound care.

flushing solution will enhance bacterial removal without being toxic to the tissues. Saline is ideal; detergents and soaps are cytotoxic as are some antiseptics. However, chlorhexidine 0.05% and povidone–iodine 0.01–1% are safe to use. In gross contamination, tap water can be used followed by a sterile lavage solution. However, topical agents such as wound powders, intra-mammary preparations, hydrogen peroxide and alcohol should not be used. These substances cause cell death, provoke a foreign body reaction and interfere with the healing process. Finally, the wound is again covered with a sterile dressing. Time spent minimizing contamination and thus preventing infection becoming established at the earliest possible stage, can significantly shorten the recovery time of wounds.

Emergency treatment of burns: Evaluation of the area of a burn is critical and so clipping the area is essential. The damage related to a burn and the surface appearance may change in the first 48–72 hours so the clipped area should be monitored. Burns may appear as reddened areas of inflamed skin with a crust or scab over the surface. The hair may fall out or be easily plucked from full thickness burns. Partial-thickness burns may be painful when touched, although full-thickness burns are often analgesic. Once the area is assessed, aggressive fluid therapy should be started if the burnt area exceeds 15% of body surface. Patients should be assessed for evidence of dehydration, anaemia and hypoalbuminaemia. Cardiovascular, pulmonary and renal function should be evaluated and monitored for several days following the injury.

The area of the burn can be cooled by lavage, and in chemical burns all residues should be washed away with copious volumes of water. Large burns should be cooled with care in order to prevent severe heat loss in a debilitated patient. Application of soaked dressings or bags of fluid at 3–10°C for at least 30 minutes are recommended. The necrotic skin in the eschar has great potential for infection and will not be penetrated by systemic antibiotics. Until this tissue can be removed, it should be protected with topical antibiotics, particularly

silver sulphadiazine in a water-soluble cream, and covered with a sterile non-adherent dressing. Definitive treatment is initiated using principles and techniques common to the management of other wounds. These are dealt with below.

Starting definitive wound treatment

Once the animal is stable and other injuries have been addressed, more definitive treatment can be instigated (Figures 13.6 and 13.7). Thorough treatment normally requires analgesia and general anaesthesia. The nature and extent of the wound should be evaluated and a plan for the subsequent preparation and treatment devised. Such a plan will depend on the nature of the wound (see Figure 13.4). Wounds should be treated in an aseptic fashion using sterile technique and sterile apparel. A large area of normal skin should be clipped to allow for a thorough inspection and for any enlargement of the surgical site, such as the use of skin flaps. The skin is scrubbed thoroughly using a proprietary scrub solution. Any exposed areas of the wound can be protected by covering them with a water-soluble gel or swabs soaked in sterile saline, which can then be lavaged away together with any debris from the clipping and preparation.

Debridement:

1. Remove all foreign debris such as gravel and superficial gun shot (the tissue should not be aggressively explored to retrieve all shot)
2. Dissect out and remove obviously necrotic tissue, especially muscle and skin (nerves, blood vessels, tendon, ligaments and bone with soft tissue attachments should be preserved)
3. Leave tissue that has a good chance of viability, especially when major structures are involved. If viability is questionable, a delayed debridement can be made several days later if necessary
4. Remove partial-thickness burn eschar by 'tangential section,' sharply cutting back the tissue parallel to the surface until healthy bleeding dermis is encountered
5. Debride full thickness burn eschar vigorously, as early as it is possible to define its extent
6. Control haemorrhage carefully, as blood provides the ideal conditions for bacterial proliferation. Use pressure and diathermy where possible, with ligation for larger vessels
7. Lavage the wound with sterile saline as described above
8. Take a swab for culture at the end of cleaning and debridement as this has been found to produce the most significant results (Merrit, 1987).

Decisions on the amount of tissue to remove can be difficult. The most common cause for delayed wound healing and infection is inadequate debridement

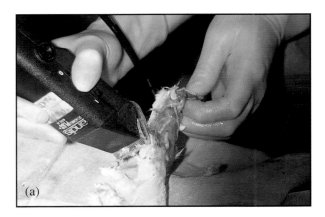

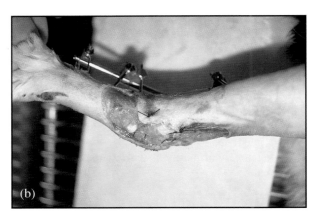

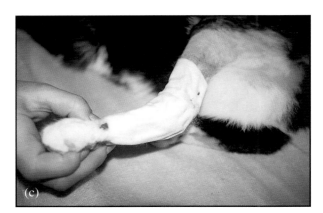

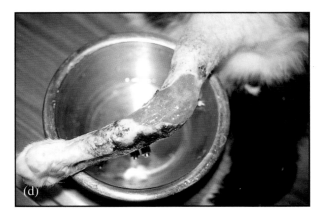

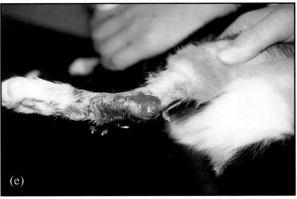

Figure 13.6: *Treatment of a wound involving considerable skin loss. (a) Using sterile technique wherever possible the area around the wound is clipped prior to debridement. (b) The wound has been debrided, cleaned and flushed, and a transarticular external fixator applied to stabilize the joint, before application of the appropriate dressing (c). Careful initial treatment will lead to uniform granulation tissue cover (d) and rapid epithelialization and cicatrix formation (e), accelerating wound healing.*

(Edlich *et al.*, 1982), so aggressive debridement, especially with expendable structures, is often the best policy. There is some variation for the different types of tissue, and the following guidelines are useful:

*   Assess skin viability based on colour, temperature, bleeding and pain sensation. Non-viable skin will appear black, blue-black or white, feel cool, lack pain sensation and not bleed. Skin of questionable viability may appear blue or purple
*   Debride muscle until it bleeds and contracts following appropriate stimuli
*   Remove small bone fragments from open fractures, as they may prevent complete granulation
*   Excise contaminated fat aggressively as it is easily devascularized, harbours bacteria and is expendable.

Other techniques that have been used to assess viability include dye injection, radiographic contrast media, transcutaneous oxygen and carbon dioxide measurements, laser and Doppler velocimetry (Bellah and Krahwinkel, 1985; Rochat *et al.*, 1993). However, visual examination is feasible in most situations and has been found to be as accurate as dye infusion in one study (Bellah and Krahwinkel, 1985).

Assessment of bacterial contamination: Wound closure and antibiotic therapy are influenced by the degree of bacterial contamination. Swabbing for culture and sensitivity at the end of debridement and lavage is sufficient for most wounds healing by second intention, as antibiotic therapy can be accurately targeted. However, infection is a significant source of morbidity in prematurely closed wounds, and further precautions may be needed if closure is contemplated. Gross inspection will not determine whether a wound is infected or not, but quantitative bacterial counts and culture can provide insights into the advisability of wound closure. If there are >10^5 organisms/g or β-haemolytic streptococci present, then the wound should not be closed (Gfeller and Crowe, 1994). The rapid slide test (RST) can be performed prior to attempting wound closure. The method involves swabbing 1 cm^2 of the deepest surface of the prepared wound with a sterile cotton-tipped swab. The swab is rubbed over 1 cm^2 of a clean microscope slide. The slide is examined under microscopy and if even one bacterium is seen, the wound should not be closed (Gfeller and Crowe, 1994).

Closure: After cleaning and debridement the wound may either be closed immediately (primary), left for 3–5 days and then closed (delayed primary), or closed after the granulating bed has matured (10 days; secondary closure), or left to heal by granulation and re-epithelialization (second intention healing). The wound should only be closed if one is confident that all necrotic tissue and debris have been removed and if closure can be achieved without excessive tension. Tension-relieving techniques such as undermining, walking sutures, subdermal suture patterns (inverted vertical mattress pattern), vertical mattress sutures, far-near-near-far and far-far-near-near suture patterns, stented sutures, relaxing incisions, bipedicle flaps, V–Y plasties or Z plasties may be useful in closing selected wounds (Swaim, 1980; Pavletic, 1993).

For wound repair, a small diameter monofilament non-absorbable suture material should be selected, although, if available, stapling is faster than suturing and is associated with a lower infection rate (Edlich *et al.*, 1987). Primarily closed wounds should be covered, as it takes 24–48 hours for a fibrin seal to form that will resist bacterial invasion, and unpublished studies demonstrate a 50% higher infection rate in uncovered wounds. For selected wounds, drainage should be provided as wound fluids and exudates interfere with normal healing. A drain can be used for dead space obliteration, to eliminate established fluid and for prophylactic prevention of fluid or air accumulation within a wound. Active suction drains are particularly useful under these circumstances (Bellah and Krahwinkel, 1985; Edlich *et al.*, 1987; Rochat *et al.*, 1993). In-depth discussions of protracted wound management and surgical reconstruction of wounds can be found in more specialized texts (Swaim, 1980; Pavletic, 1993).

Selection of antibiotics: Clean wounds primarily closed within 6–8 hours of the injury and more extensive wounds correctly treated with debridement and lavage do not need antibiotic therapy, provided tissue damage is minimal. Deep wounds involving muscle, severe tissue damage, tissue of doubtful viability left after debridement, systemic infection or an immunocompromised patient, are all indications for the

Aseptic technique
Evaluation and treatment plan
Preparation of skin and surrounding area
Debridement
Lavage
Bacterial culture and evaluation of contamination
Evaluation and execution of closure if appropriate
Administer appropriate antibiotics
Apply a sterile dressing and bandage

Figure 13.7: Summary of initial definitive wound care.

use of antibiotics. If antibiotics are given in the first 3 hours, they will contact bacteria via the fluid in the wound, before debris and fibrin surround them. To exploit this opportunity, intravenous therapy should be started as soon as possible to maximize antibiotic levels in tissue and wound fluid. As results from culture will not be available at this stage, simple guidelines are used to select a broad-spectrum antibiotic. Most wounds are exposed to contamination from *Staphylococcus* and *Streptococcus* species. Bite wounds may contain *Pasturella* and Gram-negative species such as *Escherichia coli*. Gram-negative species may be found in puncture wounds and in potentially contaminated areas such as the perineum. Cephalosporins, trimethoprim/sulphonamides, amoxycillin/clavulanate and enrofloxacin all have activity against these organisms and can be given intravenously. Where there is the possibility of extensive Gram-negative contamination, an aminoglycoside should be considered. Ampicillin and penicillin should only be used after culture, as in more than two-thirds of cases the bacteria isolated are resistant to these agents (Hirsch and Smith, 1978).

During definitive treatment, antibiotic therapy can be modified on the basis of culture and RST results. Unless there is an indication to change or extend the course, the most effective, narrowest spectrum, cheapest and safest antibiotic available should be continued by injection or orally for 5–7 days. If the appearance of the wound does not improve or the patient's systemic condition deteriorates, a change in antibiotics coupled with re-swabbing the wound is indicated.

Systemic antibiotics alone will be adequate in most situations, but heavily contaminated wounds and burns are best treated with a combination of topical and systemic therapy (Figure 13.8). Gentamicin, nitrofurazone, bacitracin/polymixin and neomycin may all be delivered to the wound via the primary dressing layer. They are particularly useful when the contaminants are resistant or difficult to treat systemically, such as *Pseudomonas* spp. Soaking the primary dressing in *tris*-EDTA also aids the control of *Pseudomonas*. Topical water-soluble silver sulphadiazine cream can be applied to the eschar in burn cases, to prevent the necrotic tissue becoming infected.

> For serious wounds start broad-spectrum intravenous therapy immediately
>
> For simple wounds, which are treated correctly, do not use antibiotics
>
> Re-assess therapy on the basis of culture, RST results, wound progress and patient's condition
>
> Once therapy is started, continue for 5–7 days
>
> Consider combinations of multiple systemic and topical drugs in heavily contaminated wounds with resistant bacterial species

Figure 13.8: *Summary of antibiotic selection.*

Dressings and bandages

Dressings are required as a primary contact layer with the wound. Maintaining the apposition of the dressing, provision for the storage of exudate and mechanical stability can be achieved using various combinations of bandages, adhesives, sutures and the external skeletal fixator. Thus the principal decision relates to the choice of a dressing. Individual bandages are dealt with in the section on musculoskeletal trauma (see Figure 13.13). Selection of appropriate dressings depends on evaluation of the state of the exposed tissue, the degree of contamination and the anticipated production of fluid from the wound surface (Figure 13.9). Ideally a dressing should:

- Prevent further contamination
- Assist the process of debridement
- Conduct fluid away from the surface preventing pooling, maceration and the formation of an environment conducive to bacterial proliferation
- Prevent desiccation and maintain a moist, well oxygenated environment to promote repair.

The primary consideration for initial management of wounds is whether to use an adherent or non-adherent dressing. Adherent dressings such as dry swabs or sterile saline-soaked swabs allowed to dry in contact with the wound (wet to dry) aid debridement. Such dressings are useful in wounds where there is a considerable amount of necrotic debris and where surgical debridement is delayed. However, they can be painful to remove, may disrupt granulation tissue and the wound surface may become desiccated if the dressing is too dry, and macerated if it is too wet. Non-adherent dressings prevent disruption and damage to epithelializing or granulating tissue at removal. They vary in their degree of absorbency, and conduct fluid away from the surface to a greater or lesser extent. In addition, some of them have interactive properties that promote the removal of necrotic debris and bacteria from the wound surface, but they are not as valuable in the process of debridement as the adherent dressings. Non-adherent dressings are easier to manage as they are less painful to change and maintain a more constant wound environment.

Ideally, initial treatment of most wounds would be with an adherent dressing to assist micro-debridement, followed by non-adherent dressings once granulation commences. However, to ease the management of dressing changes, there are many cases where non-adherent dressings can be used throughout the healing process. Recent improvement in the properties and variety of these dressings, particularly the ability of some of them to participate in microdebridement, allows selection of a dressing with properties appropriate to the stage of wound healing. Whatever dressing materials are used, a schedule for dressing changes should be devised based on the severity of the wound. Frequent dressing changes allow more accurate monitoring, but may retard healing and distress the patient. Dressings on contaminated wounds and those with severe skin loss should be changed within the first 24 hours. Dressings over simple lacerations should be changed after 48–72 hours. Removal of adherent dressings can be painful and this can be ameliorated by soaking the primary layer with sterile saline or 2% lignocaine. The protocol described for initial wound management should be followed as far as possible at dressing changes.

MUSCULOSKELETAL TRAUMA

Although they are often the most obvious and impressive part of a case, musculoskeletal injuries have a low priority in the initial handling of the trauma patient, and emergency care must be primarily directed towards systemic injuries. Even after evaluation of the major organ systems, these injuries cannot be considered in isolation. The haemorrhage and local disruption of the surrounding soft tissue may pose more problems than the injury itself, so the integrity of all tissue involved and its systemic implications must be considered before definitive fixation (Figures 13.10 and 13.11).

Definitive treatment frequently requires a prolonged period of anaesthesia to allow accurate evaluation and corrective surgery. Most definitive treatment should thus be outside the remit of emergency care. However, the emergency management of a specific injury can be important in improving the systemic condition of the animal, and can have more impact in achieving complication-free healing than definitive fixation.

Fractures and luxations

Most fracture/luxation presentations are simple, acute and have a clear history related to external trauma. Clinical signs include pain, deformity, swelling, crepitus and instability. The systemic consequences can be severe. The osseofascial haemorrhage that occurs in closed femoral and humeral fractures can result in up to 30% of circulating blood being sequestered at the frac-

Description (and proprietary examples)	Properties	Uses and contraindications
Thin perforated polyester film, backed with absorbent cotton and acrylic fibre pad (Melonin, Smith & Nephew)	Semi-occlusive Non-adherent	Clean sutured wounds, abrasions, lacerations and minor burns
Open weave gauze impregnated with paraffin jelly (Jelonet, Smith & Nephew)	Non-adherent Free draining into absorbent secondary dressing May be antibiotic impregnated	Low viscosity exudative wounds Avoid on granulating wounds as interdigitates with expanding granulating tissue which causes damage at removal
Outer polyurethane film, hydrophilic core, polyurethane wound contact layer (Allevyn, Smith & Nephew)	Non-adherent Controlled exudate absorption Absorbs 10 times its own weight Keeps wound moist	Granulating wounds with some exudation, but without necrotic debris. Can be left in position for up to 5 days
Hydrocolloid gel (Intrasite, Smith & Nephew; Granuflex E.R., Squibb)	Non-adherent Interactive conformable Waterproof	Granulating wounds including those with some necrotic debris. Can assist in microdebridement
Calcium alginate fibre (Kaltostat, Hoechst Animal Health)	Interactive ion exchange Haemostatic Absorbs 20 times weight	Bleeding and exudating wounds, dry wounds or wounds with necrotic slough
Open weave gauze saturated with sterile saline Wet to dry or wet to wet	Adherent Saline dilutes exudate and facilitates absorption Debriding – necrotic material entrapped as gauze dries, and removed at dressing change	Open degloving wounds, especially contaminated or necrotic. Use in early stages to aid debridement, soak with *tris*-EDTA and antibiotics or perfuse solutions to moisten dressing continuously

Figure 13.9: *Dressing characteristics.*

ture site. Fractures and luxations in which external trauma is clearly not involved require less consideration of systemic problems in the early phase of treatment. In these much less common cases, investigation can progress more rapidly to a definitive evaluation of the fracture and the underlying cause, once simple support and analgesia have been implemented.

Evaluation

There are numerous systems by which to evaluate and classify fractures. They are mostly used in decisions related to definitive treatment, rely on accurate imaging and are unnecessary for initial treatment. An evaluation should be made of the position of the injury, its relationship to critical structures and whether it is open or closed. The accompanying systematic examination should include a general evaluation of the extremities, assessing pulses, neurological status and the presence of wounds or devitalized skin. Oedema indicates impaired venous and lymphatic return caused by haematoma or mechanical impingement. On the basis of this information, the problem can be categorized in the following manner:

- Fractures and luxations, which require prompt treatment due to life-threatening complications (impacted cranial fractures, spinal fractures/ luxations and open fractures involving major structures)
- Fractures that will benefit from being treated immediately, provided the animal is not at increased risk from anaesthesia (open fractures and luxations)
- Fractures that should be treated within 24–48 hours for optimal results (articular and epiphyseal fractures and all other luxations) (see Figure 13.10)
- Fractures that need to be treated within 5 days of occurrence (all other fractures).

Evaluation of position: Although evaluation of abnormal range of movement, swelling and crepitus is useful, manipulation and palpation should be minimized to prevent discomfort and further damage to adjacent tissue. If the animal will lie quietly, it is often possible to take a survey radiograph to give information on the position and extent of the injury. Even though such radiographs may not be accurate enough for use in the definitive fixation, they are often the best and least distressing method of evaluating the position of the fracture.

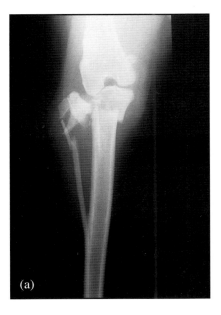

(a)

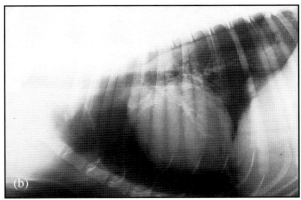

(b)

Figure 13.10: Prioritization of therapy. (a) The comminuted fracture of the proximal tibia has an articular component, which requires early treatment. (b) However, this patient had thoracic complications with a pneumothorax and ECG abnormalities, and so surgery was delayed until the 5th day after the original trauma.

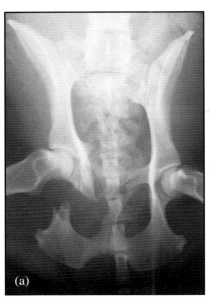

(a)

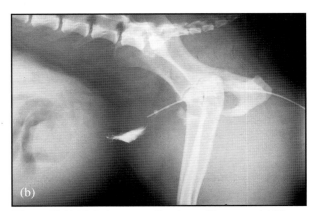

(b)

Figure 13.11: Soft tissue complications of fractures. (a) The pelvic fracture involves the ischium, pubis and the sacrum. Sacral fractures may involve the nerves which run out through the sacral foraminae, and this dog had a neurological deficit. (b) In addition, the bladder was ruptured. No fluid was collected with abdominocentesis, but leakage of positive contrast from the cystogram into the abdomen clearly demonstrates the problem.

Evaluation of open fractures: The main feature of open fractures is direct exposure of the bone to the outside environment. Evaluation along simple guidelines allows straightforward selection of therapy and an early indication of prognosis. The guidelines for evaluation are:

Grade I   Penetration of the skin by a bony fragment from the fracture. The fragment frequently retracts back beneath the skin. Prognosis is as good as a closed fracture, providing there is aseptic wound handling and early fixation

Grade II   The fracture is created by an external force, which also creates a wound. The bone is not directly exposed but there is a variable loss of skin and underlying tissue.

Prognosis depends on the degree of soft tissue loss and contamination

Grade III   Severe injuries, which are often associated with high-energy trauma. The fractures are often comminuted and there is a high degree of tissue loss, contamination and devitalization. Bony union is normally delayed and there are often complications during the healing period

The prognosis in grade III fractures is variable. In some cases it may not be possible to resolve the fracture successfully and initial treatment should be aimed towards an amputation. In humans, the grade III group has been further subdivided to help in this decision (Caudal and Stern, 1987):

Grade IIIA Adequate covering of bone despite extensive soft tissue loss and/or high-energy trauma. Fair prognosis despite extended healing time

Grade IIIB Exposure of bone and periosteal stripping often highly contaminated. Prognosis is guarded and in some cases prognosis will force amputation

Grade IIIC Type IIIB tissue damage with major arterial damage. Prognosis is poor and amputation should be considered.

Principles of emergency treatment of fractures and luxations

The principles of emergency management of fractures and luxations consist of:

- Limiting swelling
- Prevention of further compromise of blood supply
- Limiting further soft tissue damage resulting from instability
- Increasing patient comfort and minimizing movement (Figure 13.12)
- Provision of analgesia
- Treating open fractures in the same way as described for wounds.

Application of these principles is primarily dependent on the position of the injury. Some techniques for fracture management are valid for one area and wholly inappropriate for another.

Open injuries should be considered as wounds involving a fracture or luxation. The same considerations of emergency treatment, debridement, contamination, antibiotics and dressings should be applied to them as outlined earlier. The depth of tissue involved in grade II and III injuries dictates the application of maximal care to these injuries. Early stabilization, where possible, reduces discomfort and can speed recovery.

Temporary stabilization should always be considered concurrent with early treatment of the wound, as stability promotes wound-healing processes, decreases pain and reduces complications. External coaption can be used if appropriate to the site. The external fixator (ESF) is often the optimal definitive fixation for open fractures. However, the ESF should also be considered during the initial treatment, as an alternative to external coaption. The ESF can be placed rapidly in a closed fashion, and is therefore applicable during anaesthesia for wound debridement. Unlike external coaption, the ESF allows the stability of the site to be maintained during dressing changes, and the recurrent use of bandaging material is reduced. The transarticular ESF (see Figure 13.6b) can be used to control the stability of a wound over a joint, even when no fracture is present.

Selection and use of bandages

Bandages can be used to stabilize traumatized areas and to hold dressings in place. However, it can be difficult to place bandages correctly on a distressed patient and the benefit of a bandage, particularly the complex ones such as the slings and spica splints (Figure 13.13), must be weighed against the problems of correct placement. Simple bandages also have limitations. The Robert Jones bandage, when applied above the elbow or stifle, tends to slip down and form a 'pendulum' of extra weight at the joint. Thus, when considering emergency stabilization there are a number of situations where it is better not to apply an extensive bandage, but to use cage rest, analgesia and sedation to restrict further damage at the fracture site (see Figure 13.12).

There are specific situations in which certain bandage configurations are appropriate, and these are outlined in Figures 13.9 and 13.13 and in the text below. Dressings can be held in place over the body with wraps, particularly using the newer elasticated and conformable materials. The most useful general configuration is the support bandage.

Bone affected	Method of stabilization
Mandible	None or tape muzzle
Maxilla and cranium	None
Cervical spine	Neck splint
Scapula or humerus	None or full spica splint (see Figure 13.16)
Radius and ulna or tibia	Support bandage or splinted bandage
Carpus or tarsus and all bones distal	Support bandage
Thoracolumbar spine	Back splint (see Figure 13.20)
Caudal lumbar spine	None
Pelvis	None
Femur	None or a full spica splint

Figure 13.12: Emergency stabilization of fractures.

Type of bandage	Description	Uses	Comments and specific contraindications
Support (modified Robert Jones dressing)	Use deformable secondary layer applied under compression. Leave pads of middle two digits protruding to allow checking for swelling	Stable fractures distal to the elbow or stifle. Positioning of a dressing, especially over an exudative wound	Do not use in proximal limb fractures, rarely of use in elbow or stifle injuries. In these cases the bandage may slip down and become a pendulum weight
Splinted bandage	Augment a support bandage with a splint to increase rigidity without extra bulk	Unstable fractures distal to elbow or stifle	Do not use in proximal limb fractures, rarely of use in elbow or stifle injuries
Velpeau sling	Bandage placed around leg and over body to flex carpus, elbow and shoulder	Holds entire forelimb in flexion to prevent weight bearing and movement of distal limb	Provide sufficient padding to prevent sores
Carpal flexion	Figure-of-eight bandage applied over padding from distal radius to metacarpals	Flexion of carpus and prevention of forelimb weight bearing, although limb can still be moved	Do not use for antebrachial or distal injuries
Ehmer sling	Figure-of-eight bandages from metatarsals to distal femur with the bandage all medial to the tibia	Internal rotation of hip and stifle reduces the chance of re-luxation after craniodorsal hip luxation	Difficult to apply especially on cats or short-legged dogs
Hobble	Bandage connection between both distal tibiae	Prevents abduction and reduces the chance of re-luxation after reduction of ventral hip luxations	
Spica splint	Flat splint strapped from toe to dorsum. Held in place with support bandage distally and body bandage	Fractures proximal to the elbow (use in hindlimb is reported)	Not usually recommended for injuries distal to the elbow or stifle

Figure 13.13: Bandages (see also Figures 13.14, 13.16 and 13.17).

Support bandage: Support bandages minimize swelling and oedema, aid haemostasis, provide stabilization and increase patient comfort. Rarely are true pressure bandages necessary. The Robert Jones bandage is known as a pressure bandage, but with the deformable bandage materials used, pressure is generally not maintained for a significant length of time. Pressure gauges placed on the skin under such bandages soon return to normal. The bandage should be applied with a primary layer covering any wound, a secondary layer of a conformable material such as cotton wool, a tertiary layer using a tightly wound bandage and an outer protective bandage. The bandage should be placed to follow the normal aspect of the limb (Figure 13.14) and can be reinforced by a splint placed after the secondary layer has been pressurized.

Luxations

Traumatic luxations require definitive treatment as early as the systemic condition of the animal allows in order to minimize cartilage destruction, muscle contracture and periarticular fibrosis. Examination under general anaesthesia and two orthogonal radiographic views are essential to confirm the presence and direction of the luxation, concurrent periarticular injuries and pre-existing disease such as hip dysplasia, which may influence management. There will be damage to some part of the bone, muscle, tendon and ligament complex, which confer stability on the normal joint. In some joints, surgical repair of this damage, coupled with postoperative support, is indicated to maintain reduction (Figure 13.15). The hip, elbow, temporomandibular joint and occasionally the shoulder have enough inherent stability to remain reduced despite some damage, and closed reduction of these joints is indicated as a primary treatment (Figure 13.15). The Ehmer sling can be used to assist stability of the hip joint after reduction, and the Velpeau sling may be applied to support the shoulder (Figure 13.16). In general, surgical reduction and repair of any joint should be considered if:

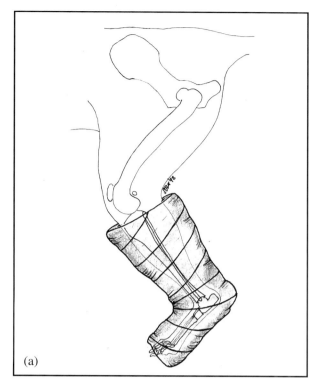

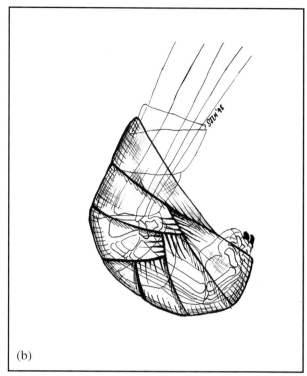

Figure 13.14: Bandaging the lower limb. (a) The Robert Jones bandage provides a column of support, but follows the basic conformation of the limb, allowing the patient to manage the limb comfortably. (b) The carpal flexion bandage prevents weight bearing but allows movement of the limb.

- Closed reduction is impossible
- The joint is still unstable or luxates easily after closed reduction
- Periarticular or articular fractures prevent reduction or require fixation
- Exploratory surgery is required to evaluate periarticular structures such as nerves
- Developmental or congenital abnormalities are present which can cause instability.

Articular fractures

Articular fractures should be definitively treated within 24–48 hours provided the animal can be safely anaesthetized. Accurate reconstruction of articular surfaces, compression and rigid internal fixation are essential. Early return to function minimizes periarticular fibrosis and joint stiffness. Bandages or splints applied prior to treatment will be beneficial in decreasing swelling and increasing comfort, but are contraindicated in some situations. Cats in particular do not tolerate bandages well and, with closed injuries, cage rest may be preferable to bandaging. In general, the joints below the elbow and stifle can be supported with a bandage or splint. The elbow and stifle can be supported if necessary using a spica splint (Figures 13.16 and 13.17). Support of either the shoulder or hip joint prior to definitive treatment is generally not necessary, as the large muscle mass surrounding these joints provides sufficient support.

Diaphyseal fractures

Fractures involving the pelvis, scapula, femur and humerus should generally be left unbandaged. The muscle mass surrounding these bones provides some support, and bandages for these areas are cumbersome and restricting. Tubular bandages are ineffective in supporting these fractures and tend to form a pendulum of extra weight swinging at the level of the fracture. Femoral and humeral fractures may be supported with spica splints for transport or if repair must be delayed. Cage rest with suitable analgesia may be preferable. Fractures of the bones below the elbow and stifle should be supported with a bandage or splint.

Spinal fractures

Spinal fractures are candidates for immediate treatment, despite the high (40–50%) incidence of concurrent problems (Selcer *et al.*, 1991). The potential for injury to the spinal cord itself is high and early intervention is essential to allow the maximum chance of conserving spinal cord function. There is a risk of further injury to the spinal cord during transport and examination of the patient. Animals should be transported on a flat board, a firm stretcher or slung in a strong blanket.

Examination: Early neurological examination is important, but extensive testing involving movement of the animal may cause further problems. Particular attention should be paid to deep pain sensation and the

Affected joint	Direction of luxation	Technique for reduction (under general anaesthetic)	Postoperative support	Comments
Temporomandibular	Rostrodorsal	Lever in mouth and close mouth	Tape muzzle 7–10 days	Associated fractures may require surgery
	Coronoid displacement	Open mouth further and move mandible towards midline	None	Partial zygomatic arch resection if recurrent
Scapulohumeral	Medial	Manipulate proximal humerus/ acromion	Velpeau 2–3 weeks	Small dogs, often congenital
	Lateral	Manipulate proximal humerus/ acromion	Spica	Large dogs, often traumatic
Elbow	Lateral	Flex elbow more than 90°, supinate antebrachium[a]	Maintain extension[a]	Very rarely medial. May need surgical reduction
Carpus	Variable	Surgical	Support bandage	Arthrodesis may be required if function is unsatisfactory
Phalangeal	Lateral or abaxial	Closed for pet animals, surgical treatment in working dogs	Support bandage	Require surgical imbrication of collaterals, or arthrodesis
Hip	Craniodorsal	Externally rotate hip, extend leg and then internally rotate hip[b]	Ehmer sling or cage rest	Surgical stabilization ultimately required in many cases (15–71%)
	Ventral	Externally rotate and abduct whilst gently pushing dorsally	Hobble	Closed reduction usually successful
Stifle	Cranial	Surgical	Spica or ESF	Repair combination injuries of collaterals and cruciates
Tibiotarsal	Variable	Surgical	Bandage, splint or ESF	Repair fractured malleoli and collateral ligaments if possible

Figure 13.15: *Management of luxations.*

[a] Technique for elbow reduction:
1. Flex elbow to >90° and abduct and pronate antebrachium whilst applying medial pressure to caudal ulna to engage anconeus
2. Extend elbow slightly and then slowly extend elbow further and pronate and adduct antebrachium whilst applying medial pressure to radial head
3. Use high support bandage or spica, to maintain extension or carpal flexion bandage to avoid weight bearing.

[b] Technique for reduction of hip luxations
When hip is craniodorsal:
1. Externally rotate femur; distract limb against counter traction
2. Adduct then internally rotate, extend and abduct limb
3. Manipulate through full range of movement to dispel clots.
When hip is ventral:
• Manipulate into craniodorsal position and then reduce as above.

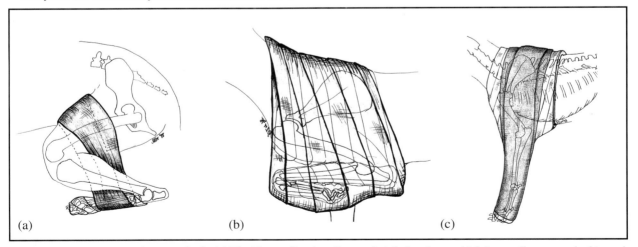

(a)   (b)   (c)

Figure 13.16: *Bandaging the upper limb. (a) The Ehmer sling is a figure-of-eight bandage, which internally rotates the hip and prevents re-luxation. (b) The Velpeau sling provides stability for the shoulder area and prevents weight bearing by limiting movement of the limb. (c) The spica splint stabilizes the elbow and humerus and can also be used in the hindlimb. The antebrachium is padded with a Robert Jones bandage and there is some padding over the scapula. A flat lateral splint (darker grey shading) is placed over the midline at the tip of the scapula and all the way down to the foot. The splint can be made from a sheet of thermosetting cast material and pleated for resistance to bending. It is held in place with adhesive tape over the Robert Jones dressing and a body bandage around the thorax.*

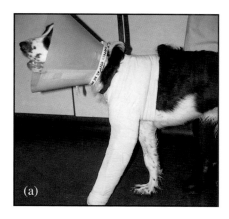

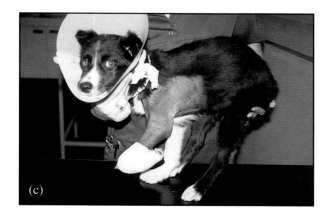

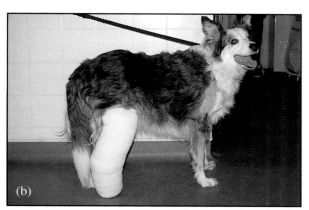

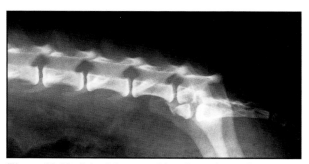

Figure 13.17: *Bandage configurations. (a) Spica splint. (b)Robert Jones dressing. (c) Carpal flexion bandage. (d) Hobbles placed on a dog while still anaesthetized after surgery.*

testing of local reflexes, where all the muscle groups should be observed acting coherently. Repeated monitoring is important to assess any change in status. Survey radiographs of the conscious patient are indicated, as muscle relaxation and positioning for radiographs may cause further damage at the site of instability. Lateral views of the entire spine are advisable as multiple fractures occur in 20% of patients. Oblique views assist evaluation of the articular process and can be taken with the animal in lateral recumbency. Positioning for dorsoventral views can be hazardous, and using a horizontal beam view is the preferred option (Wheeler and Sharp, 1994).

It is important to assess the stability of the fracture. Bending, shear, rotational and axial loading forces all act on the spine. Evaluation of the damaged areas from radiographs can indicate the residual capacity of the spine to resist these forces, and indicate the optimum fixation technique. The key areas of evaluation are the ventral spinal component, that is the vertebral body and the intervertebral discs, which resist load and bending, and the articular processes, which resist a combination of forces. If one or both of these areas are severely compromised, the fracture will be unstable and a candidate for surgical fixation. More complex systems for staging the damage in relation to stability can be consulted, but the information is often difficult to apply to commonly occurring fracture patterns (Smith and

Walter, 1985; Patterson and Smith, 1992; Shores, 1992). Stress radiography under fluoroscopy to evaluate instability should only be undertaken with extreme caution (Wheeler and Sharp, 1994).

Treatment: Owners of animals under treatment for spinal fractures need to commit themselves to a 4–6 week recovery period to allow an opportunity for return to function. Animals without deep pain sensation have a poor prognosis for any return to function. Although conservative and medical therapy coupled with contin-

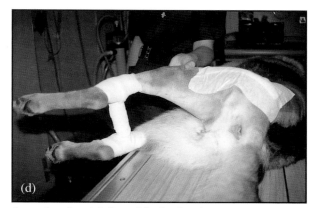

Figure 13.18: *Spinal fracture. Plain lateral spinal radiographs demonstrate an oblique fracture of L7 with considerable displacement. Despite the damage to the ventral spinal component and the accessory processes, this animal had intact neurological function and was treated conservatively. This area is difficult to splint so internal fixation would have been used if necessary.*

ual reassessment, or exploratory surgery to identify a malacic cord, are possible in these patients, euthanasia should be considered.

The treatment of spinal fractures has three components, medical therapy, stabilization and decompression (Figure 13.19). Selection of appropriate therapy is initially based on the clinical presentation. Indications for conservative treatment are:

- Animals that can walk or are paraparetic
- Animals that exhibit strong voluntary movement and have peripheral pain perception.

Major indications for surgery:

- Non-ambulatory animals
- Palpably unstable or significantly displaced injuries
- Animals that deteriorate with conservative treatment
- Animals with peripheral pain perception but no voluntary movement
- Where decompression is required for displaced spinal segments, bone fragments or extruded disc material
- Non-ambulatory animals with no deep pain.

Medical management includes appropriate analgesia once neurological evaluation is complete. Patients presented within 8 hours of acute cord trauma will benefit from methylprednisolone sodium succinate (MPSS) treatment. An intravenous bolus of MPSS should be given slowly over several minutes at 30 mg/kg. Therapy is continued with either an intravenous infusion of MPSS at 2.5–5.0 mg/kg/h for 23 hours or slow intravenous injection of MPSS at 15 mg/kg every 4–6 hours over the next 24 hours. Treatment with non-steroidal drugs during this time is contraindicated.

Stabilization can be carried out conservatively (Figure 13.20) or surgically depending on the clinical signs, radiographic indications of stability and anatomical position (see Figure 13.19). If surgery is indicated, a myelogram should be used to determine if there is a significant lesion which requires decompression. Hemilaminectomy should be used for decompression as it has minimal effect on spinal stability. Decompression should always be accompanied by appropriate internal fixation.

Compartment syndrome

Acute compartment syndrome following trauma has been reported in the dog (De Haan and Beal, 1993). Bleeding or tissue swelling into a fascial compartment can cause the rapid rise in pressure in that compartment which is responsible for the problem. The condition is common in humans, especially associated with tibial fractures. Due to the non-specific nature of the signs and the difficulty of making a definitive diagnosis, the condition may be underdiagnosed in the dog.

Pathogenesis

Physiological compartments are enclosed by skin, epimysium, fascia or bone. The term osseofascial is used to describe a compartment where bone and fascia are the barriers to swelling (Basinger *et al.*, 1987). An extraneous material, such as a dressing, or casts can also define a compartment. In dogs, osseofascial compartments have been reported in:

- Craniolateral crus
- Caudal crus
- Caudal antebrachium
- Femoral compartment (complex multifascial envelope).

If the pressure in one of these compartments rises, the veins will collapse and the local venous pressure will rise. This reduces the arteriovenous gradient, blood flow and tissue perfusion, leading to ischaemia and necrosis. Peripheral nerves and muscles have limited resistance to hypoxia and are damaged first by the rise in pressure, leading to impaired neuromuscular function (Rorabeck and McGee, 1990). As there is an inverse linear relationship between pressure and the time taken for the tissue damage to become irreversible, early treatment is essential. Reperfusion injury, for example after cast removal, may also play a part in the pathophysiology of the condition.

Pressure can increase for several reasons:

- Bleeding into the compartment after trauma
- Increased capillary permeability and swelling post-ischaemia (reperfusion injury may occur here too)
- External pressure constricting a compartment.

Normal pressures in muscle average 4 mm Hg, with a range of 0–8 mm Hg. Measurements of muscle pressure in dogs with compartment syndrome reported in the literature were 26–30 mm Hg (De Haan and Beale, 1993).

Diagnosis and treatment

Compartment syndrome should be considered in trauma patients with swollen and tense limbs, where there is little compliance to surface finger pressure and which are especially uncomfortable and resistant to analgesia. Arterial pulses are still palpable, as the pressure does not generally rise enough to stop arterial blood flow. There is decreased sensation due to nerve compression. It can be difficult to differentiate compartment syndrome from arterial occlusion and neuropraxia.

The only reliable method of diagnosis is to measure tissue pressures. Slit catheters, wick catheters, needle manometers and continuous infusion systems have been used to measure pressure. However, the simplest practical system is to use a standard CVP manometer linked to an ordinary needle and zeroed at the tip of the needle when placed in the compartment.

Treatment	Indications	Advantages	Disadvantages
Cage rest. Confine in very small space until radiographic evidence of healing	Ambulatory or paraparetic animals with stable thoracolumbar injuries	Economical. No exposure to lengthy surgery and anaesthesia	Difficult to restrict some animals. Animals may suffer prolonged discomfort, and neurological deficits may worsen or even become irreversible
Back splinting (Patterson and Smith, 1992)	Caudal cervical, thoracic and lumbar injuries	Economical. Provides better stability than cage rest. Can combine with internal fixation	Intensive nursing required especially for large dogs. Not ideal if ventral component involved
Vertebral body pinning	Lumbar fractures	Economical. Implants often readily available	Weakest form of internal fixation
Dorsal spinous process plating. Apply a metal or plastic plate to dorsal spinous processes either side of lesion	Thoracic and lumbar fractures	Effective combined with vertebral body plating in resisting bending forces	Difficult to apply to small dorsal spinous processes. Processes may fracture
Modified segmental fixation. Secure a pin or pins to two dorsal spinous processes cranial and caudal to the lesion	Thoracic and lumbar injuries in small dogs and cats	Economical. Equipment usually readily available	Articular processes may fracture. Immobilizes a long segment of spine. Ideally require intact ventral component
Vertebral body plating. Plate applied to dorsolateral vertebral bodies above transverse processes	Thoracic and cranial lumbar vertebrae (application caudal to L3 requires sacrificing nerves to the lumbosacral plexus)	Effective versus bending forces, enhanced when combined with dorsal spinous plating. Can combine with hemilaminectomy	Difficult to apply plate in thoracic region as need to disarticulate ribs. Little resistance to rotational forces
Pins or screws and polymethylmethacrylate	Any location	Very versatile technique. Provides rotational stability	Occasionally see wound infection and pin migration
Trans-illial pinning. Pin through wings of illium dorsocaudal to the bone of the dorsal spinous process of L7	Lumbosacral injuries	Can combine with dorsal spinous body plating or stapling	Pins may migrate and may provide inadequate stability if used in isolation

Figure 13.19: Treatment options for spinal fractures and luxations.

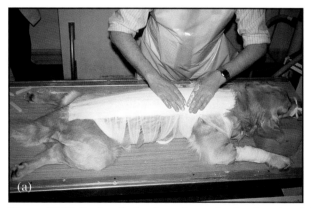 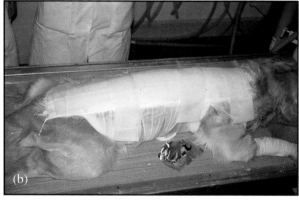

Figure 13.20: Back splinting for a thoracolumbar luxation. (a) Layers of plaster of Paris are built up to provide good conformation to the animal's back. (b) The cast is strengthened with layers of fibreglass resin cast and 'side tabs' are left in position to aid the attachment of the bandage loops which will hold the cast in place.

Compartment syndrome should be treated as an emergency. Rapid relief of the pressure is necessary to prevent irreversible damage occurring from the hypoxia and ischaemia. For cases of confirmed or suspected compartment syndrome, the treatment is to remove the barrier to swelling by cutting the skin, fascia and epimysial layer. In humans, after fasciotomy the incision is left open for delayed closure or split skin grafting 7–8 days later, but postoperative management in animals is facilitated by closure of the skin (De Haan and Beale, 1993). Fractures concurrent to compartment syndrome should be rigidly fixated to promote soft tissue healing, but this can be delayed if necessary. Removal of dressings or bivalving casts can reduce compartment pressures by 50–85% and should be considered if there is a potential for compartment syndrome to occur.

REFERENCES AND FURTHER READING

Basinger RR *et al.* (1987) Osteofascial compartment syndrome in the dog. *Veterinary Surgery* **16**, 427–434

Bellah JR and Krahwinkel DJ (1985) Xylenol orange as a vital stain to determine the viability of skin flaps in dogs. *Veterinary Surgery* **14**, 124–126

Caudle RJ and Stern PJ (1987) Severe open fractures of the tibia. *Journal of Bone and Joint Surgery* **69-A**, 801–807

DeHaan JJ and Beal BS (1993) Compartment syndrome in the dog: case report and literature review. *Journal of the American Animal Hospital Association* **29**, 134–140

Edlich RF *et al.* (1982) Technical factors in the prevention of wound infections. In: *Surgical Infectious Diseases*, eds. RL Simmons and KJ Howard, pp. 449–472. Appleton-Century-Crofts, New York

Edlich RF *et al.* (1987) Scientific basis of skin staple closure. In: *Advances in Plastic and Reconstructive Surgery*, ed. MB Habel, p. 306. Year Book Medical Publishers, Chicago

Feliciano DV (1992) Trauma to the peripheral vascular system. In: *Principles and Practice of Emergency Medicine*, eds. CR Schwartz, CG Cayten and MA Magelson, p. 1098. Lea and Febiger, Philadelphia

Gfeller RW and Crowe DT (1994) The emergency care of traumatic wounds: current recommendations. *Veterinary Clinics of North America* **24**, 1249–1274

Griffon DJ *et al.* (1994) Thoracic injuries in cats with traumatic fractures. *Veterinary Comparative Orthopaedics and Traumatology* **7**, 98–100

Hirsch DC and Smith TM (1978) Osteomyelitis in the dog. Microorganisms isolated and susceptibility to anitimicrobial agents. *Journal of Small Animal Practice* **19**, 679–687

Houlton JEF and Dyce J (1992) Does fracture pattern influence thoracic trauma? *Veterinary Comparative Orthopaedics and Traumatology* **5**, 90–92

Johnson DE (1974) Wound healing. *Archives of the Journal of the American College of Veterinary Surgeons* **3**, 30

Merrit K (1987) Factors increasing the risk of infection in patients with open fractures. *Journal of Trauma* **28**, 823

Patterson RH and Smith G (1992) Backsplinting for treatment of thoracic and lumbar fracture luxation in the dog: principles of application and case series. *Veterinary Comparative Orthopaedics and Traumatology* **5**, 179–187

Pavletic MM (1993) *Atlas of Small Animal Reconstructive Surgery.* JB Lippincott, Philadelphia

Rochat MC *et al.* (1993) Evaluation of skin viability in dogs using transcutaneous CO_2 and sensor current modification. *American Journal of Veterinary Research* **54**, 476

Rorabeck CH and McGee HMJ (1990) Acute compartment syndromes. *Veterinary Comparative Orthopaedics and Traumatology* **3**, 117–122

Selcer RR *et al.* (1991) Management of vertebral column fractures in dogs and cats: 211 cases (1977–1985). *Journal of the American Veterinary Medical Association* **198**, 1965–1968

Shores A (1992) Fractures and luxations of the vertebral column. *Veterinary Clinics of North America* **22**, 171–175

Smith GK and Walter MC (1985) Fractures and luxations of the spine. In: *Textbook of Small Animal Orthopaedics*, eds. CD Newton and DM Nunamaker, pp. 307–332. JB Lippincott, Philadelphia

Spackman EJA *et al.* (1984) Thoracic wall and pulmonary trauma in dogs sustaining fractures as a result of motor vehicle accidents. *Journal of the American Veterinary Medical Association* **185**, 975–977

Swaim SF (1980) Surgery of traumatized skin: management and reconstruction in the dog and cat. WB Saunders, Philadelphia

Swaim SF and Henderson RA (1997) *Small Animal Wound Management.* Williams and Wilkins, Philadelphia

Tamas PM *et al.* (1985) Thoracic trauma in dogs and cats presented for limb fractures. *Journal of the American Animal Hospital Association* **21**, 161–166

Tandberg D (1982) Glass in the hand and foot — will X-ray film show it? *Journal of the American Animal Hospital Association* **248**, 1872

Wheeler SJ and Sharp NJH (1994) *Small Animal Spinal Disorders.* Mosby-Wolfe, London

Whitney WO *et al.* (1987) High-rise syndrome in cats. *Journal of the American Animal Hospital Association* **191**, 1399

Wolf AW *et al.* (1978) Autosterilisation in low velocity bullets. *Journal of Trauma* **18**, 63

CHAPTER FOURTEEN

Dermatological Emergencies

Petra Roosje

INTRODUCTION

Dermatological conditions in small animals often have a chronic character and do not require emergency care. Some problems, although not requiring emergency care, may be alarming to the owner, for example hot spots. Other conditions which may not appear severe initially can prove to be fatal to the animal, e.g. toxic epidermal necrolysis (TEN).

This chapter describes a selection of acute dermatological conditions, emphasizing those which may have serious consequences for the animal's health.

JUVENILE CELLULITIS

Juvenile cellulitis (puppy strangles or juvenile pyoderma) is an uncommon disease that affects puppies between the ages of 3 weeks and 4 months. Rarely, the condition has also been described in adult dogs (Jeffers *et al.*, 1995). It can occur in numerous breeds, although Gordon Setters, Golden Retrievers and Dachshunds appear to be predisposed (Mason and Jones, 1989; Scott *et al.*, 1995).

The cause of the disease is unknown. Secondary infection with *Staphylococcus* spp. may occur.

Clinical signs

Initially, affected puppies may have a painful and swollen face. The eyelids, muzzle and lips are especially affected (Figure 14.1). Papules and pustules develop within a few days. The pinnae are also often involved, and sometimes the preputial and perianal area. Other findings often include enlarged mandibular and prescapular lymph nodes, which may become abscessed, rupture and drain in some cases. It is reported that around 50% of the puppies are lethargic, anorexic and pyrexic. A small number of affected animals show joint pain. Occasional puppies may have a concurrent sterile pyogranulomatous panniculitis.

Diagnosis

Differential diagnoses should include staphylococcal pyoderma, demodicosis, drug eruption and dermatophytosis. Multiple deep skin scrapings should be taken

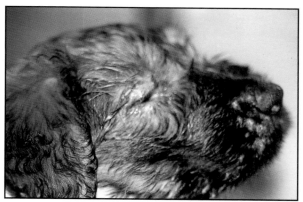

Figure 14.1: *Briard puppy with swollen eyelids, nose and pinnae due to juvenile cellulitis.*

to exclude demodicosis. A thorough history will provide information about previous drug administration. Aspirates of intact lymph nodes and pustules should be taken for cytology and bacterial culture. Cytology of intact pustules will reveal pyogranulomatous inflammation without microorganisms. Bacterial cultures of intact pustules should be negative. Skin biopsies of early lesions show multiple discrete or confluent granulomas and pyogranulomas consisting of macrophages and neutrophils. The presence of dermatophytosis (usually of dissimilar clinical appearance), should be excluded prior to treatment of juvenile cellulitis with glucocorticosteroids (see below).

Clinical management

Oral prednisone or prednisolone 1 mg/kg/day should be given until the clinical signs improve, which usually occurs within 1–2 weeks. Administration should then be tapered off and stopped. Some animals may show an improved clinical response to the administration of oral dexamethasone (0.1–0.2 mg/kg/day) (Scott *et al.*, 1995).

Concomitant administration of antibiotics is often indicated in the presence of secondary bacterial infection. Affected puppies often do not recover on antibiotics alone (White *et al.*, 1989). Cephalexin (40–60 mg/kg/day divided into two or three doses) or amoxicillin clavulanate (25 mg/kg/day divided in two doses) are the drugs of choice. Antiseptic washes or shampoos containing chlorhexidine 2–4% have been recommended, but may often cause struggling and stress in the puppies. In some cases where anorexia or fever are present, more intensive therapy is required, including the use of intravenous fluid and electrolyte administration. Rarely, euthanasia may be indicated in severe cases (Mason and Jones, 1989).

The prognosis is generally good, although permanent facial scarring can occur.

PYOTRAUMATIC DERMATITIS

Pyotraumatic dermatitis ('hot spots' or acute moist dermatitis) is a condition frequently seen in dogs and less often in cats. The condition is more commonly reported in breeds with a heavy coat such as St Bernards, Golden Retrievers, Collies and German Shepherd Dogs. Lesions may be induced within a few hours. Most occur as complications of one or more of the factors listed in Figure 14.2.

Flea bite hypersensitivity
Otitis externa
Atopic dermatitis
Foreign bodies in the coat
Food hypersensitivity
Dirty, matted, unkempt coats
Ectoparasite infestations
Painful musculoskeletal disorders
Anal sac problems

Figure 14.2: Causes of pyotraumatic lesions.

These factors can induce the itch–lick or scratch cycle that varies in intensity with individuals.

Clinical signs
These animals are presented with an acute, self-induced, erythematous, moist, exudative, alopecic and painful lesion (Figure 14.3).

Diagnosis
The diagnosis is based on clinical appearance and a history of acute onset. The lesion occurs in an area where the dog can cause self-trauma. The primary cause may not always be apparent. A true pyotraumatic dermatitis should be differentiated from a pyotraumatic folliculitis, as the former is treated with glucocorticosteroids whereas the latter should be treated with antibiotics. These diseases differ in the fact that a true pyotraumatic dermatitis is a superficial process consisting of a flat erosive or ulcerated lesion. The hair is lost from the lesion but a clear margin is present between the lesion and the normal surrounding skin. In a pyotraumatic folliculitis, the lesion is thickened, plaque-like and surrounded by satellite papules and pustules. These lesions, which

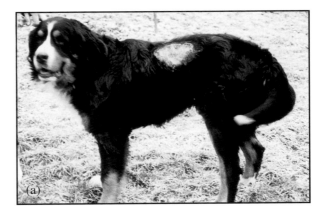

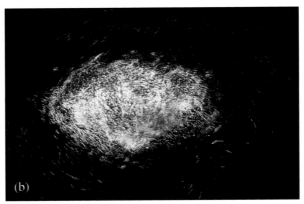

Figure 14.3: (a) A Bernese Sennen with a hot spot. (b) Hot spot with dried exudate and clear margin between affected and normal skin.

are especially common on the head and neck, are true local pyodermas. They are especially observed in young dogs and seem to be more common in St Bernards and Golden Retrievers.

Clinical management
The hair in and around the lesion should be clipped to allow a better examination of the lesion and thorough cleaning of the area. As this can be very painful to the dog, sedation or anaesthesia may be needed. Cleaning with a povidone–iodine or chlorhexidine solution is recommended. After cleaning, a drying agent should be applied two to three times daily. Most of these products are combination products that contain a local anaesthetic, antibiotics or corticosteroids. A 2% aluminium acetate solution or a combination of an aluminium acetate and 1% hydrocortisone solution gives good results. If oral use of corticosteroids is not contraindicated, most cases benefit from a short course of prednisone or prednisolone (1 mg/kg/day). Initially, an Elizabethan collar may be used in addition to prevent further trauma to the lesion. Treatment should be continued until the lesion has dried, usually 7–10 days. Flea bite hypersensitivity is often an underlying cause and therefore stringent flea control measures are advisable.

URTICARIA AND ANGIOEDEMA

Immunologically mediated urticaria, angioedema and anaphylaxis can be thought of as the same disease with a variation in severity and target organ.

Urticaria (hives) are focal superficial anaphylactic reactions visible as erythematous wheals. Possible causes are listed in Figure 14.4. Dogs are more commonly affected than cats. Urticaria often disappear within a day but may persist longer, with the development of new urticaria. A chronic form also exists.

Foods
Drugs
Antisera, bacterins and vaccines
Stinging and biting insects
Blood transfusions
Plants
Intestinal parasites
Infections (staphylococcal pyoderma, canine distemper)*
Sunlight*
Excessive heat or cold*
Oestrus*
Atopy*
Psychogenic factors

Figure 14.4: Factors reported to have caused urticaria in dogs and cats. *Reported in dogs only (Scott et al., 1995).

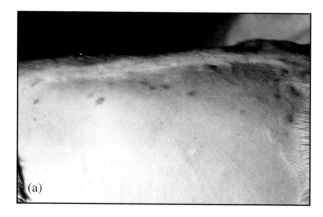

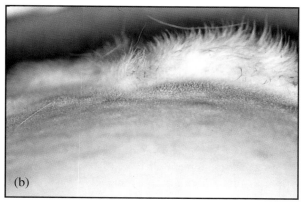

Figure 14.5: (a) Multiple urticaria that developed within 2 hours. (b) Close-up showing erythematous wheals.

In angioedema, deep blood vessels are affected. The resulting oedema causes diffuse swelling. Both diseases result from mast cell or basophil degranulation, which may have an immunological (type I hypersensitivity) or non-immunological origin. The origin of the wheal formation is often hard to find. Wheals can be irritating to the animal and there is a risk that associated swelling of the mucous membranes may obstruct the airway.

Clinical signs

Urticaria can develop within a few hours. Lesions may be single or multiple and may occur all over the body (Figure 14.5). Animals are variably pruritic. Signs of angioedema consist typically of facial swelling and sometimes swelling of the extremities. Angioedema usually does not cause pruritus.

Diagnosis

The differential diagnosis for urticaria includes folliculitis, erythema multiforme, vasculitis and neoplasia. Definitive diagnosis is based on obtaining an extensive history, and a thorough physical examination. Staphylococcal folliculitis can be mistaken for urticaria, especially in short-coated dogs, where hairs can stand out focally. In staphylococcal folliculitis lesions, hairs can be easily epilated and, compared with urticaria, lesions are more exudative. Clipping of the coat can help to identify the lesions. Skin biopsies can be helpful for differentiation when the lesions persist.

Clinical management

Therapy consists of avoidance and elimination of the aetiological factors. In cases of urticaria, the wheals will resolve within a day unless the initiating factor remains present, when new lesions may develop. If the animal is not distressed by the lesions and pruritus is minimal, therapy is not strictly necessary. It is important, however, to inform the owner of the risk of development of angioedema. The prognosis for angioedema varies with the severity and location. Angioedema of the larynx may produce potentially fatal airway obstruction.

When there is life-threatening angioedema, adrenaline (diluted 1:1000, 0.1–0.5 ml s.c. or i.m.) can be administered, while monitoring the heart rate. Corticosteroids can be given simultaneously at 1 mg/kg. In case of angioedema, administration should be by injection. In cases of pruritic urticaria, oral administration of prednisone or prednisolone at 1 mg/kg/day for 1–2 days is often sufficient.

Antihistamines are not always useful with acute urticaria. They may be useful in prevention of chronic urticaria, although it is often more useful to identify the causal factor.

CUTANEOUS DRUG REACTIONS

Drugs can induce various cutaneous adverse reactions with a wide range of clinical manifestations and can therefore mimic many other skin diseases (Figure 14.6). The severity of the lesions covers a range from a local and rather benign reaction to extensive skin lesions that may result in death of the animal. Cutaneous drug reactions can occur as the result of immunological and non-immunological mechanisms. The latter may be due to overdoses, accumulative toxicity, genetic predisposition, interaction of drugs or idiosyncratic metabolism. These reactions can be evoked by any type of drug, including topically applied drugs, shampoos and insecticides. Although drug reactions occur in a very small number of patients, the incidence is probably higher than the literature indicates (Affolter and Von Tscharner, 1993).

Vaccinations, antisera, bacterins
Blood transfusions
Antibiotics (e.g. sulphonamides, penicillins, cephalosporins, gentamycin, neomycin, tetracyclines, chloramphenicol, lincomycin)
Corticosteroids (e.g. triamcinolone)
L-Thyroxine
Aurothioglucose, cyclosporin, azathioprine, cyclophosphamide, chlorambucil, hydroxyurea
5-Fluorocytosine
Retinoids
Primidone
Griseofulvin, ketoconazole, itraconazole
Shampoos (especially insecticidal)
D-Limonene
Diethylcarbamazine, thiarsetamide
Levamisole, ivermectin

Figure 14.6: *Drugs reported as causing drug reactions in dogs and cats. (Scott et al., 1995).*

Clinical signs

Lesions can be urticarial, angioedematous, papular, exfoliative, vesiculobullous, erythrodermatous or ulcerative. Draining nodular lesions, focal or diffuse alopecia, fixed drug reaction and pseudolymphomatous changes can also be seen (Affolter and Von Tscharner, 1993). Diseases that can be caused by drug reactions include vasculopathies, panniculitis, drug-induced pemphigus foliaceous, bullous pemphigoid, superficial suppurative necrolytic dermatitis of Miniature Schnauzers, erythema multiforme (EM) and toxic epidermal necrolysis (TEN). Signs of systemic illness can accompany the cutaneous signs.

Diagnosis

In addition to an extensive history and complete physical examination, other skin disease should be excluded by means of multiple skin scrapings, bacterial culture, fungal culture and cytology. Skin biopsies may help to define a specific cause for the animal's lesions, may reduce the list of differential diagnoses and can strongly support the diagnosis of a drug reaction. It is important to take *multiple* skin biopsies from different lesion sites because disease-specific histopathological changes are sometimes apparent in a few lesions only. Although a histological pattern is not always pathognomonic for a drug reaction, the knowledge that a drug reaction can be the cause of the cutaneous lesions should lead to a careful review of the patient's history.

The following list may help in making a tentative diagnosis of a drug reaction:

- Think about a drug reaction when a skin condition worsens suddenly and unexpectedly after initiating drug therapy, or when there is a sudden deterioration after an initial improvement
- Think about a drug reaction when skin lesions occur when the animal receives treatment for a non-dermatological condition
- When observed manifestations do not resemble known pharmacological actions of the drugs
- Prior exposure to the drug may have been tolerated without adverse effects
- There is a history of exposure to the drug or related drugs
- Biopsy results indicate histological features that can be consistent with a drug eruption
- A physical examination demonstrating clinical signs consistent with a drug eruption
- Resolution of the signs occurs following withdrawal of the drug. This may take 1–2 weeks and is dependent on the severity of the initial skin lesions or possibly induced secondary infections
- A negative challenge with other concurrently used drugs and the appropriate ruling out of other causes
- The ultimate test of a causative association is to challenge with the suspect drug. This is however not without serious risk and is therefore generally not recommended.

Clinical management

The most important part of the therapy is to stop the causative drug and prevent further administration. When animals are receiving several drugs (including topical medication or shampoos) they should all be stopped at the same time. If this is not possible, the drugs that were added to the regimen last should be stopped first. Most drug reactions improve spontaneously within 7–14 days upon drug withdrawal. Complete healing may take longer and depends on the severity of the skin lesions. Reactions due to repositol or body-stored agents (i.e. gold salts) respond to withdrawal more slowly and can continue for long periods.

Supportive therapy is not necessary unless animals have a more severe form of drug reaction like EM major or TEN. If lesions have healed but animals are pruritic because of remaining crusts, a mild shampoo can be used. The choice of shampoo should be based on history of previous use. If the suspected causative agent was a sulpha-containing drug it may be safer to avoid use of a salicylic acid containing shampoo (Noli *et al.*, 1995).

To prevent future drug reactions it is important to inform the owner about the causative agent (if known). Patients allergic to penicillins should not be treated with any other drug of the penicillin group. Because cephalosporins have a β-lactam ring in common with penicillins, they should be used with care.

ERYTHEMA MULTIFORME

This disease is an uncommon, acute, sometimes self-limiting eruption of the skin and mucous membranes. In humans, a distinction is made between the mild form (EM minor) and a more life-threatening form (EM major). This distinction is less clear in animals, although the severity of the disease is also variable. EM in dogs has been associated with infection and drug administration, but may also be of idiopathic origin. In cats, EM is associated with drug administration and herpes infections.

Clinical signs
Lesions are variable but are initially characterized by an acute onset of symmetrical erythematous macules or papules that spread peripherally and clear centrally, producing annular (target) or arciform patterns (Figure 14.7). Urticarial plaques, vesicles and bullae or a combination of lesions may appear, especially later in the course of the disease.

Sometimes the animals become systemically ill (fever, anorexia and depression) with involvement of mucous membranes and mucocutaneous junctions. Ulceration of the face, pinnae and groin may be present (Figure 14.8).

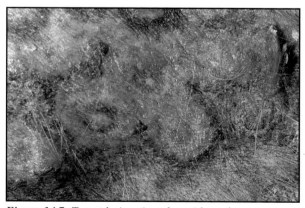

Figure 14.7: *Target lesions in a dog with erythema multiforme. The causative drug was not identified because the dog had received multiple drug therapy.*

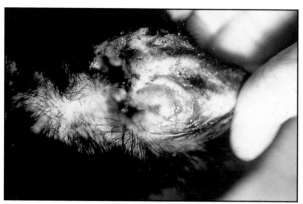

Figure 14.8: *Erosive lesion on the pinna in a cat with erythema multiforme.*

Diagnosis
The diagnosis of EM is based upon history, clinical features, exclusion of other diseases and histopathology of multiple skin biopsies. The differential diagnosis includes bacterial folliculitis, dermatophytosis, demodicosis, urticaria, toxic epidermal necrolysis and autoimmune diseases.

Some patients with EM show a positive Nikolsky's sign. This is elicited by applying pressure on a vesicle or to the edge of an ulcer, erosion or normal skin with a blunt object like a pencil. It is positive when the outer layer of the skin is easily rubbed off or pushed away. This indicates poor cell cohesion as found in EM, TEN and the pemphigus complex.

Clinical management
The disease may run a mild course with spontaneous regression of lesions within a few weeks. If possible, an underlying cause should be identified and addressed. If extensive vesiculobullous lesions or ulceration is present the prognosis is guarded. These animals may need more intensive therapy, as discussed with TEN.

TOXIC EPIDERMAL NECROLYSIS

This is a rare disease reported in humans, dogs and cats. Clinically, TEN and the severe form of EM (EM major) can be hard to differentiate in dogs and cats. In humans, TEN is currently more often associated with drug administration, whereas EM major is often associated with herpesvirus infections (Roujeau and Revue, 1994). This distinction is as yet not clear in dogs and cats; TEN has been associated with drug administration, neoplasia, toxins, infections and systemic disorders and may have an idiopathological origin.

Clinical signs
Animals show an acute onset of fever, anorexia and depression and extensive vesiculobullous lesions over the body as well as mucous membranes (including the

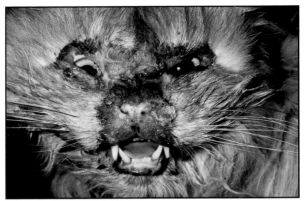

Figure 14.9: Ulcerative lesions of toxic epidermal necrolysis due to a trimethoprim-sulphadiazine reaction.

conjunctiva), mucocutaneous junctions and footpads. Ulcerations and epidermal collarettes may appear (Figure 14.9). These patients often have cutaneous pain and a positive Nikolsky's sign.

Diagnosis

The differential diagnoses include burns, autoimmune diseases, EM major and epitheliotropic lymphoma. Diagnosis is based on obtaining a thorough history, the results of physical examination and examination of multiple skin biopsies. A haemogram can reveal neutrophilia or neutropenia.

Histopathology will show hydropic degeneration of basal epidermal cells, full-thickness coagulation of the epidermis and usually minimal dermal inflammation (silent dermis). Dermoepidermal separation results in subepidermal vesicles.

Clinical management

The treatment of TEN includes elimination of the underlying cause and symptomatic and supportive measures. It is helpful to collect blood and urine samples to establish initial values. These animals may lose a considerable part of the epidermis and are comparable to second-degree burn patients, as fluid, electrolytes and proteins are lost and secondary bacterial infections occur. It is therefore imperative to handle these patients with the utmost care and keep their surroundings as clean as possible. In one author's experience the success of management of patients with TEN increased when they were not bathed or clipped (Reedy *et al.*, 1997). In addition to the skin, other organ systems may become involved during the course of the disease. Oedema may develop and many animals succumb to the development of secondary factors such as shock, sepsis or disseminated intravascular coagulation (DIC).

As well as supportive intravenous fluid administration, antibiotics are indicated to prevent secondary bacterial infection, the choice being based upon earlier drug administration. The benefits of corticosteroid administration in these cases is controversial.

The prognosis is generally guarded or poor. In humans, the extent of the skin lesions gives an indication of the prognosis. Whether this holds true for animals is not clear. Removal of the inciting agent at an early stage may be helpful.

PRIMARY IRRITANT CONTACT DERMATITIS

Irritant material coming into contact with animal skin can cause irritant dermatitis (Figure 14.10). The mechanism by which the epidermal cells are affected varies with the substance. Irritant dermatitis is therefore a heterogeneous disease with variable clinical manifestations.

Soaps
Insecticides
Topical fungicides
Shampoos
Disinfectants
Flea collars
Tar
Caustic substances

Figure 14.10: Substances that may cause irritant contact dermatitis.

A thorough history may give an insight as to what substances were used on the animal or whether there are possible agents in the environment that could cause irritant dermatitis. The location of the lesion should fit with possible contact with the agent.

Clinical signs

Environmental irritants typically produce lesions where the hair coat is thin or missing and where the body parts have contact with the irritant. Susceptible areas are the abdomen, chest, interdigital spaces, legs, axillae, scrotum and flank (Figure 14.11). Oral lesions can occur when the animal has been trying to lick the irritating

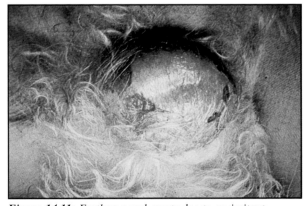

Figure 14.11: Erythema and crusts due to an irritant contact dermatitis.

lesion. When the offending agent is a liquid or a collar, the skin lesions occur where the substance touches the skin. Erythema or papules are primary lesions. In more chronic cases erosions, crusts, lichenification or ulcerations may occur. Pruritus may occur and can influence the primary lesions.

Diagnosis

A careful history and physical examination may lead to a tentative diagnosis. When the irritants are less aggressive, obtaining a definitive diagnosis is more difficult. The differential diagnoses should include atopic dermatitis, food hypersensitivity, allergic contact dermatitis, malassezia dermatitis, drug hypersensitivity and ectoparasite infestations.

Clinical management

Eliminate and avoid further contact with the causative agent. Washing of the animal may help to dilute or remove the agent. If the dog or cat tries to lick or bite at the lesion, an Elizabethan collar or bandaging of the affected area may help. With removal of the agent the lesions should heal spontaneously. When animals are very pruritic, oral prednisone or prednisolone 1 mg/kg/day for 1 week may be indicated.

CANINE UVEODERMATOLOGICAL SYNDROME OR VOGT—KOYANAGI—HARADA-LIKE SYNDROME

This syndrome occurs in many breeds but is most often seen in Arctic breeds such as Huskies, Samoyeds, Malamutes or Akita Inus. In humans, the Vogt–Koyanagi–Harada syndrome consists of three phases: (1) a meningoencephalitic phase with fever, malaise, headache, nausea and vomiting, (2) an ophthalmic–auditory phase with photophobia, uveitis, decreased eyesight and dysacousia and (3) a dermatological phase with alopecia, vitiligo and poliosis (greying). The uveodermatological syndrome in dogs rarely presents with meningoencephalitis or dysacousia. In dogs, poliosis often progresses to leucotrichia (white hairs). Although the pathogenesis is unknown, it is considered an immune-mediated disease in which the melanocytes and melanin are attacked.

Clinical signs

In dogs, the syndrome is often characterized by the acute onset of uveitis and/or depigmentation of the iris. Dermatological signs may occur concurrent or subsequent to the ophthalmological problems and include depigmentation of the nasal planum, eye rims, or mouth and erosive, crusting lesions around the eyes, muzzle and ears (Figure 14.12).

Diagnosis

After a thorough history and physical examination,

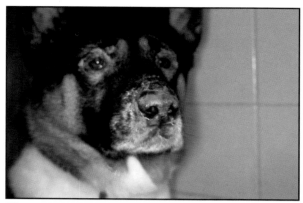

Figure 14.12: *Depigmentation of the nasal planum, perinasal and periocular erosions and erythema.*

multiple skin biopsies should be taken. Differential diagnosis should include pemphigus foliaceous, discoid lupus erythematosus, leishmaniasis, vitiligo and thallium toxicosis.

Histopathology will reveal an interface dermatitis with melanin drop-off and macrophages loaded with melanin.

Clinical management

Dogs with this disease can be considered dermatological emergency patients. Treatment of ocular pathology is required to prevent the development of a panuveitis and possible blindness. Ophthalmic examinations should be periodically performed even when the cutaneous changes are in remission. The skin lesions are treated with a combination of azathioprine 1–2 mg/kg/day and prednisone or prednisolone 1–2 mg/kg/day. Initial haematology is indicated to facilitate monitoring for azathioprine-induced bone marrow depression. Generally, azathioprine should be given at the above dosage for at least a month or until lesions have resolved, whereas prednisolone may be tapered off to an alternate day regimen after 1–2 weeks, depending on effect. Monthly rechecks and repeat haematology should be scheduled. Unfortunately, many of these animals require lifelong treatment and it is therefore important to try to taper off the medication to the lowest effective dose. Where animals respond to lower doses of treatment, the prognosis for the dermatological changes is usually good, repigmentation often occurring, although leucotrichia may remain (Figure 14.13).

BURNS

Burns may result from radiation therapy, microwave radiation and thermal or chemical insult to the skin. Thermal burns may result from the use of fires, heating pads/lamps, hair dryers, improperly grounded electro-surgical units, from fire, boiling water or oil (Figures 14.14 and 14.15). Chemical burns may result from con-

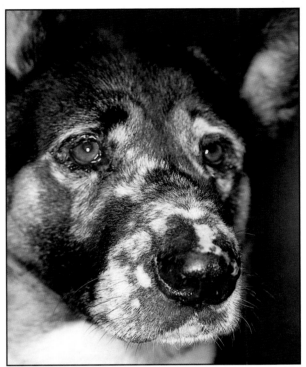

Figure 14.13: Repigmentation of the nasal planum and leucotrichia after 4 months of therapy with azathioprine and prednisolone.

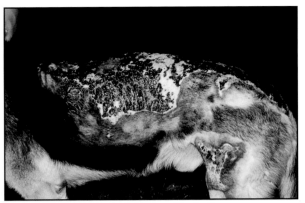

Figure 14.14: Burn wounds caused by boiling water.

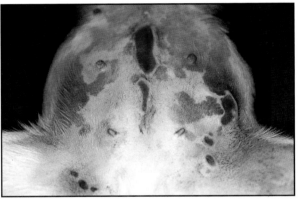

Figure 14.15: Burn wounds caused by heating lamps.

tact with caustic or acid materials. Burns are classified according to their depth.

Superficial partial-thickness burns affect only the epidermis, which becomes thickened and erythematous and ultimately desquamates. The burn usually heals by re-epithelialization in 3–6 days, and hair regrowth is likely.

Deep-partial thickness burns involve the epidermis and part of the dermis. In these cases a marked subcutaneous oedema and inflammatory response occur. These burns heal by re-epithelialization from the remnants of hair follicles and sebaceous glands and from the wound edge. Healing rate and quantity of hair regrowth depend on the depth of the burn.

In full-thickness burns, destruction of all cutaneous structures occurs and a dark brown insensitive leathery covering (eschar) is formed. After removal or sloughing of the eschar these wounds heal slowly by contraction and re-epithelialization. Hair regrowth will not occur and full-thickness burns often need surgical intervention.

Burn wounds may not only cause local tissue damage but can also cause severe systemic pathology, possibly involving the respiratory tract. Burn shock patients require intensive aggressive therapy including management of fluid and electrolyte balance, body temperature and, due to massive increases in metabolic demand, a nutritious, high-calorie, high-protein diet if liver and kidney function are adequate. Monitoring of vital signs, mental status, body weight and urine output should occur throughout treatment. Initial val-

ues of haematocrit, serum protein, haemoglobin, sodium, potassium, chloride, blood urea nitrogen, creatinine, blood glucose, albumin and blood gases (where available) should be obtained.

Clinical signs

Burns caused by microwave radiation, electric currents, chemicals, heating pads, or cage dryers may take a few days before they are visible to the owner, as they are hidden by the hairs. These lesions often feel hard and dry in the beginning. Later they may become erosive or necrotic.

Burns caused by hot metals or fire are obvious but it may take another 24–48 hours before the full extent of the lesion is visible. Chemical burns are erosive and necrotic in nature and it can take 24–48 hours before they are maximally expressed.

Diagnosis

Diagnosis is clear when the burn incident was observed, but may be less so if it was not seen, especially when the burn is superficial. A complete history and physical examination, including eyes, ears, oral cavity, respiratory tract, urogenital tract, anus and foot pads should be performed. The presence of circulatory shock and/or respiratory thermal injury should be assessed. Biopsies of different points of the lesion and especially the margins, can be helpful to discern between chemical or thermal burns and electric burns.

Clinical management of thermal wounds

The depth and the extent of burn (percentage of total body surface area, TBSA) should be assessed. A decision should be made if (a) the thermal injury is only minor requiring only local therapy; (b) local wound care and systemic therapy are indicated; or (c) the animal is burnt to such an extent that euthanasia is indicated. Euthanasia should be considered when full-thickness burns cover more than 30–50% of the TSBA or when there are severe burns of the face or genitalia with a chance of permanent deformation (Swaim and Henderson, 1997).

Evaluation of the depth of a burn may be difficult in the early stages following a burn. If hair is still present and epilates easily, it generally indicates a deep burn. Analgesia should be provided, and the patient may be sedated to facilitate treatment. Care should be taken if there is a compromise of ventilatory or cardiovascular function. Hair should be clipped from the burned surface. If the burn has just occurred, application of saline or water (3–17°C) for at least 30 minutes may relieve pain and arrest the progression of the burn. When large burns are present, care should be taken to avoid hypothermia.

Generally the following procedures can be applied:

- After the above mentioned procedures, an aloe vera cream can be applied, as it has an antithromboxane effect which helps to maintain local blood circulation (Swaim and Henderson, 1997)
- To help soften and separate viable from non-viable tissue in superficial and deep partial-thickness burns, the wound can be gently spray lavaged with warm water or a bandage wet with antimicrobial agent and kept as a wet-to-wet bandage. Necrotic tissue can be debrided from the wound after the lavage or in between the wet-to-wet bandages, which should be kept in place for several hours at a time. Between lavages, bandages with a water soluble medication should be applied. A silver sulphadiazine medication is used most commonly. Other topical antimicrobial agents that can be considered for smaller burns are gentamicin sulphate ointment or a nitrofurazone ointment

- Superficial partial thickness burns can be allowed to heal as an open wound
- In deep partial-thickness burns, the resulting wound can be allowed to heal by contraction and re-epithelialization under bandages and medication. Alternatively, a combination of reconstructive techniques and healing as an open wound may be used
- In full-thickness burns with areas of demarcated devitalized tissue, the tissue can be debrided by wound excision and eschar removal. An eschar may protect the underlying tissue from electrolyte, fluid and protein loss, but it can also harbour bacteria and influence wound contraction. Total removal of the eschar is indicated when the animal is stable enough for anaesthesia
- When all the devitalized tissue has been removed from a full-thickness burn, it should be decided if the wound can be closed by relocation of local tissue using a skin flap.

REFERENCES AND FURTHER READING

Affolter VK and Von Tscharner C (1993) Cutaneous drug reactions: a retrospective study of the histopathological changes and their correlation with clinical disease. *Veterinary Dermatology* **4**, 79—86

Jeffers JG, Duclos DD and Goldschmidt MH (1995) A dermatosis resembling juvenile cellulitis in an adult dog. *Journal of the American Animal Hospital Association* **31**, 204—208

Mason IS and Jones J (1989) Juvenile cellulitis in Gordon Setters. *Veterinary Record* **124**, 642

Noli C, Koeman JP and Willemse T (1995) A retrospective evaluation of adverse reactions to trimethoprim-sulfonamide combinations in dogs and cats. *Veterinary Quarterly* **17**, 123—128

Reedy LM, Miller WH and Willemse T (1997) *Allergic Skin Diseases of Dogs and Cats*, 2nd edn, pp. 239—245. WB Saunders, Philadelphia

Roujeau JC and Revue J (1994) Toxic epidermal necrolysis: an expanding field of knowledge. *Journal of the American Academy of Dermatology* **31**, 301—302

Scott DW, Miller WH, and Griffin CE (1995) *Small Animal Dermatology*, 5th edn. WB Saunders, Philadelphia

Swaim, ST and Henderson RA (1997) *Small Animal Wound Management*, 2nd edn, pp. 87—101. Williams & Wilkins, Baltimore

White SD, Rosychuk RAW, Stewart LJ, Cape L and Hughes BJ (1989) Juvenile cellulitis in dogs: 15 cases (1979—1988). *Journal of the American Veterinary Medical Association* **195**, 1609—1611

CHAPTER FIFTEEN

Toxicological Emergencies

Robert H. Poppenga

RECOGNITION OF THE INTOXICATED PATIENT

Given the wide range of effects caused by the ingestion of poisons, recognition of an intoxicated patient can be difficult, particularly in the absence of a history of exposure. Alternatively, animal owners are often convinced that the illness of a pet is due to malicious poisoning or exposure to an industrial or environmental poison. The clinician should not be misled by allegations of intoxication, but rather the objective historical and clinical findings should guide the case work-up.

Historical clues to possible poison exposure include recent changes in routine, such as dietary change or access to a new environment, acute illness after a period of being unsupervised, acute onset of neurological or gastrointestinal signs, and liver and/or kidney failure. Correlation of the onset of illness with recent use of pesticides or household products may be important. Illness from poisons such as lead can be associated with renovations of older buildings. Access to human medications and herbal remedies should be included in initial questioning.

Identification of affected organ systems from the initial physical examination and laboratory work-up of a patient is extremely useful in formulating a list of differentials. The occurrence of several clinical signs characteristic of a particular toxic syndrome can also be helpful. For example, muscarinic receptor overstimulation manifested clinically by DUMBELS (Diarrhoea, Urination, Miosis, Bronchospasm, Emesis, Lacrimation and Salivation) is strongly suggestive of intoxication by a cholinesterase-inhibiting insecticide. Visual examination of vomitus may reveal coloured baits or fragments of medications. Detection of specific odours may provide useful clues, e.g. many organophosphates have a garlic-like odour that might be detected in vomitus or on the skin.

MANAGEMENT OF THE INTOXICATED PATIENT

A general approach to management of the intoxicated patient should adhere to the following principles

(Beasley and Dorman, 1990; Shannon and Haddad, 1998):

- Stabilize vital signs
- Obtain a history and clinically evaluate the patient
- Administer an antidote if indicated and available
- Prevent continued systemic absorption of the poison
- Enhance elimination of absorbed poison
- Provide symptomatic and supportive care
- Closely monitor the patient.

Each situation is unique and one or more of the steps may be unnecessary. For example, there may not be an antidote for a given poison or a way to enhance its elimination once systemically absorbed.

In recently exposed animals, the severity of poison exposure must be determined in order to choose the appropriate sequence of management steps (Figure 15.1). Several factors must be considered, including the inherent toxicity of the chemical, the dose, the species and age of animal and the presence of underlying disease conditions. For example, close monitoring at home for several days may be sufficient for management of recent ingestion of an anticoagulant rodenticide at well below reported toxic doses (less than or equal to one-tenth of an LD_{50}). Ingestion of higher doses may warrant administration of an adsorbent, a cathartic and/or a specific antidote, followed by close monitoring in the clinic. If a known poison has been ingested, but information is not available about its toxicity to the particular animal species exposed, toxicity data may be extrapolated from other species. Ultimately, the advice to 'treat the patient and not the poison' is sound.

Specific approaches to stabilization of vital signs are discussed in other sections of this Manual. Attention should be paid to maintaining a patent airway and providing adequate ventilation, maintaining cardiovascular function with attention to appropriate fluid and electrolyte administration, maintaining acid–base balance, controlling central nervous system signs such as seizures and maintaining body temperature.

Once vital signs are stable, a thorough history should be obtained while the animal is being further evaluated. If blood or urine samples are obtained,

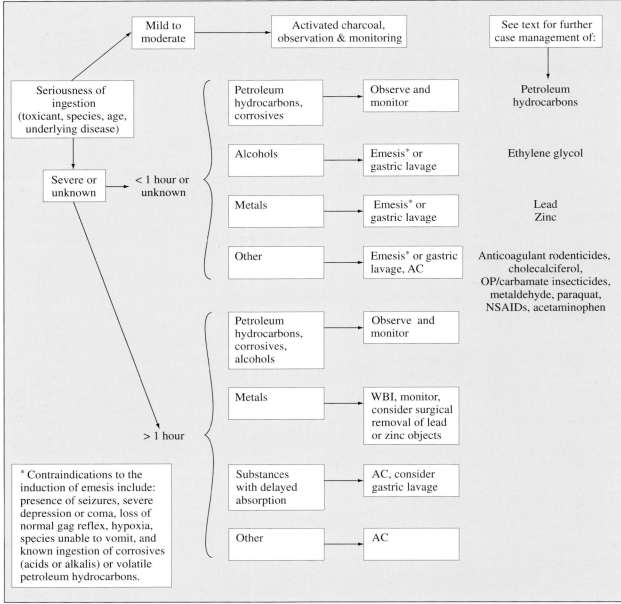

Figure 15.1: *Treatment algorithm for initial management of small animal intoxications. AC = activated charcoal, WBI = whole bowel irrigation.*

specimens should be set aside for possible toxicological testing (Figure 15.2).

Administration of specific antidotes

Antidotes should be administered if indicated and available. In some situations, it may be critical to administer an antidote quickly. For example, in suspected cholinesterase-inhibiting insecticide intoxications, administration of atropine may be critical to control life-threatening signs before proceeding with subsequent management steps.

Figure 15.3 lists antidotes that should be immediately available, based on the frequency with which intoxications occur as reported by animal poison control statistics. Figure 15.4 lists antidotes that may be

needed less frequently. A source such as a human hospital or pharmacy should be identified for obtaining the latter antidotes, prior to their need in an emergency situation.

Gastrointestinal decontamination

Gastrointestinal decontamination (GID) is a critical component of case management, which may prevent the onset of clinical signs or significantly decrease the severity or shorten the course of intoxication. GID consists of (Shannon and Haddad, 1998):

- Gastric evacuation
- Administration of an adsorbent
- Catharsis.

Sample	Amount
Whole blood	5 ml, EDTA/heparin tube, refrigerate
Serum/plasma	5–10 ml, serum clot tube or plastic vial, frozen
Vomitus, stomach contents, lavage fluid	100 g, plastic bag or vial, frozen
Liver	100 g, plastic bag, frozen
Kidney	100 g, plastic bag, frozen
Brain	Right or left half, plastic bag, frozen
Urine	5–20 ml, plastic container, frozen
Feed	1 kg, plastic container, frozen if wet food otherwise refrigerated (dry or semi-moist food)
Water	1 litre, plastic or clean glass container, refrigerated or frozen
Environmental samples (bedding, soil, paint)	Check with laboratory

Figure 15.2: Routine samples and amounts to submit for toxicological investigations.

Indication	Antidote	Dosage
Acetaminophen	*N*-Acetylcysteine	Loading dose of 140–280 mg/kg orally or 140 mg/kg in 5% dextrose/water i.v. followed by maintenance dose of 70 mg/kg orally qid for 2–3 days
Anticoagulant rodenticides	Vitamin K$_1$	1st generation anticoagulants: 1 mg/kg orally in divided doses bid to tid for 4–6 days. For 2nd generation anticoagulants: 2.5–5.0 mg/kg orally for 2–6 weeks in divided doses bid to tid
OP/carbamate insecticides	Atropine sulphate	0.1–0.2 mg/kg (given until muscarinic signs controlled), $^1/_4$ initial dose given i.v. with the remainder given i.m. or s.c. Given as needed
OP/carbamate insecticides	Pralidoxime chloride (2-PAM)	20 mg/kg i.m. or slow i.v. bid to tid
Cholecalciferol	Calcitonin	4–6 IU/kg s.c. bid to qid
Ethylene glycol – cats, dogs	Ethanol (20%)	Dogs: 5.5 ml/kg by slow i.v. infusion every 4 hours for five treatments then every 6 hours for four treatments. Cats: 5 ml/kg by slow i.v. infusion qid for five treatments then tid for four treatments
Ethylene glycol – dogs	4-Methylpyrazole (fomepizole)	Initial dose: 15 mg/kg slow i.v. in a 5% dextrose or 0.9% saline solution. This is followed by 10 mg/kg every 12 hours for four doses and then 5 mg/kg every 12 hours until ethylene glycol levels fall below 20 mg/dl
Lead, arsenic	Succimer	10 mg/kg orally tid for 5 days followed by 10 mg/kg orally bid for 2 weeks
Lead, zinc	CaNa$_2$.EDTA	25 mg/kg s.c. qid as a 1% solution (in 5% dextrose/water) for 5 days. Provide 5-day rest period between courses of treatment

Figure 15.3: Antidotes for the most common intoxications.

Indication	Antidote	Dosage
Arsenic, cyanide	Sodium thiosulphate	30–40 mg/kg of a 20% solution i.v., may be repeated
Copper, lead	D-Penicillamine	Copper: 10–15 mg/kg/day orally Lead: 110 mg/kg/divided qid orally for 1–2 weeks, re-evaluate animal 1 week after cessation of initial course
Cyanide	Sodium nitrite	16 mg/kg of a 1% solution i.v., given only once
Iron	Desferrioxamine mesylate	Not determined; for children the dose is 20 mg/kg i.m. or slow i.v. followed by 10 mg/kg at 4-hour intervals depending on clinical response. Subsequent doses of 10 mg/kg may be given every 4–12 hours
Cholecalciferol	Pamidronate	Not determined although in dogs, 1.3 mg/kg i.v. in 150 ml normal saline 1 and 8 days after ingestion of a toxic dose of cholecalciferol was effective in decreasing hypercalcaemia
Nitrites, chlorates	Methylene blue	Dogs: 8.8 mg/kg of a 1% solution given by slow i.v. drip Cats: not recommended
Opioids	Naloxone	Not determined. In children a dose of 2 mg is given i.v. If there is no response, a 2nd dose of 2 mg is given. This dose is repeated every 2 minutes until there is a clinical response or 10–20 mg has been given (if no response to this dose, opioid overdose can be ruled out)
Venomous spiders, snakes, fish and marine invertebrates	Antivenins	Follow specific antivenin recommendations
Arsenic and mercury	Dimercaprol (BAL)	2.5–5.0 mg/kg of a 10% solution in oil i.m. every 4 hours for 2 days then bid for the next 10 days or until recovery

Figure 15.4: *Less commonly used antidotes.*

Gastric evacuation

Approaches to gastric evacuation include induction of emesis with emetics such as syrup of ipecachuana, 3% hydrogen peroxide, apomorphine or xylazine (Figure 15.5) and gastric lavage. Induction of emesis is contraindicated in the presence of seizures, severe depression or coma, loss of normal gag reflex, hypoxia, species unable to vomit (e.g. rat) and known ingestion of corrosives or volatile petroleum products. Syrup of ipecachuana and 3% hydrogen peroxide are often available in the home and should be considered prior to transport to the hospital. Hydrogen peroxide can be administered relatively easily and if emesis does not occur within 10 minutes, the dose can be repeated once. Emesis is often more effectively induced when the stomach is full; therefore feeding a small amount of food prior to induction can improve efficacy. Owners may have difficulty administering syrup of ipecachuana to cats due to its objectionable taste. Other disadvantages of syrup of ipecachuana include prolonged emesis and adsorption by activated charcoal (AC). Administration of AC may have to be delayed to allow the emetic action of syrup of ipecachuana to occur.

Apomorphine is the emetic of choice for dogs (Beasley and Dorman, 1990), but it is not recommended for cats. Xylazine has been used instead as an emetic for cats (also suitable for dogs). While apomorphine and xylazine induce emesis quickly, they may also cause undesirable CNS depression.

Gastric lavage

Gastric lavage can be employed when administration of an emetic is contraindicated. In a conscious animal, gastric lavage requires anaesthesia and the airway should be protected with a cuffed endotracheal tube. The largest possible gastric tube, with terminal fenestrations, is introduced into the stomach. Tube placement is confirmed by aspiration of gastric contents or air insufflation with a stethoscope placed over the stomach. After gastric intubation, the mouth should be kept lower than the chest. Tepid tap water or normal saline (5–10 ml/kg) is introduced into the stomach under minimal pressure and is withdrawn by aspiration or gravity flow. The procedure is repeated until several lavages are clear, often requiring numerous cycles. AC (with or without a cathartic) can be administered just

Agent	Indication	Dosage
Syrup of ipecachuana	Emesis	Dogs: 1–2 ml/kg orally Cats: 3.3 ml/kg orally diluted 50:50 with water
3% Hydrogen peroxide	Emesis	1–2 ml/kg orally; if no emesis, repeat once
Apomorphine	Emesis	Dogs: 0.03 mg/kg i.v. or 0.04 mg/kg i.m. Do not use in cats
Activated charcoal (AC)	Adsorption	All animals: 1–4 g/kg orally as an aqueous slurry (~1 g per 5 ml water); may be repeated at 4–6 hour intervals
Sodium or magnesium sulphate	Catharsis	Dogs: 5–25 g mixed in AC slurry Cats: 2–5 g mixed in AC slurry Give only once
Sorbitol	Catharsis	Often included in AC formulations. If not, give 3 ml/kg orally of 70% sorbitol
Polyethylene glycol	Whole bowel irrigation	Not established for animals, however, young children are given 20–40 ml/kg per hour until clear rectal effluent noted
Sodium bicarbonate	Urine alkalinization	Generally, 1–2 mEq/kg administered every 3–4 hours; goal is to achieve urine pH of 7 or above
Ammonium chloride	Urine acidification	Dogs: 100 mg/kg orally bid Cats: 20 mg/kg orally bid

Figure 15.5: Common gastrointestinal and systemic decontamination agents.

before tube removal. The initial lavage sample should be retained for possible toxicological analysis.

Activated charcoal

AC is the only adsorbent routinely used in companion animal medicine, although others such as Fuller's Earth may be indicated rarely for specific poisons (see paraquat). AC is an effective adsorbent for most poisons, with several notable exceptions, including alcohols, corrosives and some metals such as iron and lithium (Howland, 1994). It is available as a powder, an aqueous slurry or combined with cathartics such as sorbitol. Repeated doses of AC are effective in interrupting enterohepatic recycling of several poisons, and continued presence of AC in the gastrointestinal tract may create a sink for trapping poison passing from the circulation into the intestines. Repeated administration of AC is usually safe.

Both saline (sodium sulphate or magnesium sulphate or citrate) and saccharide (sorbitol) cathartics are available (Figure 15.5). Cathartics hasten the elimination of unabsorbed poison via the stools and are safe, particularly if used only once. Repeated administration of magnesium-containing cathartics can lead to hypermagnesaemia manifested as hypotonia, altered mental status and respiratory failure, while repeated administration of sorbitol can cause fluid pooling in the gastrointestinal tract, excessive fluid losses and severe dehydration.

Recent innovations in human medicine

Recently in human medicine there has been a movement away from combining gastric evacuation with an adsorbent, toward the administration of only the adsorbent, especially in mild to moderate intoxications (Perry and Shannon, 1996). Early administration of AC alone has been shown to be as efficacious as gastric evacuation followed by AC. The case for or against inclusion of a cathartic with AC is less clear-cut, but a single dose of a cathartic along with the initial dose of AC is currently recommended. AC formulations that include a cathartic should be administered once, followed by AC alone if repeated doses are indicated.

One newer approach to human GID is whole bowel irrigation (WBI), the oral administration of large volumes of an electrolyte-balanced solution until a clear rectal effluent is produced. A polyethylene glycol solution, routinely employed to cleanse the gastrointestinal tract for surgical or radiographic procedures, is used (Perry and Shannon, 1996). WBI may be efficacious when an ingested poison is poorly adsorbed to AC, or when sustained-release medications, small metal objects or lead-based paint have been ingested. WBI is well tolerated by human paediatric patients, but its utility in veterinary medicine has not been determined.

Enhancing elimination via the urinary tract

Removal of absorbed poisons via urinary excretion may be indicated in several specific situations. For example, alkalinization of the urine to a pH above 7.0 with sodium bicarbonate enhances the urinary elimination of weak acids such as ethylene glycol, salicylates, phenobarbitone and the herbicide, 2,4-D (Beasley and Dorman, 1990). Administration of ammonium chloride to acidify the urine (pH 5.5–6.5) may enhance the elimination of weak bases such as amphetamines and strychnine. Urinary alkalinization or acidification requires close patient monitoring to avoid acid–base disturbances.

Supportive care and monitoring

Fortunately, many intoxicated patients will recover if attention is paid to appropriate symptomatic and supportive care. For example, even if GID is not possible following the ingestion of strychnine, effective control of muscle rigidity with pentobarbitone should result in complete recovery from intoxication. Other sections of this manual should be consulted for appropriate symptomatic care protocols.

USE OF A TOXICOLOGY LABORATORY

Effective use of a toxicology laboratory requires submission of appropriate ante-mortem and post-mortem samples for analysis. Appropriate samples vary depending on the poison. For example, whole blood is required for diagnosis of lead intoxication, whereas plasma, serum or urine is required for diagnosis of chocolate intoxication. Often, several samples are necessary to detect a poison; urine may contain detectable concentrations whereas plasma or serum may not. Figure 15.2 lists samples commonly used for toxicological diagnoses. Most samples can be kept frozen for extended periods of time without interfering with the analysis. Thus, histopathological examination of tissues can be performed first, perhaps suggesting an alternative diagnosis or identifying a need for specific toxicological analyses.

It is a common misconception that the clinician needs to have some idea which poison to look for before toxicological testing will be useful. In fact, many toxicology laboratories offer relatively inexpensive organic and inorganic screens that may detect an otherwise unanticipated poison. Despite the availability of screens, it remains necessary to develop appropriate differential lists based on historical or clinical findings.

In most cases, toxicological testing does not change initial clinical management, due to delays in obtaining laboratory results and the fact that relatively few poisons have specific antidotes. However, detection of a specific poison may confirm a tentative diagnosis, have prognostic value and identify human health hazards. In addition, toxicological testing may produce negative results, which may allay client fears of environmental contamination or malicious poisoning.

SPECIFIC POISONS

Anticoagulant rodenticides

The anticoagulant rodenticides are among the most common poisons of small animals, particularly dogs. Anticoagulant rodenticides derived from coumarin include warfarin, brodifacoum, bromodiolone and difenacoum. Indandione derivatives include pindone, chlorophacinone and diphacinone. New compounds such as difethialone are routinely added to those already in commercial use. Most modern 'second generation' anticoagulants are potent, single-feeding rodenticides, which have largely replaced older 'first generation' rodenticides such as warfarin, pindone, chlorophacinone, dicoumarol and valone.

Anticoagulant rodenticides competitively inhibit vitamin K epoxide reductase, which converts vitamin K epoxide to its active reduced form. Final activation of clotting factors II, VII, IX and X depends on reduced vitamin K epoxide. Coagulopathies ensue once the supply of active clotting factors is consumed, generally 1–3 days following ingestion of a toxic dose. Second generation anticoagulants such as brodifacoum are more effective at inhibiting vitamin K epoxide reductase and persist longer in the body.

Clinical signs are due to a coagulopathy. Haemorrhage can be acute and massive or slow and sustained. Subcutaneous haematomas, epistaxis, melaena and haematemesis may be readily apparent. Presenting signs also depend on the location of haemorrhage, often without external signs of bleeding. For example, haemorrhage into the central nervous system may cause ataxia, convulsions or sudden death, whereas pulmonary haemorrhage may cause respiratory distress.

Diagnosis relies on demonstrating prolonged coagulation and detection of a specific anticoagulant. Tests of coagulation such as one-stage prothrombin time (OSPT), activated partial thromboplastin time (APTT) and activated coagulation time (ACT) are affected at different times following ingestion, due to differences in the half-lives of the affected clotting factors. Since factor VII has the shortest half-life, the extrinsic coagulation pathway is affected first and OSPT is prolonged before and more severely than the APTT. OSPT should be used to monitor coagulation times in asymptomatic animals after exposure to an unknown amount of anticoagulant, when vitamin K_1 is not given prophylactically, or following cessation of vitamin K_1 therapy. All coagulation tests are likely to be prolonged in animals presenting with clinical signs.

Several veterinary diagnostic laboratories offer anticoagulant screens of whole blood or serum ante mortem, or liver post mortem. Generally, the most commonly used anticoagulants are included in the screen, but some less commonly used compounds may not be included. Analysis of stomach contents is inappropriate since exposure of a symptomatic animal was 1–3 days prior to presentation.

Vitamin K_1 is used as an antidote and the dose and duration of therapy depends on the specific compound ingested. Recommended doses for first generation anticoagulants such as warfarin are 1 mg/kg for 4–6 days. For newer anticoagulants such as brodifacoum, doses of 2.5–5.0 mg/kg, for a minimum of 2–6 weeks are suggested. When the specific compound is unknown, it should be assumed that exposure was to one of the more potent compounds. The oral bioavailability of vitamin K_1 is greatly improved if it is fed with a small fatty meal such as canned dog food. OSPT should be checked 1, 3 and 5 days after cessation of therapy to detect recurrence of a coagulopathy. Vitamin K_1 can be given subcutaneously at several sites with a small gauge needle. Intramuscular administration should be avoided due to the possibility of haemorrhage at the injection site. A delay of 6–12 hours occurs before synthesis of new clotting factors is evident. In severely symptomatic animals, plasma or blood transfusions may be necessary.

If pregnant or lactating animals are exposed to anticoagulant rodenticides, haemorrhage may occur during delivery and the toxins can be eliminated in milk (Felice and Murphy, 1995). Nursing puppies or kittens should be removed from the exposed dam and supplemented with vitamin K_1 orally for 2–3 weeks. Alternatively, nursing animals can be placed on vitamin K_1 while the coagulation status of the dam is monitored. If the dam remains normal, vitamin K_1 can then be discontinued. Anticoagulant-exposed pregnant animals should be maintained on vitamin K_1 until birth and newborns maintained on vitamin K_1 for at least one additional week or until their coagulation status can be monitored.

Cholecalciferol (vitamin D_3)

Cholecalciferol is a relatively new rodenticide, which kills rodents within 1–3 days of ingestion. After absorption, it is metabolized to 25-hydroxyvitamin D in the liver, then metabolized to the active 1,25-dihydroxyvitamin D by the kidney. Active vitamin D increases calcium absorption from the intestine, osteoclastic resorption of bone and calcium reabsorption from the renal distal tubules. Toxic doses result in hypercalcaemia, which causes cardiac conduction disturbances and metastatic tissue mineralization. Clinical signs develop 12–36 hours after ingestion of a toxic dose and include depression, anorexia, emesis, polydipsia and polyuria. Renal failure may develop with resultant azotaemia.

A presumptive diagnosis relies on detecting high serum calcium concentrations. Cholecalciferol toxicosis must then be differentiated from hypercalcaemia of malignancy, primary hyperparathyroidism and primary renal failure. Measurement of parathormone, 25-monohydroxycholecalciferol and total and ionized calcium can be used to differentiate causes of hypercalcaemia (Nachreiner and Refsal, 1990). Hyperphosphataemia is a consistent finding that may precede hypercalcaemia.

Case management is challenging, with several approaches to lowering serum calcium. Normal saline and frusemide at 1–2 mg/kg i.v. followed by 1 mg/kg tid should be given to promote calciuresis. Frusemide should not be administered if the animal is dehydrated. Prednisolone (2 mg/kg orally bid or tid) inhibits the release of osteoclast-activating factors, reduces intestinal calcium absorption and promotes calciuresis. Salmon calcitonin has been used when hypercalcaemia is severe or refractory, but is ineffective when used alone. Pamidronate disodium, a drug used to treat hypercalcaemia of malignancy in humans, shows promise for reversing cholecalciferol-induced hypercalcaemia in dogs at 1.3 mg/kg i.v. in 150 ml normal saline 1 and 8 days after cholecalciferol ingestion (Rumbeiha et al., 1997).

Cholinesterase-inhibiting insecticides: organophosphates and carbamates

While the use of organophosphate (OP) and carbamate insecticides for flea and tick control has declined in recent years, environmental exposure remains common. OPs and carbamates inhibit cholinesterase enzymes, particularly acetylcholinesterase, which breaks down acetylcholine. Acetylcholine propagates nervous impulses at a number of sites within the central and peripheral nervous systems. Overstimulation of muscarinic and nicotinic receptors causes most of the clinical manifestations of intoxication.

Clinical signs related to overstimulation of parasympathetic muscarinic receptors include diarrhoea, increased urination, miosis, bradycardia, bronchospasm and dyspnoea, emesis, excessive lacrimation and salivation. Excessive stimulation of nicotinic receptors initially results in muscle stimulation, followed by a depolarizing blockade. Death usually results from respiratory failure.

Diagnosis depends on a history of exposure, detection of a specific chemical in gastric contents and demonstration of low cholinesterase enzyme activity in whole blood ante mortem or in the brain post mortem. Enzyme activities below 50% of normal indicate exposure to a cholinesterase-inhibiting insecticide. Often, enzyme activity is depressed by more than 80%.

Early after exposure before clinical signs occur, management prioritizes decontamination. If the animal is symptomatic, atropine should be given before decontamination. Atropine specifically blocks muscarinic receptors and at high doses it can provide immediate but short-lived relief. It must be re-administered when signs begin to recur. Atropine is administered to effect and precise dosages may vary. Once signs of muscarinic overstimulation are controlled, decontamination can begin.

Pralidoxime hydrochloride (2-PAM) reverses enzyme inhibition and prevents 'ageing' following OP exposure (20 mg/kg bid to tid i.m. or slowly i.v.). Once ageing has occurred, 2-PAM is ineffective; therefore, the efficacy of 2-PAM is greatest soon after intoxication. Nevertheless, if treatment is delayed, 2-PAM therapy may still be helpful and it is continued until the patient is asymptomatic or shows no improvement of nicotinic signs after 24–36 hours of therapy (Fikes, 1990). Pralidoxime is not effective for treating carbamate intoxication, since enzyme ageing does not occur. When it is uncertain whether intoxication is due to an OP or a carbamate, however, 2-PAM should be administered. Diphenhydramine (1–4 mg/kg orally tid to qid) has been suggested to reverse signs due to nicotinic receptor stimulation, but its clinical efficacy has not been established.

Paraquat

In general, herbicides are not a significant hazard to pets. Serious intoxications of dogs most commonly involve exposure to paraquat and the related herbicide diquat. Reported LD_{50} values for dogs are 25–50 mg/kg. Both the herbicidal action and the toxicity are believed to be due to production of free radicals resulting in lipid membrane damage. Paraquat is concentrated in alveolar cells and this results in oxidant damage. Initial clinical signs following ingestion include mucosal irritation, emesis, hyperexcitability and ataxia. In dogs, proximal tubular necrosis and renal failure often occur. The hallmark of paraquat intoxication is pulmonary oedema and congestion, occurring several days after exposure and resulting in dyspnoea. Necrosis of alveolar cells occurs, resulting in scarring and fibrosis, and death due to respiratory failure. Diquat does not cause lung damage.

Management includes decontamination with bentonite or Fuller's Earth, which bind paraquat and diquat more effectively than does activated charcoal. Supportive and symptomatic care are important. Superoxide dismutase and N-acetylcysteine have been recommended and both have theoretical benefits, but their clinical efficacy for preventing oxidant damage due to paraquat has not been proven.

Metaldehyde

Metaldehyde is the active ingredient in many slug and snail baits (at 3.5–4.0%). Reported lethal doses are 100–1000 mg/kg for dogs and approximately 200 mg/kg for cats. Metaldehyde decreases brain concentrations of γ-aminobutyric acid, resulting in loss of its CNS inhibitory action. Early clinical signs include anxiety and restlessness followed by salivation, mydriasis, tremors and ataxia. Advanced signs include polypnoea, tachycardia, muscle tremors, opisthotonos, continuous seizures, cyanosis and hyperthermia. The diagnosis can be confirmed by detection of metaldehyde in gastric contents. Treatment involves GID if soon after ingestion and control of seizures with diazepam or barbiturates. Particular care should be taken to monitor and maintain appropriate acid–base status.

Non-steroidal anti-inflammatory drugs (NSAIDs)

NSAIDs are a large group of drugs that share pharmacological actions and side-effects. They are classified chemically as carboxylic acids and enolic acids. Carboxylic acids are further divided into: salicylic acid derivatives, including aspirin and diflusinal; acetic acid derivatives, including diclofenac, indomethacin, tolmetin and sulindac; proprionic acid derivatives, such as carprofen, fenoprofen, flurbiprofen, ibuprofen, ketoprofen and naproxen; and fenamic acids, including meclofenamic acid, meclofenamate sodium, flunixin meglumide and mefenamic acid. The enolic group is divided into: pyrazolone derivatives, which include phenylbutazone, dipyrone and apazone; and oxicam derivatives, such as piroxicam.

NSAIDs act by inhibiting prostaglandin synthesis, which reduces inflammatory mediators such as prostaglandins E_2 and $F_{2\alpha}$ and endoperoxides, and also causes the adverse effects noted following their ingestion. The toxicity of NSAIDs varies considerably and cats tend to be more sensitive than dogs. The most common adverse effects of NSAIDs are mild epigastric pain, erosive gastritis, peptic ulcers and haemorrhage. Anaemia and hypoproteinaemia may occur secondary to gastric and intestinal ulceration. Nephrotoxicity is manifested as acute interstitial nephritis, acute papillary necrosis, nephrotic syndrome and acute and chronic renal failure.

Single ingestions of ibuprofen of 300 mg/kg can cause acute renal failure, while repeated dosages of 8 mg/kg/day can produce gastrointestinal irritation and haemorrhage. Doses of 15 mg/kg naproxen are considered toxic to dogs and repeated dosages of 5 mg/kg cause significant gastrointestinal damage. Aspirin doses of 50 mg/kg bid cause emesis in dogs and higher dosages cause depression and metabolic acidosis. Aspirin should *not* be given to cats. In general, cats are more sensitive than dogs to the toxic effects of NSAIDs.

Diagnosis of NSAID intoxication relies on the history, detection of a specific NSAID in gastric contents, plasma or urine and compatible clinical signs. Management of acute ingestions involves GID and supportive care. Repeated doses of AC should be administered every 4–6 hours, for NSAIDs with long half-lives and significant enterohepatic recirculation (carprofen, indomethacin, piroxicam, sulindac, meclofenamic acid, meclofenamate and diclofenac). Gastrointestinal ulcers can be treated with cimetidine or ranitidine and sucralfate. Acute renal failure may be reversible while acute papillary necrosis is most likely irreversible. Fluid therapy is the most important component in treating acute renal failure. If oliguria persists after fluid therapy, frusemide, mannitol or low-dose dopamine should be initiated (see Chapter 6). Hyperkalaemia and acid–base disturbances should be corrected.

Acetaminophen

Acetaminophen is a non-opiate derivative of *p*-aminophenol, which produces analgesia and antipyresis by a mechanism similar to that of salicylates. Acetaminophen is detoxified by the liver via conjugation with glucuronide, sulphate or glutathione. Cats lack the glucuronide conjugation pathway and are quite sensitive to acetaminophen toxicity. If the conjugating ability of the liver is surpassed, N-acetyl-p-benzoquinone, a toxic metabolite, causes severe oxidative stress to hepatocytes and red blood cells. Oxidative damage to erythrocytes causes oxidation of haemoglobin to methaemoglobin and the formation of Heinz bodies. Potentially toxic doses of acetaminophen for cats are 50–100 mg/kg, while a reported toxic dose for dogs is 600 mg/kg.

Clinical signs of intoxication include depression, weakness, anorexia, emesis, tachypnoea, tachycardia and hypersalivation and facial oedema in cats. Methaemoglobinaemia imparts a muddy colour to the mucous membranes and there may be haematuria and haemoglobinaemia. Acute hepatic necrosis is the most important toxic effect in dogs.

Routine decontamination should be attempted early after a known or suspected ingestion. N-Acetylcysteine (NAC) is a specific antidote that provides one of the limiting precursors (cysteine) for glutathione synthesis. A loading dose of 140–280 mg/kg orally or 140 mg/kg i.v. in 5% dextrose/water is followed by a maintenance dosage of 70 mg/kg orally qid for 2–3 days. Although AC binds orally administered NAC, both should be administered as soon as possible after ingestion, as the recommended oral dosage of NAC provides sufficient cysteine despite reduced systemic absorption (Howland et al., 1994). Ascorbic acid can be administered (30 mg/kg orally or s.c. qid) to help reduce methaemoglobin to haemoglobin.

Chemotherapeutic emergencies

Antineoplastic drugs, including cyclophosphamide, methotrexate, 5-fluorouracil and cisplatin, may occasionally cause serious adverse effects. Antineoplastic drugs kill the actively dividing cells in malignant tumours. Unfortunately, cells such as intestinal epithelial cells, bone marrow cells, hair follicles, lymphoid cells and gonadal cells also undergo rapid division and are also susceptible to their effects. Most serious intoxications are related to haematological and gastrointestinal effects.

Leucocyte, platelet and red blood cell precursors can be damaged by antineoplastic drugs with resulting effects on peripheral blood counts depending on the circulating half-life of each cell type. Since the half-life of circulating neutrophils is the shortest (4–8 hours), neutropenia occurs first, followed by thrombocytopenia (platelet circulating half-life of 5–7 days). The most serious consequence is sepsis, which positively correlates with the severity and duration of neutropenia. Broad-spectrum, bactericidal antibiotics and appropriate fluid therapy should be instituted. Thrombocytopenia

can result in petechiae, ecchymoses and mucosal haemorrhage. If needed, platelet replacement therapy consists of either whole blood or platelet-rich plasma.

Gastrointestinal toxicity is manifested by nausea, emesis and gastroenterocolitis. Anti-emetics such as metoclopramide or butorphanol may reduce the incidence of emesis, but animals with persistent emesis may require hospitalization for fluid therapy. Gastroenterocolitis is treated symptomatically with demulcents, fluid and electrolyte therapy and, if necessary, broad-spectrum antibiotics.

Herbal remedies

A complete discussion of intoxication risks from herbal remedies is available elsewhere (Tyler, 1993; Lewin et al., 1994; Poppenga, 1995). Since there are a large number of herbs with a wide range of biologically active constituents, it is important to ask about their use when presented with an ill animal. Haematological, gastrointestinal, cardiac, neurological, hepatic and renal signs may occur. The source of the herbal remedy is important, as many imported Chinese patent medicines are adulterated with metals, pesticides and drugs such as NSAIDs and sedatives. Chinese patent medicine formulations may also contain cinnabar (mercuric sulphide), realgar (arsenic sulphide) or litharge (lead oxide). The risk of intoxication depends on the dose administered, the duration of use and the presence of pre-existing diseases. The potential for adverse drug reactions increases when herbal medicines are given concurrently with traditional pharmaceuticals.

A human poison control centre may be consulted regarding the active constituents of herbal remedies, particularly if the label is incomplete or in a foreign language. Toxicological testing of fluid or tissue samples may identify some active ingredients, although many potentially toxic constituents are not detected by routine screens. Testing for contaminants such as metals and drugs may be indicated when an imported patent remedy has been used. In general, acute ingestion of potentially toxic herbal products should be managed following standard decontamination protocols and symptomatic treatment. Decontamination may not be helpful when a herbal remedy has been given chronically.

Ethylene glycol

Ingestion of ethylene glycol (EG) remains one of the most common toxicoses of dogs and cats. It is readily consumed by animals and the incidence of toxicoses is highest in late autumn and early spring when antifreeze use increases. EG has been replaced in some antifreeze formulations by relatively non-toxic propylene glycol. EG itself is not particularly lethal. A metabolite, glycolic acid, causes severe metabolic acidosis within several hours of ingestion. In addition, another metabolite, oxalic acid, combines with calcium to form calcium oxalate crystals in blood vessels and renal tubules.

Renal tubular damage with subsequent renal failure occurs 1–3 days after ingestion.

EG toxicosis can be divided into three clinical phases. Phase 1 occurs 1–4 hours after ingestion, is manifested by ataxia, tachycardia, polypnoea, diuresis, polydipsia and dehydration. Phase 2 occurs 4–6 hours after ingestion and coincides with onset of metabolic acidosis due to EG metabolites. Clinical signs include anorexia, depression, emesis, miosis and hypothermia. Following large ingestions, severe depression, tachypnoea, coma and death ensue unless treatment is initiated. With smaller doses, clinical signs may resolve only to be followed by phase 3, characterized by oliguric renal failure.

Diagnosis of EG toxicosis can be difficult. Increased serum osmolality, metabolic acidosis and an anion gap greater than 40–50 mEq/l are often observed, but isopropanol, salicylates, methanol, paraldehyde, toluene, formaldehyde and ibuprofen toxicoses can cause similar changes. Birefringent rosette-shaped calcium oxalate crystals may be seen in urine sediment, particularly under polarized light. Laboratory detection of EG or glycolic acid in serum or urine confirms exposure. Colorimetric kits allow detection of EG in serum within 24 hours of exposure, when serum EG concentrations are high. Unfortunately, animals may recover from phases 1 and 2, only to be presented in renal failure, which is associated with a guarded prognosis.

Management depends on the time of presentation following ingestion. If an animal is presented several hours after ingestion, GID is not useful, since EG is rapidly absorbed from the gastrointestinal tract. Specific antidotes include ethanol and 4-methylpyrazole (fomepizole), which prevent metabolism of EG to toxic metabolites by inhibiting alcohol dehydrogenase. In dogs, a 20% ethanol solution is given i.v. at 5.5 ml/kg by slow i.v. infusion every 4 hours for five treatments, then every 6 hours for four additional treatments. In cats the recommended dose is 5.0 ml/kg i.v. every 6 hours for five treatments then every 8 hours for four treatments. The dose should be titrated to maintain severe depression for up to 72 hours. In dogs, 4-methylpyrazole is administered by slow i.v. infusion of 15 mg/kg as a 5% solution, then 10 mg/kg every 12 hours for four doses followed by 5 mg/kg every 12 hours until plasma EG concentrations fall below 20 mg/dl. If EG concentrations cannot be monitored, the 5 mg/kg dose should be continued for at least 24 hours. While 4-methylpyrazole has fewer side-effects than ethanol and is the antidote of choice for dogs, it is ineffective for cats. Since metabolism of EG occurs quickly, the antidotes need to be given as soon as possible after ingestion. Supportive care should be provided, specifically, correction of metabolic acidosis and maintenance of urine flow are critical to success.

Household agents

There are hundreds of chemicals in the household to which animals may be exposed and some of these are listed in Figure 15.6. Many household products are, however, generally considered to be non-toxic (Figure 15.7). The majority of toxic exposures are managed using standard GID protocols and supportive treatment.

Petroleum-based products

With the exception of petroleum distillates serving as vehicles for more toxic chemicals, ingestion of petroleum-based products is not considered to be life-threatening. Aspiration pneumonia is the most serious sequel of ingestion of volatile petroleum products such as paraffin (kerosene), naphtha or petroleum distillates. Aspiration risks increase with spontaneous or induced emesis and GID should be avoided. When co-ingestion of another toxic chemical has occurred, GID should be considered.

Chest radiographs should be considered for all patients who have ingested petroleum-based products. Those who remain asymptomatic with normal chest radiographs 4 or more hours after ingestion can be sent home after a 1-day observation period, with no further treatment. However, patients with radiographic and/or clinical evidence of pneumonitis require close monitoring, symptomatic oxygen supplementation and serial arterial blood gas determinations. Indications for antibiotic therapy include documented bacterial pneumonia, worsening of radiographic infiltrates, leucocytosis and fever after the first 40 hours. There appears to be no benefit from the administration of corticosteroids.

Illicit drugs

While the documented incidence is unknown, the widespread availability of drugs such as cocaine, narcotics and amphetamines makes exposure of pets likely. Drug sniffer dogs may be at particular risk. Most illicit drugs are rapidly absorbed and target the CNS. Therefore, illicit drug exposure should be considered in any animal with acute neurological signs.

Cocaine intoxication is manifested by CNS excitation, peripheral vasoconstriction, hyperthermia and increased muscular activity. Death results from respiratory or cardiac arrest, or hyperthermia. Narcotics such as heroin exert their effects on the gastrointestinal, cardiovascular and central nervous systems. Early clinical signs may include drowsiness, ataxia, decreased sensory pain perception, transient excitation, emesis, defecation and tachypnoea. Late clinical signs include delirium, seizures, miosis, coma, respiratory depression and hypotension. Pulmonary oedema often occurs in fatal cases and death is often attributed to respiratory arrest. Amphetamine overdoses cause restlessness, behavioural changes, hyperactivity, mydriasis, polypnoea, hyperthermia, tachycardia, tremors, respiratory depression, cardiac arrhythmias, heart block and circulatory shock.

Treatment is largely symptomatic. Early after ingestion GID should be considered. Treatment of seizures,

Product	Toxicity rating	Ingredients	Clinical presentation
De-icer	4	~75% ethylene glycol and isopropyl alcohol	Disorientation, ataxia, weakness, depression, irritation of mucous membranes and eyes
Fertilizer	2	Mainly nitrogen (e.g. potassium nitrate, urea), phosphorous, potassium; may contain small amounts of metals or pesticides	Gastrointestinal irritation, emesis, diarrhoea, methaemoglobinaemia
Fuels (cooking fuels, lighter fluid)	3	Petroleum hydrocarbons, kerosene, or methanol	Depression, coma, seizures, emesis
Glues	3–4	Carriers include aliphatic hydrocarbon solvents (e.g. petroleum solvents, acetone, toluol, toluene, methyl acetate, naphtha)	Direct irritation, depression
Paint and varnish removers	4	Benzene, acetone, toluene, methylene chloride, methanol	Direct irritation, depression
Radiator cleaners	4	Oxalic acid	Direct irritation of mucous membranes and gastrointestinal tract, muscle twitching, tetany, seizures, depression, paralysis, renal failure
Rust removers	4	Hydrochloric acid, phosphoric acid, hydrofluoric acid, naphtha and mineral oil	Necrosis
Thawing salt	2–3	Calcium chloride, sodium chloride, or potassium chloride	Erythema, exfoliation, ulceration, general irritation of the gastrointestinal tract, emesis, anorexia, diarrhoea, direct irritation of footpads, mouth, or pharynx from contaminated water
Fire extinguisher chemicals	2–4	Chlorobromomethane, methylbromide, or halogenated hydrocarbons consisting of brominated or chlorinated fluoromethanes	Irritation of the skin and eyes, emesis, CNS signs, hypotension, coma, pulmonary oedema
Fireplace colours	3–4	Coke dust, sawdust, heavy metal salts (e.g. copper, rubidium and caesium compounds, lead, arsenic, selenium, tellurium, barium, molybdenum, antimony, zinc), chloride, borate and phosphate	Severe gastroenteritis, emesis, diarrhoea, followed by depression, shock and renal failure
Fireworks	3–4	Oxidizing agents (e.g. potassium nitrate, chlorates), heavy metal salts (e.g. mercury, antimony, copper, strontium, barium, phosphorus)	Emesis, severe abdominal pain, bloody faeces, rapid shallow breathing, methaemoglobinaemia and death from respiratory or cardiac failure; other signs relate to specific effects of toxic heavy metals
Fluxes	3–4	Zinc chloride, hydrochloric acid, salts of aniline, glutamic and salicylic acid, aliphatic alcohols, terpenes, hydrocarbons, boric acid and fluorides silver solder)	Irritation of the mouth, gastrointestinal tract or skin; nausea, emesis, diarrhoea, ataxia, delirium and excitement progressing to stupor or coma
Matches	2	Potassium chlorate	Methaemoglobinaemia with cyanosis and haemolysis
Photographic developer	4–5	Boric acid, p-methyl aminophenol sulphite, ammonium thiosulphate, potassium thiocyanate, sodium hydroxide	p-Methyl aminophenol sulphite causes methaemoglobinaemia; corrosive effects may result from acids and alkalis
Bleach	3	~5% sodium hypochlorite	Acid solutions combined with hypochlorite bleaches can cause release of chlorine gas and hypochlorous acid, presenting an acute inhalation hazard characterized by pain and inflammation of the mouth, pharynx, oesophagus and stomach; oral ingestion results in irritation with oedema of the pharynx, glottis, larynx and lungs

Figure 15.6 (continued overpage)

Product	Toxicity rating	Ingredients	Clinical presentation
Drain cleaners	No rating	Sodium hydroxide, sodium hypochlorite	Necrosis and ulceration of the oral mucosa and, possibly, the oesophagus; sequelae include strictures, laryngeal or glottal oedema, asphyxiation and pneumonia
Furniture polish	3	Petroleum distillates, mineral spirits, petroleum hydrocarbons	Depression, coma, seizures, emesis
Metal cleaners, oven cleaners	3–4	Caustic soda or potash (alkaline cleaners), kerosene, high concentrations of chlorinated ethylenes or 1,1,1-trichloroethane (solvent cleaners), hydrochloric, sulphuric, chromic or phosphoric acids	Necrosis, emesis
Pine oil disinfectants	3	Pine oils (terpenes), phenols, synthetic phenol derivatives (e.g. o-phenyl phenol)	Gastritis, emesis, diarrhoea are followed by depression, unconsciousness, or mild seizures followed by depression and renal failure
Shoe polish	2	Animal, petroleum or vegetable waxes, mineral spirits, turpentine, aniline dyes; nitrobenzenes or terpenes may also be present	Large amounts could produce methaemoglobinaemia
Deodorant/ antiperspirants	3	Cream base and an antibacterial agent, antiperspirants also contain 15–20% aluminium salts (e.g. aluminium chlorohydrate, aluminium chloride); less commonly used agents include titanium dioxide, oxyquinoline sulphate, and zirconium salts	Gingival necrosis and haemorrhagic gastroenteritis, sometimes accompanied by ataxia and nephrosis, severe effects are rare unless large amounts of active ingredient are ingested
Denture cleaners	4	Perborates decompose to hydrogen peroxide and sodium borate, which are strongly alkaline and very irritating	Salivation, emesis, early stimulation of the CNS followed by depression, non-specific liver and kidney damage
Perfumes	3–4	Alcohols, essential oils (e.g. savin, rue, tansy, apiol, juniper, cedar leaf, cajupute)	Essential oils are often hepato- or nephrotoxic and may irritate the skin, mucous membranes and lungs resulting in aspiration, pulmonary oedema and pneumonitis; albuminuria, haematuria and glycosuria result from renal damage; CNS effects include excitement, ataxia, disorientation and coma
Rubbing alcohol	2–3	Ethanol or isopropyl alcohol	Disorientation, ataxia, weakness, depression, irritation of mucous membranes
Shampoos	3	Surfactants, fragrance, sodium lauryl sulphate or triethanolamine dodecyl sulphate; antidandruff shampoos contain one or more metals (e.g. zinc pyridinethione, selenium sulphide) coal tar derivatives or salicylic acid	Only mild toxicosis is expected in most cases; progressive blindness has been reported in dogs and cats ingesting zinc pyridinethione (lesions include retinal detachment and severe exudative chorioretinitis)
Suntan lotion	2	Alcohol	See Rubbing alcohol
Styptic pencil	2	Potassium alum sulphate	Corrosive lesions from sulphuric acid formed during hydrolysis of the salt

Figure 15.6: *Toxicity of common household products. Toxicity is based on a scale of 1–6, where 1 is relatively harmless (probable oral lethal dose of >15 g/kg) and 6 is extremely toxic (probable oral lethal dose <1 mg/kg).*
Reproduced from Osweiler (1996) with permission of Williams and Wilkins.

Abrasives
Adhesives
Antacids
Antibiotics
Baby product cosmetics
Ballpoint pen inks
Bath oils
Birth control pills
Bleach with <5% sodium hypochlorite
Body conditioners
Bubble bath soaps
Calamine lotion
Candles (beeswax or paraffin)
Chalk
Colognes
Cosmetics
Crayons marked AP, CP
Deodorants
Deodorizers
Elmer's glue
Fabric softeners
Fish bowl additives
Hand lotions/creams
3% Hydrogen peroxide
Incense
Indelible markers
Ink (blue and black)
Iodophil disinfectant
Laxatives
Lipstick
Lubricants
Magic markers
Mineral oil
Modelling clay
Newspaper
Pencil (graphite lead and colouring)
Perfumes
Petroleum jelly
Plant foods and fertilizers
Play-Doh
Polaroid picture coating fluid
Porous tip marking pens
Rubber cement
Sachets
Shampoos (liquid)
Shaving creams and lotions
Silica gel
Soaps and soap products
Suntan preparations
Sweetening agents
Thermometers (mercury)
Toothpaste
Vitamins (without iron)
Wallpaper paste
Washing powder (except those for dishwashers)
Watercolours
Zirconium oxide

Figure 15.7: *Household items considered to be non-toxic.*

hyperthermia, respiratory depression and cardiac arrhythmias are of primary concern. The toxic effects of most narcotic agents can be reversed by naloxone (0.01–0.02 mg/kg i.v., i.m. or s.c.) to effect; repeated doses may be needed. Chlorpromazine (10–18 mg/kg i.v.) may antagonize many of the effects of cocaine and amphetamines. Haloperidol (1 mg/kg i.v.) may be protective against the lethal effects of amphetamines. Several reference sources are available (Kisseberth and Trammel, 1990; Dumonceaux, 1995).

Plants
While scores of potentially toxic plants may be ingested, relatively few plants (Figure 15.8) account for the majority of exposures (Beasley and Trammel, 1989; Buck, 1995; Hornfeldt and Murphy, 1995).

Lead
Lead intoxication is still common, despite efforts to decrease environmental sources of exposure. The incidence is highest in young dogs and in pets kept in older houses. Sources of exposure include paint and paint residue or dust from sanding, lead objects such as curtain and fishing weights, improperly glazed ceramic food or water bowls, plumbing materials, solder, putty and linoleum.

Lead interacts with sulphydryl groups and interferes with numerous enzymes, including those involved in heme synthesis, resulting in increased fragility and reduced survival of red blood cells. Damage to CNS capillaries may account for acute CNS effects. Clinical signs are related to the gastrointestinal and nervous systems. Gastrointestinal signs are prominent in animals with chronic low-level exposure to lead and include emesis, diarrhoea, anorexia and abdominal pain. Neurological signs are more common with acute exposures and include lethargy, hysteria, seizures and blindness. Diagnosis relies on detection of clinically significant lead concentrations in whole blood. A large number of nucleated red blood cells and basophilic stippling suggests lead exposure, but their absence does not rule out lead toxicosis. Radio-opaque material in the gastrointestinal tract may be an important clue to ingestion of lead objects or paint chips.

Case management should be tailored to the individual situation. Activated charcoal is not effective in binding lead. Sodium sulphate may hasten the elimination of lead from the gastrointestinal tract by forming lead sulphate, which is not well absorbed. WBI to remove small metallic objects or paint chips seems reasonable, although such a decontamination approach has not been evaluated for efficacy. Alternatively, metal objects may be removed via endoscopy or surgery. Calcium disodium edetate ($CaNa_2.EDTA$) and succimer (dimercaptosuccinic acid or DMSA) are effective lead chelators. DMSA is relatively new and has several major advantages over $CaNa_2.EDTA$ including oral efficacy and fewer side-effects (Graziano, 1994).

Common name	Scientific name	Poison	System(s) affected	Clinical signs	Treatment
Philodendron Dumbcane	*Philodendron* spp. *Dieffenbachia* spp.	Insoluble calcium oxalate	GI, respiratory	Painful burning of lips, oral mucosa, throat; if severe, oedema, dyspnoea	Pain and oedema resolve slowly without treatment, symptomatic
Rhododendron Azalea	*Rhododendron* spp.	Andromedotoxins	GI, cardiovascular	Transitory burning in mouth followed by salivation, emesis and diarrhoea; muscular weakness; bradycardia; hypotension; coma and convulsions terminally	GID, monitor ECG, fluids, atropine for bradycardia
Easter and tiger lilies	*Lilium loniflorum* and *L. tigrinum*	Unknown	Renal	Consistent with acute renal failure: anorexia, depression, emesis	GID, treatment for acute renal failure
Marijuana	*Cannabis sativa*	Tetrahydrocannabinol (THC)	CNS	Ataxia, depression, hallucinations evidenced by barking and agitation, emesis, dry mucous membranes	GID (antiemetic properties of THC may negate emetics), place in warm quiet environment
Poinsettia	*Euphorbia pulcherrima*	Unknown	GI	Not generally toxic; emesis most severe sign	Not generally needed, symptomatic

Figure 15.8: *Most commonly implicated poisonous plants.*

CaNa$_2$.EDTA should be diluted to a 1% solution with 5% dextrose in water and administered subcutaneously at 25 mg/kg qid for 5 days (Poppenga, 1997). Animals with blood lead concentrations greater than 1 ppm often need multiple treatments separated by 5-day rest periods. Blood lead concentrations should be monitored several days after cessation of treatment to determine whether additional chelation will be necessary. Succimer is administered orally at 10 mg/kg tid for 5 days, followed by 10 mg/kg bid for 2 weeks. Extended treatment should be separated by 2-week rest periods. Seizures should be controlled with diazepam.

Zinc

Zinc intoxication may occur following the ingestion of zinc-containing objects such as coins, galvanized hardware materials or ointments containing zinc oxide. It is most frequently reported in dogs and pet birds. Zinc causes severe gastrointestinal irritation and intravascular haemolysis. Multiple organ failure, disseminated intravascular coagulation and cardiopulmonary arrest have been reported. Diagnosis relies on the measurement of elevated serum zinc concentrations. Metallic objects may be detected on abdominal radiographs and may be an important clue to zinc intoxication in patients with a haemolytic crisis.

Specific treatments for zinc toxicosis include removal of metallic objects from the gastrointestinal tract and the administration of CaNa$_2$.EDTA which chelates zinc (succimer does not chelate zinc effectively). Symptomatic and supportive care should be instituted and liver, renal, coagulation and cardiac function monitored. Removal of the source of zinc often results in gradual improvement over 48–72 hours.

REFERENCES

Beasley VR and Dorman DC (1990) Management of toxicoses. In: *Veterinary Clinics of North America: Toxicology of Selected Pesticides, Drugs and Chemicals*, ed. VR Beasley, pp. 307–337. WB Saunders, Philadelphia

Beasley VR and Trammel HL (1989) Incidence of poisonings in small animals. In: *Current Veterinary Therapy X: Small Animal Practice*, ed. RW Kirk, pp. 97–113. WB Saunders, Philadelphia

Buck WB (1995) Top 25 generic agents involving dogs and cats managed by the national animal poison control centre in 1992. In: *Current Veterinary Therapy XII: Small Animal Practice*, ed. JD Bonagura, p. 210. WB Saunders, Philadelphia

Dumonceaux GA (1995) Illicit drug intoxications in dogs. In: *Current Veterinary Therapy XII: Small Animal Practice*, ed. JD Bonagura, pp. 250–251. WB Saunders, Philadelphia

Felice LJ and Murphy MJ (1995) CVT update: anticoagulant rodenticides. In: *Current Veterinary Therapy XII: Small Animal Practice*, ed. JD Bonagura, pp. 228–232. WB Saunders, Philadelphia

Fikes J (1990) Organophosphorus and carbamate insecticides. In: *Veterinary Clinics of North America: Toxicology of Selected Pesticides, Drugs and Chemicals*, ed. VR Beasely, pp. 353–367. WB Saunders, Philadelphia

Graziano JH (1994) Antidotes in depth: 2,3-dimercaptosuccinic acid (DMSA, succimer). In: *Toxicologic Emergencies*, ed. LR Goldfrank *et al.*, pp. 1045–1047. Appleton and Lange, Norwalk

Hornfeldt CS and Murphy MJ (1995) Incidence of small animal poison exposures in a major metropolitan area. In: *Current Veterinary Therapy XII: Small Animal Practice*, ed. JD Bonagura, pp. 209–210. WB Saunders, Philadelphia

Howland MA (1994) Antidotes in-depth: activated charcoal. In: *Toxicologic Emergencies*, ed. LR Goldfrank *et al.*, pp. 66–71. Appleton and Lange, Norwalk

Howland MA, Smilkstein, J and Weisman RS (1994) Antidotes in depth: *N*-acetylcysteine. In: *Toxicologic Emergencies*, ed. LR Goldfrank *et al.*, pp. 498–500. Appleton and Lange, Norwalk

Kisseberth WC and Trammel HL (1990) Illicit and abused drugs. In: *Veterinary Clinics of North America: Toxicology of Selected Pesticides, Drugs and Chemicals*, ed. VR Beasely, pp. 405–418. WB Saunders, Philadelphia

Lewin NA, Howland MA and Goldfrank LR (1994) Herbal preparations. In: *Toxicologic Emergencies*, ed. LR Goldfrank *et al.*, pp. 963–979. Appleton and Lange, Norwalk

Nachreiner RF and Refsal KR (1990) The use of parathormone, ionized calcium and 25-hydroxyvitamin D assays to diagnosis calcium disorders in dogs. *Proceedings 8th ACVIM Forum*, pp. 251–254, Washington, DC

Osweiler GD (1996) Clinical toxicology of common household chemicals. In: *The National Veterinary Medical Series: Toxicology*. Williams and Wilkins, Baltimore

Perry H and Shannon M (1996) Emergency department gastrointestinal decontamination. *Pediatric Annals* **25**, 19–29.

Poppenga RH (1995) Risks associated with herbal remedies. In: *Current Veterinary Therapy XII: Small Animal Practice*, ed. JD Bonagura, pp. 222–226. WB Saunders, Philadelphia

Poppenga RH (1997) Lead poisoning. In: *The 5 Minute Veterinary Consult: Canine and Feline*, ed. LP Tilley and FWK Smith, Jr, pp. 760–761. Williams and Wilkins, Baltimore

Rumbeiha WK, Kruger J, Fitzgerald S, Render J, Nachreiner R, Kaneene J, Vrable R, Richter M and Chiapuzio C (1997) The use of pamidronate disodium for treatment of vitamin D_3 toxicosis in dogs. *Proceedings, American Association of Veterinary Laboratory Diagnosticians*, 40th Annual Meeting, p. 71. Louisville, KY

Shannon MW and Haddad LM (1998) The emergency management of poisoning. In: *Clinical Management of Poisoning and Drug Overdose*, ed. LM Haddad *et al.*, pp. 2–31. WB Saunders, Philadelphia

Tyler VE (1993) *The Honest Herbal: A Sensible Guide to the Use of Herbs and Related Remedies*. Pharmaceutical Products Press, New York

CHAPTER SIXTEEN

Monitoring the Critical Patient

Richard Hammond and Clare Walters

INTRODUCTION

After the initial assessment of patient status, monitoring the critical patient provides a means of continued re-evaluation of the patient's condition and response to therapy. Selection of the parameters to be monitored depends on the nature of the clinical disease process and the results of the initial evaluation. The level of monitoring and type of equipment used will depend upon equipment availability, operator experience and the need for accuracy. Often, with repeated evaluation, the most important information is provided by determining data trends. These trends may provide a better indication of patient response than the recording of accurate but infrequent measurements. It is therefore important that data are recorded in a readily accessible way that allows trends to be quickly detected.

Recently, relatively inexpensive, accurate, simple to use and advanced monitoring equipment has become widely available for veterinary intensive care. This equipment detects changes in physiological parameters, below the threshold of detection of more basic methods, i.e. has a higher sensitivity. Earlier detection of potentially significant changes allows prompt (and often therefore more effective) corrective measures. An example is measurement of pulse pressure. Mean arterial pressures below 70 mm Hg are associated with reduced tissue perfusion, yet mean arterial pressures between 70 and 150 mm Hg may feel similar on digital palpation. These are easily distinguished using a blood pressure monitor.

Good ICU monitoring consists of the measurement and recording of changes in specific, relevant parameters producing an overall picture of changing patient status. This may be helped by, but is not usually dependent on, the use of advanced monitoring equipment.

MONITORING THE CARDIOVASCULAR SYSTEM

The cardiovascular system provides tissue perfusion by maintaining a driving force for blood flow. Mean arterial pressure (MAP) is maintained by cardiac output and affected by local alterations in vascular tone. Cardiac output is the product of heart rate and stroke volume. Cardiac output may be increased by raising heart rate and stroke volume, but this must be supported by an adequate preload (circulating volume). In disease states, there is a complex interaction between compensatory mechanisms all aimed at the maintenance of tissue perfusion by supporting MAP. In terms of cardiovascular monitoring it is important to recognize the following:

- Low or falling MAP reflects a failure of the normal cardiovascular compensatory homeostatic mechanisms
- Failure to maintain MAP often indicates severe reduction in a single parameter, e.g. circulating blood volume. In serious or advanced disease, it may reflect a failure of multiple parameters, e.g. circulating blood volume and a secondary failure of myocardial contractility or vascular tone
- Individual parameters may be normal or show a compensatory change (e.g. heart rate increase) in cardiovascular failure. Data from multiple cardiovascular monitoring parameters must be assessed to understand the overall status of the cardiovascular system
- Reduction of a controlled end-point of cardiovascular function, e.g. tissue perfusion or MAP, indicates inadequacy of effective circulating volume, cardiac output or vascular tone and failure of compensation
- Often it is the failure of end-point function coupled with compensatory increases in parameters such as heart rate that are most easily detected on examination. Underlying causes must then be determined and corrected where possible.

The approach to assessing cardiovascular system status may be simplistically but usefully divided into stages as follows.

Measurement of circulating blood volume
Many critical conditions lead directly (traumatic blood loss, diarrhoea) or indirectly (decreased mentation and fluid intake) to a reduced circulating fluid volume. Effective circulating volume determines cardiac preload and consequently is a determinant of cardiac out-

put. Therefore, the ability to monitor circulating volume and effectiveness of replacement therapy is important. Increases in haematocrit and total protein may suggest haemoconcentration and can be useful in monitoring ongoing changes in fluid status, especially during replacement therapy. In addition, skin tenting may be used to suggest a reduced interstitial fluid content. Both of these techniques are prone to individual variation, are relatively insensitive and may be altered and difficult to interpret in the presence of pathology.

Central venous pressure monitoring

Central venous pressure (CVP) is a measurement of pressure in the cranial vena cava immediately proximal to the right atrium. Because the venous system is a low-pressure capacitance system, CVP reflects intravascular volume. CVP is relatively easy to measure accurately in the ICU, by placement of a catheter (usually through-the-needle) via the jugular vein into the intrathoracic cranial vena cava (see Chapter 22). Catheters are readily obtainable in a range of lengths and sizes to suit most small animals. The CVP catheter also provides a central line for the administration of fluids or emergency drugs. It is connected via a three-way tap to either a vertical column of saline or a signal amplifier via a pressure transducer (see invasive arterial pressure measurement below). Measurements are made with the three-way tap or pressure transducer level with the right atrium (zero) and are usually recorded in cm H_2O. Measurements in mm Hg may be converted to cm H_2O by multiplying by 1.36. CVP measurement is altered by animal positioning, which should be consistent when comparing multiple or sequential readings. Correct catheter placement should be ensured by measurement of the required catheter length against the body surface prior to insertion. Overlong catheters may enter the right atrium. Correct placement can be confirmed by radiography, fluoroscopy or observation of the pressure trace obtained where available. The CVP trace is characteristic (Figure 16.1).

Normal values for CVP are 0–5 cm H_2O, but are variable in individual animals, and changing trends during multiple measurements are much more important than individual values. Although it is a measurement of pressure rather than volume, a low CVP reflects low effective circulating volume; either intravascular fluid loss or decreased peripheral resistance (vasodilation). It may also be seen in potential high cardiac output states such as sepsis. Normally, increases in preload lead to compensatory increases in stroke volume (Frank Starling Law), bringing the preload back to normal. Measured increases in CVP therefore reflect possible right-sided myocardial failure, restrictive pericarditis or excessive increases in circulating volume (intravenous fluid administration). CVP is routinely used to monitor the effectiveness and rate of fluid replacement therapy. The significance of an abnormal CVP (raised or reduced) can be assessed by

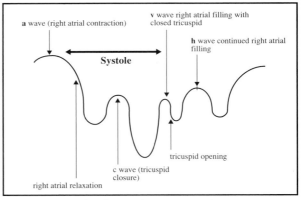

Figure 16.1: *Stylized central venous waveform characteristics, showing the determinants of individual peaks. Interpretation of the waveform allows determination of correct catheter placement and may be used as part of the diagnostic investigation in intra-cardiac disease.*

the response to a small 'test' bolus of normal saline of approximately 4–5 ml/kg. A low CVP due to reduced circulating volume will respond by a rapid but temporary increase in CVP (usually as well as MAP) towards normal. Further volume administration should then result in a sustained improvement of CVP and MAP. When CVP is raised due to primary right-sided myocardial failure or volume overload, the fluid bolus will further raise the CVP, with subsequent sustained elevation or slow decrease back to baseline. In these cases, further fluid administration should be curtailed. In cases of severe or prolonged hypovolaemia, however, CVP may be normal or raised due to myocardial failure secondary to myocardial hypoxia. In these cases, a bolus injection may actually improve cardiac output and produce an apparently paradoxical reduction in CVP.

Measurement of cardiac output

In the clinical setting, we often rely on indirect methods to detect a reduction in cardiac output. A failure of adequate cardiac output is suggested by the presence of a low MAP or inadequate tissue perfusion in organ systems that are dependent on high blood flow, such as the brain or kidney. Reduced perfusion is implied by the presence of tissue hypoxia (lactic acidosis) or reduction in organ function (e.g. reduced mentation or urine output).

Direct measurement of cardiac output

Cardiac output (with systemic vascular resistance) determines MAP and (with arterial oxygen content), tissue oxygen delivery. Measurement of cardiac output can therefore be extremely useful in the critical patient. Unfortunately, methods currently available for the measurement of cardiac output in veterinary species are invasive and require technical skill and training to provide reproducible results. The most commonly used technique is the thermodilution method. Briefly, a thermistor-tipped multi-lumen catheter is placed in the pulmonary artery. A bolus injection of iced saline is administered upstream (often into the central vein or right atrium) and the resultant temperature depression in pulmonary arterial blood is then measured. Pulmonary arterial catheterization may be associated with complications, including pulmonary arterial thrombosis, endomyocarditis, dysrhythmias and even rupture of the pulmonary artery. These problems, as well as the equipment, training and time required, mean that this technique is usually impractical for routine veterinary use.

Measurement of myocardial performance and stroke volume

Since cardiac output is the product of stroke volume and heart rate, the ability to measure these parameters would also provide some information about the cause of an apparent reduction in cardiac output. Like cardiac output, stroke volume is difficult to measure directly. Reduction in stroke volume may be caused by inadequate ventricular preload (determined by CVP and pulmonary arterial wedge pressure) or reduced myocardial performance. Although not suitable for continuous monitoring, Doppler echocardiography allows intermittent measurement of myocardial performance and may be useful in the initial assessment of cardiovascular status. M-mode echocardiography provides an indication of fractional shortening and left ventricular ejection fraction, both indicators of myocardial contractility.

Monitoring heart rate and rhythm: chest auscultation

Auscultation of heart sounds using a stethoscope, in association with palpation of the peripheral pulse, provides some indication of heart rate and rhythm. Although dependent on factors such as breed conformation and hair coat, chest wall thickness, body condition, presence of pleural or pericardial pathology and blood viscosity, a subjective finding of reduction in heart sound intensity suggests systolic dysfunction. This may reflect myocardial dysfunction or inadequate ventricular filling (e.g. inadequate preload or supraventricular tachydysrhythmia).

Monitoring heart rate and rhythm: use of the electrocardiogram (ECG)

Although the heart rate may be inferred from pulse rate or auscultation of heart sounds, the ECG provides a simple non-invasive means of continuous heart rate measurement in the ICU and shows changes in cardiac rhythm. Determination of rate and rhythm is important for two reasons. Firstly, acute cardiovascular compensatory mechanisms primarily rely on alteration of heart rate to maintain homeostasis and preserve cardiac output. The heart rate therefore provides a useful indicator of acute changes in cardiovascular function. Secondly, dysrhythmias are common in critical patients and may lead to a significant reduction in cardiac output. The pathogenesis of these dysrhythmias includes intrinsic myocardial disease, but is more likely to involve

myocardial hypoxia, hypercapnoea, myocardial trauma, severe pain or electrolyte disturbances (Chapter 4).

Practically, the ECG is used in two ways in the ICU. Often a baseline six-lead hard copy ECG is recorded as part of the initial assessment and then a single lead (usually II) is monitored continuously with an oscilloscope type display. Initial assessment includes measurement of parameters such as P-wave amplitude and duration and R–T interval from the hard copy. This may be repeated periodically. Continuous monitoring is used for the early detection of dysrhythmias, pacemaker malfunction and changes in the S–T segment, which may reflect myocardial hypoxia (Figure 16.2). The significance of ECG changes in ICU patients depends on the underlying cause, the effect on cardiac output and the likelihood of progression to a more serious dysrhythmia.

Lead placement is usually in the standard lead II position to provide the greatest P-wave voltage (therefore requiring the least amplification and associated background noise). Exact lead position is less important than consistency of position to allow detection of waveform changes. In the dog and cat, a relatively normal lead I and II trace for the hard copy evaluation can be obtained if the right arm (red) lead is placed cranial to the heart on the right side, on the neck or near the thoracic inlet, or on the right foreleg and the left leg (black) leads are placed caudal to the heart on the inguinal skin folds or on the left hindleg. The left arm lead (yellow) should be placed on the left cranial quadrant of the body or on the left foreleg. For ongoing monitoring of heart rate and rhythm, adhesive skin patch electrodes can be securely taped in place on the corresponding distal limbs and are usually tolerated well (see Chapter 21). Adequate electrode contact with the patient is very important if an artefact-free ECG is to be obtained. Ideally, the electrodes should be silver

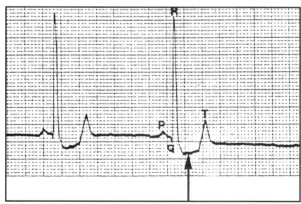

Figure 16.2: *Example of ST segment depression during anaesthesia (two lead ECG recording at 25 mm/s). Although ST segment deviation from baseline (elevation or depression) may be a relatively frequent and often incidental finding, changes with time (especially in patients during anaesthesia or in those with respiratory dysfunction) may suggest myocardial hypoxia. The presence of systemic hypoxaemia (blood gases, pulse oximetry) and the effects of increased FiO_2 (see Chapters 5 and 22) should be investigated.*

plated to avoid resistance mismatching. Crocodile clips are unsuitable for prolonged use. They may be modified to clip to adhesive skin pads or fine surgical wire skin sutures, which provide good electrical contact without discomfort.

Most electrocardiograph amplifiers and display modules can be used for both monitoring and limited diagnostic purposes. Displays using LCD technology should be avoided, as pixel density is too low for correct measurement of wave intensity, and screen refresh rate is too slow for rapid interpretation of altering waveforms. In addition, the necessity of active matrix screen technology makes these devices relatively expensive. Ideally, an ECG machine suitable for the ICU should be easy to use, inexpensive and should have:

- The ability to connect to a printer for hard copy output
- Selectable noise filtering
- User variable sensitivity
- The ability to freeze the display for dysrhythmia evaluation
- Easily replaceable leads of adequate length to allow location of the machine away from the patient.

Often a combination of physiological monitoring parameters (combined electronic units with ECG, temperature and blood pressure measurement capabilities) in a single machine reduces overall expenditure.

Measurement of arterial blood pressure

Blood pressure is the lateral force exerted on vasculature by the flow of blood. It provides the driving force for tissue perfusion. Normal values for arterial pressure are systolic 112–192 mm Hg and diastolic 56–110 mm Hg in dogs and systolic 120–170 mm Hg and diastolic 70–120 mm Hg in cats. MAP is an integrated mean of systolic (ventricular systole) and diastolic (end diastole) pressures. Measurement of MAP alone therefore does not reflect individual systolic and diastolic pressures. It is calculated from the following formula:

$$MAP = \text{Diastolic pressure} + (\text{Systolic pressure} - \text{Diastolic pressure})/3$$

Mean arterial pressures are frequently reduced in critical patients, due to low circulating blood volume (trauma, fluid loss), myocardial pump failure or lack of vascular tone. MAP values less than 70 mm Hg in small animals are associated with reduced tissue perfusion, hypoxia and failure of highly oxygen-dependent organ systems (heart, kidney and ultimately brain). MAP is therefore monitored routinely. Usually, unless there is a failure of vasomotor tone autoregulation (as is seen in sepsis), low MAPs reflect low systolic pressures and are associated with a raised diastolic pressure due to compensatory vasoconstriction. Thus, treatments to increase cardiac output (restore circulating volume and increase myocardial contractility), rather than to increase vascular tone, are used to restore a reduced MAP. When systolic and diastolic pressures cannot be measured, the presence of peripheral vasoconstriction implies failure of cardiac output. The causes (myocardial failure or inadequate preload) should therefore be investigated.

Palpation of peripheral pulses

Palpation of pulse pressure (e.g. femoral in small animals) provides limited but useful information. Pulse pressure does not truly measure MAP, but reflects the difference between systolic and diastolic pressures. It is affected by both stroke volume (affects systolic pressure) and vascular compliance (affects diastolic pressure). Wide (hyperkinetic) pulses occur when the difference between these pressures is high (e.g. patent ductus arteriosus, which may be associated with high systolic and low diastolic pressures). In contrast, narrow (hypokinetic) pulses are seen when there is low cardiac output (e.g. myocardial failure) or low cardiac output and vasoconstriction (e.g. hypovolaemia).

Palpation of beat-to-beat changes in pulse amplitude may reflect alterations in stroke volume, which may accompany dysrhythmias such as second degree heart block, atrial fibrillation or ventricular premature contractions, which lead to changes in preload. It is therefore useful to palpate the pulse synchronously, with observation of the ECG waveform. This also allows an indication of the effect of ECG changes on the pulse, and contributes to an evaluation of their clinical significance. Alterations in pulse pressure associated with respiration (sinus arrhythmia) are not normally detectable on palpation but may be exaggerated in cases of restricted right-sided cardiac filling (cardiac tamponade or restrictive pericarditis).

Although useful, pulse pressures do not directly reflect MAP. Other methods of estimation of arterial pressure are therefore necessary. Practically, they are divided into non-invasive and invasive methods.

Non-invasive blood pressure monitoring

All non-invasive techniques are based on inflation of a cuff to occlude arterial flow and detection of the pressure at which blood flow returns (systolic pressure). Non-invasive methods are not technically demanding and are associated with minimal complications. Unfortunately, both commonly used indirect methods (oscillometric and Doppler techniques) are prone to error, including operator familiarity and selection of the correct cuff size for each animal. If operators are not familiar with potential pitfalls and sources of error, data of low reproducibility may be obtained. As with other monitored parameters, data trends are more useful than absolute values. Less accurate but clinically reproducible measurements therefore often provide valid information.

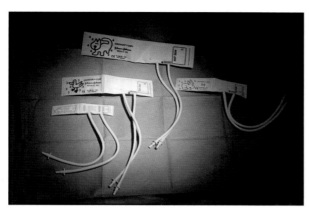

Figure 16.3: Paediatric disposable cuffs are available in a range of sizes (1–5) and all are required to cover the range of animal sizes encountered in small animal critical care. They may be re-used. The selection of the size of cuff for an individual patient is important for both patient comfort and accuracy of data obtained. Where an unexpected or abormal pressure reading is obtained using non-invasive methods, the measurement should be repeated with a different cuff size before corrective or therapeutic intervention is considered.

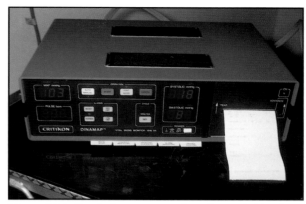

Figure 16.4: Stand-alone automated oscillometric blood pressure monitor. These are invaluable in both ICU and anaesthesia monitoring environments. With correct cuff size selection, these devices provide an acceptably accurate and repeatable estimation of mean arterial pressure.

Disposable paediatric cuffs are readily available, covering the size range required for measurement of pressures in dogs and cats of all sizes (Figure 16.3). Selection of appropriate cuff size is important. Cuffs should be 20% wider than the limb diameter to obtain correct readings. Undersized or overtightened cuffs produce artificial elevation of both systolic and diastolic pressures and *vice versa* for oversized or loose cuffs. Cuffs may be placed over any suitable peripheral artery (commonly dorsal metatarsal, dorsal metacarpal or ventral tail). The animal should be restrained so that the cuff is at the same level as the heart.

Different measurement techniques depend on the method of determining the return of arterial flow after occlusion by the inflated cuff.

Oscillometry: Oscillometry is the only non-invasive technique capable of measuring MAP. The Dinamap® (Device for Indirect Non-invasive Automatic Mean Arterial Pressure) is one of the most frequently used in veterinary medicine, but several other instruments are on the market. These devices use a single cuff, which is alternately inflated and deflated. During deflation, alterations in cuff pressure are sensed by a transducer. Oscillations are caused by pulses in the limb, and those of peak amplitude correspond to the MAP. The pressure at which oscillations are first detected is the systolic pressure and the pressure at which the oscillations decrease rapidly is the diastolic pressure. Heart rate is calculated from oscillation frequency. Although useful, as cuff inflation and readings may be automated, this method is expensive, prone to movement error and cannot operate in the presence of ventricular dysrhythmias. In addition, frequency of reading is ideally limited to greater than 5 minutes to allow inflation/deflation cycles and reperfusion of tissue distal to the cuff in the

intervening period. The accuracy is reported to be within ± 10 mm Hg in humans, but may be poor in domestic species due to variations in limb size. These devices can be incorporated into multiple parameter monitoring devices or stand alone (Figure 16.4). When purchasing new or from second-hand hospital stock for intended small animal use, these devices must be designed (or reprogrammed) for paediatric use to measure the high heart rates of small animals.

Doppler: This device uses a 10 MHz ultrasound probe to detect blood flow in the artery. The probe is placed over the artery distal to the cuff. Pressure in the inflated cuff is measured by use of a combined manometer/inflation bulb (Figure 16.5). Doppler sounds become apparent when cuff pressure falls below the systolic arterial pressure and flow in the artery returns. Diastolic pressures are implied by a change in sound to a continuous flow pattern. This method has been shown to be fairly accurate for estimation of systolic pressure but inaccurate in the estimation of diastolic pressures, and unable to estimate mean arterial pressure. Doppler

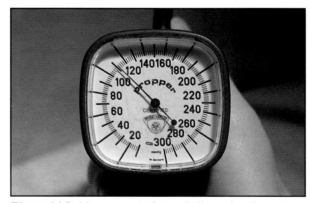

Figure 16.5: Manometer/inflation bulb used to determine pressure within a cuff positioned so as to occlude a peripheral artery. When used alongside a means of determining arterial flow distal to the cuff (e.g. Doppler ultrasound probe) this allows determination of systolic pressure.

measurement is useful when systolic pressures are low or when dysrhythmias prevent use of oscillometric techniques.

Direct invasive blood pressure measurement

The placement of an intra-arterial cannula (usually femoral or dorsal metatarsal) allows direct measurement of arterial pressure, still considered the gold standard. Arterial cannulation requires practice, but is not technically difficult. In short-term use, with the usual precautions of sterility and haemostasis, it is rarely associated with complications. Cannula placement may be achieved after intradermal infusion of a small volume of local anaesthetic to reduce response to skin penetration, although this is rarely required in critically ill patients. Sedation is seldom required. The cannula is attached to a length of fine bore, semi-rigid connecting tubing, containing heparinized saline. This may then be placed against a vertical scale (zeroed with reference to the estimated position of the tricuspid valve or heart base) and MAP measured in cm H_2O as the mid-point of oscillations at the level of the meniscus. A rough estimation of pulse pressure is provided by the range of oscillations. Pressure readings may be converted to mm Hg by division by 1.36. This simple technique requires little equipment and provides a continuous indication of MAP.

The aneroid manometer is a very simple and inexpensive instrument, which provides an accurate assessment of MAP (Figure 16.6). It is connected to the arterial catheter via a three-way tap and saline-filled tubing. A 20 ml syringe filled with heparinized saline is also connected to the three-way tap. The zero point of the manometer must be at the level of the heart. Then the three-way tap is turned so that heparinized saline from the syringe can be injected into the system, until the manometer reads more than 100 mm Hg. The tap is opened so that the manometer is connected to the arterial catheter. Saline in the tubing will flow into the artery until the pressure in the system (as measured by the manometer) is equal to the MAP. This is a very useful way of monitoring trends in blood pressure, involving inexpensive and disposable equipment that is easily portable.

Alternatively, the changes in pressure in the saline column may be converted to an electrical signal by use of a pressure transducer placed at the level of the heart, amplified and displayed as systolic, diastolic and mean pressures alongside a trace of the pressure waveform. Display of the pressure waveform may be beneficial as it provides information on individual components of the pressure wave (Figure 16.7). The costs of monitors capable of displaying invasive pressure-waveforms are now within the range of clinical practice. Disposable pressure transducers, although expensive and designed for single use in humans, may be repeatedly resterilized. These monitors may also be used for measurement of CVP.

Although blood pressure measurements made using direct techniques are accurate and reproducible, there are still several sources of error, of which the

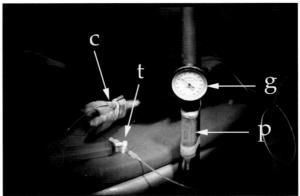

Figure 16.6: *Aneroid manometer used to measure mean arterial pressure. Changes in pressure in a column of sterile saline connected to the arterial catheter (c) are measured by connection to the manometer positioned and zeroed at the level of the heart. The saline does not enter the manometer but terminates at a flexible membrane within a Pressurveil® (p). The pressure exerted by the saline on the membrane is directly reflected by changes in air pressure distal to the membrane within the manometer. Pressure is displayed on the gauge (g). A three-way tap (t) allows flushing of the catheter and zeroing of the manometer (3-way tap positioned at level of heart base, manometer connected to room air and adjusted so that pointer reads zero, tap closed to room air so that manometer and line are in communication).*

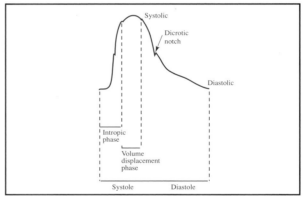

Figure 16.7: *Stylized arterial pressure trace. As with the CVP trace, individual wave components provide information as to aspects of both the recording set-up (damping, harmonic interference) and the patient's cardiovascular status (e.g. position of dicrotic notch, rate of diastolic run-off).*

operator must be aware. Firstly, partial occlusion of the cannula by thrombus formation or the presence of air bubbles within the tubing leads to signal damping, which reduces the recorded systolic value and increases the diastolic value. MAP is not affected until occlusion is near complete. A second important source of damping is the use of highly flexible (compliant) or long lengths of tubing or use of a high number of connections and three-way taps. Conversely if there is inadequate damping in the system, there may be resonance and consequent artefact in the pressure trace (e.g. position of dicrotic notch) and inaccuracy of the absolute values obtained. Frequent intermittent or continuous flushing of the cannula with heparinized saline is necessary to reduce thrombus formation and remove small air bubbles.

Functional characteristics

The most important function of the cardiovascular system is oxygen delivery to tissues. Unfortunately, physical characteristics may not directly reflect cardiovascular function, especially in the presence of disease. Oxygen delivery is the product of cardiac output and the oxygen content of arterial blood. The oxygen content of arterial blood is determined by the haematocrit and the oxygen saturation of haemoglobin. A haematocrit of greater than 25% and arterial oxygen saturation greater than 90% (equivalent to a PaO_2 greater than 70 mm Hg) will provide adequate tissue oxygen delivery if cardiac output is normal. Accurate measurement of oxygen delivery therefore depends on assessment of these factors. Haematocrit is routinely measured, and SpO_2 can be determined by pulse oximetry in most circumstances. Adequate cardiac output is more difficult to demonstrate (see above), but may be inferred by normal function of organs that are dependent on high tissue blood flow, for example the kidneys. A normal haematocrit, SpO_2 greater than 90% and urine output of 1–2 ml/kg/h therefore suggests adequate oxygen tissue delivery for most circumstances.

Failure of adequate oxygen delivery may be indicated by dysfunction in organs dependent upon a large oxygen supply. Reduced mentation, evidence of renal failure or myocardial hypoxia may therefore suggest tissue hypoxia. Acute myocardial hypoxia is indicated by electrocardiographic changes, including S–T segment depression or ventricular ectopic foci. Such findings, however, may also reflect intrinsic organ disease.

Occasionally, an apparently adequate oxygen delivery (based on arterial oxygen content and cardiac output) does not reflect the true requirements of the tissues. Diseased animals as well as those post-trauma or surgery have increased metabolism and metabolic oxygen demand. Normal levels of delivery may be inadequate to prevent anaerobic metabolism and tissue acidosis. Also, in some disease states such as sepsis, distribution of tissue perfusion may not match demand (flow maldistribution). Assessment of changes in oxygen consumption at varying levels of oxygen delivery can provide important information about the adequacy of oxygen delivery in individual patients. If oxygen consumption reaches a plateau despite increased delivery, oxygen delivery can be assumed to be adequate. Measurement of oxygen consumption is difficult, requiring analysis of pulmonary arterial blood samples and determination of cardiac output.

Clinically useful information about the balance between oxygen supply and demand may be determined by the measurement of partial pressure of oxygen in mixed venous (pulmonary arterial) or central venous blood. Low (<35 mm Hg) venous partial pressures reflect high levels of oxygen extraction or flow maldistribution, and trends of elevation can imply improved delivery. Very low levels (<20 mm Hg) are consistently associated with a very poor prognosis. Conversely, very high venous oxygen concentrations (> 55 mm Hg) can imply poor tissue perfusion and limited extraction of oxygen from blood by the tissues. In this instance, improved perfusion is accompanied by a decrease in venous oxygen concentrations.

MONITORING THE RESPIRATORY SYSTEM

Respiratory function can be divided into two parts: ventilation is the movement of gases between the alveoli and the environment, while gas exchange is the exchange of gases between the alveoli and cells of the body tissues.

Monitoring ventilation

The most important factor in the control of ventilation under normal conditions is the arterial partial pressure of CO_2 ($PaCO_2$). Central and peripheral chemoreceptors detect changes in $PaCO_2$, and ventilatory drive is varied to maintain it within the normal range of 35–45 mm Hg. This ventilatory response is reduced by drugs such as opioids and barbiturates and chronic increases in the work of breathing. If hypoxaemia develops, then hypoxic drive takes over and hyperventilation and hypocapnia may occur in an attempt to maintain normoxaemia.

Mechanical positive-pressure ventilation may be indicated in intensive care patients who are unable to maintain normal ventilation or gas exchange when breathing spontaneously. Ventilators may be categorized as pressure, time or volume limited, indicating the mechanism by which the inspiratory cycle is terminated. *Peak inspiratory pressure* should be carefully monitored in ventilated patients, particularly those with decreased lung compliance. Pressures greater than 20 cm H_2O may cause pneumothorax or pneumomediastinum in patients with pulmonary disease. Time- and volume-limited ventilators are generally fitted with pressure relief valves to avoid excessive airway pressures. All types of ventilator should have an alarm to alert operators of disconnection.

Minute volume

Ventilation is measured in terms of minute volume, which is normally about 200 ml/kg.

Minute volume = tidal volume x respiratory rate.

Respiratory rate can be measured relatively easily by observation of movement of the chest or abdominal wall. *Tidal volume* is more difficult to monitor. Observation of excursion of the chest or abdominal wall gives a rough indication of tidal volume. However, increased ventilatory effort in the presence of raised airway resistance may give a false impression of adequate tidal volume in a patient that is actually hypoventilating.

A more accurate measurement of tidal volume can be obtained using a *Wright's respirometer* in patients that are intubated or have a tracheotomy tube. This collects and measures the volume of expired gas, using a light vane that rotates within a cylinder as the air stream flows through. The rotation of the vane activates a gear chain, which drives a pointer round a dial. With appropriate calibration, the volume of gas that has passed through the meter corresponds to the volume read from the dial. In very small dogs and cats with low tidal volumes, the respirometer tends to under-read due to inertia.

Capnography

Capnography is the sampling of expired gas to determine the concentration of carbon dioxide, which may then be displayed as a capnogram. The end-tidal CO_2 (ETCO$_2$) is the partial pressure of CO_2 measured at the end of the expired tidal volume. Since end-tidal gas is virtually the same as alveolar gas, ETCO$_2$ is a very close estimation of the alveolar concentration of CO_2. Under ideal conditions, the partial pressure of CO_2 in the alveoli is equal to $PaCO_2$. However, there is usually a difference of about 5 mm Hg (with $PaCO_2$ being greater) because blood leaving ventilated alveoli mixes with blood from parenchymal lung tissue and unventilated alveoli, creating venous admixture. The normal value for ETCO$_2$ is approximately 35–40 mm Hg. ETCO$_2$ greater than 50 mm Hg indicates moderate hypercapnia and greater than 70 mm Hg indicates severe hypercapnia.

Capnography is an extremely useful, non-invasive method of monitoring, providing information on adequacy of ventilation, cardiac output and metabolism. It also provides a warning of disconnection of mechanically ventilated patients or blockage of the airway. Capnographs generally use infrared radiation projected through the expired gas mixture to measure carbon dioxide concentration. Carbon dioxide absorbs a band at 4.26 mm. A narrow band pass optical infrared filter is used to prevent the passage of radiation that would be absorbed by gases other than CO_2. Interference by elemental gases that do not absorb infrared radiation, but influence the absorption bands of CO_2 and affect the sensitivity of the infrared analyser, is compensated for electronically. In addition, water vapour can reduce the accuracy of CO_2 determination, and a narrow band filter is essential to keep this interference to a minimum.

Capnographs are either mainstream or sidestream analysers. The mainstream analyser has a sensor placed between the endotracheal tube and breathing circuit and so gives a very fast response. The disadvantage of this type is that the sensor is in a very vulnerable place — great care is vital to prevent the need for frequent

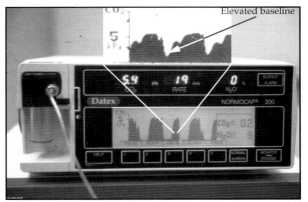

Figure 16.8: *Stand-alone capnograph (here with N_2O monitoring). Insert shows an example of raised baseline (and therefore presence of CO_2 in inspired gas). Where supplemental CO_2 is not being provided, during anaesthesia this may reflect dead space, inappropriate flow rates on breathing systems not containing soda lime, or exhaustion of soda lime where present. In a conscious patient where the capnograph probe is inserted nasally, the high anatomical dead space means that apparent re-breathing is a normal finding. In that incidence it is the value of end tidal gas, as a measure of ventilatory function, that is most useful.*

replacements. Sidestream analysers have a connector situated between the breathing circuit and endotracheal tube. The sensor is located away from the patient in the main unit. Gas is continuously aspirated from the connector and drawn into the analyser via tubing. In unintubated, spontaneously breathing patients, the tip of the sampling tube can be inserted into the nostrils. The capnogram produced in this way can appear abnormal because of the increase in dead-space and entrainment of gas from the environment. There is a short delay in display of ETCO$_2$, due to the time taken for the gas to be transported to the analyser. Accuracy and speed is improved with a short sampling tube and with the connector placed as close as possible to the tracheal tube to prevent mixing with fresh gas. High respiration rates and panting are associated with falsely low results.

Abnormalities of the capnograph:

- Raised baseline: failure of the baseline to return to zero indicates rebreathing, i.e. the inspiratory gas mixture contains some CO_2. This occurs when the fresh gas flow rate is lower than the minute volume, particularly in T-piece and Bain circuits (Figure 16.8)
- Slanted and prolonged phase II: indicates an obstruction to expiration, e.g. obstructive airway disease or a partly blocked endotracheal tube
- Biphasic or uneven plateau: this can indicate unequal emptying of the lungs due to differences in compliance from one part of the lungs to another
- Persistently high ETCO$_2$: hypercapnia, generally caused by hypoventilation

- Persistently low ETCO$_2$: this can indicate a mechanical fault such as a leak in the sampling tube or contamination of the sample with fresh gas. Falsely low values are also seen in animals with high respiration rates. Otherwise, it may indicate hyperventilation and hypocapnia
- Sudden decrease in ETCO$_2$: can occur during a severe cardiopulmonary crisis such as hypotension, pulmonary embolism or cardiac arrest and represents a decrease in pulmonary perfusion
- Absence of a capnogram trace: indicates apnoea, complete airway obstruction or disconnection. An alarm should sound if no ventilation is detected after a preset length of time.

Monitoring gas exchange

It is vital that adequate oxygen is transported by haemoglobin to the cells of the body for use in metabolic processes. Reduced (i.e. unoxygenated) haemoglobin has a blue colour that gives a cyanotic appearance to mucous membranes. Therefore examining the colour of mucous membranes can give an indication of oxygen content of the blood. However, it is very important to realize that blood must contain a high proportion of reduced haemoglobin before cyanosis is detectable. This proportion corresponds to a dangerously low oxygen saturation of haemoglobin.

Pulse oximetry

Oxygen delivery to the tissues can be more accurately monitored by pulse oximetry. This is an extremely useful, non-invasive method for monitoring critical patients; however, it has a number of limitations that must be understood if the information provided by the pulse oximeter is not to be misleading.

The pulse oximeter compares the absorption by haemoglobin of electromagnetic energy of two different wavelengths passed through an extremity. The degree of absorption changes with the percentage of oxygen bound to haemoglobin. The value of SpO$_2$ (arterial haemoglobin saturation) is determined from the ratio of the absorption of the energy at the two wavelengths. The pulse oximeter probe consists of two light-emitting diodes, which are placed in close contact with the skin surface (Figure 16.9). The light energy is detected by a sensor generally placed perpendicular to the light source, on the other side of the extremity. Pulse oximeters can distinguish arterial blood from venous or capillary blood due to a change in orientation of erythrocytes during the cardiac cycle. In systole, the erythrocytes are perpendicular to the vessel wall; in diastole, they are parallel. Therefore, absorption is greater during systole than diastole. Through this pulsatile variation in absorption, the arterial component of the signal can be differentiated from other blood flow and tissue cells.

Pulse oximeters generally display pulse rate and SpO$_2$. A beep may sound to audibly indicate pulse rate,

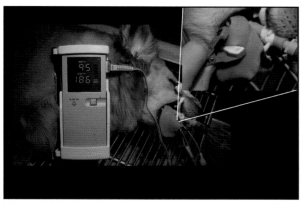

Figure 16.9: *Example of portable hand-held pulse oximeter used during anaesthesia. Insert shows detail of probe used. Although better tolerated during anaesthesia, probes placed on the tongue are most commonly used in the veterinary application. Other sites include almost any part of the body where an approximately 0.25–1 cm thick area of perfused tissue can be accessed, and include ear, prepuce, vulva and toe web. Often where a reading cannot be obtained immediately, this reflects tissue thickness. Repositioning the probe or artificially increasing thickness with dry single layered paper towel may help.*

the pitch of which may vary with SpO$_2$. The normal value for SpO$_2$ in an animal breathing room air is greater than 95%. Oxygen supplementation should be considered if SpO$_2$ is less than 92%, and values less than 90% are seriously low.

Uses and limitations of pulse oximeters:

- SpO$_2$ provides a good estimation of the oxygen saturation of haemoglobin. However, it should be realized from the sigmoid shape of the oxyhaemoglobin dissociation curve that although SpO$_2$ varies in a fairly linear way with PaO$_2$ at low partial pressures, the slope plateaus at higher partial pressures. Therefore, SpO$_2$ will be reasonably high (above 90%) until PaO$_2$ is as low as 60 mm Hg. Thus unless the pulse oximeter is reading an SpO$_2$ in the high 90s, it is impossible to know whether PaO$_2$ is at a safe level or if the animal is about to desaturate
- Pulse rate. Pulse oximeters give an accurate estimation of pulse rate unless there is movement artefact. However, they do not provide any information as to arterial blood pressure. As long as the pulse pressure exceeds 20 mm Hg, then pulse oximeters may be able to determine a pulse rate. It should be noted also that pulse oximeters amplify the signal they receive; therefore, the flashing lights vary with signal received, not arterial blood pressure
- Probe position. Transmission probes can be placed over unpigmented, hairless skin or mucous membranes. Useful sites include the tongue, toe-web, lip, ear pinnae, vulva or prepuce. Probes designed to wrap around a toenail are very useful, as they are much less susceptible to movement artefact. Reflection probes (the photodetector is

next to the light-emitting diodes) do not need two skin or mucous membrane surfaces and can therefore be placed at sites such as in the rectum. However, this type of probe has been associated with problems of inaccuracy

- Movement artefact. Movement such as shivering greatly reduces accuracy as the change in absorption of energy with each cardiac cycle is less than 2%
- Interference. Electromagnetic energy, visible light such as fluorescent lighting and surgical diathermy, may interfere with pulse oximetry
- Dyshaemoglobins. Some pulse oximeters are calibrated for human haemoglobin, for which absorption spectra may vary slightly from animal haemoglobin. Carboxyhaemoglobin produces a falsely high reading of SpO_2, as the pulse oximeter measures HbCO as fully oxygenated haemoglobin. Therefore pulse oximetry cannot be used to monitor SpO_2 in animals that may have been exposed to carbon monoxide. Methaemoglobinaemia causes pulse oximeters to indicate a low oxygen saturation of approximately 85%
- Delay. This may be physiological, i.e. the time it takes between a fall in inspired oxygen and the resultant fall in oxygen saturation at the probe site, or technical, i.e. the time taken to average and display the result
- Poor perfusion. It is often noted when using a pulse oximeter that it reads consistently for a certain length of time, but then saturation gradually falls. When the probe is removed and replaced it reads accurately again. This is because the pressure of the probe gradually compresses the tissue and then the probe needs to recalibrate in order to read accurately. Removing the probe briefly enables this to occur
- Tissue, such as cats' tongues or ear pinnae, may be too thin for probes to measure, as the probes are designed for human paediatric fingers. A folded paper towel can be placed under the probe to increase the width and compensate for the thin tissue.

Arterial blood gas analysis

Although very expensive, blood gas analysis is invaluable for monitoring trends in PaO_2, $PaCO_2$ and pH and is considered the gold standard for monitoring respiratory function. An arterial blood sample is drawn into a heparinized syringe over about four breaths, mixed thoroughly and then capped. If there is a delay of greater than 15 minutes before analysis, the sample should be kept on ice. Suitable arteries include the dorsal metatarsal, auricular and femoral in very small patients. To reduce the risk of haematoma and the pain of frequent arterial penetrations, a catheter can be placed under aseptic conditions. Arterial catheters must be flushed frequently with heparinized saline to prevent occlusion, and the first 2 ml of blood should be discarded at each sampling time.

Sources of error in blood gas analysis

- Air bubbles
- Excess heparinized saline dilutes the blood, giving a lower reading of PO_2 and PCO_2. This also decreases the pH of the sample as it is acidic, and very strong solutions may increase PCO_2 as bicarbonate is neutralized
- Not discarding the heparinized blood in the catheter
- Application of excessive negative pressure when taking the sample causes escape of gases from solution and entrainment of air into the sample
- Inadequate mixing
- Some electrodes may cause under-reading of PO_2 by 2–6%, because the electrode itself uses up oxygen in the blood in contact with it, which is not replaced due to the slow diffusion of oxygen in fluids
- Accumulation of blood proteins on the surface of the pH electrode results in inaccurate readings
- Blood gas analysers assume body temperature is 37°C. A low body temperature will result in under-reading of PCO_2 and overestimation of pH. Blood gas results should be corrected by the instrument to reflect the body temperature of the patient.

Transcutaneous blood gas monitoring

If skin is warmed to 44°C, dissolved gases in the blood diffuse through the skin. Transcutaneous blood gas analysers consist of a pH sensor, a heater and a thermistor. The thermistor and heater regulate the skin temperature below the probe to 44°C, and the probe attaches to the skin surface using a sticky patch and contact fluid. Transcutaneous PO_2 ($P_{TC}O_2$) tends to be lower than PaO_2. Carbon dioxide from the skin diffuses through a permeable membrane and combines with water to produce H^+ and HCO_3^-. The pH sensor measures the concentration of H^+ in the solution and from this derives the PCO_2. The transcutaneous PCO_2 ($P_{TC}CO_2$) is approximately 20 mm Hg higher than $PaCO_2$, and under stable conditions a change in $PaCO_2$ is followed after a delay of 3–4 minutes by a corresponding change in $P_{TC}CO_2$.

Limitations

- Trends are more useful than absolute values when using transcutaneous blood gas monitoring
- Slow response time — the probes take about an hour to warm up to a functioning temperature, and the delay in responding to change in blood gases precludes its use in emergency situations
- Transcutaneous blood gas monitoring tends to become less accurate in sick patients in whom skin perfusion is poor. Therefore the use of this monitoring method in critical patients is probably limited
- The sticky patch must be maintained on a horizontal surface to prevent the contact liquid from draining away. The technique is most useful, therefore, in patients that are immobile.

ASSESSMENT OF PAIN IN CRITICAL PATIENTS

Control of pain is vital to optimize the outcome of patients in the intensive care unit. Pain is detrimental to the patient for the following reasons:

- It causes suffering
- It may result in reduced food intake and enhance the stress response, leading to a catabolic state
- It delays wound healing
- It may impair respiration, leading to hypoxia, hypercapnoea and acidosis
- It may result in interference with the wound site, and self-mutilation.

Pain may be assessed objectively by monitoring changes in physiological parameters, or subjectively by assessing changes in behaviour. Physiological parameters that may indicate pain include tachycardia, tachypnoea, raised blood pressure and increased serum cortisol, catecholamine and glucose levels. Obviously, however, all of these parameters can also be affected by other factors. For example, hypovolaemia may cause tachycardia, decreased lung compliance may cause tachypnoea, stress will increase catecholamine and glucose levels, and so on. For this reason, physiological parameters should be used in conjunction with the clinical picture to assess the need for analgesia.

Pain may be assessed subjectively by observing for abnormal behaviour that indicates the animal is suffering. It is useful to have some experience of the animal's normal behaviour in order to assess accurately changes in behaviour due to pain. Pain-related behaviour can include:

- Vocalization: crying, whimpering, hissing or growling
- Unusual body posture: hunched, rigid, prolonged recumbency
- Restlessness: unable to settle or sleep
- Attention to wound: chewing, licking
- Change of character: aggression, fear, depression, disinterest.

Pain can be assessed more objectively by using a simple four-point numerical scale, ranging from 0 (no behavioural signs of pain and no resentment to palpation of wounds) to 3 (obvious behavioural signs of pain and serious resentment to palpation of wounds).

Pain should be assessed at set time intervals, i.e. reassess every hour and record the findings on the ICU monitoring sheet. In this way, analgesia is not forgotten and can be varied according to the animal's needs.

MONITORING RENAL PERFUSION AND FUNCTION

Practical methods for direct evaluation of renal function are limited, measurement of indirect variables such as urine volume and specific gravity is used, combined with serum chemistry, to assess adequate renal perfusion and function.

Urine volume

Urine output may be monitored as a sign of adequacy of renal perfusion, based on the assumption that patients with diminished renal perfusion excrete a low volume of concentrated urine. The rate of urine production is, however, an indirect indicator of renal function because many non-renal factors may directly and profoundly affect renal output. The presence of urine flow (regardless of the amount) indicates that there is blood flow to the kidney. Generally, a urine production rate of 1–2 ml/kg/h is considered normal. Measurement of urine production requires catheterization and connection of the urinary catheter to a sterile closed urinary collection system. This may prove difficult in the bitch and queen and may be associated with a risk of ascending urinary tract infection. In critical patients the vital information obtained using an indwelling urinary catheter is often worth the risk of infection, but these catheters are left in place for the minimum time necessary. Catheterization and maintenance of the indwelling system should be carried out in an aseptic manner.

Urine specific gravity

The urine specific gravity (USG) is a measure of the total urine solute concentration. It is very simple and relatively cheap to monitor this parameter. The isosthenuric range (USG 1.007-1.015) relates to urine of the same solute concentration as unaltered glomerular filtrate. Dogs and cats normally excrete urine which is moderately concentrated. In the presence of dehydration or hypovolaemia, the USG should increase if kidney function is adequate, as water and sodium are conserved.

Serum creatinine and urea

Repeated measurement of serum urea and creatinine is a cheap and practical method of monitoring renal function. Urea concentration increases when renal excretion is impaired, during volume depletion, following a high-protein meal or in the presence of starvation, infection or fever. Urea may decrease with factors unrelated to renal function, such as severe hepatic disease, or during treatment with anabolic steroids. Therefore, the non-renal effects on serum urea concentration limit its usefulness as a test of renal function. In contrast, serum creatinine is much less affected by diet and other non-renal factors and is therefore more reliable as an indication of renal function. Increases in serum creatinine and urea concentrations are late signs of renal dysfunction. In the absence of pre-renal disease, the glomerular filtration rate must be reduced by as much as 75% before these parameters reach abnormal levels.

MONITORING BODY TEMPERATURE

Core body temperature affects cellular metabolism, function and oxygen demand. Severe or prolonged body temperature derangements are common in critical patients and are usually due to increased heat loss or reduced functioning of homeostatic mechanisms. Reduced homeostasis reflects decreased central control (CNS depression) or reduced compensatory mechanisms (reduced muscular activity, fluid losses). Elevated body temperature (fever) reflects a re-setting of the thermoregulatory setpoint in the hypothalamus, as a response to circulating inflammatory cytokines. Rarely, increased body temperature may be present owing to increased heat production (muscle activity in tetanus or status epilepticus) or due to iatrogenic body warming (waterbed, heat lamp or enclosed oxygen cage). Prolonged or severe abnormalities in body temperature may lead to multiple organ dysfunction. Peripheral temperature monitoring may not reflect core body temperature owing to compensatory vasoconstriction.

Recently, non-invasive tympanic thermometry has become available for veterinary use. These hand-held devices evaluate tympanic temperature with a response time of 5 seconds. Caution should be exercised in their use as they may not always be able to adequately contact the tympanic membrane, depending on the conformation of the animal's ear canal. If these instruments read accurately, tympanic temperature closely reflects hypothalamic temperature (site of thermoregulatory centre) and is an accurate measure of core temperature.

More traditionally, rectal temperature may be measured with either a traditional rectal thermometer or more usefully a continuously recording indwelling rectal probe. Continuous measurement is important when patient rewarming is applied (heat pad or waterbed). Rectal measurements are prone to underestimation of core temperature due to local alterations in rectal blood flow or air in the rectum. Some electronic temperature monitors also have the ability to monitor toe-web temperature. Although less a reflection of core temperature than peripheral perfusion, when measured in combination with rectal or tympanic temperature, toe-web temperature allows assessment of core-to-peripheral temperature difference and changes in peripheral circulation with therapy.

Conclusion

Critical care monitoring provides the basis for the evaluation of the progression of a patient's disease and that patient's response to veterinary intervention and management. Recently introduced accurate and sensitive equipment is now widely available and applicable for veterinary intensive care. Its use should not, however, detract from basic monitoring skills, overall patient evaluation and measurement of less glamorous but important parameters, such as core body temperature. Good critical care monitoring does not rely on expensive equipment but on an ability to measure, interpret and appreciate the significance of trends in relevant parameters.

FURTHER READING

Hines L (1995) *Monitoring in Anesthesia and Critical Care Medicine.* Churchill Livingstone, Edinburgh

Martin L (1999) *All You Really Need to Know to Interpret Arterial Blood Gases.* Lippincott, Williams & Wilkins, Philadelphia

CHAPTER SEVENTEEN

Cardiopulmonary–Cerebral Resuscitation (CPCR) in Dogs and Cats

William W. Muir

INTRODUCTION

Cardiopulmonary–cerebral resuscitation continues to command a great deal of interest and occupy a large number of written pages in both research and clinical journals because of its catastrophic nature, the development of new treatment modalities, the clinical use of sophisticated monitoring techniques and the natural aversion to death (Niemann, 1992). Cardiopulmonary arrest is defined as an abrupt cessation of spontaneous and effective ventilation and systemic perfusion (circulation) which leads to inadequate oxygen delivery to tissues, shock and death. Common causes include anaesthetic overdose, trauma (multiple fractures, head injury, coma) with or without exsanguination, acute cardiac failure from cardiac arrhythmias or myocardial disease (cardiomyopathy, valvular insufficiency) and debilitating diseases.

Cardiopulmonary–cerebral resuscitation (CPCR) is an organized preplanned approach for providing artificial support of ventilation and circulation (basic life support) until spontaneous breathing and circulation can be restored and sustained (advanced life support). It is interesting to note, however, that regardless of the progress made in our understanding of pathophysiological processes and therapeutic potentialities, little or no improvement in long-term survival (patient leaves the hospital) following CPCR has been reported. Indeed, although several studies suggest initial survival rates ranging from 20% to 75%, most critical reviews of long-term survival following cardiopulmonary resuscitation in dogs and cats note that less than 5% of the patients resuscitated ever leave the hospital (Kass and Haskins, 1992; Wingfield and Van Pelt, 1992). There are many reasons for the discrepancies in the survival rate percentages reported, including the criteria used to determine when resuscitation should be initiated, which patients were selected for resuscitation, definitions of successful resuscitation and a host of patient-related (e.g. age, disease status), personnel (training, preparedness) and environmental (monitoring capabilities) considerations. Certainly the best method for improving patient survival is to maximize patient monitoring, have immediate access to drugs and equipment and to become familiar with the techniques and therapeutic interventions necessary to perform CPCR. Stated in different terms, 'an ounce of prevention is worth a pound of cure' and 'practice makes perfect'.

WHEN TO RESUSCITATE

The decision to begin CPCR is based upon clinical signs, consideration of the potential outcome and a previous agreement (if possible) with the animal owner (Figure 17.1). Patients that have a treatable disease should be resuscitated. CPCR should not be performed in animals in the terminal stages of an incurable disease (hepatic, renal or cardiac failure), those that have suffered severe head trauma with brain damage, where there is no reasonable chance of restoring near-normal mentation, or when the owner of the animal has instructed the veterinary surgeon not to resuscitate.

PHASES OF CPCR

Once the decision to perform CPCR has been made, basic and advanced life support should be initiated as rapidly as possible in a sequential, orderly and predetermined manner. All pertinent personnel should be prepared for and have practised appropriate CPCR techniques (Figures 17.2 and 17.3). Basic life support includes establishing and maintaining an airway (A), controlling breathing (B) and circulatory (C) support via the initiation of manual chest compression. Advanced life support includes measures that lead to the establishment and maintenance of spontaneous breathing and circulation at or above normal values via the administration of drugs (D), evaluation of the electrocardiogram (E) and treatment of cardiac arrhythmias, including ventricular fibrillation (F).

Airway

The first and most essential step in performing CPCR is the establishment of a secure and patent airway. The most effective way to achieve this goal is by endotracheal intubation with a cuffed endotracheal tube. The head should be extended and pulled forward prior to endotracheal intubation. Occasionally, animals become

Changes in the effort, rate or rhythm of breathing
Dyspnoea (abdominal breathing)
Gasps (gurgling sounds)
Tachypnoea
Bradypnoea
Apnoea
Altered patterns of breathing
    Periodic breathing
    Agonal breathing

Absence of pulse
The peripheral arterial pulse becomes difficult, if not impossible, to palpate at arterial blood pressures <40–50 mmHg

Irregular or inaudible heart sounds
Heart sounds of varying intensity suggest a cardiac arrhythmia (atrial fibrillation, ventricular tachycardia) Heart sounds become difficult to hear at arterial blood pressures <50 mmHg

Changes in heart rate or rhythm
Tachycardia
Bradycardia
Irregular rhythm

Absence of bleeding

Altered peripheral perfusion
Change in mucous membrane colour:
    Pale or white
    Blue or cyanotic: 5 g/dl of reduced haemoglobin produces a bluish discoloration of the mucous membranes regardless of the haemoglobin concentration. Anaemic animals (<5 g/dl haemoglobin) do not demonstrate cyanosis

Pupillary dilation
The pupils dilate within 1–2 minutes of cardiac arrest

Depression or coma

Figure 17.1: *Signs and symptoms of impending cardiopulmonary arrest.*

Drugs
Atropine/glycopyrrolate
Calcium chloride
Dexamethasone sodium phosphate
Adrenaline
Dopamine
Dobutamine
Frusemide
Lignocaine
Sodium bicarbonate
Lactated Ringer's solution bags

Supplies
Pressure bag
Ambu bag
Various size endotracheal tubes
Laryngoscopes
Isopropyl alcohol
Nolvasan/betadine scrub
Hypodermic needles, various sizes
Syringes, various sizes
Assorted intravenous catheters
Intravenous administrations sets
2 x 2″, 4 x 4″ gauze sponges
1/2″, 1″, 2″ tape
2″ roll of gauze
Polyethylene urinary catheters
Suture material
Stopcocks
Cut down tray with loaded scalpel
Clippers
Electrocardiogram monitor
Defibrillator
External and sterile internal defibrillator paddles

Figure 17.2: *Emergency cart supplies.*

cyanotic and subsequently unconscious because mucus, soft tissue structures (soft palate, tongue) or foreign material such as food obstruct the upper airway. Brachycephalic breeds are particularly susceptible to upper airway obstruction during recovery from anaesthesia. Excessive mucus or foreign material should be removed manually or by suction.

When airway obstruction is severe or cannot be removed, an emergency tracheostomy should be performed. A 3–5 cm incision is made on the ventral midline parallel to the trachea, 2–4 cm caudal to the larynx, on the ventral midline parallel to the trachea (Figure 17.4). The tissue over the trachea is bluntly dissected and an incision is made between the tracheal rings, through which an endotracheal tube is placed. In animals with upper airway obstruction, transtracheal catheter ventilation, an alternative to tracheostomy, is less traumatic and does not predispose to infection (Reich and Mingus, 1990). Ventilation is achieved by transcutaneously puncturing the trachea with a 14 gauge

plastic intravenous over-the-needle catheter assembly. The catheter is attached to venous extension tubing and a hand operated oxygen release valve. Oxygen flow rates are initially adjusted to 50 ml/kg. This technique has the advantage of providing 100% oxygen directly into the trachea and is relatively non-traumatic. Tracheostomy remains the technique of choice, however, when upper airway obstruction inhibits normal breathing. Tracheostomy is also preferred in conscious animals that require ventilatory assistance, because of the difficulty in maintaining orotracheal intubation (retching, gagging, vomiting).

Breathing

Controlled or assisted ventilation can be accomplished by connecting a properly placed endotracheal tube to a self-inflating bag, demand valve or anaesthetic machine (Figure 17.5). Respiratory rate should be between 6 and 12 breaths per minute. Ratios of one breath to five chest compressions or two breaths per 10–15 chest compressions are used when simultaneously performing chest compressions. The amount of gas volume delivered (tidal volume) should approximate 15 ml/kg at a peak inspiratory pressure of 20–25 cm H_2O. This volume is generally delivered with minimum expansion of the chest or movement of the

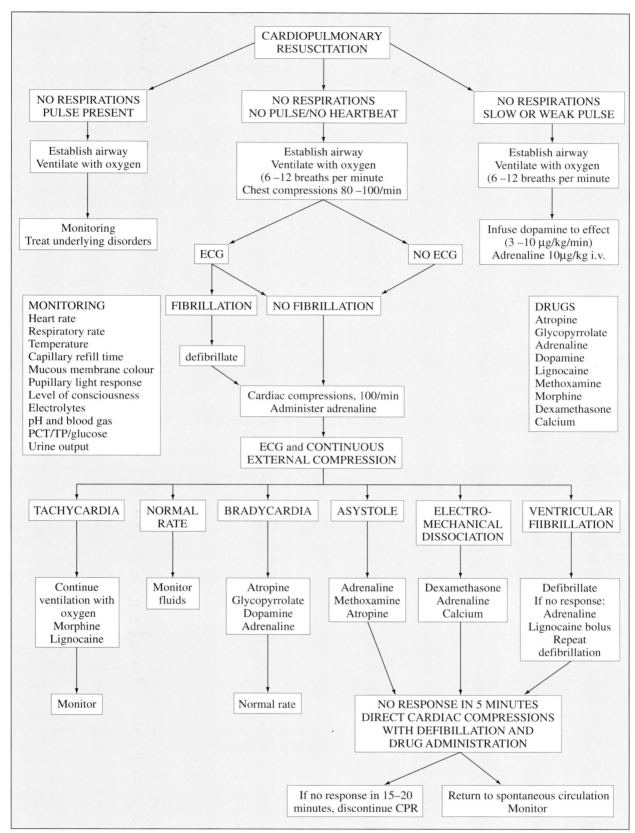

Figure 17.3: *Cardiopulmonary resuscitation flow chart.*

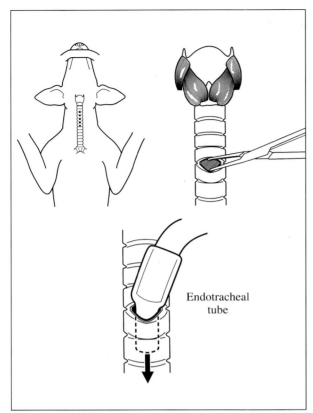

Figure 17.4: *A tracheostomy is performed as illustrated after creating a ventral midline incision.*

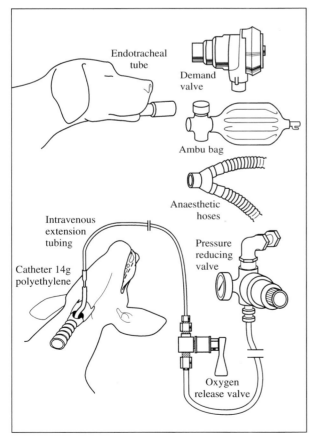

Figure 17.5: *Methods of providing oxygen.*

abdomen. The lungs of cats, neonates and patients with restrictive types of lung disease (e.g. pneumonia, adult respiratory distress syndrome (ARDS), pulmonary fibrosis, diaphragmatic hernia) are easily overinflated. Lung overexpansion can lead to pulmonary barotrauma, pulmonary haemorrhage and pneumothorax. Smaller tidal volumes (10 ml/kg) at greater respiratory rates (15–20) should be used in these patients.

Inspiratory time should be approximately 1.5 seconds. Excessively long inspiratory times (>3 seconds) or the maintenance of positive end expiratory pressure (PEEP) >10 cm H_2O) increase intrathoracic pressure, thereby decreasing venous return, cardiac output and arterial blood pressure. Small amounts (3–5 cm H_2O) of PEEP, however, are not harmful and are inconsequential when the thoracic cavity is open to the atmosphere (open thorax), as during internal cardiac massage, and may improve arterial oxygenation. Mechanical artificial respiratory assist devices, particularly pressure-cycled ventilators, perform poorly during CPCR. The intrathoracic pressure fluctuations produced by chest compression cause mechanical respirators to prematurely initiate or terminate the inspiratory cycle, resulting in inadequate ventilation.

Mouth-to-nose ventilation is performed when endotracheal tubes and ventilatory assist devices are not available. This is accomplished by cupping both hands around the animal's muzzle, placing the operator's mouth against the thumbs (attempting to produce an airtight seal) and blowing air into the animal's mouth. Inflation of the stomach with air may occur, but can be avoided by pushing the larynx dorsally in order to occlude the oesophagus. This technique is inefficient, but easily performed and can be life saving in puppies and kittens or in larger dogs and cats in acute respiratory distress situations after removal of foreign material from the upper airway.

Kinking or mucus obstruction of the endotracheal tube, oesophageal intubation and accidental intubation of one of the mainstem bronchi make it difficult to inflate the lungs (high inspiratory pressure) and frequently produce dyspnoea and cyanosis. Other conditions that restrict breathing include pleural effusions, diaphragmatic hernia and pneumothorax. Auscultation and percussion of the chest are helpful and rapid diagnostic techniques which may differentiate between these problems. Muffled heart sounds and a dull response to percussion are indicative of fluid or tissue in the thoracic cavity. Normal heart sounds and a hyper-resonant chest are indicative of pneumothorax or tension pneumothorax. A chest drain should be used to remove excessive fluid or air, particularly when tension pneumothorax is suspected.

Ventilatory support should not be stopped once signs of spontaneous ventilation begin. Intermittent positive pressure ventilation is usually necessary until the patient regains consciousness. Listening to the end of the endotracheal tube, watching for normal ventilatory movement of the chest wall and continued monitoring of mucous membrane colour and capillary refill time will help to assess the adequacy of ventilation. Nasal oxygen and oxygen cages help to maintain arterial oxygenation in conscious animals (Fitzpatrick and Crowe, 1986). The measurement of arterial pH and blood gases on a point of care analyser or non-invasive assessment of oxygen saturation using pulse oximetry (SpO_2 >90%) and end-tidal capnography ($ETCO_2$ 30–40 mmHg) are also helpful in assessing patient status.

Circulation

The restoration of normal cardiac electrical and pumping activity is dependent upon the early restoration of myocardial oxygenation and blood flow. Blood flow is initiated and supported by compressing the chest wall. Blood moves through the heart and vessels during chest compression due to direct cardiac compression in cats and narrow-chested dogs (cardiac pump mechanism), and phasic increases in intrathoracic pressure, which collapses intrathoracic veins, in larger animals (thoracic pump mechanism; Peters and Ihle, 1990). The ideal chest compression rate in dogs and cats is approximately 100 compressions per minute, devoting equal time to compression and relaxation.

Effective chest compression in small animals is accomplished by compressing the chest wall from side to side with the animal in lateral recumbency (Figure 17.6). The heel of one hand compresses one side of the chest wall while the palm of the other hand or a sand-filled pillow is placed under the opposing chest wall for support. The thumb and forefinger can be used to accomplish the same manoeuvre in cats and very small dogs. Attention should be focused upon how fast the heel of the hand compresses the thorax, not the force necessary to compress the chest, although enough force must be generated to produce an obvious indentation of the chest wall of approximately 1–3 cm depending on patient size.

The patient should be ventilated once between every fifth or sixth chest compression or 2–3 times for every 10–15 chest compressions. Blood flow to the brain and heart is more effectively maintained by administering chest compressions simultaneously with ventilation at relatively high airway pressures (30–40 cm H_2O), and simultaneous abdominal binding (Koehler *et al.*, 1983). Intermittent slow abdominal compression (counter pressure) appears to be another effective means of improving blood flow during resuscitative efforts. Abdominal counter pressure is accomplished by having a second person use the palms of both hands to compress the abdominal cavity slowly at approximately 20 second intervals. Alternatively, the abdomen may be temporarily bound during CPR with an elastic bandage or towel if extra help is not available. Signs of restoration of effective peripheral blood flow include improvement in mucous membrane colour, decrease in capillary refill time, a reduction in pupil size and the restoration of a peripheral arterial pulse. If spontaneous cardiac contraction is occurring, the peripheral arterial pulse should be evaluated during a short pause in chest compression because shock waves carried into the femoral veins during chest compression may be mistaken for an arterial pulse.

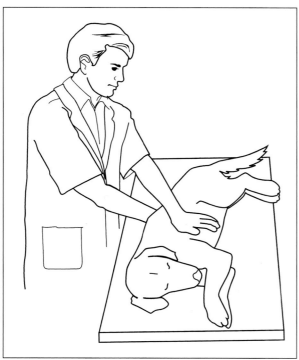
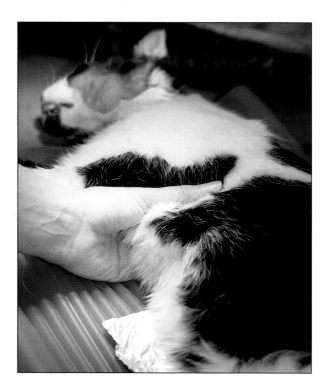

Figure 17.6: *Chest compression in the dog and cat.*

Attempts to maintain peripheral blood flow by chest compression should be evaluated within 3–4 minutes of initiation. If signs of successful resuscitation are not evident or if the patient continues to deteriorate (bradycardia or cardiac arrest), the chest should be opened and internal (direct) cardiac massage initiated. Severe chest trauma, fractured ribs, pneumothorax, haemothorax, pericardial effusion, diaphragmatic hernia and other primary thoracic diseases (neoplasms, foreign bodies) are reasons for immediately initiating direct cardiac compression. The chest is opened by making an incision from the top of the scapula to approximately 4 cm from the sternum on the left thoracic wall between the fourth and fifth ribs. The hair should be clipped and antiseptic solution applied to the skin before incision. Care must be taken not to damage the lung when entering the thoracic cavity. Once the chest is entered, the fourth and fifth ribs are spread apart and the lungs are reflected dorsally and caudally. The pericardium is grasped and opened near the apex of the heart, and reflected dorsally exposing the ventricles. The heart is grasped between the thumb and forefinger and direct cardiac massage initiated at a rate of approximately 100 compressions per minute. Excessive force during direct cardiac compression should be avoided as it can result in the development of severe cardiac trauma, cardiac arrhythmias and ventricular fibrillation. The colour, tone and rhythm of the heart can be evaluated once the chest is open. Colour can be improved by appropriate ventilation and cardiac compression. Cardiac contractile function and rhythm can be improved by normalizing acid–base and electrolyte balance and the administration of cardiotonic or antiarrhythmic drugs. In larger dogs, the aorta can be compressed dorsally against the spine with the thumb of the opposite hand, which promotes blood flow to the heart and brain. Direct cardiac compression (chest open) always produces better blood flow than chest wall compression, but does require surgical intervention and predisposes to infection.

DRUGS

No drug should be used to replace the establishment of an airway (A), breathing (B) and circulation (C). Drugs should always be administered by bolus injection and followed by 1–3 ml of crystalloid (lactated Ringer's) flush through a peripheral vein (Figure 17.7). Drug administration should occur simultaneously with chest compression, if possible, since the chest compressions are responsible for blood flow and the delivery of the drug to the heart and brain. Intravenous drug administration is preferred, although intracardiac and intratracheal (endobronchial) routes can be used when venous access is not readily available (Mazkereth et al., 1992). Using the intracardiac route, drugs are deliberately injected into the lumen of the left ventricle in order to hasten their delivery to the coronary arteries and ventricular myocardium. Intracardiac injections are easily performed during open chest resuscitation, but are not recommended prior to opening the chest, since inadvertent pneumothorax, haemopericardium, or intramyocardial injections leading to cardiac arrhythmias can occur. The intracardiac drug dose is generally one-half the intravenous dose, while the endobronchial dose is 2–3 times the recommended intravenous dose. Adrenaline, atropine and lignocaine can be administered by the endobronchial route. They are diluted in 1 ml/5 kg of saline and followed by two or three manual lung inflations in order to promote drug distribution and absorption from the lung. It is noteworthy that acupuncture stimulation of Governing vessel 26 (GV 26; Jen Chung) has been used successfully to restore respiratory and cardiac function in cats, dogs, kittens and puppies. Acupuncture therapy consists of vigorous pricking and twirling of a 25 gauge needle 2–4 mm deep in GV 26, a point located in the 'T' formed in the philtrum below the nose or in the midline of the nasolabial cleft at the level of the lower canthi with the nostrils (Janssens et al., 1979; Altman, 1997).

Adrenaline, a catecholamine, is the first drug selected for the treatment of severe bradycardia, severe hypotension and cardiac arrest. Adrenaline increases heart rate, arterial blood pressure and blood flow. Although large doses of adrenaline (0.2 mg/kg i.v.) are recommended when resuscitation is unwitnessed or delayed, smaller doses (0.01–0.02 mg/kg i.v.) should be used to treat the acute development of bradycardia or ventricular asystole (Figure 17.8; Brown et al., 1992). Adrenaline overdose can produce ventricular arrhythmias, ventricular fibrillation and cardiac contracture (stone heart).

Atropine and glycopyrrolate are anticholinergics that are particularly effective in treating bradyarrhythmias caused by increases in vagal tone. Opioids (morphine, oxymorphone, fentanyl), α_2- agonists (xylazine, medetomidine, romifidine) and occasionally inhalant anaesthetics (halothane, isoflurane) can produce bradyarrhythmias that are responsive to anticholinergic therapy. Profound bradycardia, asystole and bradyarrhythmias that are unresponsive to an initial dose of either atropine or glycopyrrolate should be treated with adrenaline. Excessive doses of anticholinergics can produce sinus tachycardia and predispose to ventricular arrhythmias. If the cause for bradycardia is unknown low doses (0.01 mg/kg i.v.) of adrenaline should be administered.

Either dopamine (3–10 µg/kg/min i.v.) or dobutamine (5–20 µg/kg/min i.v.) are used to maintain arterial blood pressure and blood flow once heart rate, rhythm and a palpable pulse have been restored. Dopamine is the preferred drug if heart rate continues to be slow while dobutamine is preferred when heart rate is within normal limits or elevated. Dopamine is more likely to increase heart rate than dobutamine, but

Drug	Indications	Dosage	Actions
Atropine sulphate	Sinus bradycardia Atrioventricular block Ventricular asystole	0.04 mg/kg i.v. 0.4 mg/kg intratracheally	Parasympatholytic
Glycopyrrolate	Sinus bradycardia Atrioventricular block Ventricular asystole	0.004–0.010 mg/kg i.v.	Parasympatholytic
Calcium chloride	Hyperkalaemia Hypocalcaemia Calcium channel-blocker toxicity Hypermagnesaemia	1–2 ml i.v. to effect; closely observe the ECG	Positive inotrope
Diltiazem	Supraventricular tachycardia Ventricular fibrillation Hypertrophic cardiomyopathy	Dogs: 0.5–1.5 mg/kg tid orally Cats: 1.75–2.4 mg/kg tid–bid orally Dogs, Cats: 0.25 mg/kg i.v. bolus, to cumulative dose of 0.75 mg/kg 5–10 µg/kg/min CRI	Calcium channel blocker
Dobutamine	Myocardial failure Low cardiac output	5–20 µg/kg/min CRI	Synthetic catecholamine Positive inotrope
Dopamine	Bradycardia Low cardiac output Low renal or mesenteric blood flow	3–5 µg/kg/min CRI for increased renal perfusion 5–10 µg/kg/min for increased cardiac output	Dopaminergic ß$_1$ agonist Noradrenaline precursor
Adrenaline	Severe bradycardia Ventricular fibrillation Ventricular asystole Electromechanical dissociation	0.01–0.2 mg/kg i.v. bolus q 3–5 min 0.04–0.4 mg/kg intratracheally 1.0 µg/kg/min i.v., CRI	α and ß-agonist
Methoxamine	Ventricular fibrillation Ventricular asystole Electromechanical dissociation	2.2–10 mg/kg i.v.	α-agonist
Frusemide	Cerebral/pulmonary oedema Congestive heart failure Hypertension Anuria/oligouria	Dogs: 2–4 mg/kg orally i.m., i.v. Cats: 1–2 mg/kg orally i.m., i.v.	Loop diuretic
Lignocaine	Ventricular tachycardia Ventricular fibrillation	Dogs: 2–8 mg/kg i.v. bolus followed by 40–60 µg/kg/min CRI	Class 1B ventricular antiarrhythmic
Magnesium chloride	Unresponsive ventricular arrhythmias Chemical defibrillator Severe hypotension	10–15 mg/kg i.v. given slowly over 5 min	Electrolyte chemical defibrillator
Mannitol	Cerebral oedema Free radical scavenger Anuria/oliguria	0.5–1 gm/kg i.v.	Osmotic diuretic
Morphine sulphate	Analgesic Vasodilator Pulmonary oedema Sedative	0.04–0.08 mg/kg i.m. i.v., s.c.	Narcotic analgesic
Naloxone	Electromechanical dissociation Narcotic overdose	0.03 mg/kg i.v. or intrathecally	Opiate antagonist
Sodium bicarbonate	Severe metabolic acidosis	0.5–1–2 mEq/kg i.v.	Alkalinizing agent

Figure 17.7: Drugs commonly employed during and following cardiopulmonary resuscitation.

Route	Dose (mg/kg)	Comments

Intravenous
    Arrest/fibrillation
    Severe hypotension
    Bradycardia
	0.01–0.05
	0.01–0.02
		Used to treat unwitnessed cardiac arrest[*]
		Used to treat witnessed cardiac arrest and bradycardia

Intracardiac	0.005–0.01	For bradycardia
Intratracheal	0.05–0.2	Dilute with 0.9% saline to 1 ml/5 kg and breathe 3–4 times following administration

Figure 17.8: *Emergency doses of adrenaline. *Note: Larger doses of adrenaline (0.1–0.2 mg/kg; i.v.) are used if arrest is unwitnessed and suspected to have been present for greater than 2–3 minutes.*

both drugs increase arterial blood pressure and systemic blood flow. As with all catecholamines, excessive doses can cause sinus tachycardia, ventricular arrhythmias and ventricular fibrillation.

Lignocaine, a local anaesthetic, possesses potent antiarrhythmic, antishock and analgesic effects. Lignocaine is particularly effective in treating ventricular arrhythmias providing the patient is not hypokalaemic (K^+ <3.0 mEq/l). Neurological side-effects (muscle twitching, seizures) may occur if excessive doses are administered, particularly to cats. Initial bolus doses should not exceed 4 mg/kg in dogs and 1 mg/kg in cats. A lignocaine infusion (40–60 µg/kg/min) is used to produce sustained effects for periods of up to 24–48 hours when necessary.

Sodium bicarbonate is used to treat non-respiratory (metabolic) acidosis. Hypoxia results in anaerobic metabolism and lactic acidosis, which is responsible for central nervous system depression, myocardial depression and the production and release of tissue destructive metabolites. Excessive sodium bicarbonate administration, however, produces alkalaemia, decreases serum ionized calcium and impairs the release of oxygen from haemoglobin. The initial dose of sodium bicarbonate should not exceed 1 mEq/kg unless there is evidence for severe non-respiratory acidosis (dehydration, diarrhoea, acid–base values). Subsequent doses (0.5 mEq/kg i.v.) of sodium bicarbonate should be administered every 10 minutes until the circulation is restored or resuscitative efforts are terminated.

Atropine and glycopyrrolate are anticholinergics that are particularly effective in treating bradyarrhythmias caused by increases in vagal tone. Opioids (morphine, oxymorphone, fentanyl), α_2- agonists (xylazine, medetomidine, romifidine) and occasionally inhalant anaesthetics (halothane, isoflurane) can produce bradyarrhythmias that are responsive to anticholinergic therapy. Profound bradycardia, asystole and bradyarrhythmias that are unresponsive to an initial dose of either atropine or glycopyrrolate should be treated with adrenaline. Excessive doses of anticholinergics can produce sinus tachycardia and predispose to ventricular arrhythmias. If the cause of bradycardia is unknown, low doses (0.01 mg/kg i.v.) of adrenaline should be administered.

Other drugs that have been used for the acute treatment of cardiac arrest include calcium chloride, diltiazem, magnesium chloride and methoxamine (see Figure 17.7; Redding *et al.*, 1983; Capparelli *et al.*, 1992). None of these drugs has been shown to improve long-term outcome, although the administration of calcium containing solutions is therapeutic in patients that are hypocalcaemic, hyperkalaemic, or that have been administered an excessive dose of a calcium channel blocking drug (verapamil, diltiazem).

ELECTROCARDIOGRAPHY

An electrocardiogram is essential for accurate diagnosis of cardiac rhythm disturbances and provides valuable insight as to appropriate drug selection. A normal electrocardiogram, however, does not ensure that cardiac contractile function is adequate to maintain arterial blood pressure or adequate peripheral blood flow (Figures 17.9 and 17.10).

Pulseless electrical activity (PEA) is a catch-all term used to describe patients that have electrocardiographic evidence of a cardiac rhythm, an auscultatable heartbeat, but a very weak or non-palpable peripheral arterial pulse. Clinically, patients in normal sinus rhythm but with a systolic arterial blood pressure below 50 mmHg are considered to be demonstrating PEA. If not treated, this condition deteriorates to ventricular asystole or ventricular fibrillation due to poor myocardial perfusion, hypoxia and acidosis. Either dopamine or dobutamine and intravenous fluids are therapeutic if treatment is initiated immediately. Once severe bradycardia occurs, adrenaline is the drug of choice.

Bradyarrhythmias (sinus bradycardia, third degree heart block, ventricular escape rhythm) are a potential cause for cardiac arrest or fibrillation and are a common occurrence in anaesthetized and toxic patients (pyometra), or immediately after successful cardiopulmonary resuscitation. Sinus bradycardia and junctional escape rhythms are frequently observed prior to ventricular asystole or fibrillation, while junctional and ventricular (idioventricular) escape rhythms develop after defibrillation (Figure 17.10). These rhythm distur-

Cause	Peripheral pulse	Auscultation of heart sounds	ECG	Visual observation of heart
Pulseless electrical activity (PEA)	Very weak or absent	Normal, muffled or none	Normal P–QRS–T; rapid, normal or slow heart rate	Weak cardiac contractions; poor cardiac filling
Bradycardia (supraventricular or ventricular)	Slow, may be irregular	Normal or muffled; infrequent	Infrequent P–QRS–T or ventricular complexes; junctional or ventricular escape complexes	Infrequent co-ordinated ventricular contractions
Supraventricular tachycardia	Rapid, may be weak, pulse deficit	Normal or muffled intensity; may be irregular	Normal QRS–T; may have inverted or abnormal P waves, P wave is buried in previous T wave	Rapid, occasionally irregular, heart rate
Ventricular tachycardia	Weak, rapid pulse deficit; may be irregular	Muffled; may be variable intensity	Wide QRS–T complexes; absence of P–QRS relationship; large T waves	Disorganized, rapidly beating heart
Ventricular asystole (cardiac arrest)	None	None	Absence of QRS–T complexes; straight flat-line ECG	No cardiac movement
Electromechanical dissociation (EMD)	None	None	Normal P–QRS–T or ventricular complexes	Weak or absent cardiac contractions; no peripheral pulse
Ventricular fibrillation	None	None	Absence of QRS–T complexes; fibrillation waves	Fine to coarse rippling of the ventricular myocardium

Figure 17.9: *Distinguishing characteristics of several types of cardiac rhythm or arrest disorders.*

bances are impossible to distinguish from one another without an electrocardiogram. Their haemodynamic consequences are similar, resulting in hypotension and poor systemic blood flow. Patients that present with slow junctional or idioventricular escape rhythms should be suspected of suffering from severe hypoxia, hyperkalaemia or systemic toxicity. Therapy includes anticholinergics (atropine, glycopyrrolate), adrenaline or specific techniques to lower serum potassium. Saline, sodium bicarbonate, calcium chloride and hyperventilation are therapeutic when acute hyperkalaemia is responsible for the bradyarrhythmia. When the cause for the acute onset of bradycardia is unknown, the first steps should be to administer oxygen, begin chest compression and administer adrenaline and/or atropine. Adrenaline should also be administered intravenously when the heart rate is rapidly slowing and peripheral pulses are not palpable.

Ventricular tachycardia may be difficult to distinguish from sinus tachycardia without the aid of an electrocardiogram, since both can produce a weak peripheral pulse. Lignocaine is the drug of choice for the treatment of most ventricular arrhythmias and is administered intravenously as a bolus or infusion. Intravenous procainamide (5–10 mg/kg, i.v.) can be used as an alternative if lignocaine is not effective in restoring normal sinus rhythm. The serum potassium concentration should be determined and normalized (4–5 mEq/l), since most anti-arrhythmics are ineffec-

tive in hypokalaemic patients and toxic in hyperkalaemic patients. If the peripheral pulse remains weak after normal sinus rhythm has been restored, infusions of fluids, dopamine or dobutamine can be administered to improve cardiac contractile force, increase arterial blood pressure and enhance peripheral perfusion once normal sinus rhythm is restored, if the peripheral pulse remains weak. Alternatively, low intravenous doses of adrenaline can be administered. In the post-arrest patient, intravenous sodium bicarbonate (0.5 mEq/kg i.v.) can assist with restoration of normal sinus rhythm. Ideally, sodium bicarbonate administration is based upon arterial pH and blood gas determination.

Ventricular asystole is difficult, if not impossible, to distinguish from ventricular fibrillation without an electrocardiogram (Figure 17.10). This distinction is helpful, since ventricular asystole may respond to chest compression and the administration of adrenaline, while ventricular fibrillation requires electrical defibrillation. In either case, an airway should be established, and breathing and chest compression should be instituted immediately. All anaesthetic drugs should be discontinued. Adrenaline and sodium bicarbonate should be administered intravenously. Adrenaline can be readministered at 3–5 minute intervals if asystole persists. External electrical defibrillation is required if asystole deteriorates to ventricular fibrillation. Dopamine or dobutamine are administered by infusion once heart rhythm is restored. Ventricular asystole usu-

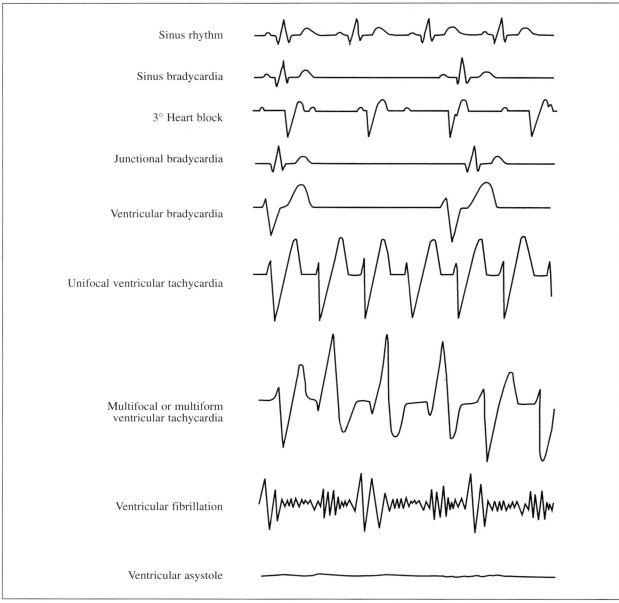

Figure 17.10: Cardiac rhythms observed during CPR in the dog and cat.

ally results from severe myocardial depression and is associated with a poor prognosis.

Electromechanical dissociation (EMD) cannot be distinguished from ventricular fibrillation or asystole without an electrocardiogram. EMD is characterized by electrocardiographic evidence of organized electrical activity (sinus or ventricular rhythm), but absence of effective myocardial contraction. Anaesthetic overdose, acute hypoxia, severe acidosis, systemic toxicity and cardiogenic shock are potential causes of EMD. Severe hypovolaemia, tension pneumothorax and pericardial effusions can mimic EMD and must be ruled out prior to therapy. Ventilation, chest compression, correction of acidosis, adrenaline and calcium chloride should be administered immediately.

FIBRILLATION AND DEFIBRILLATION

Ventricular fibrillation is an irregular quivering motion of the ventricles caused by continuous disorganized electrical activity. The ECG demonstrates fibrillatory waves (no QRS complexes) and no blood is pumped (pulselessness). Lignocaine cannot convert ventricular fibrillation to normal sinus rhythm, but can be used to prevent ventricular arrhythmias following defibrillation. The inability to convert ventricular fibrillation to sinus rhythm, or the recurrence of ventricular fibrillation after restoring cardiac rhythm, are indications of myocardial hypoxia, acidosis, depression or severe systemic disease. The adequacy of ventilation, chest or cardiac compression and initial therapies should be re-evaluated. Intravenous or intracardiac adrenaline should be administered prior to repeated attempts to defibrillate the heart. Once a stable cardiac rhythm is produced, dobutamine or dopamine can be used to maintain arterial blood pressure and systemic blood flow. Occasionally, drugs are deliberately injected into the left ventricle (intracardiac) in order to hasten their delivery to the coronary arteries and ventricular myocardium. Intracardiac injections are easily performed during open chest resuscitation, but are not recommended prior to opening the chest, since inadvertent pneumothorax, haemopericardium or intramyocardial injections leading to cardiac arrhythmias can occur.

Electrical defibrillation remains the method of choice for the conversion of severe unresponsive ventricular arrhythmias or ventricular fibrillation to sinus rhythm (Figure 17.11). Electrical defibrillation should be performed as soon as ventricular fibrillation is diagnosed, because survival decreases linearly with increasing time to defibrillation. Adrenaline (0.01–0.05 mg/kg i.v.) should be administered and defibrillation repeated if initial attempts to restore a perfusing cardiac rhythm are unsuccessful. No clinically effective chemical methods for producing defibrillation are currently available.

Ventricular tachycardia with severe hypotension or ventricular fibrillation

Direct-current fibrillators
    Internal: 0.5–2.0 watt-seconds (Ws/kg)
    External: 5–10 Ws/kg
        Small patient (<7 kg)
            Internal: 5–15 Ws
            External: 50–100 Ws
        Large patient (>10 kg)
            Internal: 20–80 Ws
            External: 100–400 Ws
Alternating-current defibrillators
    Small patient
        Internal: 30–50 V
        External: 50–100 V
    Large patient
        Internal: 50–100 V
        External: 150–250 V

Unresponsive ventricular fibrillation
Evaluate ventilation
Evaluate thoracic wall or cardiac compression
Evaluate fluid therapy
Repeat and increase dose of adrenaline
Repeat sodium bicarbonate administration
Administer lignocaine for ventricular arrhythmias
Repeat electrical defibrillation (direct-current; see above)

Figure 17.11: *Defibrillation techniques. Modified from Muir and Bonagura (1985).*

MONITORING

Proper post resuscitation monitoring and therapy is as critical as the resuscitation period itself if the patient is to survive. The period of hypoxia and ischaemia, regardless of how brief, results in metabolic acidosis, an increase in capillary and blood–brain barrier permeability and intense peripheral vascular constriction. These effects can lead to temporary or permanent blindness, neurological deficits, cerebral or pulmonary oedema, gastrointestinal mucosal sloughing, renal failure, hypothermia and shock. Careful monitoring of central nervous system signs (mental status), heart rate and rhythm (ECG), the peripheral pulse (arterial blood pressure), packed cell volume, acid-base (pH, PO_2, PCO_2) and electrolytes (Na$^+$, K$^+$, iCa^{2+}), urine volume (1–2 ml/kg/h) and ventilation (15 ml/kg) must be continued for many hours post resuscitation in order to enhance success. Infusions of dopamine or dobutamine are useful in maintaining cardiac contractile force and peripheral blood flow during the post-resuscitation period. Judicious use of polyionic salt solutions containing lactate (10–20 ml/kg/h), with frequent auscultation of the chest and measurement of arterial and central venous pressures and urinary output, help to prevent pulmonary or cerebral oedema (Fischer and Hossmann, 1996).

BRAIN ISCHAEMIA

The clinical consequences of partial or complete brain ischaemia include sensory deficits, blindness, cerebral oedema, seizures and coma culminating in respiratory arrest and cardiovascular collapse. These signs can be used to determine the progression of neurological status and emphasize the importance of monitoring the patient's level of consciousness, voluntary and involuntary body movements, extraocular reflexes, pupil position and response to light, respiratory rate and pattern and heart rate and rhythm. Bilateral pupillary constriction is an early response to brain ischaemia and suggests interruption of sympathetic tracts. Altered patterns of breathing, including Cheyne–Stokes respiration, suggest respiratory centre depression. Loss of corneal reflexes and widely dilated pupils indicate brainstem herniation and are usually followed by respiratory arrest.

Long-term recovery of normal brain function is possible after resuscitation if resuscitative efforts are initiated early (within 1–3 minutes) and optimized. Clinical signs of neurological injury, however, may not become apparent for several hours after successful resuscitation and often do not develop for 4–12 hours post-resuscitation (White *et al.*, 1983). The delay in onset of clinical signs is difficult to explain and suggests that the transient restoration of near normal brain function followed by gradual deterioration may be due to the maturation or continuation of mechanisms responsible for poor brain blood flow. Brain ischaemia causes cytotoxic or cellular oedema due to failure of cell membrane pumps (Na^+–K^+; Ca^{2+}). Relatively short periods of hypoxia can cause disruption of the blood–brain barrier, which in conjunction with increases in intracranial pressure caused by chest compression, promotes increased transfer of water and protein across the blood–brain barrier predisposing the patient to cerebral oedema. Cerebral oedema caused by the net gain in brain water may eventually impede cerebral blood flow, causing delayed clinical signs. Capillary vasospasm and abnormal vasoconstrictive activity due to the local release of prostaglandins and calcium from damaged cells are responsible for large increases in post-ischaemic vascular resistance. Highly tissue-destructive oxygen free radicals are produced following resuscitation and the re-introduction of oxygenated blood. These pathological consequences of brain ischaemia and reperfusion are responsible for the delayed onset of hypoperfusion of the brain and the neurological signs following cardiac arrest and resuscitation in dogs and cats.

TREATMENT OF POST-RESUSCITATION BRAIN ISCHAEMIA

The prevention of post-resuscitation neurological abnormalities is dependent upon the rapid re-establishment of brain blood flow, the control of intracranial pressure and inhibition of the products and detrimental processes triggered by brain ischaemia and reperfusion (Figure 17.12). The duration of circulatory arrest prior to the initiation of CPCR and the time required to re-establish normal haemodynamics and breathing are paramount in limiting complications and determining outcome. If resuscitation takes longer than 10–15 minutes when conventional closed-chest cardiac massage is used, neurological prognosis is poor. The reason for this is that closed chest compression techniques do not provide adequate brain blood flow. The intravenous administration of adrenaline (0.01–0.02 mg/kg) concurrent with ventilation, abdominal compression or abdominal binding helps to maintain higher levels of blood flow to the brain. If CNS injury is to be avoided, CPCR should begin promptly at chest compression rates of approximately 100/min. Abdominal compression or binding produces the best brain blood flow and does so without significantly elevating venous pressures (Koehler *et al.*, 1983). The administration of adrenaline during CPCR significantly improves myocardial and brain blood flow by intensely vasoconstricting peripheral vascular beds, thereby centralizing blood volume.

Problem	Therapy/Drug	Dose
Hypotension	Lactated Ringer's 6% Dextran 70; Hetastarch 7% NaCl 7% NaCl in 6% dextran 70 Dopamine Dobutamine	35–70 ml/kg i.v. 10 ml/kg i.v. 5 ml/kg i.v. 5 ml/kg i.v. 3–10 µg/kg/min i.v. 5–20 µg/kg/min i.v.
Seizures	Pentobarbitone Thiamylal, thiopentone Diazepam Propofol	1–3 mg/kg i.v. 1–3 mg/kg i.v. 0.1–0.2 mg/kg i.v. 1–3 mg/kg i.v.
Cerebral oedema or increased ICP	Oxygenation Hyperventilation Frusemide Mannitol Methylprednisolone sodium succinate	PaO_2 >80 mmHg $PaCO_2$ 25–35 mmHg 1 mg/kg i.v. 0.5–1.0 g/kg i.v. 5–10 mg/kg i.v.
Cerebral vasospasm	Diltiazem	2–3 mg/kg tid orally, 5–10 µg/kg/min CRI
Toxic cellular products[*]	Desferoxamine Superoxide dismutase Dimethyl sulphoxide Allopurinol	10–15 mg/kg i.v. slowly 5–50 mg orally 250–500 mg/kg i.v. 10 mg/kg orally

***Figure 17.12:** Brain-oriented resuscitation. Modified from Muir (1989). *These therapies await clinical verification of efficacy.*

Fluids must be administered judiciously with close patient monitoring during and following CPCR. The administration of crystalloids or colloids during resuscitative efforts improves arterial blood pressure and blood flow, but can also cause dramatic increases in intracranial pressure (ICP) if given at shock doses (20–40 ml/kg i.v.). The increase in interstitial fluid volume and ICP occurs because venous return may be hampered by resuscitative efforts and because the brain lacks a lymphatic drainage system. Hypertonic saline (5 ml/kg 7% NaCl, i.v.) produces rapid, but transient restoration of haemodynamics, increases cerebral blood flow (CBF) and decreases ICP. The administration of hyperoncotic or hyperosmotic solutions (5 ml/kg of 7% NaCl in 6% dextran 70) also minimizes increases in ICP. Mannitol, a hyperosmotic inert sugar, removes water from the brain by creating an osmotic gradient between the intravascular and extravascular compartments. Dosage recommendations range from 0.5 to 1.0 g/kg administered twice 1–2 hours apart. Additional benefits of mannitol infusions include increases in CBF, haemodilution and scavenging of oxygen and hydroxyl free radicals.

Brain blood flow is increased by increases in $PaCO_2$ and decreases in PaO_2. Maximal vasodilation occurs when $PaCO_2$ is greater than 60 mmHg, while PaO_2 values less than 50 mmHg are required to increase brain blood flow. Increases in brain blood flow increase the vascular to interstitial compartment fluid flux, thereby increasing ICP and predisposing to or causing cerebral oedema. Nasal oxygen or oxygen cages are helpful in maintaining PaO_2 above 100 mmHg (Fitzpatrick and Crowe, 1986). Ventilation using an inflatable bag, anaesthetic machine or respirator will help to prevent potentially detrimental increases in brain blood flow by normalizing $PaCO_2$ and maintaining PaO_2 values above 110 mmHg (FiO_2 = 50–90%). Head elevation and neck extension during spontaneous or controlled ventilation may help to alleviate increases in ICP and ensure a patent airway. After extubation, nasal oxygen or oxygen cages are helpful in maintaining PaO_2 above 100 mmHg (Fitzpatrick and Crowe, 1986). When pH and blood gases can be measured, blood $PaCO_2$ values between 30–40 mmHg and PaO_2 values greater than 100 mmHg are recommended. The determination of pH and blood gases ($PaCO_2$, $PaCO_2$, PaO_2) using a point of care blood analyser is the most practical and accurate method of assessing pH and blood gas disorders. Central venous blood samples are superior to arterial blood samples when assessing the severity of the acid–base abnormality, while arterial blood samples provide more information about lung function. Empirically, the administration of 0.5–1.0 mEq/kg of sodium bicarbonate for every 10 minutes of resuscitation effort has proven satisfactory for normalizing acid–base disorders due to metabolic acidosis.

Care must be taken not to overventilate the patient. Overventilation ($PaCO_2$ < 20 mmHg) can cause cerebral hypoxia and increases in CSF lactate concentrations. Large increases in tidal volume during controlled ventilation also increases intrathoracic pressure, which increases cerebral venous pressure causing disruption of the blood–brain barrier. High tidal volumes also lead to decreases in venous return to the heart, thereby decreasing and systemic blood flow.

Loop diuretics (frusemide, bumetanide) and osmotic diuretics (20% mannitol) are capable of rapidly decreasing ICP. Frusemide inhibits Cl^- and Na^+ reabsorption in the ascending limb of the loop of Henle, producing immediate large volume diuresis, and redistributes blood to peripheral vascular beds by dilating venules. The net effect of diuresis and redistribution of blood favours the movement of fluid from the brain (or lung) to the intravascular space, decreasing brain water and ICP. Frusemide also inhibits carbonic anhydrase, decreasing Na^+ uptake by the brain, which decreases brain swelling. Frusemide is initially administered at 1 mg/kg i.v. or 2 mg/kg i.m., followed by 0.5 mg/kg i.v. every 2–4 hours, if required. Although, frusemide has the potential to produce hypokalaemic metabolic alkalosis, this is generally not a concern during acute administration.

Mannitol produces an osmotic diuresis and establishes an osmotic gradient that moves water from the brain to the intravascular space. This effect, combined with its ability to promote reperfusion and scavenge oxygen free radicals, makes it an excellent choice for the prevention and treatment of increases in ICP and cerebral oedema. As previously detailed, dosages of 0.5–1.0 g/kg i.v. are recommended and repeat doses of 0.5 g/kg i.v. may be given at approximately 4 hours.

Diazepam and midazolam (0.1–0.2 mg/kg) are centrally acting muscle relaxants that produce mild calming effects and help to prevent seizures post resuscitation. If anaesthesia is required, low dosages of either sodium pentobarbitone (3–5 mg/kg i.v.) or sodium thiamylal (2–5 mg/kg i.v.) given to effect will help limit CNS damage and control seizures. Benzodiazepines and barbiturates decrease cerebral metabolic rate (O_2 consumption) by decreasing neuronal activity, protect membranes from free radicals and other excitatory neurotransmitters, decrease intracranial blood volume and ICP and increase tolerance to brief periods of complete brain ischaemia. Isoflurane, ketamine and propofol have been advocated as alternatives to barbiturates for acute seizure control in dogs and cats. Propofol (1–3 mg/kg) may be an excellent alternative to the barbiturates for seizure control in dogs. Finally, lignocaine administered by infusion (40–60 µg/kg/min) significantly reduces brain metabolic rate and stabilizes cell membranes.

Calcium entry blockers are believed to produce beneficial effects by preventing or reducing large increases in the concentration of intracellular iCa^{2+}, thereby inducing vasodilation and increases in brain blood flow. Diltiazem 5–10 µg/kg/min produces long-term increases in brain blood flow and improves outcome (Figure 17.8; Capparelli *et al.*, 1992). Blood pressure should be monitored during infusion, since calcium entry blocking drugs can produce hypotension due to their vasodilatory and negative inotropic effects.

CONCLUSION

Clinical experience suggests that when complete brain ischaemia lasts for longer than 5 minutes and the cardiac resuscitative effort lasts in excess of 10–15 minutes, neurological outcome is worsened and long-term survival is reduced. Age, concurrent disease and current medical or surgical complications are all important factors in determining outcome. Important prognostic indicators include the level of consciousness, pupil, eyelid and upper airway reflexes, breathing patterns and the ability to maintain a normal body temperature. The use of the oculocephalic (doll's eye) and oculovestibular (caloric) reflexes are useful indicators of prognosis, but are suppressed by sedatives, anaesthetics and hypothermia. These reflexes are generally absent when body temperature falls below 36 °C in the dog and cat. Rapid recovery of eyelid, pupillary and swallowing reflexes, resumption of a normal arterial pulse and breathing pattern, increasing levels of consciousness and the maintenance of normal body temperature are considered good prognostic signs. Most dogs and cats that show signs of recovery within 5 minutes of restoration of spontaneous circulation will recover with normal brain function. Progressive mental deterioration, seizures or unconsciousness, particularly after initial partial recovery, dilated fixed pupils, loss of eyelid and swallowing reflexes, prolonged respiratory arrest and gradual decreases in body temperature are poor prognostic signs. An inability to maintain a strong arterial pulse, normal heart rate and resume breathing regardless of specific therapies is an excellent indicator of impending death. Close monitoring should be continued for at least 24 hours after cardiorespiratory function is restored.

REFERENCES

Altman S (1997) Acupuncture as an emergency treatment. *California Veterinarian* **33**, 6–8

Brown CG, Martin DR, Pepe PE, Stueven H, Cummins RO, Gonzalez E and Jastremski M (1992) A Comparison of standard-dose and high-dose adrenaline in cardiac arrest outside the hospital. *New England Journal of Medicine* **327**, 1051–1055

Capparelli EV, Hanyok JJ, Dipersio DM, Kluger J, Fieldman A and Chow MS (1992) Diltiazem improves resuscitation from experimental ventricular fibrillation in dogs. *Critical Care Medicine* **20**, 1140–1145

Fischer M and Hossmann KA (1996) Volume expansion during cardiopulmonary resuscitation reduces cerebral no-reflow (review). *Resuscitation* **32**, 227–240

Fitzpatrick RK and Crowe DT (1986) Nasal oxygen administration in dogs and cats: experimental and clinical investigations. *Journal of the American Animal Hospital Association* **22**, 293–300

Janssens L, Altman S and Rogers PAM (1979) Respiratory and cardiac arrest under general anaesthesia: treatment by acupuncture of the nasal philtrum. *Veterinary Record* **105**, 273–276

Kass PH and Haskins SC (1992) Survival following cardiopulmonary resuscitation in dogs and cats. *Journal of Veterinary Emergency and Critical Care* **2**, 57–65

Koehler RC, Chandra N, Guerci AD, Tsitlik J, Traystman RJ, Rogers MC and Weisfeldt ML (1983) Augmentation of cerebral perfusion by simultaneous chest compression and lung inflation with abdominal binding after cardiac arrest in dogs. *Circulation* **67**, 266–275

Mazkereth R, Paret G, Ezra D, Aviner S, Peleg E, Rosenthal T and Barzilay Z (1992) Adrenaline blood concentrations after peripheral bronchial versus endotracheal administration of adrenaline in dogs. *Critical Care Medicine* **20**, 1582–1587

Muir WW (1989) Brain hypoperfusion post-resuscitation. *Veterinary Clinics of North America: Small Animal Practice* **19**, 1151–1166

Muir WW and Bonagura JD (1985) Cardiovascular emergencies. In: *Medical Emergencies*, ed. RG Sherding, p. 90. Churchill Livingstone, New York

Niemann JT (1992) Cardiopulmonary resuscitation (review). *New England Journal of Medicine* **327**, 1075–1080

Peters J and Ihle P (1990) Mechanics of the circulation during cardiopulmonary resuscitation — pathophysiology and techniques (part I). *Intensive Care Medicine* **16**, 11–19

Redding JS, Haynes RR and Thomas JD (1983) Drug therapy in resuscitation from electromechanical dissociation. *Critical Care Medicine* **11**, 681–684

Reich DL and Mingus M (1990) Transtracheal oxygenation using simple equipment and a low-pressure oxygen source. *Critical Care Medicine* **18**, 664–665

White BC, Winegar CD, Jackson RE, Joyce KM, Vigor DN, Hoehner TJ, Krause GS and Wilson RF (1983) Cerebral cortical perfusion during and following resuscitation from cardiac arrest in dogs. *American Journal of Emergency Medicine* **1**, 128–138

Wingfield WE and Van Pelt DR (1992) Respiratory and cardiopulmonary arrest in dogs and cats: 265 cases (1986–1991). *Journal of the American Veterinary Medical Association* **200**, 1993–1996

CHAPTER EIGHTEEN

Anaesthesia and Analgesia for the Critical Patient

Daniel J. Holden and Richard Hammond

INTRODUCTION

Most critically ill patients will need sedation, analgesia and often anaesthesia at some point during their hospitalization. Anaesthesia may be required to allow elective diagnostic, therapeutic or emergency procedures to be undertaken, and therefore requires careful consideration.

Neural and hormonal responses in the critically ill or injured patient will act to preserve circulation to essential organs, including the brain and myocardium. This effectively centralized circulation may make the patient more susceptible to the adverse effects of any anaesthetic agents used. This effect may be exacerbated by the concomitant presence of factors such as hypothermia, hypoalbuminaemia and acid-base and electrolyte disturbances. It should be remembered that few procedures require general anaesthesia to be performed on an emergent basis. Careful preoperative assessment, stabilization of vital parameters and attention to detail are essential if perioperative crises are to be avoided.

In most critical patients, the establishment of a patent protected airway with provision of increased inspired oxygen concentration and the potential for ventilatory support, is usually associated with a better outcome than a period of heavy sedation. Therefore the commonly held belief that 'sedation is safer than anaesthesia' does not always apply in patients with critical disease.

PREOPERATIVE ASSESSMENT AND STABILIZATION

When assessing the patient for anaesthesia, it is useful to adopt the 'A, B, C' approach of body system evaluation. This forms a structured and prioritized checklist of potential problems that may arise during the perianaesthetic period. Awareness of these potential problems allows preparedness and, where required, further pre-induction stabilization and support. It also forms the basis for the choice of anaesthetic protocol.

The assessment may be summarized as:

- A – Airway
- B – Breathing
- C – Circulation

plus

- D – Drugs.

Airway

The patient's ability to maintain a patent airway pre- and postoperatively should be carefully assessed:

- Can the patient maintain an airway?
- Is there a potential need for tracheotomy?
- Will patency be lost at induction (e.g. brachycephalic airway obstruction syndrome, BAOS)?
- Is there a need or potential need for airway clearance (i.e. suction)?

Any potential airway obstruction involving (or rostral to) the larynx (e.g. laryngeal trauma/paralysis/ BAOS) may effectively be resolved by orotracheal intubation. In such patients, rapid establishment of an airway at induction is therefore indicated, and excessive sedation prior to induction should be avoided. Patients at risk of airway obstruction should be carefully monitored post-premedication.

The potential for failed intubation in these patients must, however, be considered and alternative techniques for securing the airway (including tracheostomy) must be available.

Obstruction of the airway between the larynx and carina presents a considerable problem and is unlikely to be resolved by normal endotracheal intubation techniques.

Patients at risk of aspiration or obstruction due to the presence of fluid and/or debris in the pharynx may require clearance using suction techniques. Prolonged suction quickly leads to marked arterial desaturation, and intermittent supplementation of FiO_2 is mandatory.

Breathing and gas exchange

The patient's ventilatory drive, tidal volume, pulmonary gas exchange and blood oxygen-carrying capacity should be assessed as far as possible.

- Is the patient dyspnoeic and/or tachypnoeic?
- Is oxygen supplementation required to maintain normal arterial oxygen saturation at rest (SaO_2)?
- Can the patient maintain an adequate arterial oxygen content (importance of haematocrit and circulating haemoglobin levels)?

Evaluation of the dyspnoeic patient

Once the involvement of airway obstruction has been eliminated, the presence of disease affecting either the pleural space or the lung parenchyma should be determined. Where intrathoracic disease is suspected or suggested from the history or initial physical examination, survey thoracic radiographs should be obtained. Any air or fluid within the pleural space should be removed by needle thoracocentesis or placement of a chest drain.

Evaluation of the patient's ability to oxygenate may be determined by other techniques such as pulse oximetry and arterial blood gas analysis where available.

As arterial oxygen content also depends heavily upon haemoglobin concentration; the patient's haematocrit (and if possible haemoglobin concentration) should be measured. Patients with acute falls in haematocrit to below 20% will require transfusion if severe tissue hypoxia is to be avoided during anaesthesia.

Increasing the fraction of inspired oxygen (FiO_2)

There is a range of techniques for increasing inspired oxygen. Use of any of these should be balanced against the potential for stressing the patient, which will increase oxygen demand and may precipitate a crisis.

Techniques include:

- Flow-by oxygen
- Oxygen mask
- Nasal or nasopharyngeal oxygen
- Trans-tracheal oxygen
- Oxygen cage/incubator.

Details on these techniques are found in Chapters 5 and 22.

Circulation

The adequacy of circulation and tissue perfusion must be ensured. Questions that should be addressed include:

- Is the patient's circulating volume adequate?
- Is heart rate normal at rest?
- Is there a dysrhythmia likely to result in a reduced cardiac output?
- Does the type or frequency of the patient's dysrhythmia preclude general anaesthesia?
- Does the patient have adequate tissue perfusion to vital organ beds?

Assessment of circulating volume

Adequacy of circulating volume can largely be assessed by means of physical examination and history.

Pulse pressure is not a reliable indicator of the status of circulatory volume, although absence of a peripheral pulse suggests reduced peripheral perfusion. Capillary refill time is a poor indicator of circulating volume.

Central venous pressure is considered the most reliable method of assessing both circulating volume and response to the administration of intravenous fluids.

Circulating volume should be optimized prior to premedication by the use of intravenous crystalloids and colloids as appropriate. Rates, routes and choices of fluid are discussed in Chapter 2.

Although heart rate may be deduced from the clinical examination, true electrical activity can only be assessed by means of an ECG. Dysrhythmias are common in any patient with illness or major injury and can be broadly classified into brady- and tachydysrhythmias. Indications for therapeutic intervention include:

- Heart rate >160 or <60 beats per minute
- Multifocal ventricular premature complexes (VPCs)
- Runs of more than five VPCs
- Evidence of 'R on T' phenomenon
- Any dysrhythmia producing clinical signs of reduced cardiac output.

In all cases, anaesthesia should be delayed if possible and therapy directed at the underlying cause (e.g. electrolyte disturbances, hypoxia, cardiac disease, hypercapnoea, pain); agents known to precipitate dysrhythmias (α_2-agonists, barbiturates, halothane) are best avoided.

Adequate perfusion of vital organs is essential during anaesthesia, and it should be remembered that normal blood pressure does not always reflect adequate perfusion. Examination of mucous membranes and capillary refill time may be helpful, but results are often subjective. Measurement of urine output provides a useful index of renal perfusion; values below 0.5 ml/kg/h require intervention. Pulse oximetry relies on adequate peripheral perfusion, and readings taken in the presence of a poor pulse signal may not be reliable.

Drugs – the significance of pre-existing therapy

Patients may be presented with long-term ongoing drug regimens. The direct and indirect effects of these agents on the anaesthetic protocol must be considered.

Significant therapies include:

- Diuretics (hypovolaemia, hypokalaemia, acid-base disturbances)
- Non-steroidal anti-inflammatory drugs (NSAIDs) (gastrointestinal ulceration, renal damage, increased potential for overdose through altered protein binding)
- Anticonvulsants (altered protein binding, liver enzyme induction)

- Steroids (interaction with NSAIDs)
- Antibiotics (potentiation of neuromuscular blockade with aminoglycosides and macrolides)
- β-Blockers (lack of response to inotropes).

In most cases, drugs should not be withdrawn prior to anaesthesia, as this may increase the potential for complications.

SEDATION AND PREMEDICATION

In order to reduce stress associated with restraint during the induction period (which may precipitate catecholamine release) and to minimize required doses of induction agents, adequate sedative premedication is advisable. Choices of sedative agent include:

- α$_2$-Agonists
- Phenothiazines
- Benzodiazepines.

The profound respiratory and cardiovascular depressant effects produced by the α$_2$-agonists effectively preclude their use in patients with significant disease.

Of the phenothiazines, acepromazine is the most commonly used. The sedative effects are potentiated by combination with an opioid. Hypotension may be seen in hypovolaemic patients or when higher doses (>0.03 mg/kg) are used. Low doses can produce selective arteriolar vasodilation, thereby reducing afterload, which may improve cardiac output in some patients. Acepromazine has been shown to protect the heart from the arrhythmogenic effects of adrenaline. Use of the drug in patients with head trauma has been questioned, as it purportedly reduces the threshold at which seizures occur, although this is controversial.

Benzodiazepines possess minimal cardiovascular and respiratory depressant properties and may significantly reduce the induction dose requirement. Sedation is less reliable than with acepromazine, but is often more profound in debilitated patients. The two most commonly used agents are diazepam and midazolam (neither of which hold a veterinary license); both can be used at doses ranging from 0.1 to 0.25 mg/kg. Diazepam also exists as an emulsion preparation, which is only effective by the intravenous route. Midazolam is a water-soluble preparation that can be used by any parenteral route. To avoid potential dysphasia, either drug may be given intravenously immediately prior to induction. Benzodiazepines also possess excellent muscle relaxant properties, which make them a valuable adjunct to ketamine anaesthesia.

Use of anticholinergic agents in compromised patients may be detrimental, as the resultant tachycardia will increase myocardial oxygen demand and may precipitate dysrhythmias. Should significant bradycardia occur in the peri-anaesthetic period, judicious doses of anticholinergic may be employed:

- Atropine 0.02–0.04 mg/kg i.v. slowly
- Glycopyrrolate 0.005–0.01 mg/kg i.m. or i.v.

Glycopyrrolate may induce less tachycardia than atropine but has a slower onset of action.

Opioids form a major component of the premedication protocol; their indications and use will be discussed later in this chapter.

INDUCTION PERIOD

The aim of induction is to produce a smooth passage to the unconscious state with minimal compromise of ventilatory or cardiovascular function. Induction allows a secure patent airway to be obtained.

Pre-oxygenation is recommended in all patients where possible, and is mandatory in patients with respiratory compromise if it can be achieved without undue patient stress. This helps to reduce desaturation associated with induction apnoea. To be effective, pre-oxygenation must be performed for a period of at least 5 minutes. High flow rates are indicated to maximize FiO_2.

Choices for the method of induction of anaesthesia include:

- Mask induction
- Rapid intravenous bolus
- Combinations of the above.

Mask induction

Advantages

- Permits provision of a high FiO_2
- Obviates the need for the use of intravenous agents and their associated unwanted effects
- Useful where protein binding or total protein is reduced, making estimation of the dose of usually heavily albumin-bound intravenous agents difficult.

Disadvantages

- Often stressful to the patient
- Does not allow rapid control of the patient's airway.

Due to the unpleasant odour, mask inductions with isoflurane are often not significantly quicker than those with halothane, as breath-holding may occur.

Nitrous oxide may be a useful adjunct to mask induction, as the second gas effect allegedly reduces induction time by hastening the uptake of the volatile agent. Use of nitrous oxide will reduce the FiO_2. Mask induction should be *avoided* in:

- Patients with upper airway obstruction
- Patients at risk of regurgitation/reflux
- Patients with severe dyspnoea and/or intrinsic pulmonary disease
- Patients with reduced pulmonary blood flow.

Intravenous induction

Frequently used agents for the production of anaesthesia in small animals include:

- Barbiturates (methohexitone, thiopentone)
- Propofol
- Ketamine
- Alphaxalone/alphadalone
- Etomidate.

Barbiturates

Although barbiturates are frequently used to induce anaesthesia in fit healthy patients, in haemodynamically unstable patients they may have a profound effect upon cardiac output, preload and myocardial contractility. Although many of these effects can be minimized by haemodynamic support, administration to patients with severe cardiovascular compromise should be avoided. Dysrhythmias are also common during the induction phase of barbiturate anaesthesia. Although apnoea is a common occurrence immediately post-induction with barbiturates, its duration is usually no longer than that seen with other agents (including propofol).

Propofol

Propofol produces a very rapid smooth induction of anaesthesia that is usually accompanied by apnoea unless the drug is administered slowly to effect. It is essentially non-cumulative and may be used to maintain anaesthesia by incremental dosage or continuous infusion. It is a potent venodilator and its effects upon the baroreceptor reflex mean that the hypotension produced (which is often marked) is not offset by a compensatory reflex increase in heart rate. The drug is strongly protein-bound, making estimation of dose requirement difficult in hypoalbuminaemia, renal disease and geriatric patients (altered protein binding kinetics).

Propofol is easily cleared by both hepatic and extrahepatic mechanisms and is the induction agent of choice in dogs with hepatic dysfunction. Cats do not possess the same ability to metabolize phenolic compounds and therefore care should be exercised when using propofol in cats with hepatic disease.

Ketamine

In normal patients, ketamine is associated with minimal cardiovascular and respiratory depression. In patients with high resting sympathetic drive, its effects on the cardiovascular system may be less predictable. Indirect sympathomimetic effects include an increase in heart rate, which may be detrimental in hypertrophic cardiomyopathy and ischaemic heart disease. It should be avoided in patients with head trauma, as it may produce increases in cerebral blood flow, causing intracranial hypertension. The drug also possesses active metabolites and should be used with caution in patients with hepatic or renal dysfunction. Ketamine is the only induction agent with any recognized analgesic properties and is best used in combination with a benzodiazepine to provide adequate muscle relaxation. Doses of 3–10 mg/kg are used in both dogs and cats.

Alphaxolone/alphadolone

Alphaxolone/alphadolone (Saffan) at 2–4 mg/kg produces anaesthesia of short duration in the cat. Its cardiovascular effects are not dissimilar to those of the barbiturates, but its non-cumulative pharmacokinetic profile means that it can be used to maintain anaesthesia by infusion or incremental dosage. The drug combination's effects on the lower oesophageal sphincter predispose patients under anaesthesia to gastro-oesophageal reflux.

Etomidate

Etomidate is not licensed for veterinary use in the UK. It frequently causes pain and phlebitis on intravenous injection, owing to its high osmolarity, and is expensive. Although its cardiovascular and respiratory effects are minimal, the drug causes profound and long-lasting suppression of adrenocortical activity, which could be detrimental in patients with critical illness.

Combinations

The combination of the above agents with potent opioids and/or benzodiazepines to induce anaesthesia allows the use of lower doses of individual agents, thereby minimizing unwanted side effects. In severely debilitated patients, the combination of a benzodiazepine and a potent opioid such as fentanyl may be sufficient to allow endotracheal intubation. Administration of potent opioids such as fentanyl or alfentanyl may cause marked vagally mediated bradycardia and coadministration of atropine is recommended.

Suggested combinations include:

- Diazepam 0.2 mg/kg + fentanyl 5–10 µg/kg + thiopentone/propofol to effect (often only 2–3 mg/kg needed)
- Alfentanyl 10 µg/kg + propofol/thiopentone to effect
- Midazolam 0.2 mg/kg + thiopentone/propofol to effect.

MAINTENANCE OF ANAESTHESIA

Anaesthesia may be maintained by the use of intravenous agents, volatile inhalational agents or a combination of the two.

Intravenous infusions

Maintenance of anaesthesia by intravenous infusion of a sole agent may be performed where the agent has suitable pharmacokinetics (e.g. propofol). Practically, production of a stable plane of anaesthesia is difficult to obtain in all but prolonged procedures. In addition, infusion of agents such as propofol is associated with a greater incidence of unwanted effects such as hypotension as compared to use as a single bolus.

The use of rapid onset, short duration, highly potent opioids such as fentanyl or alfentanyl as an adjunct to general inhalation anaesthesia has found favour in human trauma anaesthesia. These agents are very powerful analgesics and will usually ablate the patient's response to noxious surgical stimuli. As such, although not holding a veterinary licence, the rapid onset and short duration of these agents make them suitable for intraoperative management of the response to surgical stimulus (as inferred from changes in cardiovascular parameters). At 1 μg/kg body weight, fentanyl (used during general anaesthesia maintained by inhalational agents) produces a change in ventilatory drive, often manifested as a reduction in ventilatory rate. Although

not usually warranting use of IPPV, facilities for assisted ventilation should be available.

Use of inhalational agents

Volatile inhalational agents still form the mainstay of anaesthesia maintenance in critical patients.

Sevoflurane and desflurane

Agents more recently introduced into human anaesthetic practice include sevoflurane and desflurane. These agents hold no veterinary licence at the time of writing. Although these agents possess valuable pharmacokinetic properties, their expense currently precludes their use.

Isoflurane

The advantages and disadvantages of isoflurane compared with halothane for anaesthesia of critical patients are shown in Figure 18.1.

If isoflurane is unavailable, halothane may be used for production of anaesthesia in critical patients. Use of potent narcotic analgesics as an adjunct is recommended, to allow the reduction of the required inspired halothane concentration.

Nitrous oxide

Nitrous oxide can be used as part of the carrier gas combination for the induction and maintenance of general inhalational anaesthesia. The beneficial and potential detrimental effects of its use in critical patients are shown in Figure 18.2.

Advantages
As a di-substituted ether, isoflurane sensitizes the myocardium to the dysrhythmogenic effects of adrenaline less than halothane
Lower blood gas partition coefficient means more rapid uptake and elimination and more rapid induction and recovery phases
Cardiovascular depressant effects are due to vasodilation rather than direct myocardial depression; thus they can in part be negated by support of effective circulating volume
Disrupts the normal homeostatic autoregulation of organ blood flow less than halothane
Undergoes minimal hepatic metabolism (0.2%); therefore recovery is not prolonged by hepatic dysfunction
Disadvantages
Until surgical stimulation, isoflurane produces greater ventilatory depression than halothane
Reflex response to vasodilation may result in a detrimental tachycardia

Figure 18.1: Advantages and disadvantages of isoflurane compared to halothane in critical patients.

Beneficial effects
Second gas effect: reduces the time of onset of induction with inhalational agents by promoting uptake of the volatile agent
Provides intraoperative analgesia
Relatively devoid of unwanted respiratory and cardiovascular effects
Low blood gas partition coefficient: rapid uptake and elimination from the body
Detrimental effects
Must be used at inspired concentrations of ≥50% to provide analgesia; therefore lowers the maximum FiO_2 that can be used
Diffuses into air-filled spaces and may increase their effective volume
Prolonged exposure leads to inhibition of hepatic methionine synthase. Efficient active scavenging systems must be in place

Figure 18.2: Beneficial and detrimental effects of nitrous oxide in critical patients.

NEUROMUSCULAR BLOCKING AGENTS

Neuromuscular blocking agents can be invaluable in anaesthesia of patients with major disease or trauma as they facilitate intermittent positive pressure ventilation (IPPV) and allow reductions in the dose of intravenous and volatile agents, thereby facilitating use of a balanced anaesthetic technique. It should be remembered that neuromuscular blocking drugs possess no anaesthetic or analgesic properties, and the importance of ensuring lack of awareness and insensibility to pain cannot be overemphasized. Facilities for IPPV are also mandatory. Non-depolarizing agents are the most frequently used; of the currently available drugs, probably the most suitable are vecuronium and atracurium. Vecuronium is a short-acting and relatively non-cumulative agent which has minimal cardiovascular effects and produces paralysis for approximately 25 minutes when used at a dose of 0.1 mg/kg i.v. Atracurium is unusual in that it is degraded by a process independent of enzymatic function and is therefore indicated in neonates and patients with significant hepatic or renal dysfunction. The potential for histamine release exists at higher dose rates, but at clinical doses (0.25 mg/kg i.v. produces 20–30 minutes of paralysis) this does not appear to be a major problem. It is worth noting that several factors capable of altering the duration of action of muscle relaxants (hypothermia, acid-base and electrolyte disturbances) are likely to be present in critically ill patients.

Although not always considered necessary, reversal of paralysis produced by non-depolarizing muscle relaxants may be advisable in diseased patients with potential respiratory muscle paresis. Reversal may be achieved by the use of neostigmine at a dose of 0.05 mg/kg, combined with 0.02 mg/kg of atropine sulphate.

MONITORING AND INTRAOPERATIVE SUPPORT

General aspects of critical monitoring are covered in Chapter 16. Specific considerations for monitoring during general anaesthesia of critical patients include cardiac rate and rhythm, and fluid status.

Cardiac rate and rhythm

Use of a continuous waveform ECG to allow early detection of life-threatening dysrhythmias is strongly recommended. Specific therapy of individual dysrhythmias is described in Chapter 4. It should be remembered that the presence of a normal cardiac rhythm does not necessarily indicate that cardiac output is normal.

Fluid input, fluid loss and volume status

The rate and type of fluid support must take into account:

- Pre-existing cardiovascular function
- Type and rate of ongoing fluid loss
- Acid-base and electrolyte disturbances
- Rate and volume of intraoperative blood loss.

For normal intraoperative support, infusion of a balanced electrolyte solution with composition similar to that of extracellular fluid (e.g. lactated Ringer's solution) at a rate of 10–15 ml/kg/h is adequate. If the patient is hypoproteinaemic or if blood losses exceed 10% of blood volume, infusion of colloids (gelatins, hetastarch or dextrans) may be indicated to maintain intravascular volume. Acute severe blood losses (>15% of blood volume) or instances where the patient's PCV falls below 20% require the transfusion of fresh whole blood or packed red cells. Blood loss can be quantitatively evaluated by weighing swabs (1 ml of blood weighs 1.3 g) and by estimating losses from the suction reservoir if one is used.

Tissue and organ perfusion

Tissue perfusion can be assessed qualitatively by regular palpation of peripheral pulses and evaluation of mucous membrane colour and capillary refill time, although these are all notoriously subjective phenomena. Urine output is a valuable indicator of renal perfusion, and an indwelling catheter and closed collection system can be used throughout the perioperative period to monitor output. Mean arterial pressure should be maintained above 60-70 mmHg to ensure perfusion of vital organs.

Oxygenation and ventilation

Pulse oximetry provides a continuous indication of the degree of saturation of arterial blood with oxygen. As accurate readings rely on the maintenance of peripheral perfusion and blood flow, changes in the status of these parameters will adversely affect accuracy. Pulse oximetry therefore provides an indicator of the presence of peripheral pulses and tissue perfusion, and an assessment of the patient's ability to oxygenate blood. It does not reflect arterial oxygen content or tissue oxygen delivery. False readings will also be obtained in the presence of certain disease states, including carbon monoxide poisoning (smoke inhalation), methaemoglobinaemia (paracetamol poisoning) and conditions resulting in venous pulsatile flow (severe right-sided myocardial failure). Although blood gas analysis represents the 'gold standard' for respiratory function monitoring, cost precludes this from being widely available.

Capnography

This is the most useful non-invasive estimation of the adequacy of ventilatory function, although its accuracy during intrathoracic procedures has recently been questioned. Measurement of expired carbon dioxide also provides an indication of the adequacy of cardiac output, and therefore estimations of ventilatory function based on capnography should be made in the light of cardiac functional status.

The rapid response time of the capnogram is of use in alerting the anaesthetist to potential disasters, including:

- Cardiopulmonary arrest
- Patient disconnection from the breathing system
- Unrecognized oesophageal intubation
- Venous air embolism.

Depth of unconsciousness

Depth of unconsciousness is particularly difficult to assess in the pharmacologically paralysed patient but is facilitated by more advanced monitoring. Signs of awareness during anaesthesia and paralysis include:

- Changes in heart rate and blood pressure unassociated with haemorrhage or drug administration
- Changes in pupil size
- Lachrymation and tongue curling (late signs).

Body temperature

Maintenance of an adequate body temperature is mandatory to prevent a prolonged recovery and its attendant complications. Many critically ill patients are hypermetabolic and rely heavily on ambient temperature to maintain core body temperature. Drugs involved in sedation and anaesthesia disrupt normal thermoregulatory mechanisms, and the respiration of cold dry gases significantly contributes to intraoperative heat loss, as do evaporative losses from exposed organs and tissues during major surgery. In the postoperative phase, muscle activity such as shivering will increase endogenous heat production at the expense of an increased oxygen demand, which may not be tolerated by a compromised patient. Hypothermia produces a plethora of adverse effects including:

- Peripheral vasoconstriction and increased vascular resistance
- Increased coagulability
- Predisposition to dysrhythmias
- Reduction in cerebral blood flow
- Reduced effectiveness of analgesics
- Derangements in substrate metabolism
- Reduced ventilation and elimination of volatile agents.

The importance of active warming processes cannot therefore be overemphasized. Methods include:

- Use of re-breathing systems (promotes inspiration of warm moist gases)
- Use of heat and moisture exchangers (artificial nose)
- High ambient temperatures in the operating theatre and recovery area

- Patient insulation (e.g. foil wrap, water beds)
- Avoidance of excessive preparation of surgical site
- Expedient surgery
- Warmed intravenous fluids
- Post-surgical use of warmed isotonic enemas and urinary bladder lavage.

IMMEDIATE POST-ANAESTHETIC PERIOD

Patient support in terms of monitoring, intravenous fluids, body temperature management, analgesia and careful observation must not stop at the door of the operating theatre. Aggressive, selected monitoring and recording should continue until the patient's vital signs have reached appropriate levels. A prioritized approach should be adopted:

- Airway (maintenance – re-intubation and/or intermittent suction clearance may be required)
- Breathing (postoperative hypoventilation)
    Incomplete reversal of paralysis
    Opioid-induced ventilatory depression
    Hypothermia-induced ventilatory depression
    Chest wall pain
    Pneumothorax/haemothorax
- Circulation (bleeding due to poor surgical technique or coagulopathy, sepsis/hypotension).

ANALGESIA IN CRITICAL PATIENTS

Recognition of pain

In recumbent debilitated or heavily sedated patients, normal behavioural responses to nociceptive stimulation may be obscured. The clinician must be more vigilant when managing pain in the critical patient. If it is unclear from an animal's behaviour whether it is experiencing pain, ethical considerations require that analgesics should be administered.

Patients experiencing pain, rapidly become catabolic and more prone to complications inherent in critical illness, e.g. delayed wound healing, sepsis and nosocomial disease. Effective analgesia therefore makes therapeutic sense. A multi-modal and pre-emptive approach to analgesia not only provides more effective relief, but also facilitates the use of balanced anaesthetic techniques.

Any analgesic protocol must also include nursing considerations such as:

- Effective immobilization of soft tissue and orthopaedic injuries
- Adequate bedding and a warm environment
- Bladder emptying
- Physiotherapy
- Effective nutritional support
- Tender loving care.

Therapeutic options for analgesia in critical patients include:

- Opioid analgesics
- NSAIDs
- Local analgesics.

Opioid analgesics

These agents form the cornerstone of any analgesic protocol. A full discussion of the pharmacology of opioid analgesics is beyond the scope of this chapter and is adequately covered in many other texts.

The drugs may be broadly classified as agonists, partial agonists, antagonists and agonist/antagonists according to their effect at the μ-receptor. 'Potency' refers purely to receptor occupancy and may bear no relationship to clinical analgesic efficacy. On a clinical level, the μ-receptor agonist agents are considered to have the greatest analgesic efficacy.

Opioids potentiate the sedative effects of acepromazine and are often used as part of a premedication combination, not only for this reason but also due to their relative lack of cardiovascular side-effects. Including an opioid analgesic in the premedication protocol will often produce a calm sedated patient and significantly reduce the dose of induction agent required to achieve intubation.

Of the available opioid analgesic agents, only pethidine, buprenorphine and butorphanol are licensed as sole agents for use in the U.K. Fentanyl is licensed in combination with fluanisone.

These drugs fall into either Schedule 2 (pure agonists) or Schedule 3 (partial agonists) of the Misuse of Drugs Act 1971. Their side-effects include:

- Respiratory depression
- Vagally mediated bradycardia
- Dysphoria
- Miosis/mydriasis (species-dependent)
- Vomiting.

These effects may be less apparent in patients with pain at the time of administration and should not preclude the judicious use of these agents in most patients.

Morphine

Morphine is a Schedule 2 Controlled Drug. It is a powerful analgesic which, despite its lack of a veterinary licence, is widely utilized due to its considerable efficacy and reliability. Systemic administration at doses of 0.1–0.4 mg/kg s.c. or i.m. produces analgesia of 4 hours' duration. The duration of effect depends on the level of painful stimulus and the dose. Morphine is also effective if administered orally or rectally. The time to onset is 15 minutes, even after intravenous injection.

Morphine is well absorbed from most routes, though less well from oral administration due to the first-pass hepatic metabolism. It is eliminated by glu-

curonidation; therefore elimination is slow in cats. Metabolites are eliminated by the kidney.

Pethidine

Pethidine (meperidine, USA) is a Schedule 2 drug licensed for veterinary use in the UK. It has a very rapid onset and short duration of effect (2 hours maximum). Pethidine has minimal vagal effects but does have a potential for histamine release when given by the intravenous route. Pethidine is used at a dose of 2–5 mg/kg i.m. Its short duration of effect makes it less suitable for prolonged postoperative analgesia. Pethidine may be the opioid of choice in pancreatitis as it does not cause spasm of smooth muscle sphincters such as the sphincter of Oddi.

Methadone

Methadone is a Schedule 2 drug. Doses of 0.25 mg/kg produce moderate analgesia with variable sedation in dogs and cats. Lack of a veterinary licence and relatively poor analgesic efficacy mean that methadone has little practical place in veterinary critical care.

Papaveretum

Papaveretum is an unlicensed Schedule 2 drug that contains alkaloids of opium. It provides effective sedation in aggressive dogs when combined with acepromazine and has fewer unwanted gastrointestinal effects than morphine. The dose for dogs and cats is 0.1–0.4 mg/kg. Peak effects occur after 30 minutes. The duration of effect depends on the level of painful stimulus and the dose, but is typically 1–2 hours. The compounds are conjugated in the liver and there is some unchanged renal excretion.

Fentanyl

Fentanyl is a Schedule 2 drug that is not licensed for veterinary use. It is a very potent agonist, approximately 50 times more effective than morphine, but with a rapid time of onset (2–7 minutes) and short duration of effect (15–20 minutes). The dose in dogs and cats is 1–10 μg/kg i.v.

Fentanyl is used primarily for intraoperative analgesia as part of a balanced anaesthetic protocol. Normal doses produce profound respiratory depression or apnoea. Provision for IPPV must be available. The short duration of action is mainly due to redistribution rather than elimination; there is therefore a risk of cumulation or prolonged respiratory depressant effects.

Alfentanyl

Alfentanyl is a Schedule 2 drug that is not licensed for veterinary use. Although a quarter as potent as fentanyl, alfentanyl has a much shorter time to onset of action (1–2 minutes). The dose for dogs and cats is 10 μg/kg i.v. Its rapid metabolism suggests it is suitable for infusion, although some studies indicate cumulation.

Apnoea is usual at clinical doses. Alfentanyl must

be given in conjunction with, or following, atropine. It is often administered as part of an induction protocol in high-risk patients as it markedly reduces the requirement for intravenous induction agents.

Buprenorphine

Buprenorphine is a Schedule 3 drug that is licensed for veterinary use. A partial agonist at μ-receptors, this drug has a slow onset of action when given by any route (35–45 minutes) but a long duration of effect (6–8 hours). It is useful for the management of moderate pain. The dose-response 'plateau' exhibited by the drug means that if breakthrough pain occurs, further doses of buprenorphine will not further increase analgesia. In addition, due to the nature of its receptor binding, any μ-receptor agonists subsequently given will be relatively ineffective. Clinical doses range from 6 to 10 μg/kg.

Butorphanol

Butorphanol is a Schedule 3 drug that is licensed for veterinary use. It is most suitably classified as an agonist/antagonist. Butorphanol possesses excellent sedative properties when used at a dose of 0.05–0.3 mg/kg in combination with acepromazine. Its use as an analgesic is controversial, not only because of its questionable efficacy, but also because of the wide availability of agents with a longer duration of effect and proven clinical efficacy.

NSAIDs

Although these are valuable adjuncts to any analgesia protocol, the critical patient is more susceptible to the toxic effects of NSAIDs because of the greater potential for hypovolaemia, adverse interactions with pre-existing drug therapy, and alterations in gastrointestinal and renal blood flow. The advent of newer agents such as carprofen and meloxicam has, however, helped to minimize these problems. Although its exact mechanism of action remains unclear, carprofen forms a valuable component of any perioperative analgesic regimen, and its use should be considered in all patients.

Local anaesthetic agents

Local and regional anaesthetic techniques are a valuable and often under-used modality in small animal anaesthesia. They are especially useful in patients with major trauma or severe disease, as they are capable (when used appropriately) of providing almost total analgesia without significant cardiovascular, respiratory or central nervous system depression.

Of the available agents, the most commonly used in small animals are lignocaine (lidocaine, USA) and bupivicaine. Bupivicaine has a slower onset of action (approximately 30 minutes depending on the site of use) but a longer duration of effect (6–8 hours) than lignocaine (1.5–2 hours). Lignocaine plus bupivicaine

mixtures can be used to offset the latency of bupivicaine. Overdose or inadvertent intravenous administration of local analgesics can result in central nervous system disturbances (including seizures) and cardiovascular depression.

Numerous local analgesic techniques have been described in small animals, and for detailed accounts the reader should consult other texts including the *BSAVA Manual of Small Animal Anaesthesia and Analgesia.* Probably the most valuable techniques in critical patients or those with major trauma include intercostal and intrapleural analgesia and lumbosacral epidural analgesia.

Intercostal nerve blockade

Analgesia for thoracotomy incisions, rib fractures, chest wall injuries or placement of chest drains can be achieved by intercostal nerve blockade. The nerves run segmentally in a neurovascular bundle along the caudal border of each rib, and can be desensitized by the injection of 0.5–1 ml of either 2% lignocaine or 0.5% bupivicaine immediately caudal to the rib surface (the needle can be gently 'walked off' the caudal aspect of the rib). Aspiration should be performed to avoid intravascular injection. Prolonged analgesia post-thoracotomy can be achieved by instillation of a local analgesic drug into the pleural space either via a dedicated catheter or via the indwelling chest drain. Care should be taken to avoid overdose, as both of these techniques will result in relatively high plasma levels of the drug (maximum total doses for lignocaine and bupivicaine are 10 mg/kg and 2 mg/kg, respectively).

Epidural analgesia

Lumbosacral epidural techniques can be used to provide analgesia for all structures caudal to the umbilicus. Excessive doses of epidural local analgesic can cause profound hypotension, due to blockade of splanchnic sympathetic innervation, and respiratory failure caused by intercostal paralysis but, if care is taken, these complications are rare. No more than 1 ml/5 kg of 0.5% bupivicaine or 2% lignocaine (preservative free) should be administered epidurally.

The lumbosacral space lies immediately caudal to a line joining the cranial aspects of the wings of the ilia and is best approached with the patient in sternal or lateral recumbency with the spine ventroflexed. Sedation or, in some cases, light general anaesthesia may be required, as immobility is essential.

1. Following aseptic preparation, a spinal needle is introduced in the midline at 90° to the skin surface and gently advanced until a popping sensation is felt.
2. To ensure correct needle position, gentle injection should be attempted; absence of resistance indicates correct placement. Alternatively, a drop of saline

can be placed on the needle hub; the negative pressure inside the epidural space will cause the bleb of fluid to be aspirated upon entry of the needle tip.

3. An epidural catheter can be inserted to allow repeated injection or infusion of analgesics. The effects of these drugs upon motor nerve function may mean that some hindlimb weakness or paresis may be evident, but at lower doses this problem is minimized.

The poor lipid solubility of morphine makes it suitable for prolonged analgesia when used epidurally as the preservative-free preparation at 0.1 mg/kg. Onset of analgesia may be slow but it may persist for up to 24 hours. The lack of effect of opioids on motor or autonomic nerve function make these drugs eminently suitable as epidural agents for analgesia in patients likely to suffer prolonged pain (e.g. orthopaedic procedures, pancreatitis), and their effects are potentiated by combination with local analgesics. For prolonged administration, placement of an epidural catheter is appropriate where sterility and catheter maintenance can be ensured.

FURTHER READING

Seymour C and Gleed R (1999) *Manual of Small Animal Anaesthesia and Analgesia.* BSAVA, Cheltenham

CHAPTER NINETEEN

Nutritional Support of the Critical Patient

Karyl Hurley and Kathy Michel

INTRODUCTION

In the critical patient, once major fluid and electrolyte deficits have been addressed and the patient has achieved a degree of haemodynamic stability, time should be taken to consider whether nutritional support is indicated as part of the patient's treatment programme. After all, the point of supporting cardiopulmonary function and vascular perfusion is to ensure adequate tissue oxygenation. The reason tissues require oxygen is to generate energy efficiently from the metabolism of nutrients.

This chapter provides an overview of the potential benefits of nutritional support for the critical patient; demonstrates how to assess whether a patient should be considered a candidate for nutritional support; illustrates methods of providing nutrition to patients unable or unwilling to nourish themselves and suggests methods for monitoring these patients to avoid or address complications.

RATIONALE FOR NUTRITIONAL SUPPORT

Any fasting animal must rely on its endogenous energy and nutrient stores until it is able to nourish itself again. A healthy animal deprived of food will undergo metabolic adaptations that improve its chances of survival by limiting the extent of tissue catabolism. The most critical of these adaptations are the ones that act to preserve endogenous proteins. Carbohydrate, fat and protein can all be utilized as sources of energy. Carbohydrate energy reserves are stored as glycogen in liver and muscle tissue, and fat is stored as triglycerides in adipose tissue. There are, however, no storage forms of protein. All endogenous proteins therefore serve some functional purpose as structural proteins, enzymes, carrier proteins and so forth.

When an animal is deprived of food, glycogen is broken down to maintain blood glucose levels. Once the glycogen reserves have been depleted (within 24 hours) glucose must be synthesized from lactate, glycerol and certain amino acids in order to provide fuel for those tissues that preferentially or obligately use glucose for energy production. In the case of a simple fast, metabolic adaptations occur over the course of days and weeks that act to decrease tissue demands for glucose and thus spare amino acids.

Metabolic adaptations do not occur in the critical patient, however, even though these patients are often in both negative caloric and nitrogen balance. The metabolic milieu of critical illness is very different from that of a simple fast. The substances that mediate the metabolic state, glucocorticoids, catecholamines, cytokines and other hormones, are released in response to tissue injury, infectious agents and inflammation as opposed to a simple lack of food. While some of the amino acids derived from the catabolism of endogenous proteins are either directly oxidized or converted to glucose, a significant portion are utilized for new protein synthesis. In the fasting critical patient it is not the lack of calories, but the lack of amino acids that is more likely to be life threatening. Amino acids are necessary for the synthesis of vital host defence proteins such as immunoglobulins, clotting factors and acute phase reactants.

Providing an exogenous source of amino acids, calories and other nutrients will not eliminate this catabolic response, but can blunt it to some extent and act to support the patient's response to disease and injury while preserving endogenous tissues.

In the case of a patient that has already experienced a significant degree of malnutrition, nutritional support may be essential for survival.

NUTRITIONAL ASSESSMENT: WHO AND WHEN TO FEED

With the greater availability of tubes, catheters and nutrient formulae specifically tailored to veterinary patients, providing nutrition, even to the most critically ill dog or cat, has become increasingly feasible (Figure 19.1). Careful patient selection is required, as nutritional support may have disadvantages. These include an increased risk of morbidity and even mortality, prolongation of hospitalization and additional cost of treatment. It is therefore important to reserve the more aggressive forms of intervention, such as tube feeding or parenteral nutrition, for those patients for whom lack of nutrition will most likely have a negative impact on their clinical outcome.

Medical history
Changes in type of diet
Reduction in food intake on a voluntary and/or non-voluntary basis
Extent and time course of weight loss
Effects of malnutrition on functional status
Underlying disease
Physical examination
Wasting of muscle mass
Wasting of adipose tissue
Presence of oedema or ascites
Evidence of micronutrient deficiencies
Ability to prehend, masticate and swallow normally
Evidence of physical trauma, in particular facial injuries
Evaluation of current intake
Calorie count
Estimation of caloric needs

Figure 19.1: Nutritional assessment.

Traditionally, the types of tests and techniques that have been used for nutritional assessment have been directed at the identification of malnourished patients. These include body condition scoring, assessment of weight loss, measurement of serum proteins, functional tests such as intradermal skin tests and sophisticated body composition analysis (e.g. dual X-ray absorptiometry, bioelectrical impedance). While the severely malnourished individual is easily identified, the diagnostic accuracy of these techniques remains unknown in less obvious cases as there is no universally accepted 'gold standard' of malnutrition against which these tests can be compared.

A system of subjective evaluation of a patient's history and physical examination has been developed for use in humans and has been shown to be accurate in predicting which patients are at risk of developing nutrition-associated complications such as infections or poor wound healing. Whilst this technique has not been validated in veterinary patients, it is a straightforward approach, organizing information that a clinician is likely to already have in his or her possession, with the objective of classifying the patient's nutritional status as normal, marginal (slightly malnourished) or severely malnourished.

Taking the history

A medical history should always include specific questions about the patient's diet and feeding behaviour. It is important to find out whether the current diet and food intake is normal or has changed. Particular attention should be paid to recent reductions in intake on both a voluntary or involuntary basis. Weight loss

should be evaluated with respect to the extent of loss and duration of time over which it has occurred. Loss of the same amount of body mass over a 2-week period can be far more significant than the same loss over a 2-month period, since a greater proportion of the tissue lost is likely to be lean tissue. A history may also reveal information about the impact of malnutrition on functional status as revealed by weakness and exercise intolerance. Finally, the underlying disease process affecting the patient will indicate whether continued deterioration or restoration of nutritional status is to be anticipated.

The physical examination

A number of systems for scoring canine and feline body condition have been published in recent years. None of the systems is ideal for evaluation of the hospitalized patient, since they do not reflect the type of alterations in body composition seen in the acutely critical patient. As previously discussed, the critical patient is often in a state of accelerated catabolism and lean tissue wasting will outstrip adipose tissue breakdown in these circumstances. A more appropriate approach is to evaluate caloric. and protein 'reserves' separately by assessing adipose tissue and skeletal muscle mass, respectively.

In addition to assessment of body condition, other features of the physical examination may indicate a state of malnutrition including oedema, ascites and skin and hair coat lesions which are specific for micronutrient deficiencies.

Selection of patients for nutritional support

Once a patient has been classified as being normal, mildly malnourished or obviously malnourished, it is necessary to decide whether that patient is a candidate for nutritional support (Figure 19.2). At this point, it is essential to have an accurate assessment of the patient's food intake. In cases where the patient appears to have a diminished appetite but is still voluntarily consuming food, it may be necessary to measure food intake for a day or two in order to determine if consumption is adequate. This assessment method requires the estimation of an 'ideal' caloric intake for the patient. Methods for the calculation of energy requirements of hospitalized patients will be discussed in the next section. Ideally, the patient should be consuming a diet balanced for all its nutritional needs. Often, palatable table foods are substituted for pet foods when animals are ill. If the patient refuses to take in at least 50% of its calories in the form of a pet food for more than a few days, efforts should be made to ensure that essential nutrients such as protein- and water-soluble vitamins are being adequately supplied.

For the patient in whom estimated food intake falls short of its ideal, it must be decided whether the lack of optimal nutrition will have an impact on clinical outcome. This is not always an easy judgement. Some general

Patients who were significantly malnourished before the onset of their current illness

Patients who are anticipated to be NPO (nil by mouth) for more than 3–5 days

Previously well nourished patients who develop or are likely to develop serious complications (e.g. septic peritonitis, open discharging skin wounds, aspiration pneumonia)

Figure 19.2: *Selection of patients for nutritional support.*

guidelines are listed in Figure 19.2. Patients assessed as obviously malnourished who have a serious illness should be considered automatic candidates for nutritional support if their voluntary food intake is below estimated goals. Normal or mildly malnourished critical patients, however, can also be at risk of nutrition-associated complications, since their nutritional status can deteriorate rapidly in the face of suboptimal intake. It has been established in human clinical trials that patients do better when nutritional support is initiated early on in their illness. The art of nutritional assessment is therefore to select patients that are likely to have a severe and complicated clinical course and prolonged partial or total anorexia. Furthermore, nutritional support should be initiated as soon as clinically feasible.

NUTRITIONAL REQUIREMENTS OF CRITICAL PATIENTS

Energy requirements

The calculation of energy requirements of critical patients is a subject of some controversy. Much of what has been published in the veterinary literature on this subject was based on human literature that is outdated and has been called into question. The daily energy requirements of an individual reflects the energy required for basic life processes (often referred to as resting energy requirement or RER), a small amount of energy used for the assimilation of nutrients, a variable amount of energy expended during thermogenesis, and the energy expended in physical activity. Generally, the more sick the patient, the more likely it is that RER will approximate that patient's total energy expenditure. The controversy involves the issue of how much the RER of critical illness differs from that of a well individual. It was previously thought that RER was often significantly elevated in critical illness, possibly as much as twice what would be expected under normal circumstances. This was the rationale for the IER (illness energy requirement) approach to estimating the energy requirements of hospitalized patients. That method involved multiplying RER by 'illness factors' ranging from 1.1 to 2.0. Clinical experience and mea-

surements of the energy expenditure of actual patients using indirect calorimetry suggests that the RER of the majority of critical patients, both human and veterinary, is at most only modestly elevated. In addition, feeding excessive calories to critical patients may cause a number of untoward effects including gastrointestinal problems, electrolyte disturbances, hyperglycaemia, hepatic dysfunction and respiratory distress.

Consequently, the current recommendation for estimation of the caloric requirements of critical veterinary patients is to use one of the formulae for RER (Figure 19.3). Using RER as a caloric goal either for patients whose voluntary food intake is being assessed or for patients that will be nutritionally supported, is a reasonable and safe starting point. The amount fed to a given patient can always be increased if that patient experiences weight loss.

Interspecific formulae*
$RER = 70 (Wt_{kg})^{0.75}$
$RER = 30 (Wt_{kg}) + 70$

Feline formula
$RER = 40 (Wt_{kg})$

Figure 19.3: *Calculation of RER for dogs and cats. *These formulae tend to overestimate feline energy requirements.*

Protein requirements

While it does appear that most hospitalized patients do not have resting energy requirements that differ greatly from normal, their protein requirements can be significantly greater during critical illness. The amount of protein an animal requires in its diet is a reflection of amino acid needs for protein synthesis and replacement of degraded or lost amino acids. Cats also have an obligatory need for amino acids for energy production. The nature of the protein source will also affect the amount required in the diet, since some protein sources are limiting in one or more essential amino acids.

Ideally, the dietary source of protein used for critical patients would be highly digestible and contain all the essential amino acids in appropriate amounts. As a rule, animal sources of protein, in particular, egg and milk proteins, meet these criteria. For patients receiving enteral nutrition, protein should comprise at least 20–30% of calories (2–3 g/kg body weight) for dogs and >30% of calories (3 g/kg body weight) for cats. There are veterinary products designed for the nutritional support of veterinary patients that meet these guidelines (Figures 19.4 and 19.5).

Some critical patients with kidney or hepatic dysfunction may not tolerate this quantity of protein. These patients do not have decreased protein requirements; rather, they have impaired ability to eliminate nitrogen byproducts of protein metabolism (e.g. urea and ammonia). Therefore feeding strategies for these patients should involve supportive therapies that

Characteristics	Whiskas Feline Concentration Diet	Pedigree Canine Concentration Diet	a/d	Eukanuba Nutritional Recovery
Energy density	1.2 kcal/ml	1.4 kcal/ml	1.3 kcal/ml	2.1 kcal/ml
Protein	37%	29%	34%	29%
Fat	60%	49%	53%	66%
Carbohydrate	3%	22%	13%	5%
Tube suitability	> 8 Fr	> 8 Fr	> 8Fr	> 8 Fr
Manufacturer	Waltham	Waltham	Hill's Pet Nutrition, Inc.	Iams

Figure 19.4: Tube feeding diets for cats and dogs.

Characteristics	Whiskas Feline Liquid Concentration Diet	Pedigree Canine Liquid Concentration Diet
Energy density	1.2 kcal/ml	1.5 kcal/ml
Protein	37%	38%
Fat	41%	35%
Carbohydrate	22%	27%
Tube suitability	All types	All types
Manufacturer	Waltham	Waltham

Figure 19.5: Liquid diets for cats and dogs.

improve the elimination of protein metabolic waste products (i.e. fluid diuresis for renal failure, oral lactulose for hepatic failure) thus allowing as much protein intake as possible.

Micronutrient requirements

In addition to water, calories and protein there are at least 25 other essential nutrients, including fatty acids, minerals and vitamins. It is not known how critical illness might affect a patient's micronutrient requirements. Current recommendations are to provide amounts that meet at least normal adult maintenance requirements (Figure 19.6). Often a patient will have adequate endogenous stores of most of these nutrients to survive weeks or in some cases months of reduced food intake. A number of these nutrients, in particular, the water-soluble vitamins, are, however, very labile and a patient may become significantly depleted in a short period of time.

Depending on a patient's nutritional status at the time of presentation, it may be already suffering from deficiencies of one or more B vitamins or electrolytes. Most veterinary enteral products are nutritionally bal-anced, so barring problems with nutrient assimilation; deficiency states should not arise. Electrolyte deficiencies are generally secondary to excessive fluid losses as opposed to malnutrition and are addressed in Chapter 12. In the case of severe protein–calorie malnutrition, extreme imbalances of potassium, phosphorus and magnesium may occur. This situation, known as 'refeeding syndrome,' will be discussed in more detail in the section on complications of nutritional support.

ROUTES OF NUTRITIONAL SUPPORT

Enteral nutrition

The age-old adage 'if the gut works, use it' still holds true. The intestinal epithelium requires glutamine and regular access to nutrients to maintain the health of enterocytes, including the height of the villi, the function of brush border enzymes and the maintenance of other neuroendocrine exchanges between the pancreas, stomach and small intestine. The nourishment provided via enteral feeding, therefore, helps to protect against bacterial translocation, absorption of endotoxin and the development of sepsis in critically ill patients unwilling or unable to maintain their own nutrient intake. Fortunately, the enteral route is also more economical, easier to implement and associated with fewer complications than parenteral feeding. Methods of enteral feeding include assisted feeding, chemical stimulation of appetite and infusion of nutrients via feeding tubes within the gastrointestinal tract, bypassing the oral cavity (Figure 19.7). Deciding which method to use is dependent upon several factors, including the animal's current nutritional status and general state of health, the estimated length of required nutritional support, the animal's tolerance for general anaesthesia, the experience of the clinician and the associated costs of the procedures.

AAFCO nutrient profiles

Nutrient	Units/ 1000 kcal ME	Adult dog		Adult cat	
		Minimum	Maximum	Minimum	Maximum
Protein	g	51.4		65	
Arginine	g	1.46		2.6	
Taurine	g			0.5	
Linoleic acid	g	2.9		1.25	
Arachidonic acid	g			0.05	
Phosphorus	g	1.4	4.6	1.25	
Potassium	g	1.7		1.5	
Zinc	mg	34	286	18.75	500
Vitamin A	IU	1429	71,429	1250	18,750
Vitamin D	IU	143	1429	125	2500
Vitamin E	IU	14	286	7.5	
Thiamin	mg	0.29		1.25	
Riboflavin	mg	0.63		1	
Pantothenic acid	mg	2.9		1.25	
Niacin	mg	3.3		15	
Pyridoxine	mg	0.29		1	
Folic acid	mg	0.05		0.2	
Vitamin B_{12}	mg	0.006		0.005	

Figure 19.6: *Micronutrient requirements of dogs and cats.*
ME: metabolizable energy.

Method	Advantages	Disadvantages
Assisted feeding	Simple, less stressful	Not effective in many animals
Chemical stimulants	Simple, 'reminds' patients of the taste of foods	May induce sedation Short term (2–3 days)
Naso-oesophageal tube (3.5–5 Fr; cats) (3.5–8 Fr; dogs)	Easy to place, least invasive, low cost Requires minimal sedation, if any Use up to 1 week	Not well tolerated by some patients Must use an E-collar Requires liquid diet
Pharyngostomy tube (8–14 Fr; cats) (12–18 Fr; dogs)	No special equipment required Can be used long term	Requires general anaesthesia Malpositioning can lead to aspiration Used only in large dogs
Oesophagostomy tube (8–18 Fr)	No special equipment required Can be used long term	Requires general anaesthesia Infection of wound may occur
Gastrostomy tube (14–20 Fr)	Easy to maintain, few complications Can be used for months	Requires general anaesthesia Specialized equipment needed
Enterostomy tube (5–8 Fr)	Bypasses pancreas and dysfunctional gastrointestinal tract	Requires general anaesthesia Liquid diet constantly infused for minimum of 7 days Requires intensive care

Figure 19.7: *Routes of enteral nutritional support.*

Assisted feeding

Assisted feeding is a sensible and easily applied method of nutritional support and may be adequate for the partially anorexic patient. This method is directed at encouraging voluntary intake and does not imply force feeding. Force feeding should be avoided, as it increases the stress of an already compromised patient, increases the likelihood of aspiration and injury and more commonly results in the topical, rather than enteral, application of nutrients. Gently tempting the patient with small, frequent meals of a highly palatable diet consisting of wet, odiferous, warm food, in a quiet environment may stimulate self-feeding. Home-prepared chicken, fish or red meats are often successful menu choices. If the patient does not voluntarily eat what is offered, gently syringing a soft or liquid diet into the corner of the mouth may stimulate the animal to eat on its own.

Chemical stimulation of appetite

If an adequate intake is not attained by the above methods, chemical stimulants such as diazepam (0.05–0.4 mg/kg i.v., i.m. or orally once daily) may be used to increase the appetite and 'remind' a patient of the taste of food, encouraging them to eat voluntarily. Application of these drugs may result in the consumption of 25% of the daily requirement in responsive cats (Figure 19.8). This option should be reserved, however, as a short-term 'kick-start' in patients likely to recover in a short time period and is not a good option for the long-term anorexic or inappetent patient. The side effects of benzodiazepine appetite stimulants may include drowsiness, excessive sedation or even hepatic necrosis in cats (diazepam), limiting their usefulness.

Tube feeding

In many critically ill animals, the *best* way to ensure that adequate nutritional intake is achieved is to place a feeding tube and deliver food and water according to the calculated requirements. Several types of feeding tubes have been described and will be reviewed here. In general, the more proximal the feeding tube, the more physiologically appropriate the feeding regimen and the less likelihood a gastrointestinal upset will occur. The authors prefer the use of naso-oesophageal tubes for the short-term feeding of critically ill patients and oesophagostomy or percutaneously placed gastrostomy tubes for periods longer than 7 days.

Naso-oesophageal tubes

These are the simplest, least invasive and most commonly used feeding tubes and are excellent choices for the short-term feeding of hospitalized patients. Owners will rarely opt to maintain these tubes in the home environment, but it can be done. Soft flexible polyvinyl feeding tubes are easily placed into the nostril with a topical anaesthetic and minimal sedation (Figures 19.9 and 19.10). They should terminate just short of the lower oesophageal sphincter rather than in the stomach, to avoid inducing gastro-oesophageal reflux. The largest tube diameter that fits snugly in the internal nares should be used to maximize the feeding capacity. Naso-oesophageal feeding tubes are contraindicated in those patients that have severe facial trauma involving the nares and nasal turbinates, those that are experiencing protracted vomiting and/or regurgitation, those that are semi- or unconscious and those that have pharyngeal, laryngeal or oesophageal physical or functional abnormalities.

Once in place, these tubes may be used intermittently, dividing the total daily intake into small frequent meals, or less commonly, a liquid diet may be given as a continuous infusion. Complications that can arise with the use of these tubes may include rhinitis, vomiting or regurgitation. Aspiration of oesophageal contents

Drug	Dose	Side effects
Diazepam	0.05 – 0.15 mg/kg i.v., i.m., or 1 mg orally sid	Sedation, idiosyncratic hepatic necrosis
Oxazepam	5–10 mg orally bid	Same as diazepam
Cyproheptadine	8 mg/m^2 or 2–4 mg/cat orally sid–bid 5–20 mg/dog orally sid–bid	Excitability, aggression, vomiting
Others:		
Nandrolone	5 mg/kg i.m. weekly; dogs	Uncommon
Stanozolol	1–2 mg orally bid; cats 1–4 mg orally bid; dogs	
Prednisolone	0.5–1 mg/kg sid–bid	PU/PD, decreased wound healing, may interfere with therapy for disease
Megoestrol acetate	5 mg/cat orally sid x 3–4 days then eod x 5 days, then twice weekly	PU/PD, diabetes mellitus, stump pyometra, adrenocortical suppression, hepatotoxicity

Figure 19.8: *Chemical stimulation of appetite.*
eod: every other day, PU/PD: polyuria/polydipsia.

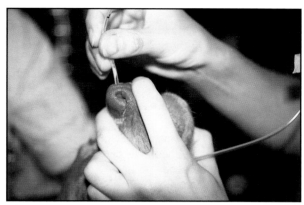

Figure 19.9: *Placement of a nasogastric tube in a 5-month-old dog. A 5 Fr naso-oesophageal tube has been measured to the 9th rib space and marked with a piece of white tape, and a topical anaesthetic has been placed in the left nostril. To facilitate passage into the ventromedial nasal meatus, the nares are directed upwards.*

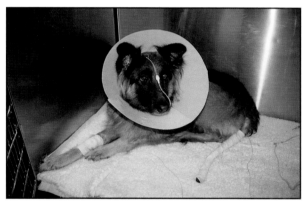

Figure 19.10: *German Shepherd Dog with a naso-oesophageal tube. Once in place, the tube is secured to the external nares with 'super-glue', or preferably a small suture passed retrogradely through a 24 gauge needle. Two more sutures secure the tube to the dorsum of the nose and top of the head, out of the dog's direct line of vision. An Elizabethan collar prevents the dog from bothering the tube.*

is more likely if the animal is very weak or suffering neurological deficits and is fed, or remains in prolonged lateral recumbency after feeding.

Oesophagostomy tubes

Oesophagostomy tubes are variably sized tubes which are easily placed under light anaesthesia with minimal equipment requirements (Crowe, 1990). The only major associated complication (rare) is the development of infection at the entry site, and meticulous care of the surgical wound is essential to maintain the tube. With the advent and increasing awareness and familiarity with the placement and use of gastrostomy tubes, the smaller oesophagostomy and pharyngostomy tubes are infrequently used. Larger bore oesophagostomy tubes may, however, be an ideal option for the general practice environment, as they are relatively simple to place and can be maintained for months.

Pharyngostomy tubes

In contrast to a naso-oesophageal tube, a pharyngostomy tube is of a larger bore. In animals with nasal disease or intolerance of naso-oesophageal tubes, a pharyngostomy tube may be preferable. The patient must be anaesthetized and the area prepared for surgery. An incision is made caudal to the hyoid bone in order to insert the tube into the pharynx. The tube is threaded into the distal oesophagus (Crowe, 1990; Simpson and Elwood, 1994). Problems associated with the placement and maintenance of these tubes include incorrect placement, interference with laryngeal function, aspiration, vomiting of the tube and production of cellulitis or infection surrounding the skin incision. Placement is difficult in small dogs and only larger breeds should be considered as candidates.

Gastrostomy tubes

Gastrostomy tubes have become invaluable for the long-term nutritional support of critically ill or recovering patients. Gastric feeding tubes may be placed surgically, endoscopically or by a 'blind' placement technique. Surgical placement of gastric feeding tubes is convenient when an abdominal surgery is warranted for other purposes such as obtaining organ biopsies or removal of masses. These tubes may be 'pexyed' in position and tightly sealed with omentum to prevent leakage. Balloon-tipped Foley catheters meant for use in the urinary tract should be avoided owing to the possibility of balloon rupture and displacement of the catheter, increasing the risk of peritoneal cavity contamination.

In our experience, an easier and less invasive means of gastric tube placement is by use of an endoscope (Figures 19.11–19.21). Tubes may be placed efficiently within 10–15 minutes under general anaesthesia, the limiting factors being accessibility and endoscopic experience. The most economical type of feeding tube is fashioned from a mushroom-tipped catheter in which only minor alterations are needed. The tip can be removed to add a feeding conduit and the widened catheter-end is then cut to form two stents which are placed on either side of the positioned tube to anchor the tube in place and to prevent its inadvertent removal. The benefit of using this type of tube is that when the animal no longer requires nutritional support, the tube is simply pulled firmly and the stents slip off allowing complete removal of the tube. The internal stent is usually small enough to be passed in the faeces and rarely ever requires a second anaesthetic for endoscopic retrieval. The disadvantage of these tubes is that they may be inadvertently removed by a strong tug.

A simpler, yet more expensive system, is the use of pre-packaged human enteral feeding tubes. We currently use a commercially available 15 Fr polyurethane tube (Fresenius). The advantage of these kits is that they contain all that is necessary to place the tube, they are suitable for use in cats and dogs and they are difficult to remove inadvertently. The disadvantage is that a second anaesthetic is required to remove the solid plastic disk that keeps the tube anchored internally, preventing its removal. Once the external tube is cut away, this disk is not easily passed along the gastrointestinal tract and may result in a foreign body obstruction if not retrieved endoscopically. 'Blind' tube placement, without direct visualization of the site of internal insertion, is facilitated by the use of a long rigid stylet passed via the oesophagus and palpated through the stomach wall (Torrance, 1996). This is an excellent technique available to practitioners when endoscopic or surgical placement is not possible. Care must be taken not to lacerate the spleen or oesophagus during placement, and it is advised to verify tube placement radiographicaly postprocedure.

Gastric feeding tubes may be used for periods up to one year if carefully maintained (Figure 19.22). Most patients tolerate the tubes quite well, although body wraps are advised to prevent the wound from becoming soiled. In the overly enthusiastic patient, an Elizabethan collar may be necessary to prevent the patient from chewing or removing the tube. Fortunately, complications are uncommon and might include splenic laceration as discussed during placement, infection or cellulitis at the site of exit from the body wall, vomiting due to slippage of the tube back into the gastric lumen, or peritonitis from contamination of the peritoneal cavity.

In the future, low-profile enterostomy 'button' devices, which occupy the fistula between the gastrointestinal tract and the body wall, now used in human medicine, may become more widely available for use in veterinary patients. These 'button' devices may be left in place long term with minimal complications.

Enterostomy tubes

Placement of feeding tubes beyond the stomach is rarely indicated, but in cases of pancreatitis, diffuse gastric mucosal disease, protracted vomiting or delayed gastric emptying, an enterostomy tube may be life saving. Enterostomy tubes are most commonly placed

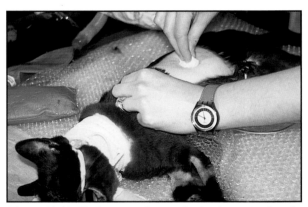

Figure 19.11: Under general anaesthesia, the cat is placed in right lateral recumbency and an area (~10cm x 10cm) just behind the rib cage is clipped and surgically prepared. A mouth gag is used to protect the teeth from damaging the endoscope. The stomach is insufflated with air to move all other abdominal contents, specifically intestines and spleen, away from the body wall.

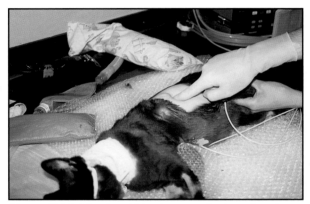

Figure 19.12: The site within the stomach where the tube will be anchored is chosen with the aid of an assistant, who wears sterile gloves and indents the surface of the prepared skin just caudal to the rib cage and directed caudally.

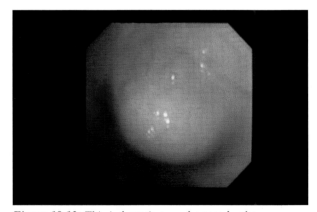

Figure 19.13: This indentation can be seen by the endoscopist, who then directs the assistant to an area well away from the pyloric outflow tract into the fundus of the stomach where the tube is to be situated.

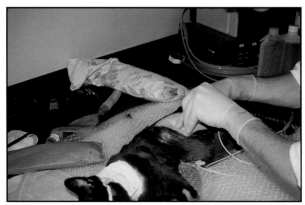

Figure 19.14: A small, ~2 mm, incision is made in the skin just over this site.

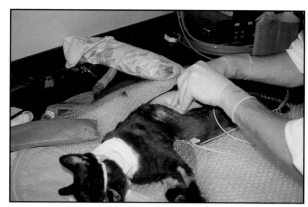

Figure 19.15: *An 18 gauge catheter (dogs and cats) is sharply introduced.*

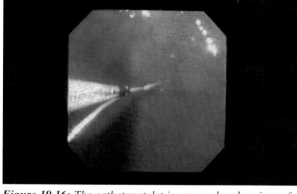

Figure 19.16: *The catheter stylet is removed and a piece of suture material is passed into the stomach. Biopsy forceps are then used to retrieve the end of the suture, which is pulled into the endoscope as it is removed from the patient. The assistant must allow the suture to thread easily into the stomach, and the catheter can then be removed.*

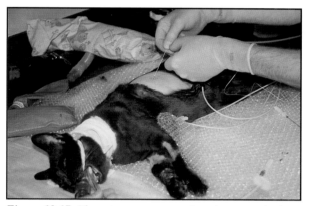

Figure 19.17: *The suture now passes into the stomach via the body wall, extends up the oesophagus and out of the mouth. In human enteral feeding tubes such as this one (Fresenius), the tip is narrowed to pass through the body wall. When using a mushroom-tipped pezzar catheter, a small pipette tip is placed on to the end of the suture (tip threaded first!), and the suture is then fixed to the tube with multiple knots.*

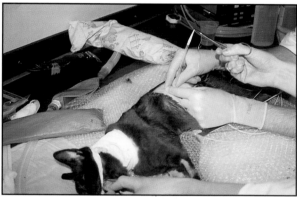

Figure 19.18: *The assistant slowly retracts the suture, exiting the body wall until the tip of the pipette can be palpated. The stomach is held in place while the tube is pulled through the gastric mucosa and exits the body wall. A haemostat clamp can be used to grab hold of the pipette tip and exert an even upward pressure. Simply pulling the suture may result in breakage.*

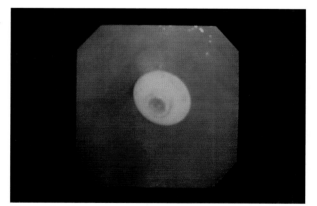

Figure 19.19: *Once the tube has been pulled into place, it is important to go back and look in the stomach to verify that the tip is not stuck at the lower oesophageal sphincter and the tube is in an appropriate position, away from the pyloric outflow tract.*

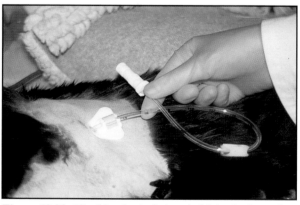

Figure 19.20: *Flexible plastic fittings hold the feeding tube in place. Tight placement may result in pressure necrosis and increase the incidence of infection. The tube site is then wrapped in sterile material.*

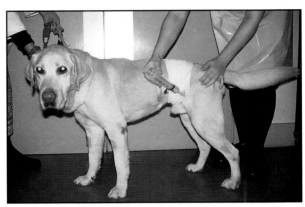

Figure 19.21: A percutaneously placed gastric tube in a 3-year-old Labrador with megaoesophagus.

surgically, or they may be introduced via a gastric tube and then directed through the pylorus with an endoscope. At surgery, a flexible, small bore tube is threaded into the proximal jejunum or late duodenum and secured with a purse string. The delivery end is exited through an abdominal stab incision and fixed to the abdominal wall (Simpson and Elwood, 1994). Feeding through an enterostomy tube must be carefully controlled since the diets are often concentrated in order to supply enough calories and may lead to osmotic overload and diarrhoea. As with other 'ostomy' tubes, these must remain in place for a minimum of 7–10 days to allow a seal to form with the abdominal wall. Continuous infusion of a dilute liquid diet is the preferred method of use, therefore the patient must remain hospitalized while the tube is in place, which limits their long-term employment.

Parenteral nutrition

Parenteral nutrition (PN) is nutrition delivered by the intravenous route. It can be lifesaving for patients who cannot tolerate enteral feeding. However, because there are numerous drawbacks associated with this form of nourishment, it should be reserved for those patients for whom no other feeding option exists and for whom the need for nourishment is felt to be a critical factor in their recovery. Generally, these are patients for whom enteral feeding is contraindicated or hazardous.

Special solutions are used for intravenous feeding and must be mixed aseptically and in a specific order. PN is best delivered continuously (although this is not absolutely necessary); therefore 24-hour nursing care is desirable. Also, many of the potential complications of PN (sepsis and various electrolyte disturbances) can be life threatening, so careful monitoring of the patient is mandated. Finally, a consequence of the intensive care and special supplies required to deliver PN to a patient is a significant increase in the cost of care.

Venous access

Ideally, a catheter should be dedicated for PN infusion alone. The reason for this is the increased risk of catheter sepsis associated with the infusion of a nutrient-rich solution. By dedicating a line to PN alone and observing strict aseptic care of the line and its connections, the potential for bacterial contamination is reduced. Central venous access is preferable to peripheral access, since PN solutions are hyperosmolar and associated with the development of thrombophlebitis. However, PN solutions can be diluted adequately to permit peripheral infusion as long as the patient is not at risk of fluid volume overload. PN solutions infused via peripheral catheters should not exceed 800 mOsm/l and if possible should be less than 600 mOsm/l. In addition, use of fine bore polyurethane or silicone elastomer cannulae will greatly reduce the risk of thrombophlebitis.

1. Don't use the tube for the first 24 hours. This will allow a primary seal to form between the stomach and body wall.

2. Start with small amounts of water; 5 ml/kg, to flush the tube.

3. Feed only one-third of the calculated daily caloric requirement the first day. This is divided into small (20–30 ml) frequent (5–6) feedings.

4. The food is warmed to body temperature and injected into the stomach over several minutes. If the animal begins to retch or swallow, slow down or stop altogether and try again the next feeding.

5. Aspirate the contents of the stomach with an empty syringe prior to each feeding. If gastric emptying is delayed and there is more than half the previous meal in the stomach, skip the feeding and consider motility modifiers such as metoclopramide.

6. ALWAYS FOLLOW BASIC TUBE ETIQUETTE: FLUSH before and after feedings with 5–10 ml of water, to clear debris and maintain tube patency.

7. On the second day of use, the feeding is increased to two-thirds the calculated caloric intake and then up to full feedings if tolerated by the third day.

8. Change sterile bandage every 2–3 days after initial placement, check placement of tube and clean wound.

Figure 19.22: General guidelines for the use of gastrostomy tubes.

PN solutions

Basic PN is composed of a protein source (crystalline amino acid solutions), a carbohydrate source (dextrose) and a fat source (lipid emulsion). Vitamins, electrolytes and trace minerals can also be added so that the resulting solution is complete and balanced, at least according to standards for healthy dogs and cats.

Because most veterinary patients receive PN for limited periods of time (often a week or less), the focus should be on providing protein, calories and the more labile vitamins (water-soluble vitamins). Electrolyte supplementation is managed as a component of fluid therapy as opposed to PN. Providing more complete nutrition to a patient parenterally is problematic due to compatibility problems between various nutrients and nutrient formulations, as well as expense. If the patient is not on a balanced enteral diet within a week of starting PN, fat-soluble vitamins are supplemented separately (intramuscularly or subcutaneously) on a weekly basis. Parenteral trace mineral supplements are also available.

PN solutions should be made fresh daily and must be mixed in a specific order under aseptic conditions. Special PN compounding bags can be used, or solutions can be prepared in evacuated glass containers. In general, amino acid and dextrose solutions are mixed first and then electrolyte and mineral solutions are added. Great care must be taken when adding combinations of electrolytes, especially phosphorus and calcium, because precipitates can easily form. Next, multivitamins are added and finally the lipid emulsion. The lipid emulsion is fragile and the suspended triglyceride particles can coalesce or even precipitate. Precipitation of lipid emulsions can be detected by visual inspection after the solution has been sitting for a while. There should not be any indication of separation or layering of the final solution.

Prescription formulation

Figure 19.23 shows a worksheet and a sample calculation for formulating PN. Because of the limited discussion of PN in this chapter the reader is encouraged to seek a more detailed review of this technique. There are several guidelines for formulating PN for small animals in the literature (Lippert *et al.*, 1989; Lippert, 1992; Hill, 1994).

Monitoring and treating the complications of nutritional support

The monitoring required of nutritional support in the critically ill patient is typically no different from what might be expected for any critical patient; routine physical examinations, body temperature, heart rate and respiratory rate, twice daily weight measurements, assessment of hydration status and general demeanour. Laboratory values frequently assessed include total proteins, albumin, packed cell volume, electrolytes and blood urea nitrogen. Alterations in these parameters may indicate improved patient status due to correction and support of the underlying disease or, conversely, may signal early warnings of complications associated with nutritional support. In a recent study of anorexic cats, high creatinine kinase (CK) activity was found exceeding an average of 250 times that of normally nourished cats (Fascetti *et al.*, 1997). In response to nutritional intervention, the CK activity decreased and eventually returned to normal. CK may prove to be a useful marker of nutritional status in the clinical setting.

Complications associated with enteral nutrition fall into the categories of mechanical, gastrointestinal or metabolic. Mechanical complications most commonly encountered include obstruction of the feeding tube, dislodgement of a tube, or infection/cellulitis at the site of tube entry. Obstruction of feeding tubes may be minimized by the use of foodstuffs of the appropriate consistency in relation to the tube size. Those tubes of 5 Fr diameter and smaller should only ever admit liquid diets, whereas larger sized tubes may admit thoroughly blenderized diets but still risk blockage if the diets are not properly diluted and the tubes are not flushed after feeding. Ideally, to minimize the chances of blockage and to prevent wear, tubes should be used solely for feeding purposes and not for the administration of medications. Should a tube become clogged and unresponsive to hydrostatic pressure, cola or, alternatively, Viokase powder mixed in sodium bicarbonate can be left in the tube overnight to help dissolve the offending material. If neither is successful, the tube requires replacement.

Gastrointestinal complications are, unfortunately, common and typically manifest as nausea, vomiting and diarrhoea. These may be avoided by a slow introduction to feeding and by administering dilute solutions to avoid a sudden intraluminal hypertonicity. The first day of feeding should begin with incremental amounts of water and one-third of the daily caloric requirements divided into five or six feedings. Two-thirds of the calculated caloric intake is given on the second day and full feedings on the third. Prior to each feeding via a gastrostomy tube, the tube is aspirated to ensure that the stomach has emptied from the previous meal. If not, the amount remaining is subtracted from the current feeding. Diarrhoea may occur despite these precautions due to villus atrophy of prolonged anorexia, intolerance of the chosen diet, antibiotic-induced alterations in intestinal flora, or as a manifestation of the underlying illness. Treatment with motility-modifying drugs, the addition of fibre, or a change to parenteral nutrition may be necessary.

Metabolic derangements resulting from enteral nutritional support are rare. The duration of illness and the severity and nature of the underlying disease may predispose some patients to glucose intolerance (and hence hyperglycaemia or glucosuria), hyperlipidaemia or electrolyte disturbances. These are more commonly encountered in patients receiving PN. Correction of

Day 1 goal: 50% RER
Day 2 goal: 100% RER

(see Figure 19.3 for RER formulae)

Protein calories: Dogs: 15–25% of RER
                               Cats: 25–35% of RER

Select % protein calories based on the patient's protein status and ability to tolerate dietary protein.

Non-protein calories: 30–60% from lipid
                               40–70% from dextrose

Dogs: provide 50% of non-protein calories from lipid and 50% from dextrose unless there is pre-existing hyperlipidaemia or hyperglycaemia.

Cats: provide 60% of non-protein calories from lipid and 40% from dextrose unless there is pre-existing hyperlipidaemia or hyperglycaemia. Cats are more likely to become hyperglycaemic, which is why more calories are provided as lipids as a rule.

Solutions:

1. Amino acids

   1 g of amino acids provides approximately 4 kcal

   Use solutions containing 3.5–5% amino acids (350–500 mOsm/l).
   Use solutions without additional electrolytes to simplify management of electrolytes with fluid therapy.

2. Dextrose

   10% dextrose contains 500 mOsm/l and provides 0.34 kcal/ml.
   20% dextrose contains 1000 mOsm/l and provides 0.68 kcal/ml.

3. Lipid emulsions

   Use 20% lipid emulsions, which contain 268–340 mOsm/l and provide 2 kcal/ml.

4. Phosphorus

   Use standard parenteral potassium phosphate solutions.

5. B vitamins

   Use standard parenteral B complex solutions.

Example calculations: a 17.5 kg dog without hypoproteinaemia

RER = $70(17.5)^{0.75}$ = 600 kcal/day
Goal calories for day 1 = 0.5(600) = 300 kcal

1. Amino acids

(0.15)(300 kcal) = 45 kcal from protein
45 kcal ÷ 4 kcal/g = 11.25 g
4.25% amino acid solution = 0.0425 g protein/ml
therefore you need *265* ml 4.25% amino acid solution
(x ml = 11.25 g ÷ 0.0425 g/ml)

2. Non-protein calories

(0.85)(300 kcal) = 255 kcal from lipid and dextrose
(a) 20% lipid emulsion to provide 50% non-protein
   calories = 127.5 kcal
   20% lipid emulsion = 2.0 kcal/ml
   therefore you need *64* ml 20% lipid emulsion
   (x ml = 127.5 kcal ÷ 2.0 kcal/ml)
(b) 20% dextrose to provide 50% non-protein calories
   = 127.5 kcal
   20% dextrose solution = 0.68 kcal/ml
   therefore you need *188* ml 20% dextrose solution
   (x ml = 127.5 kcal ÷ 0.68 kcal/ml)

3. Potassium phosphate

dosed at 8 mM/1000 kcal delivered
therefore you need *2.4* mM potassium phosphate
x mM = (8 mM)(300 kcal) ÷ (1000 kcal)

4. Vitamin B complex

dosed at approximately 2 ml/l infused
total infusate for day 1 = 518 ml
therefore *1.0* ml B complex should be sufficient

5. Infusion rate

518 ml/24 h = *22* ml/h
The osmolarity of this solution is approximately 625 mOsm/l.

Day 2 calculations
Same as day 1, but substitute 600 kcal for 300 kcal.

Figure 19.23: Worksheet for peripheral parenteral nutrition.
RER: resting energy requirement.

these abnormalities requires manipulation of the fluid regimen and dietary components and appropriate therapy for the underlying disorder. Persistent hyperglycaemia may infrequently require the use of insulin. In human medicine, a phenomenon known as 'refeeding syndrome' has been described whereupon initiation of nutritional support to malnourished patients, severe metabolic derangements occur, the most significant of which is hypophosphataemia. A similar syndrome has been recently described in association with enteral feeding in cats. Refeeding produced hypophosphataemia and haemolysis in a small number of cases within 12–72 hours. Cats with diabetes mellitus or high liver enzyme activities, hyperbilirubinaemia and weight loss seem to be at increased risk, and these patients should be closely monitored for the development of low serum phosphorus and subsequent haemolytic anaemia when initiating nutritional support (Justin and Hohenhous, 1995).

Complications of PN are more common than those of enteral support and are either associated with the mechanics of administration, sepsis, or metabolic derangements, the occurrence of which depends upon the components and proportions administered. Mechanical complications are frequent and include broken, chewed, obstructed or dislodged administration lines and catheters. They rarely have an effect on the patient, but do increase the possibility of sepsis. PN should be supplied via dedicated fluid lines to centrally placed catheters, the meticulous care of which is essential. To avoid contamination and potential sepsis, the ports must be tightly secured and wrapped with disinfectant-soaked swabs. The site of catheter placement should be inspected daily, gently scrubbed and wrapped aseptically. Patients receiving PN should be closely monitored for the development of fever, depression and leucocytosis, which signal probable sepsis. When these signs are recognized, the catheter is removed, the tip is cultured and aggressive fluid and broad-spectrum antibiotic therapy is instituted.

Metabolic derangements occur frequently in patients receiving PN but rarely result in clinical signs. Common abnormalities found include hyperglycaemia, glucosuria, azotaemia, lipaemia and electrolyte changes such as hypokalaemia, hypomagnesaemia and hypophosphataemia. Cats and some dogs readily develop glucose intolerance and may require insulin therapy. Azotaemia and lipaemia are likely to be a result of the highly concentrated intravenous infusions of amino acids and lipid emulsions, which overwhelm the body's capacity for utilization or storage. Electrolyte disturbances occur most frequently in patients that are vomiting and are easily addressed with appropriate fluid

therapy. The key to minimizing metabolic abnormalities is early detection. Frequent haematological and biochemical profiles are indicated to allow prompt correction of fluid electrolyte concentrations. In addition, antiemetics should be administered, infusion rates adjusted and proportions of components modified.

In conclusion, nutritional support is rapidly becoming a primary concern rather than an afterthought for our critically ill veterinary patients. As we become more experienced in the application of nutrition, we are increasingly aware of its benefits in shortening recovery time and decreasing morbidity and mortality experienced by our patients. The time and effort expended in stabilizing the critical patient is well spent if we do not allow that patient's nutritional status to become a limiting factor in its recovery.

REFERENCES AND FURTHER READING

Abood SK and Buffington CT (1992) Enteral feeding of dogs and cats: 51 cases (1989–1991). *Journal of the American Medical Association* **201**, 610–622

Crowe DT (1990) Nutritional support for the hospitalized patient: an introduction to tube feeding. *Compendium on Continuing Education for the Practicing Veterinarian* **12**, 1711–1720

Fascetti AJ, Mauldin GE and Mauldin GN (1997) Correlation between serum creatinine kinase activities and anorexia in cats. *Journal of Veterinary Internal Medicine* **11**, 9–13

Hill RC (1994) Critical care nutrition. In: *The Waltham Book of Clinical Nutrition of the Dog and Cat*, ed. JM Wills and KW Simpson, pp. 39–61. Elsevier Science, Oxford

Justin RB and Hohenhous AE (1995) Hypophosphatemia associated with enteral alimentation in cats. *Journal of Veterinary Internal Medicine* **9**, 228–233

Lippert AC (1992) The metabolic response to injury: enteral and parenteral nutritional support. In: *Veterinary Emergency and Critical Care Medicine*, ed. RJ Murtaugh and PM Kaplan, pp. 593–617. Mosby, Boston

Lippert AC, Faulkner JE, Evans AT *et al.* (1989) Total parenteral nutrition in clinically normal cats. *Journal of the American Veterinary Medical Association* **194**, 669–676

Lippert AC, Fulton RB and Parr AM (1993) A retrospective study of the use of total parenteral nutrition in dogs and cats. *Journal of Veterinary Internal Medicine* **7**, 52–64

Michel KE (1997) Practice guidelines for gastrostomy tubes. *Compendium on Continuing Education for the Practicing Veterinarian* **19**, 306–309

Simpson KW and Elwood CM (1994) Techniques for enteral support. In: *The Waltham Book of Clinical Nutrition of the Dog and Cat*, ed. JM Wills and KW Simpson, pp. 63–74. Elsevier Science, Oxford

Tennant B (1996) Feeding the sick animal. In: *Manual of Companion Animal Nutrition and Feeding*, ed. N Kelly and J Wills, pp. 181–187. BSAVA, Cheltenham

Tennant G and Willoughby K (1993) The use of enteral nutrition in small animal medicine. *Compendium on Continuing Education for the Practicing Veterinarian* **15**, 1054–1068

Torrance AG (1996) Intensive care — nutritional support. In: *Manual of Companion Animal Nutrition and Feeding*, ed. N Kelly and J Wills, pp. 171–180. BSAVA, Cheltenham

Wheeler SL and McGuire BH (1989) Enteral nutritional support. In: *Current Veterinary Therapy X*, ed. RW Kirk, pp. 30–37. WB Saunders, Philadelphia

CHAPTER TWENTY

Drug Therapy in the Critical Patient

Reid Groman and Dawn Merton Boothe

The critical patient presents with numerous physiological and pathological changes, which profoundly affect drug disposition and response. These patients are also likely to receive more than one drug simultaneously, predisposing to negative drug interactions.

ADVERSE DRUG REACTIONS

Type A reactions are exaggerated, but otherwise normal and expected pharmacological (or toxic) responses to a drug. They occur because plasma drug concentrations have entered the toxic or subtherapeutic range and thus are predictable and largely avoidable. Drugs that target the cardiovascular and central nervous system (CNS) present the greatest risk, as adverse responses in either of these systems are often rapidly fatal. In addition, many critical patients are predisposed to reactions in these body systems because of physiological consequences of illness, such as hypotension. Failure to respond to a life-saving drug might also be considered a type A reaction, which can be life-threatening (e.g. antibiotic therapy in a potentially bacteraemic situation). Type A adverse reactions are less likely with drugs characterized by a wide safety margin (e.g. most antibiotics), if the clinical response is easily detected (e.g. gas anaesthetics or resolution of seizures) or if the drug can be monitored to ensure that concentrations are within the therapeutic range (e.g. selected antibiotics, cardiac drugs and anticonvulsant drugs).

Many type A adverse reactions can be avoided by choosing alternative, safer or more effective drugs, or by modifying the dosing regimen of a drug to accommodate disease or drug-induced changes in drug disposition. Modification of dosing regimens requires a fundamental knowledge of drug disposition and its role in determining a dosing regimen. A focus on antimicrobial therapy in the critical care setting provides an opportunity to exemplify important points.

In contrast, type B ('bizarre') adverse reactions are unexpected aberrant responses, which are unrelated to the drug's pharmacological effects (Figure 20.1). They are not dose-dependent, are unpredictable and occur in a very small percentage of the population receiving the drug. Although critical patients are probably not more predisposed, they are more likely to be affected adversely by the negative consequences of a type B reaction.

DRUG DISPOSITION AND TYPE A ADVERSE REACTIONS

The magnitude of a pharmacological response to a drug (and thus the risk of therapeutic failure or 'toxic' response) reflects the drug concentration at the tissue site, which in turn tends to be linearly related to the plasma drug concentration (PDC). Drug doses are intended to achieve but not exceed the targeted therapeutic range in tissue. As such, dosing regimens are designed to maintain peak (maximum effective) PDC and not drop below trough (minimum effective) PDC during a dosing interval. Plasma peak and trough drug concentrations following administration of a drug are determined by the factors that control drug disposition. These factors include absorption from the site of administration into the systemic circulation, distribution from circulating blood to the body tissues and back again to the circulation and metabolism and/or excretion from the body. The extent to which each of these

Anaphylactoid reaction	
Radiocontrast material	
Amphotericin B	
Thioacetarsemide	
Snake venom	
L-Asparaginase	
Doxorubicin	
5-Fluouracil	

Allergic drug reactions	
Diazepam	Cholestasis, hepatic necrosis
Carprofen	Hepatic necrosis
Sulphonamide drugs	Multiple target tissues, eye
5-Fluouracil	Erythemic pruritus
Phenobarbitone	Bone marrow dyscrasias
Recombinant erythropoietin (human)	Decreased PCV, WBC

Figure 20.1: Drugs associated with type B adverse reactions. Cats appear more susceptible to anaphylactoid reactions, i.e. those which are associated with mast cell degranulation, which, in contrast to allergic drug reactions, are not antigen-mediated.

factors determines the disposition of a particular drug is determined by the chemistry of the drug (e.g. its lipid or water solubility, molecular size and pKa) and various local environmental conditions (e.g. barrier to passive diffusion, environmental pH, presence of protein and excretory capacity of selected organs).

Drug distribution

Gastrointestinal absorption is determined by gastrointestinal pH, motility, epithelial permeability, surface area and blood flow. The rate and extent of intramuscular or subcutaneous absorption reflects drug molecular weight and lipid solubility and regional blood flow to the site of administration. Drugs must be distributed from the central 'compartment' to extracellular (and sometimes intracellular) tissues and then back. Both rate and extent of drug distribution are affected by the size of the compartment to which the drug will be distributed (the volume of distribution, Vd), the extent of drug binding to plasma proteins (principally albumin), regional blood flow to organs and binding of drug to tissues.

Drug elimination

Drug elimination is accomplished by metabolism and/or excretion. The major site of drug metabolism is the liver. Hepatic blood flow, intrinsic (cytochrome P450) metabolism and binding to plasma proteins variably impact drugs metabolized by the liver. Drug metabolism chemically alters lipid-soluble drugs such that they become more water-soluble, rendering them more conducive to excretion. Most drug metabolism occurs in two phases, each catalysed by specific enzymes. Phase I enzymes chemically change and often inactivate a drug, but some drugs become more active following phase I metabolism. Of greater concern is the formation of reactive metabolites that may be more toxic than the parent drug. Accumulation of toxic phase I metabolites predisposes the liver to drug-induced toxicity. Phase II drug metabolizing enzymes (glucuronidases, glutathione transferases) generally inactivate a drug and often are important for removal of toxic drug metabolites.

Renal excretion represents the most important mechanism by which drugs or metabolites are irreversibly cleared from the body. Renal excretion is determined by renal blood flow, glomerular filtration (a passive, inefficient process), protein binding (protein-bound drugs are not filtered), active tubular secretion (a very rapid process that is not affected by protein binding) and passive tubular resorption of the drug back into the circulation. Passive resorption prolongs drug half-life and is determined by lipid solubility and drug ionization, which in turn depends on urinary pH and drug pKa. A drug that is un-ionized (e.g. a weakly acidic drug in an acidic environment) is more diffusible and more likely to be reabsorbed. In the case of antimicrobials, the un-ionized drug is more effective than the ionized drug because of better penetrability of bacteria. Biliary drug excretion is an inefficient route of drug excretion but is clinically relevant because of the potential of the drug to undergo enterohepatic circulation. The gastrointestinal tract is therefore re-exposed to the drug multiple times and drug elimination is slowed.

Dosing regimens

A dosing regimen, comprised of a route, dose and interval, is designed to achieve and maintain targeted PDC throughout the dosing period. The drug dose necessary to achieve a given target is determined by the volume of tissue that will dilute the drug (Vd) and for non-intravenous drugs, the bioavailability of the drug (how much of the drug reaches the systemic circulation). For intravenous drugs, dose modification in critical patients can be directly based on changes in Vd. If Vd increases (or decreases), the dose must also be increased (or decreased) proportionally if targeted PDC are to be achieved but not exceeded.

The interval of a dosing regimen is based on the acceptable change in PDC (that is, how low can PDC drop during a dosing interval without leading to therapeutic failure?) and the rate of drug elimination from the body. For drugs whose pharmacological effects require the presence of the drug (e.g. anticonvulsants, opioid analgesics, time-dependent antibiotics), the dosing interval is largely based on the elimination half-life, or the time necessary for 50% of a drug to be eliminated from the blood. For drugs characterized by 'residual' pharmacological effects, the dosing interval generally surpasses the drug elimination half-life. Residual effects occur when the response to a drug persists despite the absence of the drug, such as might occur if enzyme action is irreversibly inhibited (e.g. non-steroidal anti-inflammatory drugs), with hormones (e.g. glucocorticoids), or dose-dependent antibiotics (e.g. aminoglycosides or fluorinated quinolones).

Drug elimination half-life is determined by the rate of drug removal by the liver or kidney. However, because the drug must be in circulation to be removed by the liver or kidney, the Vd of a drug also impacts elimination half-life. A drug with a large Vd will be distributed to tissues and cannot be accessed, prolonging elimination half-life. It is common practice for clinicians to decrease the dose of a drug in patients for which elimination half-life has been prolonged. However, for most drugs, decreasing the dose will increase the risk of therapeutic failure, since PDC at the beginning of the dosing regimen may not reach therapeutic concentrations, although the lower PDC will be present for a longer period of time. Thus, for many drugs, accommodation for an increase in elimination half-life should occur through prolonging the interval.

An exception occurs for drugs that accumulate in normal animals. Accumulation occurs when a drug is given at a dosing interval that is shorter than its elimination half-life. In such cases, at least half — and often much more — of the previous dose remains in the body by the time the next dose is given. For example, if a drug is given at an interval that equals the half-life, 50% of the previous dose is still in the body when the next dose is given. The drug will accumulate until ultimately, at steady state, PDC will be twice what it was following the first dose. The magnitude of drug accumulation depends on how much longer the half-life is compared to the dosing interval. The longer the elimination half-life compared to the dosing interval, the greater the drug accumulation, the less each daily dose contributes to the total amount of drug in the body, and the greater the caution should be taken when using the drug. For drugs that accumulate, a decrease (or increase) in PDC requires a proportional change in dose or interval.

Full response to a drug will not occur until steady state, which for all drugs, is 3–5 drug half-lives. At steady state, drug elimination and drug dosing are equal and maximum accumulation of the drug has occurred. For drugs with a short elimination half-life compared to the dosing interval, the concept of 'steady state' is probably inappropriate, since no drug accumulates. For drugs with a long half-life, therapeutic response or risk of toxicity cannot be fully evaluated until steady state has been reached. Because the time to steady state may be unacceptably long (anticonvulsants), a loading dose might be given in order to achieve targeted PDC rapidly. However, if the maintenance dose is inappropriate, PDC achieved by the loading dose will not be maintained and this will not become evident until another 3–5 drug half-lives have elapsed. Maintenance doses of drugs with long-elimination half-lives are designed such that concentrations will be therapeutic at steady state. However, each daily dose of the drug may actually contribute very little to the total amount of drug in the body. Increasing PDC in such cases will actually require multiple daily doses or a 'mini-loading' dose. Likewise, decreasing PDC (in order to resolve a toxic response) in such cases may require one (50% decline) or more drug half-lives.

CHANGES IN DRUG DISPOSITION IN THE CRITICAL PATIENT

Changes in drug disposition in the critical patient that may result in adverse drug reactions must also take into account species differences. Differences in physiology render the cat more susceptible than the dog to a number of drug adversities, which must be taken into account as drugs and dosing regimens are selected for feline critical patients.

Changes in drug absorption

Decreased longitudinal smooth muscle motility (peristalsis) will decrease movement of drug into the intestine and thus prolong time to peak absorption. The extent of drug absorption is not likely to be affected. Because the surface area of the small intestine is so large, increased peristalsis affects the rate or extent of drug absorption minimally. However, drugs that slow peristalsis or enhance segmentation (e.g. opioid analgesics) may enhance the absorption of luminal contents. Undesirable toxins or degradation products (e.g. parvovirus, bacterial diarrhoea) may subsequently be absorbed. Changes in permeability (as might occur with any inflammatory disease of the gastrointestinal tract) may increase drug absorption, resulting in higher peak PDC. Drugs that normally are not absorbed (e.g. aminoglycosides) may reach the systemic circulation in such cases and caution is recommended when administering such potentially toxic drugs orally. Permeability changes may be sufficient to present a barrier to drug diffusion (e.g. oedema, inflammatory debris), resulting in decreases in both rate and extent of drug absorption. Doses may require elevation to assure adequate movement of drug across the barrier and, even then, drug movement may be insufficient. Drug-induced increases in gastric pH lead to decreased absorption of a number of weak acids and sucralfate may not be maximally activated. Bacterial overgrowth or rebound hypersecretion upon discontinuation of an antisecretory drug may complicate therapy.

Parenteral administration is often the preferred route in the critical patient. Most drugs that can be given intramuscularly can be given subcutaneously. Many, but not all (e.g. imipenem), drugs that are given intravenously can also be given intramuscularly or subcutaneously. Pain and precipitation at the site of injection limits intramuscular or subcutaneous administration of some intravenous drugs. Absorption from subcutaneous sites is generally slower than from intramuscular injection, with lower peak concentrations. Drug absorption from intramuscular and subcutaneous routes can be profoundly impacted by decreased regional blood flow associated with poor peripheral perfusion (e.g. dehydration or other causes of hypovolaemic shock, cardiogenic shock) or hypothermia (e.g. puppies). Volume replacement and normothermia is needed before drug absorption from peripheral sites is reliable. Rectal administration can be a viable route of administration for many drugs. Advantages include easy access and bypassing (to a large degree) first pass metabolism associated with oral drugs. However, the drug must be delivered as a solution or rectal suppository and may require reformulation for rectal administration. Intrathecal administration is a rarely used method of direct drug delivery to cerebrospinal fluid, but drugs do not necessarily access brain tissue with this route. Bypassing the blood–cerebral spinal fluid barrier renders the patient at greater risk to drug-induced neurological toxicities. Aerosolization can be a powerful tool for facilitating drug distribution to the upper airways or lungs, but aerosolizers must generate particles of the proper size necessary for deposition in the targeted airways. Aerosolization always should be accompanied by systemic therapy.

Drug distribution

Drug distribution and thus PDC can be affected in the critical patient by changes in Vd or protein binding. Accumulation of fluid (oedema, ascites) or loss of fluid (due, for example, to dehydration, hyponatraemia) and subsequent resolution of the problem, can cause the body tissues to which drug will be distributed (Vd) to fluctuate by more than 30%. As Vd changes, doses must change proportionately in the same direction. However, the impact of changes in Vd on PDC varies with lipid versus water-soluble drugs, since the tissues to which the drugs distribute vary. Lipid-soluble drugs distribute to all body compartments and dosing on a mg/kg basis will avoid generation of PDCs that are toxic or sub-therapeutic.

Dose modification for water-soluble drugs, however, is more complicated. Fluid shifts can be profound in states of hypovolaemia, when there is a reduction in total body water with marked contraction of the extra-cellular fluid (ECF) compartment. If ECF is contracted more than total body water, PDC of water-soluble drugs, distributed only to ECF, will be higher unless the mg/kg dose is decreased. Physiological responses during hypotension cause more blood (and thus drug) to be delivered to the brain and heart, increasing the risk of cardiac or neurological adverse drug reactions, again requiring a decrease in dose. Fluid accumulation (oedema, paediatric patients, fluid therapy) will require the opposite response. Thus, for water-soluble drugs, the mg/kg dose generally should be increased (up to 30%) to compensate for increased fluid volumes. One notable exception exists: accumulation of fluids in discrete compartments such as in ascites, as water-soluble drugs may not be distributed to the ascitic compartment. Increasing the dose of drug to accommodate this compartment, or failure to dose on lean body weight (excluding the compartment) may result in drug over-dose. Because Vd affects elimination half-life directly (and proportionately), dosing intervals also may need to be decreased or prolonged by 25%, depending on the fluid shift.

Changes in protein binding can have a variety of effects on the critical patient. Highly protein bound drugs (greater than 80% bound) often do not distribute as rapidly as unbound drugs and response to therapy may be prolonged (e.g. anticonvulsants). Weak acids tend to be bound to albumin. Disease-induced decreases in serum albumin or the presence of endogenous compounds (e.g. bilirubin, uraemic toxins) or exogenous compounds (i.e. other highly protein-bound drugs) can cause displacement of drugs from binding sites. The greater the normal percentage binding of the drug, the greater the risk of toxicity if the percentage that is bound changes, and doses of highly protein-bound drugs may need to be decreased. For example, displacement of only 1% of a 99% protein-bound drug doubles the pharmacologically active concentration of the drug. For some drugs, clearance (e.g. hepatic or glomerular filtration) of the displaced drug may increase, ultimately normalizing PDC. However, even for these drugs, an initial period of increased risk of toxicity may occur.

Cranial trauma causes unique changes in drug distribution, as the blood–brain barrier becomes permeable to small molecules normally excluded by the brain. Maximal permeability occurs several days after the injury and increased drug distribution into the brain increases the risk of neurological adverse drug reactions. Drugs might exacerbate the pathophysiological sequelae of cranial trauma by contributing to haemorrhage (e.g. mannitol), hypoxia (sedatives) or hyperglycaemia (e.g. glucocorticoids).

Drug metabolism

The liver is the predominant site of drug metabolism. As with other hepatic functions, drug metabolism appears to be preserved until moderate to severe liver disease has developed. Generally, if liver dysfunction is sufficient that serum albumin and urea nitrogen concentrations are decreased and serum bile acids are increased, a proportional decrease in drug metabolism should also be anticipated. Prolongation of the dosing interval is the most appropriate modification in the dosing regimen, although a decrease in dose might also be indicated for drugs that accumulate. Patients with portosystemic shunting present unique considerations regarding drug administration. Hepatic drug metabolism is likely to be decreased in such patients and longer dosing intervals are indicated. Drugs characterized by high hepatic extraction largely bypass the liver, depending on the fraction of blood shunted past the liver. Intervals of such drugs should be prolonged, but because the drugs normally are very rapidly eliminated, doses might also need to be decreased. Drugs characterized by first-pass metabolism and administered orally will reach higher PDC than in normal patients. The proportional increase is determined by the fraction of blood shunted around the liver and doses of potentially toxic drugs should be accordingly decreased.

Drug interactions can impact upon liver function and such drugs should be avoided in critical patients if possible (Figures 20.2 and 20.3). In particular, drugs that inhibit hepatic metabolism should be avoided. Inhibition of drug metabolizing enzymes can occur rapidly, negatively impacting hepatic clearance of other drugs. Drug-induced inhibition of metabolism is a therapeutic benefit in acetaminophen toxicity in cats: cimetidine, a potent inhibitor of hepatic drug metabolizing enzymes, decreases the formation of toxic phase I metabolites. Induction of drug metabolizing enzymes is of less concern in critical animals, unless the patient enters the hospital already receiving the inducing drug

Drug or drug class	Incompatible drugs	Other risks
Aminoglycosides	Beta-lactams, heparin	Adsorbs to glass
Aminophylline	Do not mix with other drugs	
Amphotericin B	Any diluent except 5% dextrose	Light exposure
Bicarbonate	Many drugs	
Blood, red blood cells	Any i.v. solution except 0.9% saline	
Diazepam	Cloudiness when mixed with other drugs; clinical relevance not known	Adsorbs to i.v. tubing, protect from light
Dobutamine	Alkaline solutions	Discoloration: check label
Dopamine	Alkaline solutions	
Flunixin meglumine	Most solutions	
Frusemide		Strongly acidic solution; discoloration
Heparin	Many drugs	Binds to and causes precipitation in strongly acidic solution
Insulin	Check package label regarding diluents and refrigeration needs	Binds to i.v. tubing
ß-Lactams [Cephalosporins] [Penicillins]	Aminoglycosides	Individual drug idiosyncrasies; check each label or package insert
Metronidazole		Light sensitive, do not freeze
Pentobarbitone	Alkaline-labile drugs; acid pH	
Procainamide		Discoloration: check label

Figure 20.2: *Examples of intravenous drug incompatibilities.*

(e.g. phenobarbitone). In contrast to inhibition, induction generally takes multiple doses (several weeks) before a maximum inducing effect occurs. Hepatic induction is likely to cause rapid clearance of drugs metabolized by the liver (thus therapeutic failure). More importantly (and often overlooked), hepatic induction may increase the production of toxic drug metabolites, overwhelming the normal protective mechanisms of the liver. Potentially hepatotoxic drugs should be avoided in patients receiving a drug which induces drug metabolizing enzymes. Because glutathione is a component of phase II drug metabolizing enzymes responsible for scavenging toxic metabolites, treatment with acetylcysteine (a precursor to glutathione) or ascorbic acid might be considered in patients that are subject to drug-induced hepatotoxicity.

Drug excretion

Conditions accompanied by decreased renal blood flow (dehydration, hypovolaemia, cardiac dysfunction) result in decreased glomerular filtration and active tubular secretion. Dosing intervals of potentially toxic, renally excreted drugs should be prolonged.

ANTIMICROBIAL THERAPY IN THE CRITICAL PATIENT

Care of the patient with a potentially life-threatening bacterial infection depends on the appropriate choice and judicious use of an antimicrobial agent. Drug selection is simplified if a pathogen is identified and susceptibility data are available to guide drug selection. Once samples have been collected for culture, in critical patients therapy should begin immediately with an empirically selected antibiotic (Figure 20.4). The spectrum of the initial antibiotic should include the pathogens likely to be responsible for the infection, but the drug may need to be changed once culture and susceptibility data are available. Initial antimicrobial selection is found to be inappropriate close to 50% of the time in the critical patient.

Drug 1	Drug 2	Type	Interaction
Aminoglycosides	ß-lactams NSAIDs, ACE inhibitors	A C	Chemical inactivation Enhanced nephrotoxicity due to impaired renal prostaglandin synthesis
Atropine	Oral drugs Cisapride Metaclopramide Opioid anti-diarrhoeals	A C C C	Impaired motility prolongs gastric retention Anticholinergic effects decrease efficacy Anticholinergic effects decrease efficacy Anticholinergic effects decrease efficacy
Chloramphenicol	Hepatically metabolized drugs	B	Impaired clearance due to impaired metabolism
Cimetidine	Oral drugs Sucralfate Hepatically metabolized drugs	A C B	Decreased absorption of weak acids Decreased activation Impaired clearance due to impaired metabolism
Enrofloxacin	Theophylline	B	Impaired clearance due to impaired metabolism
Ketoconazole	Hepatically metabolized drugs	B	Impaired clearance due to impaired metabolism
Phenobarbitone	Hepatically metabolized drugs	B	Increased clearance due to increased metabolism
Rifampin	Hepatically metabolized drugs	B	Increased clearance due to increased metabolism

Figure 20.3: Examples of drug-to-drug interactions.
A = Pharmaceutical interaction, occurring prior to or during drug administration
B = Pharmacokinetic interaction, occurring as drug is being absorbed until it is excreted
C = Pharmacodynamic interaction, occurring at the receptor site

Antimicrobial selection should be based on host factors and is more successful if the site of infection is identified. Normal flora are common pathogens when they reach sites that are usually sterile. For example, intra-abdominal infections commonly reflect the large number of anaerobic and Gram-negative organisms that inhabit the colon. Normal flora also cause respiratory, skin and other infections, particularly when normal host defence mechanisms are compromised.

Often, critical patients are unable to tolerate oral medications because of vomiting, and oral bioavailability may be reduced due to pathological conditions (e.g. shunting of blood away from the gastrointestinal tract in hypovolaemic patients). The oral route is therefore reserved for patients with relatively mild infections, in whom absorption is not thought to be compromised. Many drugs (e.g. aminoglycosides) are not bioavailable following oral administration. The intravenous route is more appropriate in the critical care setting for several reasons. Intravenous therapy ensures rapid achievement of effective PDC and thus the highest concentration in tissues, thereby facilitating the achievement of therapeutic concentrations at the site of infection. After intravenous administration, bioavailability is 100% and peak serum concentrations occur shortly after the end of injection (Figure 20.5). Complications of indwelling lines (infection, occlusion) and drug interactions may confound therapy, however. Drugs are often 100% bioavailable following intramuscular administration, but this route is not widely used, in part due to pain associated with intramuscular injections. Once the life-threatening risk associated with infection has been reduced, selected antibiotics can then be given orally. The subcutaneous route of antimicrobial administration is discouraged in critically ill patients, largely due to erratic and unpredictable absorption.

Cultures of bacterial pathogens may be performed on body fluids (urine, blood, pleural fluid, joint fluid, bile, peritoneal fluid, cerebrospinal fluid (CSF)), aspirates of abscess contents, transtracheal aspirates and biopsies of normally sterile organs. Blood and urine should be submitted for culture in patients with suspected bacteraemia or sepsis. As a general rule, the best samples for the microbiology laboratory are liquid specimens. Swabs should be avoided whenever possible, since these tend to dry out and swab fibres may be deleterious to some bacteria. Avoidance of contamination, adequacy of sampling and preservation of viability are critical factors in specimen collection and handling. Urine (and stool) should be transported in sealed sterile containers and refrigerated if not processed within 1 hour of collection. Blood and CSF should be incubated if processing is delayed. All other specimens may be kept at room temperature. The recognized spectrum of disease associated with anaerobic bacteria has broadened as improved techniques for isolation have been developed. Fluid specimens that may harbour pathogenic anaerobic bacteria should be collected in a syringe, from which air is immediately expressed and the end of the needle plugged with a

Common pathogens	Suggested therapy	Comments
Pneumonia *Streptococcus* spp. *Mycoplasma* *Enterobacter* *Klebsiella* *Staphylococcus* spp. *Escherichia coli*	One of: cefazolin ampicillin ticarcillin/clavulanate AND one of: amikacin gentamicin enrofloxacin	Whether antibiotics should be given by aerosol for documented respiratory infections is still unproven. If used, aminoglycosides and other antibiotics given by the airway route should be selected according to sensitivity testing
Septic peritonitis *E. coli* *Enterococcus* *Streptococcus* spp. *Proteus* spp. *Pseudomonas aeruginosa* *Enterobacter* Anaerobes	Ticarcillin/clavulanate and cefoxitin OR ampicillin and amikacin AND metronidazole if patient is bacteraemic or anaerobic organisms are isolated	Peritoneal irrigation with any antibiotic solution has been abandoned as it has been incriminated as damaging to peritoneal host defence mechanisms
Bacterial meningitis Staphylococci Streptococci *Pasteurella* *Actinomyces* *Nocardia*	Potassium penicillin Chloramphenicol Cefotaxime Ceftriaxone Enrofloxacin	Chloramphenicol if anaerobic or rickettsial organism suspected
Urinary tract infections *E. coli* Staphylococci *Proteus* *Enterococcus* *Pseudomonas*	Ampicillin Cefazolin Amikacin Enrofloxacin Chloramphenicol	In intact male dogs with recurrent urinary tract infection or urosepsis, always assume prostatic involvement

Figure 20.4: Common pathogens and empirical antibiotic choices in selected bacterial syndromes. (Note: empirical antimicrobial selection should always be accompanied by appropriate bacterial culture and sensitivity testing and the selection modified based on the results).

rubber stopper. Alternatively, the contents of the syringe can be injected into an anaerobic transport tube. Tissue specimens should be placed in anaerobic transport containers.

The time needed to grow, isolate and identify different organisms varies considerably. The most common aerobic pathogens grow rapidly and preliminary reports can be expected from the laboratory within 24 hours. Anaerobes generally grow more slowly and plates are usually not examined for 48 hours. A common method of susceptibility testing in the clinical laboratory is the disk-diffusion, or Kirby–Bauer method. This method is well suited for screening large numbers of organisms but provides only semi-quantitative information and is not applicable to slowly growing or fastidious organisms. Quantitative antibiotic susceptibilities may also be determined by either the agar or broth dilution technique. A standard inoculum of bacteria is added to serial dilutions of each antibiotic and allowed to incubate. The lowest concentration of antibiotic in which there is no visible growth is considered the minimum inhibitory concentration (MIC). Bacteria are usually considered susceptible to a drug if the achievable

peak serum concentration exceeds the MIC by at least fourfold. The breakpoint is the concentration of the antibiotic that separates susceptible from resistant bacteria and generally is the concentration of drug that will be achieved in plasma following administration of the recommended (labelled) dose. The spectrum of an antibiotic is based on the breakpoint. If a majority of the isolates of a given bacterial species are inhibited at concentrations below the breakpoint, the species is considered to be within the spectrum of the drug. The basis for determining antimicrobial susceptibility is the comparison of the MIC of an organism cultured from a patient to the breakpoint. If the MIC necessary to inhibit the organism is well below breakpoint, the organism is considered susceptible (S). As the MIC approaches breakpoint, the organism is considered to have intermediate (I) susceptibility. The organism is considered resistant (R) to the drug if the MIC equals or surpasses breakpoint because it is unlikely that effective concentrations of the drug will be achieved in plasma or tissue.

Data that include MIC values (rather than simply an S, I or R designation) can be particularly helpful in assessing the degree of susceptibility of an organism to

Potassium penicillin	30,000–50,000 IU/kg i.v. every 4–6 h
Ampicillin	22 mg/kg i.v. every 6–8 h
Clindamycin	5–10 mg/kg i.v. every 8 h
Cefoxitin	20 mg/kg i.v. every 6 h
Cefotaxime	40 mg/kg i.v. every 6–8 h
Imipenem—cilastatin	5–7 mg/kg i.v. every 6–8 h, slow infusion
Chloramphenicol	35 mg/kg i.v. every 8 h
Gentamicin	6 mg/kg i.v. every 24 h
Amikacin	13–15 mg/kg i.v. every 24 h
Metronidazole	5–10 mg/kg i.v. every 8 h, slow infusion
Enrofloxacin	10–16 mg/kg i.v. every 24 h, dilute 1:1 with saline – give slowly
Cefazolin	22 mg/kg i.v. every 6–8 h
Ticarcillin (± clavulanate)	50 mg/kg i.v. every 8 h

Figure 20.5: Doses of antibiotics commonly used in critical patients.

a drug. The further the MIC of the organism is from the breakpoint, the more likely effective concentrations of the drug will be achieved in plasma. The distance between the MIC of the organism and breakpoint becomes even more important when infections are located in tissues other than blood or urine, particularly in tissues that are difficult to penetrate (i.e. prostate, eye, CNS) or when host responses negatively impact antimicrobial efficacy. Examples include marked inflammatory debris, fibrosis or an anaerobic environment. A large difference between breakpoint MIC and organism MIC (inhibitory quotient) is also important for antibiotics whose efficacy is concentration dependent. For such antibiotics, including the aminoglycosides and fluorinated quinolones, efficacy is enhanced with inhibitory quotients that are 4 –10. For time dependent antibiotics, such as the ß-lactams and bacteriostatic drugs, efficacy is more dependent on how long drug concentrations stay above the MIC. For such drugs, dosing interval is particularly important. Ideally, time dependent antimicrobials are administered every half-life, since the risk of serum concentrations dropping below the MIC of the organism increases with each drug half-life.

Pharmacodynamic parameters that appear to correlate with reduction in the number of bacteria include the ratio of the peak antibacterial concentration to the MIC (especially for the aminoglycosides and quinolones) and the length of time that concentrations exceed the MIC (especially for ß-lactams). However, antimicrobials may still be effective even if PDC drops below the MIC. Many antibiotics exhibit a post-antibiotic effect (PAE), such that bacterial growth is inhibited after a brief exposure to the drug. For some drugs, such as the aminoglycosides, it is not necessary to maintain serum concentrations above the MIC for the entire dose interval.

The *in vitro* conditions under which susceptibility data is collected may vary considerably from those existing at the site of infection. Thus, MIC should be viewed as a rough guide to the likelihood of success or failure of treatment for that particular organism. Several other factors can cause failure to respond to antimicrobial therapy. The most obvious cause is misdiagnosis: either identification of the wrong pathogen, or treatment of a disorder that is not caused by a bacterial agent. The microbe may be resistant to the antibiotic and resistance may develop during the course of therapy, necessitating reassessment of *in vitro* susceptibility testing. Empirical changes in antimicrobial therapy should be made when valid cultures are not available and the initially chosen antibiotic appears to be ineffective. The drug may be effective *in vitro* but may not reach the site of inflammation, or may be neutralized or inactivated at the site of infection by ionization, binding to inflammatory debris, destruction by microbial enzymes and/or an anaerobic environment. Surgical drainage or other methods of debridement may be critical to successful antimicrobial therapy, especially for patients with closed-space infections or infections associated with foreign objects or obstructive lesions. Many causes of antimicrobial failure can be minimized with the use of an appropriate dose, interval and route of administration. This may be especially significant when antibiotics with a low therapeutic index (e.g. aminoglycosides) are administered at subtherapeutic dosages. Lastly, superinfection may contribute to therapeutic failure. Superinfection develops as resistant microorganisms proliferate and is more likely to occur with broad-spectrum regimens, due to loss of microbes which otherwise keep the proliferating microorganisms in check. A typical characteristic of superinfection is initial response by the patient, followed by deterioration, associated with infection by *Pseudomonas aeruginosa* and other resistant Gram-negative pathogens. Appropriate management of pain, fever, acidosis and electrolyte disturbances is important to antimicrobial success. Likewise, maintenance of perfusion, oxygenation and nutritional status will decrease the morbidity and mortality associated with septic processes.

CHOICE OF ANTIBACTERIAL THERAPY

ß-Lactams

The ß-lactams include the penicillins and cephalosporins. The advantages of ß-lactams include their safety, spectrum, and synergistic actions when used in combination with many other antimicrobials. Penicillins were among the first antibiotics to be developed and remain the most widely used group. They are generally well tolerated and are bactericidal against a broad range of pathogens. Many penicillins are destroyed by ß-lactamases, enzymes produced by both Gram-positive and Gram-negative aerobic and anaerobic organisms. The spectrum of penicillin G includes spirochaetes (*Borrelia* and *Leptospira*), streptococci, enterococci, a few staphylococci and many anaerobes (including *Bacteroides* and *Clostridium*). Penicillin also has some activity against Gram-negative organisms, including *Pasteurella*. The penicillins penetrate well into interstitial fluids of all body tissues except uninflamed meninges.

The spectrum of the aminopenicillins ampicillin and amoxicillin is extended to include some Gram-negative rods, such as isolates of *Escherichia coli*, *Proteus* and *Salmonella*. The extended spectrum or antpseudomonal penicillins (ticarcillin, piperacillin) are effective against *Pseudomonas aeruginosa* as well as enteric Gram-negative bacilli such as *E. coli*, *Klebsiella*, *Proteus* spp. and anaerobic organisms such as *Bacteroides fragilis*. However, the susceptibility of these penicillins to ß-lactamase markedly limits their utility when infections caused by Gram-negative enteric organisms are suspected. The addition of ß-lactamase inhibitors (clavulanic acid or tazobactam) to ticarcillin or piperacillin extends the spectrum of these agents to include many organisms that are resistant by virtue of ß-lactamase production.

The cephalosporins share many of the properties of the penicillins, including bactericidal activity based on the ß-lactam ring. They are generally well tolerated and are excreted by the kidneys. Separation into first, second and third generation cephalosporins is of chronological importance only. Two of the seven available first generation cephalosporins (cephalothin and cefazolin) have been used reliably as parenteral therapy in small animals. Their spectrum is similar to that of the aminopenicillins, with some enhanced coverage of Gram-negative pathogens. Notably, the cephalosporins are more resistant than the penicillins to ß-lactamase destruction. Cefazolin has several pharmacological advantages over cephalothin, including the production of higher, more prolonged blood levels when administered intravenously and is the preferred first-generation cephalosporin in most clinical situations.

The parenteral second-generation cephalosporins extend the Gram-negative spectrum of the first-generation compounds although efficacy against Gram-positive and anaerobic organisms is often less than for first-generation cephalosporins. An exception is cefoxitin, which has enhanced efficacy against anaerobic organisms, particularly *Bacteroides fragilis*.

Third-generation cephalosporins are much more effective against Gram-negative bacteria than first- and second-generation cephalosporins. In addition, they generally are more resistant to degradation by ß-lactamases. The spectrum of each third-generation cephalosporin is sufficiently variable that each drug should be reviewed prior to use to assure the targeted organism is included in the spectrum. With the exception of ceftazidime and cefoperazone, many have poor activity against *Pseudomonas aeruginosa*. In general, they have poor efficacy against anaerobes and are often less active than first-generation agents against Gram-positive organisms. Cefotaxime and ceftriaxone, the most widely used third-generation cephalosporins, are highly active against most streptococci. Because of its excellent Gram-negative spectrum, its long serum half-life and its high serum and CSF levels, ceftriaxone has become one of the drugs of choice for presumptive therapy of bacterial meningitis. In all other cases, the use of these agents should be guided by susceptibility testing. Ceftiofur, a broad-spectrum third-generation cephalosporin marketed for therapy of bovine respiratory disease, has received a great deal of attention from small animal practitioners. Compared with other third-generation cephalosporins, it is a significantly less costly drug, which can be frozen in aliquots. Ceftiofur, administered subcutaneously, is approved for the treatment of urinary tract infections caused by *E. coli* and *Proteus mirabilis* in dogs. The labelled dose (2.2 mg/kg) of ceftiofur achieves supra-MIC concentration for bacteria in urine for at least 24 hours, but the plasma concentration of ceftiofur and its metabolites is above *E. coli*'s MIC of 4.0 mg/l for only 3–4 hours. Studies to determine the efficacy and safety of ceftiofur for treatment of systemic infections at off-label doses have not been reported.

Imipenem is a carbapenem, which is marketed in combination with the renal dipeptidase inhibitor cilastatin. Cilastatin enables imipenem to escape renal inactivation, thus avoiding toxic metabolites, while increasing the elimination half-life and urinary levels of the drug. The spectrum of imipenem is excellent against virtually all bacterial pathogens and, among the ß-lactams, imipenem is associated with the least endotoxin release. Limitations to its use are its relatively low concentration in selected tissues (which may be adjusted by increasing the dose), short serum half-life and cost. Because of its broad spectrum of activity, imipenem can be used as presumptive therapy for serious nosocomial infections thought to be caused by multiple bacterial species or multi-resistant organisms.

Aminoglycosides

The aminoglycosides are rapidly bactericidal *in vitro* at low concentrations, with activity limited to Gram-negative bacteria and staphylococci. Because they require active transport into the microorganism, they are inactive against both anaerobic and facultative anaerobic bacteria. As weak bases, they are less effective in an acidic than in an alkaline environment. The aminoglycosides remain among the drugs of choice for any suspected Gram-negative bacteraemic infection and are associated with minimal endotoxin release. Aminoglycosides act synergistically with ß-lactams and are often combined with an aqueous penicillin for treating Gram-negative bacteraemia. Major limitations to aminoglycoside use are renal toxicity and relatively poor distribution to some tissues (e.g. abscesses and the central nervous system). Bacterial resistance due to enzymatic destruction has limited the use of gentamicin but is less important for amikacin. Gentamicin and netilmicin have a similar spectrum of activity. Amikacin is often more effective against Gram-negative organisms, in part because it is more resistant to bacterial destruction. Both amikacin and netilmicin may be less nephrotoxic in dogs than other aminoglycosides.

Monitoring serum concentrations can enhance therapeutic success by maximizing both safety and efficacy. In contrast to the ß-lactams, the efficacy of aminoglycosides is concentration dependent. As the inhibitory quotient increases, the rate and extent of bacterial killing are also increased. Aminoglycosides have a long enough PAE to allow for once-daily dosing. Because of their antimicrobial characteristics, amino-

glycosides are most effective and safe when given once daily, since nephrotoxicity can be directly correlated to trough PDC. The usual total daily dose (2 mg/kg tid) is administered as a single dose (6 mg/kg sid). Once daily aminoglycoside dosing may also provide more rapid killing and a decrease in the emergence of aminoglycoside resistant sub-populations. Nephrotoxicity of any aminoglycoside can be minimized by assuring that the patient is well hydrated and avoiding nephrotoxic or nephroactive drugs (e.g. non-steroidal anti-inflammatories, diuretics such as frusemide). Ideally, patients should be on intravenous fluids when aminoglycoside therapy is instituted. Urine should be monitored for the appearance of casts and serum creatinine should be followed closely, although it is important to realize that renal damage will continue for a time after the aminoglycoside is discontinued. Compelling evidence exists to support the need to measure aminoglycoside serum concentrations frequently in critically ill patients to monitor the changing pharmacokinetics of the drug and ultimately its pharmacodynamic effect. Concentrations should be monitored at 1 hour and 4–6 hours post-administration. Following administration of gentamicin (6 mg/kg sid), peak serum concentration 1 hour after dosing should be 12–20 µg/ml (4–8 x the MIC) and trough levels at 6 hours should ideally be <2 µg/ml. Samples should be collected in plastic rather than glass tubes since glass binds the aminoglycoside.

Fluoroquinolones

The fluoroquinolones have excellent activity against most aerobic and facultative Gram-negative rods, fair activity against staphylococci, variable to poor activity against streptococci and minimal activity against obligate anaerobes. *Chlamydia*, *Mycoplasma* and *Rickettsia* are also susceptible to the quinolones. Plasmid-mediated resistance against the fluorinated quinolones has not been detected, but nonetheless clinically relevant resistance is emerging in some strains of *Pseudomonas aeruginosa*, other Gram-negative organisms and *Staphylococcus* spp.

The pharmacodynamics of the fluoroquinolones support their use in the critical patient. Among the favourable characteristics are safety, rapidly bactericidal effects at low concentrations (for most organisms), a unique mechanism of action (inhibition of DNA gyrase), intracellular accumulation in white blood cells and a large volume of distribution. This latter characteristic supports their use for infections that are difficult to reach with water-soluble drugs such as ß-lactams and aminoglycosides. Both ciprofloxacin and enrofloxacin are available for parenteral use. Although only ciprofloxacin is labelled for intravenous use, enrofloxacin can be used intravenously without complications. In order to minimize or avoid nausea associated with the alkaline carrier solution, dilution in saline is recommended.

Like the aminoglycosides, the bactericidal effects of

the fluorinated quinolones are concentration-dependent and efficacy is enhanced against organisms with a high MIC (i.e. most *Pseudomonas* spp.) by using a large, once daily dose. The fluorinated quinolones are associated with less endotoxin release than the ß-lactams (except imipenem) but more than the aminoglycosides. Because of the risk of cartilage defects, fluoroquinolones should be avoided in growing animals.

Chloramphenicol

Chloramphenicol is a broad-spectrum antibiotic that is active against Rickettsiae, chlamydiae, mycoplasms, spirochaetes and most Gram-positive and Gram-negative bacteria, including anaerobes. Its spectrum generally does not include virulent Gram-negative pathogens such as *Pseudomonas aeruginosa*. In contrast to the previously discussed *bactericidal* antimicrobials, chloramphenicol is classified as *bacteriostatic*. Bactericidal drugs should be used in preference to bacteriostatic drugs in patients with compromised host defence mechanisms or diseases such as endocarditis. The difference between the designations 'bactericidal' and 'bacteriostatic' is determined by the drug concentrations that can be safely achieved in the patient, but also may vary with the organism. For example, chloramphenicol is bacteriostatic for *E. coli*, but bactericidal for *Streptococcus pneumoniae*.

Lincosamides

The only parenteral lincosamide commonly used in veterinary medicine is clindamycin. It has a broad spectrum of activity against Gram-positive and anaerobic bacteria, but development of resistance during therapy limits its use as empirical therapy for infections caused by Gram-positive cocci. Clindamycin is one of the drugs of choice for anaerobic infections because of its broad spectrum of activity against strict anaerobes. In contrast, clindamycin has no clinically significant activity against facultative Gram-negative enteric bacilli.

Clindamycin achieves particularly high concentrations in bone and has been suggested as a useful agent in the treatment of osteomyelitis. Similarly, an important characteristic of clindamycin is its ability to achieve effective concentrations in walled-off abscesses, surpassing concentrations achieved by chloramphenicol and penicillins. Clindamycin is actively accumulated by phagocytic leucocytes, reaching concentrations 5- to 50-fold greater than serum concentrations, so bacteria sequestered in white blood cells are not protected. Few other antibiotics (except enrofloxacin and perhaps chloramphenicol) are capable of penetrating into white blood cells.

Metronidazole

Metronidazole is a concentration-dependent bactericidal agent with a spectrum limited to anaerobic bacteria and thus it is ineffective as a single agent for mixed aerobic/anaerobic infections. The drug diffuses well into tissues and body fluids, including the CSF and bile. Effective tissue penetration and consistent bactericidal activity make metronidazole the drug of choice for severe anaerobic infections, including intra-abdominal abscesses, endocarditis and osteomyelitis. A combination of metronidazole and a third-generation cephalosporin is an appropriate choice for intra-abdominal infections. The combination of metronidazole, an aminopenicillin and either an aminoglycoside or a fluoroquinolone remains a time-honoured 'gold standard' for four-quadrant therapy in sepsis.

CHAPTER TWENTY ONE

Emergency and Critical Care Nursing

Elisa A. Petrollini and Dez Hughes

INTRODUCTION

Advanced veterinary nursing is an integral and essential part of the management of the critically ill patient. In addition to providing advanced traditional nursing care, most intensive monitoring is also performed by the veterinary nurse. Indeed, the ability to detect early and subtle changes in an animal's clinical status is one of the hallmarks of a true critical care nurse. The critical care nurse must be able rapidly to assess several animals, quickly identify the most unstable and be able to prioritize care to the sickest patients first.

This necessitates a full understanding of how to perform and interpret a clinical examination. It also demands in-depth familiarity with the specialized equipment (see Chapter 16) used in monitoring the critically ill patient and some expertise in recognizing which abnormalities should be addressed by a veterinary surgeon. In addition to monitoring, patient care with sophisticated therapeutic and supportive modalities, such as positive pressure ventilation and peritoneal dialysis, requires very specialized knowledge regarding their application and complications.

The workload inherent in the provision of critical care demands changes in the traditional role of the veterinary nurse as care and comfort provider. There is simply too much work for all treatments and monitoring to be performed by a veterinary surgeon. Critical care requires a team approach and the critical care nurse fills a unique role that greatly extends and supplements the capabilities of the veterinary surgeon. Because critically ill patients require continuous 24-hour care, it is virtually impossible to perform critical care without proficient, round the clock nursing coverage.

Major body systems are those that perform functions vital to the immediate survival of the animal, i.e. the cardiovascular, respiratory, central nervous and urinary systems. Changes in a major body system can have immediate and life-threatening consequences, so intensive monitoring is used to detect signs that may predict a problem before it becomes serious. The critically ill patient is sufficiently fragile that worsening of problems affecting one major body system can easily be fatal. The early prediction and prevention of possible complications is, therefore, a fundament of critical care. A convenient and helpful approach to critical care nursing is to consider the monitoring and nursing care applicable to each major body system. When examining a critically ill patient, the deleterious effects of stress on the animal cannot be overemphasized. Manipulating some patients, especially those with severe respiratory compromise, can be fatal.

Examples of basic and advanced critical care nursing orders are given in Figures 21.1 and 21.2.

MONITORING AND NURSING CARE OF THE CARDIOVASCULAR SYSTEM

Cardiovascular assessment involves evaluating mucous membrane colour, capillary refill time (CRT) and vigour, pulse quality and heart rate.

Mucous membranes and CRT

The oral mucous membrane colour is usually easiest to assess and the best site to use for CRT is the gingiva above the canine tooth. A normal animal should have pink mucous membranes with a vigorous capillary refill that takes $1-1^1/_4$ seconds. Mucous membranes in normal cats are significantly paler than in dogs. Pale, white, grey or muddy mucous membranes usually indicate poor perfusion or anaemia. Red or injected membranes may be associated with excitement, fever or the systemic inflammatory response syndrome (SIRS) seen with sepsis, severe pancreatitis, metastatic neoplasia or other causes of severe and extensive tissue damage. Cyanosis (blue or purple colour) indicates severe and life threatening arterial hypoxaemia necessitating immediate oxygen supplementation. Icterus may be due to increased red blood cell destruction, liver disease or obstructions to bile flow. Other rare abnormalities of mucous membrane colour include the brown membranes seen with paracetamol poisoning in cats and the cherry red colour from carbon monoxide poisoning. A slow CRT indicates a reduction in blood flow through the membrane and this occurs most commonly with hypovolaemia and heart failure. A fast CRT can be seen in excited animals, with fever and SIRS, and following mild to moderate haemorrhage when the cardiovascular system can still compensate for the blood loss.

Rectal temperature every 4–12 hours

Mucous membrane colour, capillary refill time, pulse quality and heart rate every 2–12 hours

Respiratory rate and effort, auscultation of the lungs every 2–12 hours

Note urine output or palpate bladder every 2–6 hours

Note mentation and neurological status every 2–6 hours

Note the presence of vomiting, regurgitation or bowel movements every 4–8 hours

Assess comfort and adequacy of pain control every 2–4 hours

Turn from side to side if recumbent or stand and walk the patient every 4 hours

Lubricate eyes with artificial tears if the animal is sedated and unable to blink, every 2–4 hours

Offer water and/or food (specify food type and amount unless 'nil by mouth') and record volumes ingested

Check oxygen supplementation percentage every 2–4 hours

Check that intravenous fluids are at the correct rate and on time every 2 hours

Check position, degree of tightness, adequacy of venous drainage and cleanliness of all bandages every 4–8 hours; replace if necessary

Heparinize and evaluate patency of all intravenous catheters every 4–6 hours

Packed cell volume, total solids, dipstick blood glucose and dipstick blood urea nitrogen estimation every 2–24 hours

Figure 21.1: Basic nursing monitoring orders applicable to most critically ill dogs and cats should include most of the above parameters. The frequency and interval of monitoring will depend on the severity of illness, the rate at which the patient's condition is changing and the type of disease.

Continuous or intermittent electrocardiography (ECG) ; note arrhythmias

Blood pressure monitoring (direct or indirect) continuous or every 2–12 hours

Central venous pressure monitoring every 2–6 hours

Pulmonary artery or pulmonary capillary wedge pressure monitoring continuous or every 2 hours

Pulse oximetry every 2–12 hours

End-tidal capnography every 2–12 hours

Arterial blood gas analysis every 2–24 hours

Urine output quantitation via closed collection system every 2–4 hours

Intra-abdominal pressure monitoring every 2–6 hours

Electrolyte measurement every 4–24 hours

Colloid osmometry every 4–24 hours

Nebulize and coupage 10–20 minutes every 4–6 hours

Check and clean inner cannula of tracheostomy tube every 2–4 hours

Aspirate chest tubes every 2–4 hours, record volumes of air/fluid obtained

Record mechanical ventilator settings, airway pressures and tidal volume every 2 hours

Peritoneal dialysis: infuse dialysate, dwell and drain every 1–2 hours, record volumes and quality of fluid obtained

Figure 21.2: Advanced nursing monitoring and treatment orders applicable to critically ill dogs and cats could include many of the above parameters. The frequency and interval of monitoring will depend on the severity of illness, the rate at which the patient's condition is changing and the type of disease.

Pulses

Both femoral and metatarsal pulses should be carefully palpated. This is usually more difficult in cats than in dogs and takes a great deal of practice. Femoral pulses are usually the easiest to feel; however, familiarity with how to feel a metatarsal pulse can be extremely helpful. The metatarsal pulse is palpated from the dorsal pedal artery on the craniomedial aspect of the proximal metatarsus (Figure 21.3). This pulse is lost before the femoral pulse in animals with poor perfusion, so it can provide a rough estimate of blood pressure. If the metatarsal pulse cannot be palpated, the animal should be evaluated for the presence of shock (see Chapter 3). Palpation of the metatarsal pulse is also useful in animals in which the femoral pulse is difficult to feel, such as obese or heavily muscled breeds. Fractious animals and animals with femoral or pelvic fractures will often tolerate palpation of a metatarsal pulse but not a femoral pulse.

Normal pulses are synchronous with the heartbeat and should not vary in strength. Asynchronous pulses or variations in pulse strength usually indicate the presence of a cardiac arrhythmia and should be evaluated via an electrocardiogram (ECG).

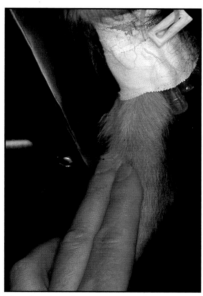

Figure 21.3: The dorsal metatarsal pulse is palpated on the craniomedial aspect of the hind leg below the hock. It can be a useful means of assessing the cardiovascular status of critically ill dogs. Inability to feel this pulse can indicate the presence of shock and hypotension. Note that an intravenous cannula has been placed in the saphenous vein of this patient.

Heart rate and rhythm

The vast majority of unstressed dogs have a heart rate of 80–120 beats per minute in the setting of an emergency clinic. The effect of body size on heart rate has been somewhat overemphasized. Normal heart rate in cats usually varies from 170 to 200 beats per minute.

Animals with abnormalities of heart rhythm should

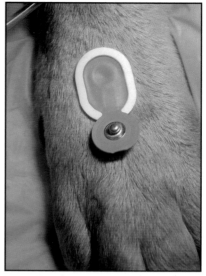

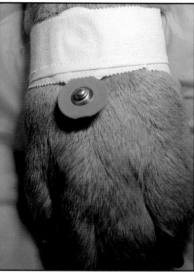

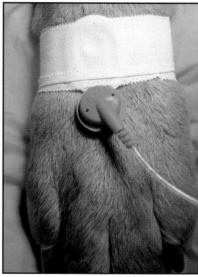

Figure 21.4: Adhesive patches are available for ECG lead attachment for continuous monitoring of critically ill patients. The skin is clipped and cleaned, then the adhesive patch is applied to the skin and taped in place. Specialized ECG leads can be obtained to attach to the patches.

be monitored with a continuous ECG. Adhesive patches (Figure 21.4) for the ECG leads are often tolerated much better than clips; however, the skin must be clipped, cleaned with alcohol, then dried to ensure good contact. The adhesive patches may dessicate over time and usually require changing every day to maintain good skin contact. Specialized ECG leads are available to attach to the pads, or alternatively alligator clips can be attached directly to the contact button of the adhesive patch. After applying the skin contacts, it is often wise to let the animal settle in the cage before attaching the leads. Any abnormalities noted on the ECG should be recorded for review by a veterinary surgeon. In cases with cardiac disease or anuria requiring fluid therapy, it is helpful to measure central venous pressure (CVP) to avoid fluid overload (see Chapters 4 and 22). In addition, the respiratory rate and effort should also be closely monitored.

MONITORING AND NURSING CARE OF THE RESPIRATORY SYSTEM

When dealing with a patient with respiratory compromise, one must remain acutely aware of the fragility of the dyspnoeic patient, and the risks of any procedure must be carefully weighed against the potential benefits. The stress of restraint for placement of an intravenous catheter can prove fatal, especially in cats. Consequently, the physical examination and diagnostic tests may need to be performed in stages. Handling and manipulation of the patient should be kept to a minimum and the animal should be given ample time to rest between procedures. Most dyspnoeic cats will benefit from a period in a high concentration of supplemental oxygen in an oxygen cage or incubator prior to a complete evaluation.

Examination

Evaluation of the respiratory system usually includes respiratory rate, respiratory effort and auscultation of the lungs. A normal animal should have a respiratory rate of 15–30 breaths per minute and very little apparent chest movement because the major contribution to a normal inspiration comes from diaphragmatic contraction. During normal inspiration, diaphragmatic contraction displaces abdominal viscera in a caudal direction and the abdominal wall moves out. Animals in respiratory distress will exhibit postural indications of dyspnoea which include standing rather than sitting, abducted elbows, increased abdominal movement, extended neck and open mouth breathing. Paradoxical abdominal movement can also occur as dyspnoea worsens. Increased intercostal movement draws the diaphragm and abdominal viscera cranially on inspiration and the abdominal wall moves in. Some of the postural manifestations of dyspnoea can vary between dogs and cats. Dogs prefer to stand with abducted elbows, while cats tend to sit in sternal recumbency. Constantly changing body position in cats implies a much worse degree of dyspnoea than it

does in dogs. Lateral recumbency and open-mouthed breathing caused by dyspnoea is a serious sign in a dog and often means impending death in a cat.

In a dyspnoeic animal the respiratory pattern can help localize the site of disease in the respiratory tract in two common situations. An upper airway obstruction is usually associated with a prolonged inspiratory time with inspiratory stridor or stertor and a short expiration. If possible without undue stress to the patient, body temperature should be measured as soon as possible. Because the main thermoregulatory mechanism in the dog is panting, upper airway obstruction can be associated with dangerously high body temperatures. Small airway disease, such as feline asthma, often has a longer expiratory phase with increased abdominal effort. Most other causes of dyspnoea are associated with mixed respiratory patterns. Pulmonary auscultation in the dyspnoeic patient is difficult to master. The easiest way to ensure a complete auscultation is to divide the chest into a noughts and crosses board, then auscultate each square (Figure 21.5). Lung sounds are normally slightly louder and coarser in the cranioventral lung fields compared to the caudodorsal fields. Lung sounds should be symmetrical when the same area is compared on both sides of the chest. Pleural space disease such as pleural effusion or pneumothorax causes muffling of lung sounds, whereas small airway or parenchymal disease usually makes them louder.

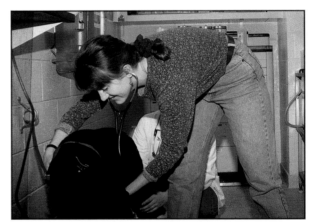

Figure 21.5: Auscultation is a vital part of monitoring the respiratory system.

Oxygen therapy

Oxygen therapy is often necessary in the patient with respiratory disease. Oxygen can be supplemented using an oxygen cage, oxygen mask or via an intra-nasal tube (see Chapters 5 and 22). An oxygen cage allows the inspired oxygen concentration to be closely controlled (between room air and 100%) and it is the least stressful method of administration. The inaccessibility of animals in an oxygen cage is often suggested as a drawback of this method of oxygen delivery; however, the reduced manipulation can be to their benefit.

Opening the door to the cage should be avoided and the small access ports should be used whenever possible to avoid rapid changes in oxygen concentration. Oxygen masks can be useful when a procedure must be performed on a dyspnoeic animal; however, many dyspnoeic animals will not tolerate a mask. In these cases, simply holding the oxygen tubing in front of the mouth and nose can suffice ('flow-by' oxygen, see Chapter 5). Intra-nasal oxygen delivery is convenient for longer-term supplementation of lower concentrations of oxygen. It requires the placement of an intra-nasal catheter or nasal prongs (see Chapters 5 and 22), which may not be tolerated by some animals. Placement can be greatly facilitated by instillation of local anaesthetic into the nostril 10 minutes prior to the procedure. Placement of an intra-nasal catheter is often too stressful for a severely dyspnoeic animal, especially one that has just been presented to the veterinary surgeon as an emergency. Ideally, all methods of oxygen supplementation should include some form of humidification of the inspired gas. Humidification consists of the saturation of the inspired oxygen with water vapour, which helps to prevent damage to the airway mucosa by dry air.

When there is evidence of lung disease on clinical examination, lung function should ideally be assessed using arterial blood gas analysis, which measures the arterial partial pressure of oxygen (PaO_2), and/or pulse oximetry, which measures haemoglobin saturation (SpO_2) (see Chapters 5 and 16). Pulse oximetry is non-invasive, requiring only that a light transmitting and receiving probe be placed on the animal. The tongue, ear, lip and inguinal skin fold can all be used as measuring sites. Unfortunately, the accuracy of the pulse oximeter can be significantly affected by movement of the animal, inadequate clipping of the placement site, poor perfusion or pigmented mucous membranes. Failure to achieve a good signal strength or waveform on the instrument display should lead one to question the accuracy of the results. Arterial blood gases are usually obtained from the femoral or dorsal pedal artery and allow measurement of the partial pressure of oxygen, carbon dioxide and pH. If infrequent samples are anticipated, the samples can be obtained by puncture with a fine (25 or 26 gauge) needle (Figure 21.6). If repeated sampling is likely to be necessary, it is often safer and less stressful on the animal to place a catheter percutaneously into the dorsal metatarsal artery (see Chapter 22).

The goal of oxygen therapy is to maintain a PaO_2 of at least 60 mm Hg, which corresponds to SpO_2 values greater than 90%. At partial pressures of oxygen below 60 mm Hg, there is a rapid fall in haemoglobin saturation. It is therefore often better to aim for a PaO_2 in the range of 70–80 mm Hg to provide a margin of safety should the lung disease worsen. Ideally, the patient should receive the minimum inspired oxygen concentration required to maintain an adequate PaO_2 or SpO_2, to avoid the risks of oxygen toxicity caused by high inspired oxygen concentrations. If blood gas analysis or

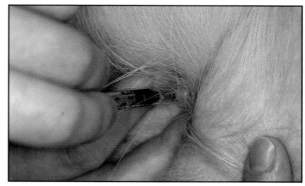

Figure 21.6: *Samples of arterial blood are obtained by percutaneous puncture of the femoral (shown here) or metatarsal arteries. Specialized pre-heparinized syringes are available or alternately standard 1 ml syringes can be flushed with heparin.*

pulse oximetry is not available, the inspired concentration is titrated to the clinical response. In emergency patients, initially 100% oxygen should be given, then the concentration should be gradually reduced to the lowest level at which the animal breathes comfortably. Oxygen concentrations of >50% for more than 12 hours or >60% for 18 hours have been suggested to cause oxygen toxicity. Ideally, an inspired oxygen concentration of 40% is recommended for long-term therapy. Maintaining an adequate PaO_2 is essential for life, so in animals with severe pulmonary parenchymal disease the guidelines for oxygen therapy may have to be exceeded in spite of the risk of oxygen toxicity.

Nebulization and coupage is used to facilitate the mobilization of respiratory secretions, usually in animals with pneumonia. Nebulization consists of the production of tiny droplets (ideally 3–7 µl) of water or saline, usually by an ultrasonic or oxygen-driven nebulizer (Figure 21.7). The mist of water droplets is infused into a closed cage every 4–6 hours and is inhaled to shower out in the small airways, moistening respiratory tract secretions to facilitate their movement out of the chest by the mucociliary escalator. Concurrently, the chest is patted firmly (coupaged) to stimulate coughing, which further assists airway clearance. In some circumstances, nebulization can be used to administer antibiotics or other respiratory medications.

MONITORING AND NURSING CARE OF THE NEUROLOGICAL SYSTEM

Since critical illness is often associated with significant muscle weakness and central nervous system depression, nursing evaluation of the central nervous system (CNS) often amounts to deciding whether the abnormalities of mental status and gait are appropriate for the other problems identified in the major body system assessment. Abnormalities of mental status include dullness/depression, stupor and coma, hyperexcitability,

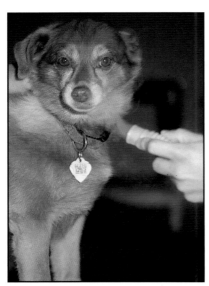

Figure 21.7: *Nebulization consists of the generation of tiny droplets of water or saline, which are inhaled and then deposit in the airways, moistening airway secretions. Since the saline or water remains in the liquid phase, nebulization differs from humidification, which is the saturation of inspired gases with water vapour (gas phase).*

hysteria and seizures. Depressed mentation is often associated with abnormalities of other body systems, such as hypoperfusion, renal failure and liver failure. When the degree of depression is greater than expected from the other disease processes present, this should raise the suspicion of primary CNS disease or CNS complications due to metabolic disorders such as hepatoencephalopathy. In any patient with abnormal mental status the blood glucose concentration should be checked immediately; hypoglycaemia is a possible underlying cause that is easily and rapidly reversible, but which can cause irreversible neurological damage if left untreated. Seizures are a common emergency problem and can be due to intracranial or extracranial causes. The body temperature of an animal presenting with seizures should be taken immediately, as hyperthermia due to muscle activity can occasionally be life threatening.

Precautionary measures are often instituted in animals with presumed brain disease or head trauma, to treat and avoid increases in intracranial pressure. Elevation of the head to an angle of approximately 30 degrees can be used to facilitate venous return and reduce intracranial pressure. It is important to place the entire animal on a board, rather than try to elevate the head alone. Care should be taken to avoid occluding the jugular veins and jugular venepuncture should be avoided. Procedures that may result in coughing should also be avoided as coughing can result in large increases in intracranial pressure. Neurological parameters monitored in the patient with neurological disease include the pupillary light response and pupil sizes, the palpebral or blink reflex, the menace reflex, the presence or absence of strabismus, and the general mental status.

Spinal cord injury or disease is the other main category of neurological injury. There are only a limited number of underlying causes of acute onset paresis or paralysis of the hind limbs or all four limbs (see Chapter 7). Intervertebral disc prolapse is, by far, the most common cause in the emergency practice. Others include spinal fractures and luxations, tumours, fibrocartilaginous emboli and discospondylitis. In addition to causing paralysis of the limbs, cervical spinal cord injury can also impair the function of the phrenic and intercostal nerves, leading to inadequate ventilation requiring mechanical ventilation. Arterial blood gas analysis and/or end-tidal capnography (see Chapter 16) allow the veterinary surgeon to monitor the partial pressure of carbon dioxide to determine whether artificial ventilation is needed. When spinal cord injury is present, progressive loss of neurological function is manifested as ataxia, loss of proprioception, followed by loss of voluntary motor activity, then extensor tone and, lastly, deep pain sensation. Deterioration in the patient's ambulatory status should be brought to the attention of a veterinary surgeon, as emergency surgical intervention may be necessary.

MONITORING AND NURSING CARE OF THE URINARY SYSTEM

Urine output is used as one of the most important indicators of renal function in the dynamic critically ill patient; however, clinicopathological tests such as blood urea nitrogen, creatinine and potassium concentration should also be monitored. In addition to intrinsic renal disease, urine output can fall due to pre-renal or post-renal causes. The fall in urine output seen with pre-renal causes of azotaemia, such as dehydration or hypoperfusion, is physiologically appropriate, as the body attempts to retain water and sodium, and should be associated with concentrated urine (high specific gravity) if renal function is normal. Post-renal azotaemia and subsequent decreases in urine output may occur with blockage of the urethra due to calculi and rupture of the bladder, urethra or ureter resulting in uroperitoneum. With urethral obstruction a large painful bladder can often be palpated. Monitoring urine output is especially important in patients at risk for acute renal failure or in animals that have sustained abdominal or pelvic trauma which can be associated with rupture of the bladder or urethra.

Indwelling urinary catheters with a sterile closed collection system are placed to measure urine output accurately and sometimes to prevent urine scalding in the recumbent patient. Indiscriminate use should be avoided as they are a potential route for bacterial infection and also result in urethral trauma. If a catheter is necessary, it should be placed using sterile equipment and aseptic technique (see Chapter 22). In a female, hair should be clipped around the perineum followed by a full surgical scrub. The urinary catheter can be placed blind, by palpation of the urethral orifice with a sterile gloved finger, or the urethral meatus can be visualized using a speculum. In the male, an assistant should extrude the penis and the catheter should be placed without allowing the catheter to come into contact with the prepuce.

If acute changes are anticipated, urine output should be measured every 2–4 hours. Normal urine output is 0.5–2 ml/kg/h; however, the appropriate urine output in a critically ill animal can vary widely. If a reduction in urine output is detected, the bladder should be palpated and the catheter should be flushed with warm saline to ensure that there is no mechanical obstruction due to catheter kinking, blood clots or calculi. To avoid potential bacterial contamination, a system which allows the urine collection bag to be emptied without disconnecting the inflow line is preferred. In systems that necessitate disconnecting the tubing, care should be taken to prevent the ends coming into contact with foreign material. The collection bag should be kept below the patient to facilitate urine drainage, but ideally not on the floor. Any changes in the appearance or odour of the urine should be noted. If a urinary catheter is not placed, manually palpating the bladder, noting its size and/or weighing absorbent cage material before and after urination, are approximate methods of assessing urine production.

PAIN DETECTION AND ANALGESIA IN THE CRITICAL PATIENT

Pain recognition
The assessment of pain can be difficult in the critically ill animal as many have abnormal mental status due to their underlying disease processes. Indicators of pain can be quite subtle and many animals do not exhibit obvious signs such as crying. It is especially difficult to recognize pain in cats, in which a crouched posture can sometimes be the only sign. In dogs, pain may be manifest as restlessness, reluctance to lie down, hypersalivation, tachypnoea or tachycardia. Some stoical dogs may show only a worried facial expression or a grimace with their lips drawn back.

Analgesia
Analgesic medications should be given as soon as possible, in adequate doses, because many analgesics are more effective when given before pain is severe. Furthermore, analgesics can sometimes effectively prevent pain but do not completely eliminate it once it has begun.

Many analgesic medications (see Chapter 18) used in critically ill animals also result in sedation and dysphoria. This can complicate subsequent clinical evaluations and the interpretation of pain status in that animal. Analgesic drugs can also have deleterious effects on the cardiovascular, respiratory and neurological systems and the side-effects of analgesic medication must be weighed against humanitarian concerns for pain relief. Furthermore, sedation, which occurs with some pain medications, can mask serious deterioration in the status of the animal. Changes in behaviour, mental status or respiratory pattern are some of the earliest signs of problems in a critically ill patient and they can be extremely difficult to interpret following sedation. Consequently, the major body systems must be closely monitored following administration of pain medication and sedation.

NURSING CARE OF THE RECUMBENT PATIENT

The comfort and welfare of the critically ill animal should be paramount in the mind of all critical care personnel. Veterinary critical care entails supporting very sick animals and it is incumbent upon all veterinary surgeons and nurses to ensure that the level of discomfort is kept to a minimum. The level of discomfort that is acceptable must be assessed on an individual basis and weighed against such factors as the likelihood of survival, the anticipated duration of survival, and the expected quality of life following successful treatment. The critical care nurse plays a vital role in the care of the critically ill patient, most of which are recumbent for at least some period during hospitalization. The care of the animal that cannot move around or clean itself is an important part of critical care nursing.

Respiratory problems
The most important short-term effect of prolonged recumbency is impairment of respiratory function and subsequent hypoxia due to atelectasis, aspiration pneumonia and ventilation–perfusion mismatching. Atelectasis, or collapse of lung lobes, occurs when a patient lies in lateral recumbency on the same side for an extended period of time. Atelectasis tends to be most common in large breed dogs. Frequent turning of the patient (every 4 hours) or maintaining the patient in a sternal position will avoid atelectasis and promote appropriate alveolar ventilation and perfusion of the lungs. Aspiration pneumonia is a relatively common complication in the recumbent patient, especially if the animal is vomiting or regurgitating frequently. Regurgitation and aspiration can occasionally occur with no clinical signs associated with the regurgitation episode.

Decubital ulcers
Recumbent patients (Figure 21.8) are at risk of developing decubital ulceration, but this is an unusual complication unless the patient is recumbent for a prolonged period of time. Persistent localized pressure on the same area of the body impairs circulation, which eventually results in necrosis. Decubital ulcers extend through the skin and underlying subcutaneous tissue

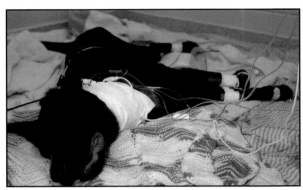

Figure 21.8: Patients that are recumbent for prolonged periods are at risk for pulmonary atelectasis, aspiration pneumonia, decubital ulcers and urine scalding. Important nursing strategies for these animals include frequent turning from side to side, physical therapy and limb massage to ensure good blood flow, and careful frequent cleaning of all excreta.

and even through muscle to bone in severe cases. They occur most commonly over the greater trochanter, ischial tuberosity and lateral aspect of the elbow. Healing of decubital ulcers is extremely slow and difficult, so prevention is far superior to cure. Frequent turning of the patient and soft bedding are the best ways to avoid decubital ulcers.

Hygiene

Close attention should be paid to the hygiene of recumbent patients. Bedding should be kept clean and dry and all faeces and urine should be promptly removed. Failure to keep the patient clean can result in urine scalding and perineal dermatitis and can contaminate urinary and intravenous catheters. Clipping the hair from the perineal area and the use of topical medications can help to prevent perineal dermatitis. Urinary catheterization or manually expressing the bladder may be indicated for some patients.

Physical therapy

Many recumbent patients require physical therapy to maintain joint mobility; however, this should be kept to a minimum in the unstable critically ill patient. If the patient is ambulatory, short walks may be appropriate.

NURSING CARE OF INTRAVENOUS CATHETERS

Intravenous catheters are essential in the care of the critically ill patient to administer intravenous medication and fluid therapy. In addition, central venous catheters can be used to monitor central venous pressure, while arterial catheters are used directly to measure arterial blood pressure and blood gases. Venous and arterial catheters can also be used for blood sampling, thus avoiding the risks and discomfort of serial venepuncture. This is especially beneficial when fre-

quent blood sampling is anticipated, such as might be needed for blood glucose monitoring in a diabetic animal. When obtaining blood samples from an indwelling arterial or venous catheter, the catheter should be flushed and, using a syringe containing 0.5–1 ml heparinized saline to prevent clotting, an adequate pre-sample (2–6 ml blood) withdrawn to avoid dilution of the test sample with flush solution remaining in the catheter. The test sample is then obtained and the pre-sample can be re-injected back into the animal via a venous catheter.

Intravenous access may be established via a peripheral vein, such as the cephalic or saphenous vein, or via a central vein, such as the jugular or medial femoral vein. In smaller dogs, central venous access can also be established by placing a long catheter into the cephalic or saphenous veins. In very small patients, such as neonates, a needle inserted into the medullary cavity of a bone (usually the femur) can be used to administer fluids and medications. When placing catheters, all hair should be clipped from the site, which should be scrubbed using standard aseptic technique (Figure 21.9). Following placement, the catheter should be securely taped or sutured in place and covered by a wrap to keep the site clean and dry.

Catheter patency is maintained by flushing with heparinized saline (1 unit heparin per ml of 0.9% NaCl) every 6 hours. The catheter site should be evaluated frequently for any swelling, reddening or pain suggestive of phlebitis and if the wrapping becomes dirty or wet it should be replaced immediately. If signs of local inflammation are seen or the animal develops an otherwise unexplained fever, the catheter should be removed.

Although routine removal and replacement of intravenous catheters has been advocated every 72 hours, studies have shown that removal of otherwise functional catheters in the absence of clinical signs of thrombophlebitis is probably unnecessary (Mathews *et al.*, 1996). Vascular access may become a limiting factor for care of critically ill dogs and cats, particularly those

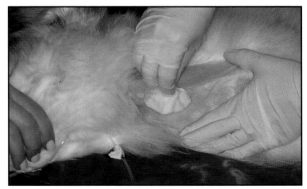

Figure 21.9: Careful catheter site preparation is one of the most important factors in preventing infections and thrombophlebitis. In this patient, the jugular vein has been clipped and draped, and the area is being scrubbed for placement of a central venous catheter.

of small body size, that are hospitalized repeatedly or for prolonged periods of time. Clinical experience has confirmed that it is best to maintain catheters in place for the longest possible time, as long as they are patent, uninfected and not associated with thrombophlebitis. Peripheral catheters usually require changing more often than central venous catheters.

The size of the catheter selected will depend upon the size of the patient and the anticipated rate of fluid infusion. Flow through a catheter is proportional to the fourth power of the radius, i.e. halving the radius of the catheter will reduce the flow by 16 times. If rapid fluid administration is required for systemic hypoperfusion or if blood products are to be given, the largest bore catheter possible should be used (e.g. an 18 gauge catheter or greater should be used in any dog over 20 kg). It is also best to place a second intravenous catheter in dogs heavier than 20 kg requiring rapid intravascular volume expansion. This ensures that an adequate rate of fluids can be given and provides a backup if one catheter comes out or does not flow well. Because of their higher viscosity, it is also best to give blood products through a separate catheter.

The dorsal pedal artery is the most common site used for arterial access. In all but the smallest animals, a 22 gauge catheter is placed percutaneously into the artery. Paradoxically, placement of a metatarsal arterial catheter is often associated with fewer bleeding complications in high-risk animals than arterial puncture using a needle. Arterial catheters are used to measure direct blood pressures and to obtain blood samples to measure arterial blood gases. Fluid therapy and medications should never be administered via an arterial line. Because of the potential for rapid exsanguination if the catheter becomes disconnected, an animal with an intra-arterial catheter must be kept under close supervision.

REFERENCES AND FURTHER READING

Burrows CF (1982) Inadequate skin preparation as a cause of intravenous catheter-related infection in the dog. *Journal of the American Veterinary Medical Association* **180**, 747–749

Johnson JA and Murtaugh RJ (1997) Preventing and treating noscomial infection. Part I. Urinary tract infections and pneumonia. *Compendium on Continuing Education for the Practicing Veterinarian* **19**, 581–586

Lees GF (1996) Use and misuse of indwelling catheters. *Veterinary Clinics of North America: Small Animal Practice* **26**, 499–504

Manning AM, Rush J and Ellis DR (1997) Physical therapy for critically ill veterinary patients. Part I. Chest physical therapy. *Compendium on Continuing Education for the Practicing Veterinarian* **19**, 675–688

Manning AM, Rush J and Ellis DR (1997) Physical therapy for critically ill veterinary patients. Part II. The musculoskeletal system. *Compendium on Continuing Education for the Practicing Veterinarian* **19**, 803–806

Matthews KA, Brooks MJ and Valliant AE (1996) A prospective study of intravenous catheter contamination. *Journal of Veterinary Emergency and Critical Care* **6**, 33–43

Nicoll SA and Remedios AM (1995) Recumbency in small animals: pathophysiology and management. *Compendium on Continuing Education for the Practicing Veterinarian* **17**, 1367–1374

Powell S and Petrollini E (1998) Emergency and first aid. In: *Comprehensive Review for Veterinary Technicians*, ed. MM Tighe and M Brown, pp. 327–337. Mosby Year Book, St Louis

Thelan LA, Urden LD, Lough ME and Stacy KM (1998) *Critical Care Nursing: Diagnosis and Management, 3rd edition.* Mosby Year Book, St Louis

CHAPTER TWENTY TWO

Emergency Techniques

Robert N. White

INTRODUCTION

This chapter describes the majority of commonly required techniques utilized in the emergency situation. For ease of use, the techniques have been broadly categorized to correspond with the other chapters of the manual.

RESPIRATORY SYSTEM TECHNIQUES

Clearance of the airway obstructed by foreign material

Direct vision of foreign material obstructing the larynx can be achieved in the unconscious individual with the aid of a laryngoscope.

Technique — ventral recumbency

1. Align the head and neck in the optimal airway position with the head pulled forward
2. An assistant is required to take the weight of the animal's head by holding the lateral aspects of the nose or, in smaller individuals, supporting the skull by the zygomatic arches
3. Open the mouth, grasp the tongue and pull it forwards
4. The frenulum of the tongue is protected from the lower incisors with the rescuer's fingers
5. Insert the laryngoscope with the blade aiming towards the midline at laryngeal level
6. Ventral depression of the laryngoscope tip will reveal the pharynx, epiglottis and larynx
7. Under direct vision, fluid material can be cleared with suction aspiration, and solid material can be removed either with protected fingers or with forceps.

Technique — dorsal recumbency

This technique can be carried out by an unassisted individual.

1. Align the head and neck in the optimal airway position with the head pulled forward
2. Introduce the laryngoscope into the corner of the mouth with the blade aiming towards the midline at

laryngeal level
3. Lift the handle of the laryngoscope upwards and forwards, taking great care not to damage the lower incisors or to damage the tongue on the lower incisors
4. Under direct vision, fluid material can be cleared with suction aspiration, and solid material can either be removed with protected fingers or with some form of forceps.

Suction apparatus

Effective suction apparatus is a vital piece of equipment in resuscitation to clear the oropharynx of secretions, blood, regurgitated gastric contents and vomitus. In human hospitals, a suction source is generally available in all patient areas and is supplied from a central vacuum unit or from a Venturi device associated with a gas pipeline. An installation of this sophistication is rarely available in veterinary hospitals and portable apparatus is more commonly utilized. Portable suction units generally fall into two groups: electrically powered and hand- or foot-powered. Electrically powered devices are used primarily in the operating theatre and are used for resuscitation only in the emergency situation. Hand- or foot-powered devices have the advantage that they do not depend on an electrical or mechanical source. Foot-powered models leave the hands of the rescuer free for other tasks. Hand-powered models require the operator to power the device and manipulate the suction end in the pharynx with one hand, and therefore they must be very lightweight. Both forms of device must be capable of generating adequate vacuum and flow rate to ensure easy aspiration of semi-solid tenacious material.

Endotracheal intubation

Although a clear airway can generally be maintained without artificial aids on a short-term basis, there are numerous occasions when endotracheal intubation is necessary. Endotracheal intubation provides a reliable, clear and secure airway through which effective positive pressure ventilation can be readily applied. It should be performed as soon as possible in all cases of cardiorespiratory arrest. Little equipment is required for effective endotracheal intubation, and all members of the nursing staff should be comfortable which the intubation technique.

Equipment required for endotracheal intubation

- A selection of cuffed endotracheal tubes of varying diameters from 2.5 to 14. Uncuffed examples of sizes from 2.5 to 5 should also be available. All tubes should be cut to the correct length, with connectors to fit the ventilating apparatus
- A laryngoscope with a range of appropriate sized blades
- A cuff inflator or syringe to inflate the cuff if fitted
- A clamp for the cuff
- Flexible stylets that fit the inner diameter of at least the smaller of the tubes
- Lubricating jelly
- Bandage or tape to secure the tube in place
- Scissors to cut tubes to required length
- 2% lignocaine without adrenaline for desensitizing the cat larynx.

Endotracheal intubation is generally carried out via the orotracheal route in small animals. The use of a laryngoscope cannot be over-emphasized when performing this procedure, especially in the emergency situation (Figure 22.1). It can sometimes prove difficult to direct the tip of the endotracheal tube through the rima glottidis. This process can be facilitated by using a rigid stylet, which is passed into the trachea. The endotracheal tube is then passed over the stylet, which guides it through the larynx into the trachea.

In the smallest cats, it may be necessary to place an uncuffed endotracheal tube. This will allow a greater internal diameter tube to be placed into the small feline trachea than can be achieved when a cuffed endotracheal tube is used. A seal preventing aspiration can be achieved by placing a wad of gauze within the oropharynx. In the emergency situation, where the cat has lost consciousness, laryngeal reflexes will not be present making it unnecessary to desensitize the larynx with a local anaesthetic spray to prevent laryngeal spasm.

Assessment of correct tube placement

It is very important to ensure that endotracheal and not oesophageal tube placement has been achieved. This is optimally determined by direct visualization using a laryngoscope. Alternatively, a very simple and safe method for assessment of correct tube placement is the oesophageal detector device. The device simply consists of a 60 ml syringe, with a catheter tip that is attached to a standard catheter mount with a 15 mm fitting (Figure 22.2). The attachment must be airtight. Once the tracheal tube is in place, the 15 mm fitting is attached to it and the syringe plunger withdrawn. An easy flow of air with minimal resistance indicates that the tube is in the trachea. Resistance to aspiration indicates that the tube is in the oesophagus because the non-rigid walls collapse and occlude the lumen. Various other configurations of this system using smaller syringes and components can be devised for more convenient use in smaller dogs and cats.

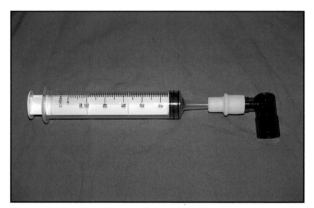

Figure 22.2: Oesophageal detector device.

Retrograde intubation

The technique of retrograde intubation involves cricothyroid membrane, thyrotracheal membrane or transtracheal puncture, with a needle directed in a rostral direction (Figure 22.3). A guide wire is then passed through the needle so that it passes through the rima glottidis and can be retrieved in the mouth. A suitably sized endotracheal tube is then passed over the wire and advanced, with rotation if necessary, until it passes through the rima glottidis to lie within the trachea. The wire can then be removed and the tube advanced further to achieve complete intubation. The technique is sometimes described as 'railroading' the endotracheal tube into the trachea. With practice, the technique can be performed with relative speed, although in the emergency situation it may be advisable to obtain control over the airway distally (e.g. needle tracheotomy) prior to embarking on the intubation.

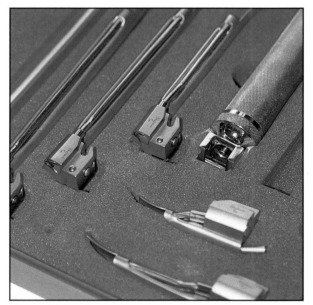

Figure 22.1: A laryngoscope set consisting of various length Miller laryngoscope blades and handle power source. Straight blades are, in general, more easy to use compared with curved blades.

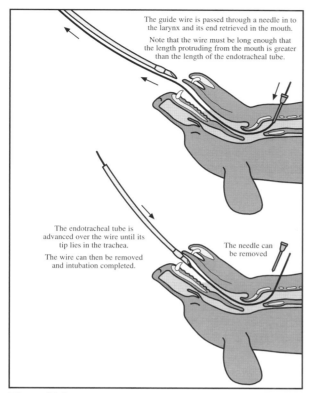

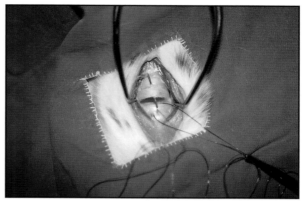

Figure 22.4: Tracheotomy – a 40% circumferential incision has been made into the trachea, and guide loops are being placed around tracheal rings on both sides of the incision.

2. Place the animal in dorsal recumbency with hyperextension of neck
3. Always have a tracheostomy kit available
4. Make a longitudinal skin incision caudal to the larynx
5. The incision is extended through the paired sternohyoideus muscles, revealing the trachea
6. The trachea is incised circumferentially at the 3rd/4th or 4th/5th ring level (40% circumference) preserving both recurrent laryngeal nerves (Figure 22.4)
7. 2-0 or 3-0 monofilament suture is passed into the trachea on both sides of the incision and tied to make guide loops for the placement of the tracheostomy tube
8. The tracheostomy tube is placed
9. The wound is loosely closed and dressed
10. The tube is secured with umbilical tapes.

Tracheostomy tube and site care

* Postoperative care is as important as the surgery
* Humidify the inspired air; either nebulize water into the cage or instil 1–3 ml of sterile saline into the trachea every 4–6 hours
* Cleanse the wound and tracheal tube frequently (every 2 hours)
* The traction sutures allow the easy removal and replacement of the tube
* Ideally, tubes should have an inner sleeve that can be removed for cleaning purposes (Figure 22.5)
* A soft urethral catheter will allow suctioning of the trachea and large bronchi, but to minimize airway trauma, this is only performed when there are excessive secretions obstructing the airway
* Tracheostomy wounds should be allowed to heal by second intention.

The technique of tracheostomy tube placement is relatively straightforward and, although nursing staff are unlikely to perform the procedure, they should be fully acquainted with the operative technique. In the non-emergency situation, the technique is the same

The guide wire is passed through a needle in to the larynx and its end retrieved in the mouth.

Note that the wire must be long enough that the length protruding from the mouth is greater than the length of the endotracheal tube.

The endotracheal tube is advanced over the wire until its tip lies in the trachea.

The wire can then be removed and intubation completed.

The needle can be removed

Figure 22.3: Retrograde direction of the endotracheal tube.

The technique will prove unreliable in individuals with laryngeal obstructive disease.

Tracheotomy and percutaneous dilatational cricothyrotomy

In a number of cases, endotracheal intubation will prove impossible or inappropriate due to extensive maxillofacial injury or severe anatomical abnormality. In these cases, tracheotomy or percutaneous dilatational cricothyrotomy may be the only method of establishing a clear airway.

Equipment required for emergency tracheotomy

It is essential to have a tracheotomy kit always available. The components of this kit should be maintained in a sterile state. A number of human paediatric/child tracheotomy kits are available, which are sold complete and sterile and comprise:

* Scalpel handle and blade (no. 10 or 15)
* Dissecting thumb forceps
* Two or three pairs of haemostat forceps
* 2-0 or 3-0 monofilament sutures
* Fenestrated surgical drape
* Range of tracheostomy tubes
* Umbilical tape to secure the tube
* Surgical swabs.

Tracheotomy — emergency technique

1. No time for surgical preparation

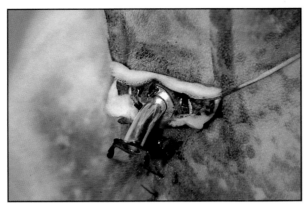

Figure 22.5: Some tracheostomy tubes have an inner sleeve that can be removed for cleaning. This allows the outer tube to remain in situ, *thus minimizing airway interference during the cleaning procedure.*

although the preparation of the surgical site should be more thorough and the technique should be performed in an aseptic manner.

Percutaneous dilatational cricothyrotomy or thyrotracheotomy — technique

1. Align the head and neck in the optimal airway position with the head pulled forward
2. A needle is introduced through the cricothyroid or thyrotracheal membrane and a Seldinger wire passed caudally into the trachea
3. The needle is removed and a skin and platysma muscle incision made across the wire large enough to accommodate a 6.5 mm tracheal tube
4. Successive dilators are passed over the wire, the final dilator being sheathed with the tracheal tube, which is railroaded into the trachea.

Purpose-designed equipment by Melker (1988) is available (Figure 22.6).

Needle tracheotomy

Needle tracheotomy is a very simple technique for

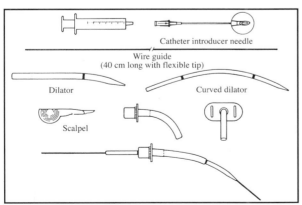

Figure 22.6: Melker percutaneous dilatational cricothyrotomy kit.

rapidly alleviating an upper airway respiratory obstruction proximal to the trachea (Figure 22.7).

1. Place the animal in dorsal recumbency with hyperextension of neck
2. A hypodermic needle or catheter-over-needle (16–18 gauge for cats, 10–16 gauge for dogs) is advanced in the ventral midline through the skin and through the tracheal wall. The trachea is stabilized with the free hand
3. An airway is now established, although its diameter will obviously depend on the size of the needle or catheter used
4. The needle or the catheter is then attached to a breathing circuit via a suitably sized 15 mm endotracheal tube connector, and oxygen flow is established.

Supplemental respiratory oxygen therapy

There are a number of techniques available for supplementing oxygen in small animals. Each technique has its advantages and its disadvantages; no one technique can be said to be appropriate in all circumstances. Therefore, an understanding of each technique will allow an informed decision to be taken when deciding which technique to use in a particular instant. It is important to remember that during normal respiration an inspiratory

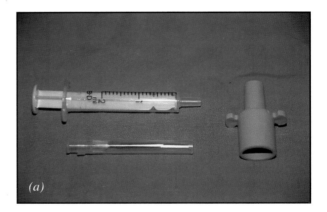

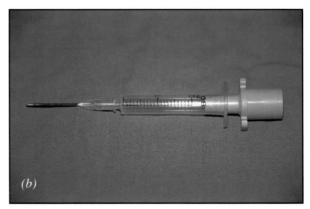

Figure 22.7: (a) Components of a needle tracheotomy set; a 18 gauge needle, a 2.5 ml syringe barrel and a suitably sized 15 mm endotracheal tube connector (8 mm).
(b) Needle tracheotomy components assembled for use.

flow rate of approximately 30 litres per minute is generated. Obviously, anaesthetic machine flow meters will not achieve such high flow rates, and therefore if the inspired gas for oxygen support is not supplied in a reservoir of at least the animal's minute volume, the animal must be diluting the inspired supplemental gas with atmospheric air to achieve its tidal volume. This phenomenon is commonly the explanation for the various inspired oxygen concentrations (FiO_2) achieved with each of the oxygen supplementation systems.

Oxygen cage

Most oxygen cages cannot raise the oxygen concentration within the cage above approximately 50%. Their size may make observation of the patient difficult. Opening the cage door drops the FiO_2 to atmospheric concentrations almost immediately.

Face mask

A close-fitting face mask connected to an anaesthetic circuit (Figure 22.8) is a means of effectively increasing the FiO_2 (70–90%). This system is obviously labour intensive and may not be tolerated by the distressed individual. In certain circumstances, it is an extremely effective technique for rapidly increasing the FiO_2.

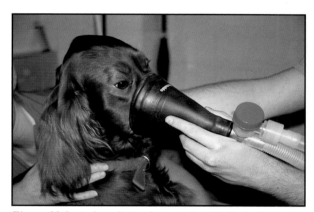

Figure 22.8: *A close-fitting face mask will effectively increase the* FiO_2.

Elizabethan collar and cling film cover

An oxygen pipe from an anaesthetic machine can supply oxygen (5–8 l/min) to this form of oxygen hood to provide a high FiO_2 (50–70%). This system is very well tolerated in both dogs and cats (Figure 22.9) and is useful for both short-term and long-term oxygen supplementation.

Nasal catheter

A nasal catheter (Figure 22.10) can be passed through the nose following instillation of a few drops of local anaesthetic (proxymetacaine). The catheter is generally held in place with superglue or sutures in butterfly tapes. The tip of the catheter should lie within the cranial nasopharynx. This system will allow the supplied oxygen to be humidified. Oxygen flow rates and the resulting FiO_2 are listed in Figure 22.11.

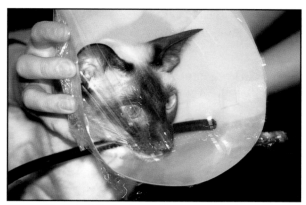

Figure 22.9: *An Elizabethan collar and cling film bag is well tolerated by both dogs and cats. Increasing the* FiO_2 *is achieved by supplying oxygen to within the collar via an anaesthetic pipe.*

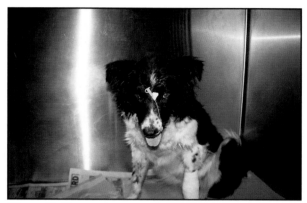

Figure 22.10: *Nasal catheterization for oxygen supplementation therapy. Butterfly tapes have been used to hold the nasal catheter in place.*

Weight (kg)	Inspired oxygen concentration		
	30–50%	**50–75%**	**75–100%**
0–10	0.5–1	1–2	3–5
10–20	1–2	3–5	>5
20–40	3–5	>5	?

Figure 22.11: *Approximate oxygen flow rates (l/min) for nasal catheter administration. Data derived from Fitzpatrick and Crowe (1986).*

Transtracheal catheter

A long intravenous catheter can be placed into the trachea following the instillation of surface local anaesthetic. Humidified oxygen is supplied at similar flow rates to those used with the nasal catheter. This system may be especially useful in individuals with laryngeal or upper tracheal obstruction.

Incubator

Incubators can often be obtained from local hospitals and provide a means of effectively increasing the FiO_2 whilst still clearly being able to observe and treat the patient. They commonly incorporate a system for humidifying the inspired gases and for warming the patient.

Nasal catheterization for oxygenation – technique

1. Infuse local anaesthetic (proxymetacaine) into the nare and elevate the muzzle
2. Pre-measure the catheter (5–10 French) between the medial canthus of the eye and the nare, and mark it at the level of the nare
3. Lubricate the tip of the catheter
4. Insert the catheter into the ventromedial aspect of the nare (below the alar fold) and advance it aborally in the ventral meatus to the pre-determined length (this may be aided by pushing the external nares dorsally as the tube is advanced beyond the external nares)
5. Secure the catheter to the face between the eyes by means of adhesive glue or butterfly tapes and suturing, thereby avoiding the whiskers
6. Secure a more proximal portion of the catheter to the skin on the forehead
7. Attach the syringe barrel to the proximal end of the catheter, using an adapter
8. Connect the syringe to the humidified oxygen source
9. Select an appropriate flow rate.

Ventilation of the lungs using basic life support techniques

Effective ventilation of the lungs can be provided by expired air respiration (EAR) using a mouth-to-mouth, mouth-to-nose or mouth-to-endotracheal tube technique. This technique should be used in all apnoeic patients unless advanced equipment is immediately available.

Mouth-to-mouth method

This method is often the first choice in the human field. Unfortunately, the disparity in mouth size and conformation between most small animals and humans makes the technique difficult to perform effectively.

1. The animal can be placed in dorsal, lateral or ventral recumbency
2. Align the head and neck in the optimal airway position with the head pulled forward
3. Press the thumb and forefinger of the same hand over both of the animal's nostrils
4. The rescuer inhales, opens their own mouth wide and seals it over the animal's mouth, and blows until the chest rises as with a normal breath
5. Once inflation has occurred, the rescuer removes their mouth, allowing complete passive exhalation to occur in the victim, then inhales again and repeats the process

6. If inflation is difficult, causes of airway obstruction should be investigated
7. The rescuer should distinguish a normal chest inflation from abdominal distension caused by stomach inflation.

Mouth-to-nose method

This method is more easily performed than the mouth-to-mouth technique, but would be considered just as unhygienic. Problems may occur with the mouth-to-nose method in patients with nasal obstruction and in nasal or maxillary injury.

1. The animal can be placed in dorsal, lateral or ventral recumbency
2. The head and neck are aligned in the optimal airway position with the head pulled forward
3. The hand of the rescuer is used to seal the lips of the animal
4. Inflation of the lungs is applied by the rescuer inhaling, sealing their mouth around the animal's nose and blowing to achieve normal inspiratory chest expansion
5. Once inflation has occurred, the rescuer removes their mouth, allowing complete passive exhalation to occur in the victim, inhales again and repeats the process
6. Passive exhalation may be helped by opening the animal's mouth during this phase.

Mouth-to-endotracheal tube method

By definition, this technique should be included within the advanced life support techniques because it involves the use of an endotracheal tube. It has been included within the basic techniques as a form of EAR. It is probably the most acceptable and effective technique, since inappropriate oesophageal inflation is unlikely to occur following correct tracheal intubation.

1. The animal is intubated as previously described
2. Inflation of the lungs is applied by the rescuer inhaling, sealing their mouth around the end of the endotracheal tube and blowing to achieve normal inspiratory chest expansion
3. Once inflation has occurred the rescuer removes their mouth, allowing complete passive exhalation to occur, then inhales again and repeats the process
4. In small individuals great care must be taken not to over-inflate the lungs and cause barotrauma.

Rates, volumes, flow rates and pressure with EAR

Rates

Respiratory rates equivalent to or above normal physiological rates for the patient should be applied during EAR. Very approximately, this means a rate of 15–20 breaths/min for large dogs, 20 breaths/min for medium dogs, and 30–40 breaths/min for small dogs and cats.

Volumes

Tidal volumes slightly above normal physiological values should be the goal. The chest movement expected in normal spontaneous ventilation in that particular patient is a good guide. Care should be exercised in small individuals not to over-inflate the lungs, which may lead to barotrauma and pulmonary oedema. A suitably sized, uncuffed endotracheal tube will allow adequate chest inflation to be performed in small patients and has the advantage that excessive inflation pressures cannot be generated making over-inflation of the lungs less likely, although there is a higher risk of aspiration because the airway is not fully protected by the uncuffed tube.

Flow rates

Inspiratory flow rates should mimic normal values of around 30 l/min. Inflation times should be gauged to normal respirations, usually about 1 second. An inspiratory/expiratory ratio of 1:2 or 1:3 is ideal. This regimen should minimize the effects of positive intrathoracic pressure on venous return to the heart.

Pressures

Excessive inflation pressures can occur with high flow rates, large tidal volumes and respiratory rates that do not allow sufficient time for complete exhalation. High inflation pressures (>20 cm H_2O), especially in the presence of an even slightly imperfect airway alignment, may lead to gastric inflation and a high probability of regurgitation and pulmonary inhalation in the individual that is not intubated.

Cricoid pressure

The possibility of gastric inflation and regurgitation of stomach contents can be substantially reduced during ventilation of the unprotected airway by an assistant who applies cricoid pressure, to obstruct the lumen of the oesophagus dorsal to the larynx and ventral to the cervical vertebral bodies.

- Consistent pressure is applied towards the cervical vertebrae, with the thumb and forefinger of one hand applied to either side of the thyroid cartilage
- Counter pressure may be applied to the dorsal neck with the other hand.

Ventilation of the lungs using advanced life support techniques

By definition, these methods are classified as advanced life support techniques as they require equipment, but they are easily capable of being carried out by trained lay members of staff. They have a number of advantages over direct mouth-to-mouth, mouth-to-nose and mouth-to-endotracheal tube ventilation:

- They avoid aesthetic concern about direct contact between rescuer and animal, especially in the presence of vomit or blood

- With certain appliances oxygen can be added to the delivered inspired air.

The self-inflating bag/valve device

The self-inflating bag/valve device is designed to inflate the patient's lungs with room air or an air-oxygen mixture if an oxygen supply is readily available. It has a clear advantage over expired air techniques in that a higher FiO_2 can be provided. The self-inflating bag is fitted at one end with an inlet valve to entrain air or an air-oxygen mixture into the bag as it re-inflates during the expiratory phase (Figure 22.12). During compression of the bag the air or air-oxygen mixture inflates the patient's lungs through the patient valve. This valve diverts the expired air into the atmosphere. The valve may be attached to an endotracheal tube or tracheostomy tube via a 15 mm fitting.

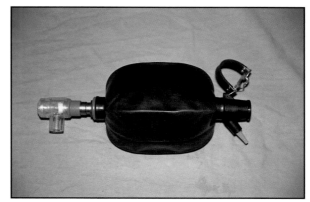

Figure 22.12: *A self-inflating bag/valve device (Ambu), which can be used to ventilate the lungs with either atmospheric air or an oxygen-enriched mixture.*

Addition of oxygen

Oxygen can be added to the bag either via a nipple, a reservoir bag or a length of reservoir tubing. Best results are achieved using a reservoir bag (less bulky) or a length of reservoir tubing. With these additions, inspired oxygen concentrations of 90% can be achieved with oxygen flow rates of 8–10 l/min. The inlet valve of bags incorporating an oxygen reservoir bag or tubing must be so designed that air will be entrained if the oxygen supply runs out. The addition of oxygen through a nipple on the bag, without a reservoir, is much less efficient. To achieve a high inspired oxygen concentration, the flow rates of oxygen must be comparable with the inspiratory flow rate (approximately 25–30 l/min). Such high flow rates over-fill the bag during inspiration, jamming the patient valve in the inspiratory position and preventing expiration through the valve. If no reservoir system is available, the added oxygen flow rate must not exceed 5–6 l/min (which will only achieve inspired oxygen concentrations of 40–50%).

Positive end expiratory pressure

Positive end expiratory pressure (PEEP) can be provided

with a self-inflating bag if a special PEEP valve is attached at the patient end. PEEP can be applied most effectively if the bag is attached to a cuffed-up endotracheal tube or a cuffed-up tracheostomy tube. In the emergency situation, the use of PEEP is not often indicated, but it is particularly valuable in individuals with pulmonary oedema or haemorrhage, those that have aspirated or inhaled irritant chemicals and victims of near drowning.

1. Apply the bag to the 15 mm endotracheal tube or tracheostomy tube fitting and PEEP valve
2. Compressing the bag inflates the patient's lungs
3. Release of the bag results in refilling and simultaneous passive exhalation through the expiratory port of the patient valve
4. Add oxygen if available (8–10 l/min if a reservoir is fitted; 5 l/min if a nipple only is fitted) if available
5. Compress and release with an inspiratory/expiratory ratio of 1:2 or 1:3, achieving normal chest movements at a normal rate for the animal's size.

Intermittent positive pressure ventilation using an anaesthetic breathing system

IPPV can be easily applied to the intubated individual, who is attached to an anaesthetic breathing system. Most current anaesthetic literature uses the following definitions and classifications for methods of delivery of inhalation agents.

Breathing systems

A breathing system (not a circuit) now describes both the mode of operation and the apparatus by which inhalation agents are delivered to the patient.

Rebreathing

Rebreathing in anaesthetic systems refers to the rebreathing of some or all of the previously exhaled gases, including carbon dioxide and water vapour.

Apparatus dead space

This refers to that volume within the apparatus that may contain exhaled patient gas and that will be rebreathed at the beginning of a subsequent inspiratory breath.

Functional dead space

Some systems may have a smaller 'functional' dead space owing to the flushing effect of a continuous fresh gas stream at the end of expiration, replacing exhaled gas in the apparatus dead space.

Classification of breathing systems

Breathing systems are classified according to function:

- Non-rebreathing systems (with unidirectional flow of gas within the system)

- Systems where rebreathing is possible, although not intended (bi-directional gas flow within the system)
- Non-rebreathing systems utilizing carbon dioxide absorption
     (a) unidirectional (circle) systems
     (b) bi-directional (to-and-fro) systems.

Attachments or circuits

Ayre's T-piece with Rees modification (Mapleson F breathing system): This circuit is generally suitable for individuals weighing up to approximately 10 kg. The corrugated tubular expiratory limb portion of the circuit should contain a volume of gas that is approximately the same as the patient's tidal volume. A fresh gas flow rate of approximately 2.5 times the patient's minute volume is required to prevent rebreathing.

1. The open end of the bag is partially or totally occluded by the fifth finger during the inspiratory phase, while the bag is squeezed between the other fingers and thumb
2. The fifth finger is relaxed during expiration
3. Squeeze and release with an inspiratory/expiratory ratio of 1:2 or 1:3, achieving normal chest movements at a normal rate for the animal's size.

Bain (Mapleson D breathing system): This circuit is generally suitable for individuals weighing between approximately 10 and 30 kg. To prevent rebreathing during controlled ventilation with this circuit, a fresh gas flow rate of approximately twice the patient's minute volume is required. The longer the expiratory pause, the more efficiently the circuit will be purged of the previously expired gases, making it less likely that rebreathing will occur during inspiration.

1. The adjustable pressure-limiting valve is partially closed so that sufficient pressure can develop in the system to inflate the lungs
2. Inspiration is produced by squeezing the reservoir bag with one or both hands
3. Squeeze and release with an inspiratory/expiratory ratio of 1:3, achieving normal chest movements at a normal rate for the animal's size.

Magill, Lack co-axial and parallel Lack (Mapleson A breathing system): This circuit is generally suitable for individuals weighing between approximately 10 and 30 kg. The flow characteristics of these circuits are such that to prevent rebreathing the fresh gas flow rate required during controlled ventilation is higher than that required during spontaneous respiration. This is usually of the order of two times the patient's minute volume. Like the Bain system, the longer the expiratory pause, the more efficiently the circuit will be purged of the previously expired gases, making it less likely that rebreathing will occur during the following inspiration.

The technique is the same as described for the Bain system.

To-and-fro and circle (vaporizer out-of-circle) circuits: These circuits are generally suitable for individuals weighing above approximately 10–15 kg, during spontaneous respiration. The problems of circuit resistance may be of less importance during controlled ventilation. A disadvantage of the 'to-and-fro' circuit during controlled ventilation is the closeness of the soda lime canister to the patient's endotracheal tube. Artificial ventilation by squeezing the rebreathing bag is likely to flush soda lime dust into the patient's respiratory tract. Cotton wool filters may be inserted in the patient end of the canister to prevent this. This disadvantage of the proximity of the soda lime canister to the patient is avoided in the circle breathing system by the canister being separated from the patient by corrugated hoses.

1. The adjustable pressure-limiting valve is partially closed so that sufficient pressure can develop in the system to inflate the lungs
2. Inspiration is produced by squeezing the reservoir bag with one or both hands
3. Squeeze and release with an inspiratory/expiratory ratio of 1:3, achieving normal chest movements at a normal rate for the animal's size.

Positive end expiratory pressure and continuous positive airway pressure

Positive end expiratory pressure (PEEP) and continuous positive airway pressure (CPAP) are two techniques that can be used to prevent and manage the condition of alveolar collapse or atelectasis. Atelectasis is commonly associated with parenchymal lung disease, pulmonary trauma, hypoventilation, abnormal posture and high concentrations of inspired oxygen. Atelectasis results in increased intrapulmonary blood flow shunting and therefore hypoxia.

PEEP applies a resistance to expiration so that airway pressure is maintained slightly positive during the expiratory phase. Simple PEEP valves, which are applied to the expiratory limb of the breathing system, can be obtained commercially. PEEP is applied during IPPV. CPAP uses the same valve applied to the breathing system, but the patient is allowed to breathe spontaneously.

When using either technique, the minimum increase in airway pressure which produces a PaO_2 within normal limits should be used since both techniques will compromise circulatory function.

Humidification

Humidity is the term used to describe the amount of water vapour present in air or oxygen. The amount of water that a gas can carry depends upon its temperature. Inspired air is normally heated and humidified by the nasopharynx and turbinates so that alveolar air is 100% humidified at body temperature. This system is bypassed by endotracheal intubation and many of the supplemental oxygenation techniques. Consequences of under-humidification include:

* Energy use by the patient to saturate and heat inspired gases. This may result in a marked drop in body temperature especially in smaller individuals
* A net water loss from the patient in exhaled saturated gas
* Drying of the lower respiratory tract mucosa resulting in inflammation, excess mucus production and decreased or absent mucociliary clearance.
* Lung compliance will fall.

The four most commonly used types of humidifiers are:

* An ambient temperature water vapour supplier (in simple terms, a water reservoir through which a gas is bubbled)
* Heated water vapour supplier
* Heat and moisture exchanger
* Nebulizer (devices which produce droplets of water rather than water vapour).

Ambient temperature water vapour suppliers or bubble humidifiers function by simply bubbling the inspired gases through a container of water. The water vapour content achieved using this method is only marginally higher than that of room air.

Heated water vapour suppliers can produce inspired gases at low flows that are 100% humidified at body temperature. They are usually incorporated into the inspiratory limb of a breathing system and have temperature sensors to ensure that the inspired gas temperature cannot inflict a thermal injury to the patient's airways.

Heat and moisture exchange units (HMEs) are disposable devices that are attached directly to the endotracheal or tracheostomy tube. The purpose of the HME is to conserve the patient's own heat and moisture without an external energy or water supply. Presently, the majority of systems trap warm expired water on a hygroscopic surface. The dry cold inspired gases pass through this surface and are both warmed and humidified. This system increases airway resistance and respiratory dead space. Both these factors are not clinically significant in the majority of dogs, but may cause further breathing difficulties in small dogs and cats suffering from respiratory compromise.

Nebulizers may be used to administer a fine mist of water droplets into the inspiratory limb of the breathing apparatus. They are very efficient and can achieve an inspired humidity close to 100% without the need to heat the inspired gases. In fact, they are so efficient that patient over-hydration and airway flooding may occur with inappropriate use.

Techniques for drainage of the pleural cavity

The technique of needle thoracocentesis can be used for both diagnostic and therapeutic purposes. The technique is generally without complication and is quick and easy to perform. It should, therefore, be considered a primary investigative technique whenever pleural disease is suspected.

Longer term management of pleural effusive diseases and pneumothoraces requires the placement of a thoracic drain. This allows complete drainage of the pleural cavities on separate occasions and the instillation of pleural lavage solutions if required.

When managing a pneumothorax, it is very important to remember that a simple pneumothorax may be converted to a tension pneumothorax by positive pressure ventilation, particularly if PEEP is applied.

Needle thoracocentesis

1. Insert a 14–16 gauge intravenous cannula or an 18–21 gauge needle through the 7th or 8th intercostal space at the lateral point of the thorax. The insertion point is high on the chest wall if air is anticipated and more ventral if fluid is expected
2. Local anaesthetic infiltration of the skin can be performed if necessary, but this is rarely required
3. Remove the needle from inside the cannula and aspirate air or fluid with a syringe attached to a three-way tap, until negative pressure is reached
4. If the end-point of negative pressure is not reached, or if air re-accumulates quickly, a thoracostomy tube should be placed.

Chest drain placement — using a drain with a trocar

Support ventilation during the procedure as required.

1. Place the animal in lateral recumbency with the side for drain placement uppermost
2. Widely clip and aseptically prepare the central and caudal aspects of the lateral chest wall
3. Infiltrate local anaesthetic as an intercostal nerve block in the intercostal space through which the tube will be passed (7th or 8th interspace) and, in addition, in one intercostal space both cranial and caudal to the above.
   or
   Infiltrate local anaesthetic locally at the site of the intercostal space where the tube is to pass into the thoracic cavity (Figure 22.13)
4. Infiltrate the skin with local anaesthetic two or three intercostal spaces caudal to the intercostal block (10th interspace) at the site of skin entrance of the tube
5. Wait several minutes for the local anaesthetic to take effect
6. Make a skin incision with a blade at the site of the skin anaesthetic block

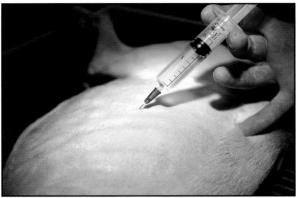

Figure 22.13: Infiltration of local anaesthetic prior to the placement of a thoracic drain.

7. Place the thoracostomy tube with the trocar in place through the skin incision and direct in a cranial direction (Figure 22.14)
8. Advance the tip of the trocar to the intercostal space where the tube is to enter the chest and lift the drain into a vertical position
9. The thumb and forefinger of one hand should grasp the drain firmly 1–2 cm from its tip to prevent the drain penetrating too deeply into the thoracic cavity (Figure 22.15)

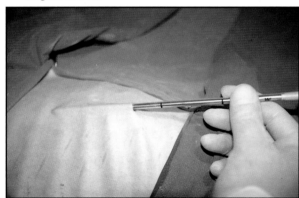

Figure 22.14: The trocar thoracostomy tube has been placed through a skin incision (10th interspace) and is being directed subcutaneously in a cranial canal.

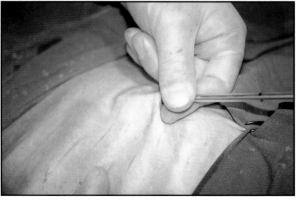

Figure 22.15: The thumb and forefinger of one hand grasp the drain firmly 1–2 cm from its tip to prevent iatrogenic damage to intrathoracic structures during drain placement.

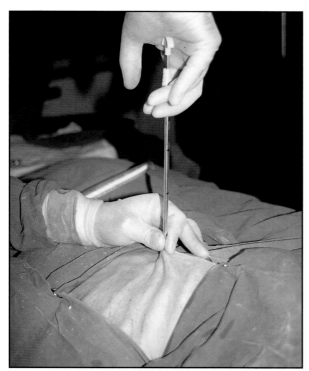

Figure 22.16: Entrance to the pleural cavity is achieved with a firm but controlled push to the trocar handle.

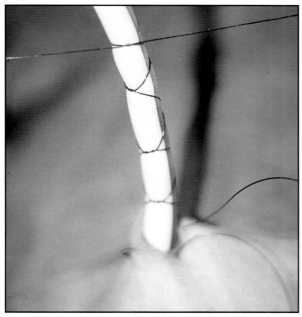

Figure 22.17: The drain should be securely fixed in place. In this case, a 'Chinese finger trap' suture is being placed to anchor the drain. A mattress suture has also been pre-placed around the drain skin wound. This will be used as a skin suture when the drain is removed.

10. A firm push with the palm of the other hand on the trocar will advance the drain through the intercostal space and enter into the pleural cavity (Figure 22.16)
11. Once the trocar is removed the pleural cavity should be evacuated using syringe suction on the thoracostomy tube
12. Secure the tube firmly to the skin with sutures

(ideally 'Chinese finger trap') (Figure 22.17)
13. The tube should be attached either to an underwater seal or should be closed in two places (usually a gate clamp and a spigot).

Chest drain placement — using a drain without a trocar
The procedure is similar to that for the trocar technique up to incision of the skin (steps 1–6, above). If the animal is anaesthetized, support ventilation during the procedure as required.

7. Probe incision with blunt forceps or scissors in a cranial direction to the level of the intercostal space where the drain will enter the thoracic cavity
8. A path can be created with the forceps or scissors into the pleural cavity
9. The thoracostomy tube should be clamped (gate clamp or spigot) prior to its placement
10. Grasp the thoracostomy tube with long curved forceps (e.g. Lahey forceps) and use the forceps to pass the tube cranially through the skin incision (Figure 22.18)
11. Pass the forceps and drain through the intercostal penetration so that they enter the pleural cavity (Figure 22.19)

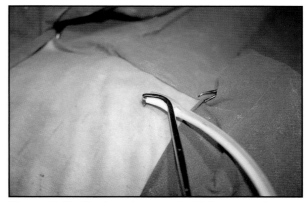

Figure 22.18: The drain is grasped with long curved forceps so that the tips of the forceps protrude beyond the end of the drain. This prevents damaging the drain during the insertion procedure.

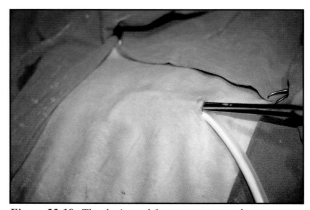

Figure 22.19: The drain and forceps are passed subcutaneously in a cranial direction prior to intercostal penetration.

12. Hold the tube at the skin incision while the forceps are removed, to prevent it leaving the pleural cavity
13. Advance the tube so that all fenestrations are within the pleural cavity
14. Evacuate the pleural cavity using syringe suction on the thoracostomy tube
15. Secure and maintain the tube as described above.

Translaryngeal and transtracheal wash

1. Allow the conscious animal to sit or lie in sternal recumbency (sedation may be required)
2. The unconscious animal should be positioned in sternal recumbency
3. The neck should be extended and the ventral midline clipped and aseptically prepared
4. The site of proposed incision (cranial-mid third of the ventral neck including the larynx for translaryngeal approach or mid-caudal third of ventral neck for transtracheal approach) should be anaesthetized in the conscious individual using a skin bleb of local anaesthetic agent
5. The neck is extended and dorsiflexed.

Transtracheal approach for large dogs

1. The needle of a through-the-needle catheter (12–18 gauge) is advanced through the midline towards the trachea, which is immobilized with the other hand
2. The trachea is penetrated between tracheal rings at the junction of the middle third and distal third of the cervical trachea (if there is doubt of tracheal lumen placement, the needle should be aspirated; resistance suggests improper placement, whereas easy aspiration of air suggests the bevel is within the tracheal lumen) (Figure 22.20)
3. The catheter is advanced through the needle as far into the airway as possible
4. The needle is removed leaving the catheter in place
5. The sampling solution (the preferred solution is warmed sterile normal saline) is instilled and then aspirated; 2–5 ml aliquots in cats and between 2 and 15 ml per aliquot in dogs; up to three aliquots used in total)
6. Between 5% and 20% of the instilled solution can be retrieved
7. Solution instillation will commonly induce coughing, which may assist retrieval of material
8. Sampled material is pooled and aliquots are made for cytological and microbial analysis
9. After withdrawal of the catheter and needle, digital pressure may be applied to the site for approximately 2 minutes.

Translaryngeal approach for smaller dogs

• The procedure is similar to the transtracheal approach; in this case the catheter is passed through the skin at the level of the larynx
• The larynx is stabilized with the other hand and the needle is advanced through the cricothyroid ligament in the ventral midline (see Figure 22.20)
• The remainder of the procedure is as described previously for the transtracheal approach.

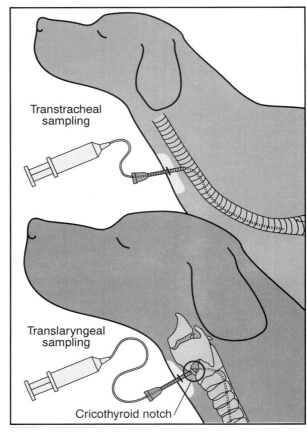

Figure 22.20: *Anatomical drawings illustrating the methods for translaryngeal (cricothyroid ligament) and transtracheal wash.*

Reproduced from the BSAVA Manual of Small Animal Cardiorespiratory Medicine and Surgery, with the permission of Vicki Martin Design.

CARDIOVASCULAR SYSTEM TECHNIQUES

Intravenous catheter placement

1. An area of hair over a peripheral vein (generally a cephalic or lateral saphenous vein) is clipped
2. The site is prepared by scrubbing with a dilute solution of chlorhexidine solution, followed by wiping with 70% isopropyl alcohol
3. The vein is raised by an assistant
4. The skin is held taut to stabilize the underlying vein and an over-the-needle catheter (20–22 gauge in cats and small dogs, 16–20 gauge in dogs) is advanced through the skin and, generally, directly into the vein
5. Nicking the skin with a no.11 scalpel blade may be required to allow the catheter to pass through the

cutis without damage, but with practice this is generally not required

6. Once the vein is penetrated, blood will commonly appear in the hub of the catheter. The stylet should now be immobilized while the outer catheter is advanced into the vein lumen

7. The assistant now occludes the vein lumen at the level of the catheter's tip while the stylet is removed

8. The catheter is now capped with either an injection cap or, if intravenous fluids are to be administered, a T-connector (Avon). Both capping devices should be pre-flushed with sterile heparinized saline

9. The catheter and capping system are then flushed with a small volume of sterile heparinized saline to ensure correct placement and maintain patency

10. The catheter and capping system are secured in place using adhesive tapes

11. Ideally, a transparent adhesive dressing should be placed over the skin entry site to maintain asepsis

12. If access to the catheter is not required immediately, the catheter and capping system should be covered with a light bandage to keep the site clean and to prevent patient interference.

When not in use, the catheter should be flushed with heparinized saline (1 IU heparin/ml) every 4–6 hours. The catheter should ideally be removed after 3 days and an alternative site should be utilized. In critical patients, however, when vascular access is limited or challenging, intravenous catheters can be maintained for longer than 3 days as long as the vascular access site appears healthy. All materials and procedures associated with the catheter placement and maintenance should be aseptically managed.

Surgical cutdown for peripheral venous catheter placement

In certain circumstances, for example, for deep vessel catheterization or in states of cardiovascular collapse, conventional catheterization techniques are ineffective. Very occasionally, direct percutaneous peripheral or central venepuncture may prove impossible because of unavailable sites or lack of appropriate operator skill. In such cases venous access can be secured using a surgical cutdown method. The external jugular, the lateral saphenous or the cephalic veins are most commonly used.

Technique

1. If possible, identify the vein by circumferential compression of the limb or neck proximal to the site

2. Prepare the skin with clipping and an antiseptic solution as previously described

3. Drape the site

4. Make a longitudinal incision in the skin over the vein

5. Probe the incision with blunt forceps to identify the vein and free it from the subcutaneous tissues

6. Pass a suture beneath the vein using forceps

7. Divide the suture to form loops proximally and distally around the proposed venepuncture site

8. Maintaining tension over the distal loop, make a 2 mm incision in the vein

9. Probe this incision with the tip of fine-artery forceps to confirm access inside the vein lumen

10. Insert the venous cannula

11. Tie the proximal loop over the cannula

12. Attach the primed giving set and confirm free flow

13. Remove the distal suture loop

14. Suture the skin incision

15. Secure the cannula hub and giving set with an adhesive dressing or tape.

Seldinger technique for introducing catheters

Percutaneous vascular catheterization, as described by Seldinger (1953), has been used successfully for many years. The technique allows entry into an area without a cutdown and, because small gauge needles are used, there is minimal trauma to surrounding tissue. The technique is applicable for the introduction of catheters into numerous sites, although the following information describes the introduction of a catheter into a peripheral vein. The technique can also be applied to a wide range of catheter types, including multi-lumen catheters.

1. The proposed insertion site is prepared in a similar manner to that described for conventional intravenous catheterization (Figure 22.21a)

2. Make a small stab incision with a no. 11 scalpel blade into the skin over the vessel at the proposed catheterization site

3. Introduce a percutaneous entry needle into the vessel (Figure 22.21b)

4. Pass a wire guide through the needle; advance a portion of the wire guide length into the vessel (Figure 22.21c)

5. Leaving the wire guide in place, withdraw the needle (Figure 22.21d)

6. Enlarge the puncture hole into the vessel wall by passing a dilator down the guide wire and into the vessel lumen (optional in some instances), and then removing the dilator, leaving the wire in place (Figure 22.21e)

7. With a twisting motion, advance the catheter over the wire guide and into the vessel (Figure 22.21f)

8. After the catheter is in position, remove the wire guide (Figure 22.21g)

9. The catheter can now be flushed, capped, sutured to the skin and dressed in a standard fashion.

Sheath needle technique for introducing catheters

A catheterization system is now available which involves the use of a Peel-away® (Cook®) sheathed needle. One advantage of this system is that different

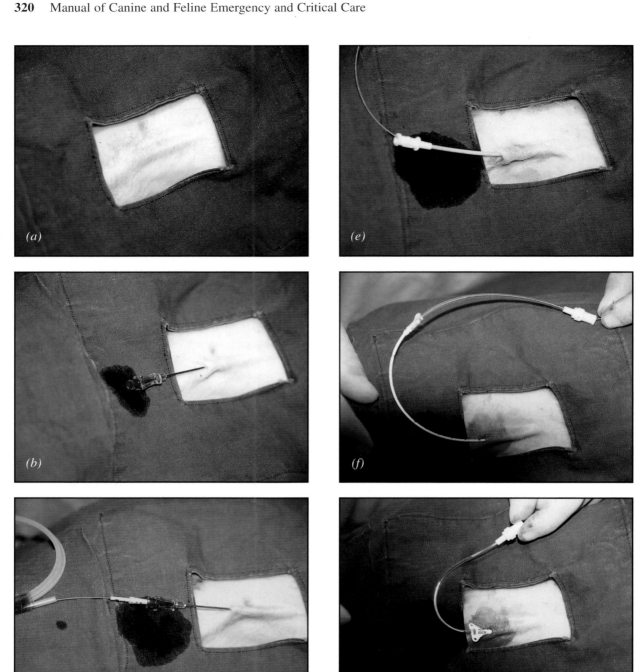

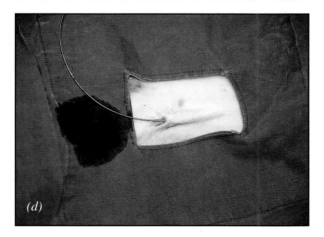

Figure 22.21: *(a) The proposed insertion site (in this case, the left external jugular vein) is surgically prepared and draped. (b) A percutaneous entry needle is introduced into the vein (in this case, in a caudal direction). (c) A guide wire is passed through the needle and into the lumen of the vein. (d) The needle is removed, whilst the guide wire remains in place. (e) A dilator is passed over the guide wire and into the vessel wall to enlarge the puncture. (f) The catheter is advanced overthe needle and into the lumen of the vessel. (g) Once the catheter is in position, the guide wire can be removed.*

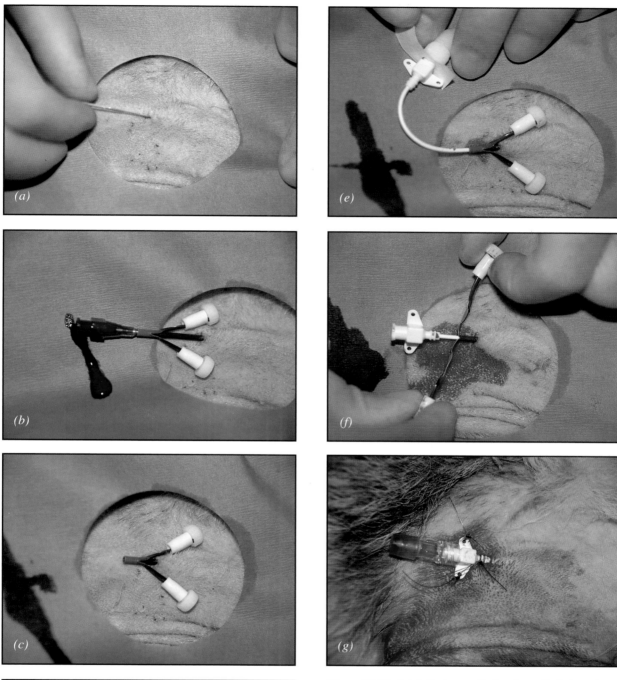

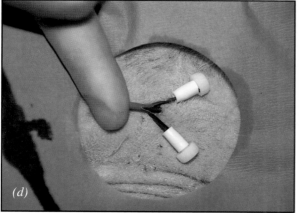

Figure 22.22: *(a) A Peel-away® sheath needle is introduced into the vein (in this case, in a caudal direction into the left external jugular vein). (b) Entrance into the vein lumen is confirmed by bleeding from the needle hub following manual distal occlusion of the vein. (c) Once the sheath has been advanced into the lumen of the vein, the needle is removed. (d) Air embolization is a potential risk at this point in the catheterization procedure. This can be minimized by occluding the cuffed proximal end of the sheath with a gloved finger. (e) The catheter is passed through the sheath's lumen and advanced to lie within the vein. (f) The sheath is peeled apart by grasping the two knobs and pulling outward and upward at the same time. (g) Once finally placed, the catheter should be flushed, capped and sutured in place.*

sizes of the sheath needle and the catheters can be purchased separately. Therefore, the user can choose a combination of sheath needle and catheter which best suits the individual being catheterized. A disadvantage of the system is that blood spillage and/or air embolization are possible during the placement procedure.

1. The proposed insertion site is prepared in a similar manner to that described for conventional intravenous catheterization
2. The sheathed needle is inserted into a vessel in a similar fashion to an over-the-needle catheter (it may be necessary to make a small stab incision with a no. 11 scalpel blade into the skin over the vessel at the proposed catheterization site) (Figure 22.22a,b)
3. Once within the vessel lumen the needle is removed (Figure 22.22c) and the actual catheter to be introduced is passed through the sheath's lumen
4. To minimize the potential risk of inadvertent air embolization, a sterile gloved thumb or finger can be placed over the cuffed proximal end of the sheath after removal of the needle (Figure 22.22d)
5. The catheter is advanced into position (Figure 22.22e)
6. By grasping the two knobs of the sheath and pulling outward and upward at the same time, the sheath can be peeled away from the catheter (Figure 22.22f)
7. The catheter can now be flushed, capped, sutured to the skin and dressed in a standard fashion (Figure 22.22g).

Intraosseous infusion techniques

Bone marrow access sites in the dog and cat include:

- The trochanteric fossa of the proximal femur
- The flat medial aspect of the proximal tibia at a site that is distal to the tibial tuberosity and the proximal tibial growth plate
- The cranial aspect of the mid-diaphyseal ulna
- The cranial aspect of the greater tubercle of the humerus.

In general, the first two of these are preferred for intraosseous fluid therapy. Various infusion needles or catheters can be used for intraosseous injection. In the very young animal, the cortical bone may be soft enough to allow the use of an intravenous over-the-needle catheter or needle. Most commonly, either a spinal needle or a commercially available intraosseous needle (Figure 22.23) is used.

1. At one of the above chosen sites, the skin is clipped and prepared aseptically
2. A bleb of local anaesthetic agent is injected into the skin and the periosteum
3. An assistant should stabilize the limb while a small stab incision with a no. 11 scalpel blade is

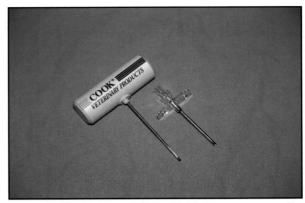

Figure 22.23: *A commercially available intraosseous needle.*

made in the skin
4. The needle is inserted, pointing in a distal direction, and it is rotated with firm pressure until it enters the near cortex (if properly seated, it will feel firm and stable)
5. The stylet is removed and the needle should be aspirated and flushed with sterile heparinized saline
6. Once an infusion set or T-connector has been attached, the needle hub should be securely fixed in place and bandaged
7. It is suggested that flow rates under gravity should not exceed 11 ml/min
8. When using pressurized infusion systems (up to 300 mm Hg), the flow rate should not exceed 24 ml/min.

The intraosseous system can be managed in a similar manner to an intravenous catheter. When not in use, the needle should be flushed every 6 hours with heparinized saline. A new needle should be placed into a different bone every 72 hours. The same bone can be reused at another location once the original site has occluded and healed. This will occur after approximately 36 hours.

Complications include:

- Infection
- Fat embolization
- Damage to the growth plates
- Leakage of administered fluids into the surrounding tissues following poor needle placement technique.

Intra-arterial catheter placement

Cannulation can usually be achieved percutaneously and the commonest site for cannulation in the dog is the dorsal metatarsal artery on the mediodorsal aspect of the hind foot. In some instances, the femoral artery may be preferred, but, with practice, the dorsal metatarsal artery can be readily cannulated in both the dog and the cat. Strict asepsis should be maintained during the procedure of arterial cannulation.

1. The proposed cannulation site should be clipped of

hair and the skin surgically cleaned

2. With the animal in lateral recumbency, the dorsal metatarsal artery on the lower limb will be most amenable to cannulation

3. If the limb is held, care must be taken not to occlude the arterial supply to the foot, otherwise, palpation of a pulse in the dorsal metatarsal artery will prove difficult

4. It is generally unnecessary to nick the skin with a blade prior to introduction of the catheter

5. A 3 cm 20–22 gauge over-the-needle type of catheter is adequate for catheterization in small animals

6. The position and course of the artery should be assessed by gentle palpation of the site whilst maintaining an aseptic technique (Figure 22.24a)

7. The skin is penetrated with a firm but controlled stab and the needle is advanced until the arterial wall is penetrated and arterial blood appears in the hub of the catheter (ideally, this penetration should occur in line with the course of the artery thus ensuring that when the catheter is advanced it remains within the lumen of the artery) (Figure 22.24b)

8. The catheter is fully advanced off the needle, into the arterial lumen, and the needle is then removed (loss of blood at this time can be prevented by occlusion of the artery proximal to the catheterization site) (Figure 22.24c)

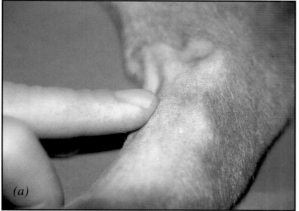

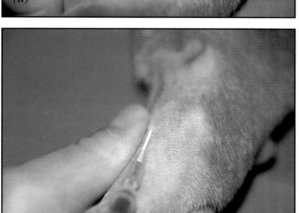

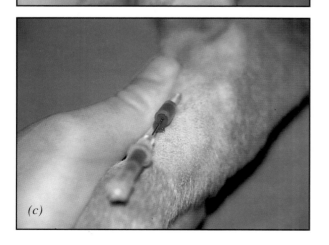

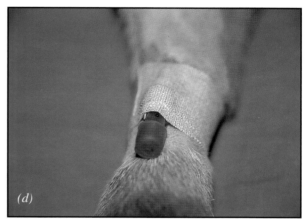

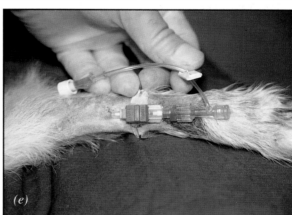

Figure 22.24: *(a) The position of the dorsal metatarsal artery can be palpated as it courses over the mediodorsal aspect of the foot. (b) The catheter is advanced into the artery in a similar manner to that employed for percutaneous venepuncture. (c) Once the catheter and needle have been advanced a short distance into the arterial lumen, the needle can be removed whilst advancing the catheter fully into the artery. (d) The catheter can be taped in place and capped with a heparinized saline-filled injection cap. (e) Alternatively, commercially available arterial catheters can be sutured in place. In this case, the catheter has been capped with a heparinized saline-filled T-connector.*

9. A heparinized saline-filled injection cap or T-connector (Avon) can be attached to the catheter, and the hub of the catheter can be taped to the skin in a manner which does not kink the catheter at the skin-air interface (Figure 22.24d,e)
10. The whole system should now be flushed with heparinized saline.

A similar technique can be applied to the catheterization of the femoral artery. In this instance, the medial aspect of the thigh should be aseptically prepared. A small stab incision in the skin with a No.11 scalpel blade at the proposed catheterization site may be required. The femoral artery is more mobile than the dorsal metatarsal artery and the operator's other hand should be used to stabilize the structure prior to penetration. Unlike the dorsal metatarsal artery catheterization technique, it is often easy to penetrate the skin and subcutaneous tissues as a separate procedure to the penetration of the femoral arterial wall. The Seldinger technique also may be applied to the catheterization of a peripheral artery (see previously).

Complications of arterial catheterization are rare in small animals, but theoretically, at least, include local ischaemia, thrombosis, infection and bleeding. With proper sterile technique, the risk of infection from cannulation of an artery is minimal. If the artery is punctured without proper catheter penetration during the process of cannulation it is common for a haematoma to form which will prevent further attempts at cannulation at that site. The artery will also locally constrict on direct physical stimulation, which also makes further attempts at cannulation very difficult.

On withdrawal of the catheter from either the dorsal metatarsal artery or the femoral artery, digital pressure should be applied to the cannulation site for at least 5 minutes so that the likelihood of haematoma formation is minimized. The dorsal metatarsal artery site is often best managed by placing a tape bandage at the site of catheterization.

Surgical cutdown for arterial catheter placement

In certain circumstances, an artery may need to be approached via a surgical cutdown procedure. A standard approach will be described and this can be applied to the majority of arteries.

1. The skin over the proposed arterial site is prepared with clipping and an antiseptic solution as previously described
2. Drape the site
3. Make a longitudinal incision in the skin over the artery
4. Use a combination of sharp and blunt dissection to approach the artery (it should be clearly identified from any veins or nerves) and free it from the surrounding tissues

5. Pass a ligature beneath the artery using forceps
6. Divide the ligature to form proximal and distal loops around the proposed incision site
7. Maintaining tension over the distal loop, make a 2 mm incision in the artery
8. Probe this incision with the tip of fine-artery forceps to confirm access inside the arterial lumen
9. Insert the venous cannula
10. Tie the proximal loop over the cannula
11. Attach the primed giving set and confirm free flow
12. Remove the distal suture loop
13. Suture the skin incision
14. Secure the cannula hub and giving set with an adhesive dressing or tape.

Central venous pressure

Classically, central venous pressure (CVP) measures the pressure of the blood in the right atrium, although the term CVP may equally be applied to the luminal pressure of the vena cava. It is affected by one or all of the following:

* Circulating blood volume
* Venous tone
* Right ventricular function
* Intrathoracic pressure.

The placement of a CVP catheter is indicated in any individual in which the right ventricular preload requires monitoring. The measurement of CVP will allow an estimation of the animal's intravascular fluid status and fluid requirements and will allow the effects of fluid replacement to be monitored accurately. The placement of a CVP catheter will also provide a central line for the administration of fluids and emergency drugs.

Access to the central veins and the right atrium is achieved via the external jugular vein in the small animal species. There are a variety of catheters available for the purpose and they can broadly be placed into one of four categories; over-the-needle, through-the-needle (Figure 22.25), peel-away sheath (see Figure 22.22) or over-the-wire (Seldinger technique) (see Figure 22.21).

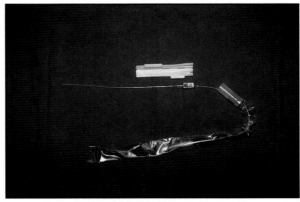

Figure 22.25: *An example of a through-the-needle central venous catheter. The white needle guard is shown next to the needle.*

1. The neck is closely clipped and aseptically prepared
2. If a very large bore catheter is to be placed, the skin directly over the jugular vein can be locally anaesthetized by placing a bleb of local anaesthetic prior to aseptic skin preparation (this will allow a small nick to be made in the skin prior to placement of the catheter, so that it will freely pass without damage or fraying to the tip over the catheter).

Placement of over-the-needle catheters in the jugular vein

1. While the vein is occluded distal to the cannulation site, the stylet or needle penetrates the vessel in a distal (caudal) direction and is advanced a small distance to ensure that the catheter tip enters the vessel lumen
2. The catheter is then advanced over the needle into the vessel lumen until the catheter hub reaches the skin
3. The stylet is held stationary in its original position inside the vessel until the catheter is fully threaded into the vessel; premature withdrawal of the stylet may cause the catheter to bend or kink and prevent complete insertion of the catheter into the vessel
4. Once the catheter is successfully threaded into the vessel, the stylet is removed and the catheter can be capped, flushed with sterile heparinized saline and secured in place.

A disadvantage of over-the-needle catheters is that although they are available in large diameters, the catheter length is often limited so that the tip of the catheter does not reach the right atrium. As long as the tip lies within the intrathoracic cranial vena cava, it can be classed as a central line and pressure measurements will compare very closely to those found within the right atrium.

Placement of through-the-needle catheters

1. Placement is achieved by penetration of the vein with the needle in a distal direction
2. Once blood is seen to flow back into the hub, the needle should be advanced a short way into the lumen of the vein to ensure proper placement
3. The catheter can now be advanced through the needle until its hub reaches the hub of the needle (Figure 22.26)
4. The needle can subsequently be removed from the vein lumen and the skin
5. Obviously, the needle cannot be completely removed from the cannulation without also removing the catheter. Therefore, it is supplied with a protective cover, which prevents it from cutting into the catheter passing through it
6. The needle and its protective guard can be sutured to the adjacent skin to secure the unit in place

7. The catheter is capped and flushed with heparinized saline.

The advantage of through-the-needle catheters is that the catheter can be of any length and is made of softer, more flexible material than that of an over-the-needle catheter. A major disadvantage of through-the-needle catheters is that their diameter is limited by the size of the needle through which they pass. The problem of catheter diameter size can be overcome by using the over-the-wire system.

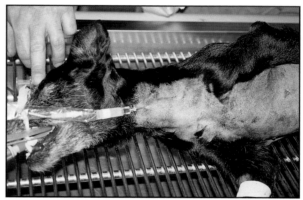

Figure 22.26: *Placement of a through-the-needle central venous catheter. The catheter is advanced through the needle until its hub reaches the hub of the needle.*

Placement of catheters in the jugular vein using a peel-away sheath needle
This technique is described above for intravenous catheter placement.

Placement of catheters in the jugular vein over a guide wire
This technique is described above as the Seldinger placement technique. There are many human and veterinary commercially available central venous catheter systems. Many of the human systems can be readily used in the dog and cat. These systems are often available as single, double or triple lumen systems. The presence of more than one lumen will allow the infusion of intravenous fluids at the same time as the continuous measurement of the CVP.

In cats and very small dogs, venous access is often best achieved via the external jugular vein, especially if intravenous fluids are to be administered. This is because patency of cephalic and saphenous vein cannulation is often very dependent on the position of the individual's limbs; flexion will often lead to occlusion. This problem does not commonly occur following jugular cannulation. Jugular cannulation in the cat is best achieved once sedation or anaesthesia has been induced. Therefore, if anaesthesia is to be induced with an intravenous agent, a cephalic vein will be cannulated first to give venous access for these anaesthetic agents.

Pulmonary artery pressure and pulmonary capillary wedge pressure

If a central venous catheter is advanced further than the right atrium, it will pass through the right ventricle and will come to lie in the pulmonary artery (PA). At this site the catheter can be used to measure the PA pressure. Simple advancement of a straight catheter will rarely achieve placement in the pulmonary artery; the catheter will either continue to lie in the central vein and end up either in the azygos vein or caudal vena cava, or it will enter the right ventricle only to become snagged against the ventricle wall. In an attempt to aid placement in the pulmonary artery, specific PA catheters are manufactured with a small balloon at their tip, which can be inflated with air or carbon dioxide (Figure 22.27). These catheters are named after Swan and Ganz, who introduced the flow-directed balloon catheter in human medicine in 1970. The air-filled balloon will be taken by the flow of blood so that it tends to enter the right ventricle. During right ventricular systole, the flow of blood will again tend to force the catheter tip to enter the pulmonary artery.

The PA pressure reflects right ventricular function, pulmonary vascular resistance and left atrial filling pressure. The PA pressure is normally 20–40 mm Hg systolic, 5–10 mm Hg diastolic and 10–20 mm Hg mean.

If the balloon remains inflated and the pulmonary artery catheter is advanced further, the balloon will 'wedge' in a distal pulmonary artery. This will produce a valveless hydrostatic column of blood between the distal port of the wedged pulmonary catheter and the left atrium. The pressure of this column of blood is the pulmonary capillary wedge pressure (PCWP). The PCWP is used as a measure of the left atrial filling pressure. Once the procedure of jugular vein catheterization is mastered, the technique of PA pressure and PCWP measurement is relatively easy to perform. In general, 5–7 French catheters are adequate. The Swan–Ganz catheters are supplied with various sampling ports along their length, so that once they are in place blood sample and pressure measurements can be taken from the right atrium, right ventricle and pulmonary artery as well as PCWP measurements without further moving the catheter. When the PCWP is not being measured the balloon is deflated so that there is no interference with pulmonary blood flow. The PCWP is normally 3–8 mm Hg.

Pericardiocentesis

Pericardiocentesis can be used as both a diagnostic and therapeutic procedure for cases of pericardial effusion. It involves the introduction of a needle or catheter into the pericardial sac. Sedation may be required for the procedure to be carried out safely, but in the majority of cases this is not necessary.

1. An area is clipped on the right side from the sternum to the costochondral junction, which encompasses the 3rd to the 7th intercostal spaces (pericardiocentesis is usually performed just below the costochondral junction at the 4th, 5th or 6th intercostal space) (Figure 22.28)
2. The area is scrubbed and aseptically prepared
3. The ECG is continuously monitored so that any dysrhythmias produced as a result of epicardial interference can be detected
4. The procedure may be performed with the animal standing or maintained in left lateral recumbency
5. The procedure should be undertaken in an aseptic manner

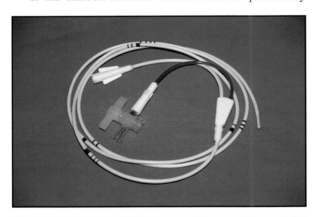

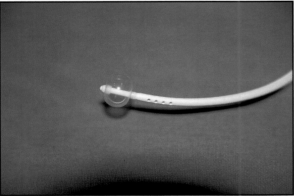

Figure 22.27: *(a) An example of a Swan–Ganz catheter. The red port allows insufflation of the catheter's balloon.*
(b) Pulmonary artery placement is achieved by air or carbon dioxide inflation of the small balloon at the tip of the catheter.

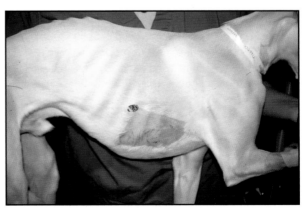

Figure 22.28: *An area is clipped on the right hand side from the sternum to the costochondral junction, which encompasses the 3rd to the 7th intercostal spaces.*

6. Local anaesthetic is infiltrated into the intercostal muscles at the proposed puncture site
7. A large bore (14–18 gauge), long (5–15 cm) over-the-needle catheter is inserted through a stab incision in the skin
8. A syringe is attached to the needle and catheter/needle are advanced through the thoracic wall towards the heart
9. A slight negative pressure is placed on the syringe so that once the pericardial sac is entered pericardial fluid will be aspirated
10. The catheter can then be advanced over the needle into the pericardial sac (if the catheter or needle touch the epicardium, changes such as ventricular premature complexes will be seen on the ECG and the movement of the heart will be felt through the syringe)
11. Once the catheter is correctly placed in the pericardial sac, the needle can be completely removed and a three-way tap and extension set attached (Figure 22.29)
12. As much pericardial fluid as possible is removed (samples of the fluid should be collected for laboratory analysis including cytology, culture and sensitivity).

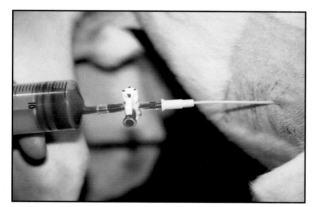

Figure 22.29: *Once the catheter is well placed within the pericardial sac, the needle can be removed and a three-way tap and syringe attached.*

Pericardiocentesis catheter systems are commercially available which are specifically designed for pericardiocentesis in small animals. In general, these systems are placed with the aid of a guide wire using the Seldinger technique.

GASTROINTESTINAL TECHNIQUES

Pharyngostomy

The technique of pharyngostomy tube enteral feeding became popular when the technique was described by Böhning and others (1970). Problems with airway obstruction and aspiration were commonly encountered and a more caudal placement site was advocated by Rawlings (1979).

1. The animal is anaesthetized, or local anaesthetic agents may be used in the severely debilitated individual
2. The animal is placed in lateral recumbency and an area extending from caudal to the angle of the mandible to the thyroid cartilage is clipped and prepared aseptically (either the right or left pharynx can be used)
3. The mouth is held open with a mouth gag, and a gloved index finger is inserted into the pharynx near the base of the tongue (it should be possible to feel the epiglottis and hyoid apparatus even in the intubated individual)
4. Feel the epihyoid bone and put the finger above the epiglottis, feeling the lateral wall of the pharynx caudodorsal to the hyoid apparatus (pressure is gently applied to the lateral wall of the pouch so that a bulge is externally visible)
5. An incision is made in the skin directly over the bulge, and curved forceps (e.g. Kelly) are used to bluntly dissect towards the finger
6. Alternatively, forceps may be placed in the pharynx and firmly forced outwards through the incision to the external surface (Figure 22.30a)
7. The feeding tube is grasped with the forceps and drawn into the pharynx through the pharyngostomy incision (the length of tube required should be determined by the distance from between the canine teeth to mid-thoracic oesophagus so that when placed the tube will lie in the caudal oesophagus) (Figure 22.30b)
8. The tube is then directed down the oesophagus and fixed in place to the skin of the neck (e.g. butterfly tapes sutured to the skin) (Figure 22.30c,d)
9. The tube should be capped when not in use and the skin wound should be regularly inspected and cleaned
10. On removal, the wound is allowed to heal by second intention.

Pharyngostomy tube placement has fallen out of favour over the past few years. Reasons for this include the requirement of anaesthesia for the placement procedure and the technique's unacceptably high association with haemorrhage, infection and airway aspiration (Crowe and Downs, 1986). This technique cannot, therefore, be recommended as a procedure for the enteral feeding of a compromised individual.

The pharyngostomy incision can also be used to place an endotracheal tube when surgery on the oral cavity, mandible and/or the maxilla is undertaken.

Oesophagostomy

Oesophagostomy techniques have been investigated and developed in an attempt to produce an enteral feeding tube system without the complications associated with a pharyngostomy. Two recognized techniques are

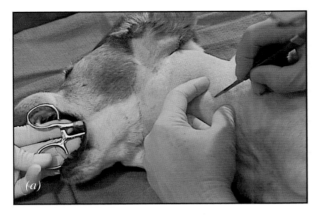
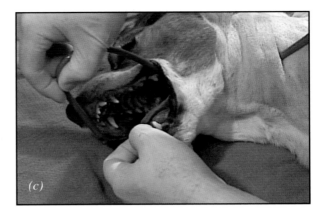
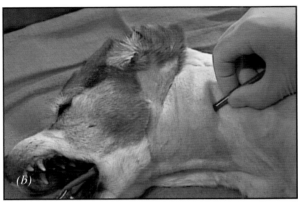
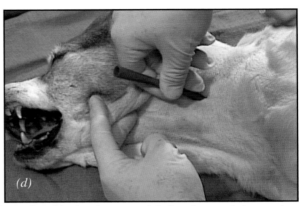

Figure 22.30: *Pharyngostomy tube placement. (a) Forceps have been placed in the pharynx and their points are being used as a guide for the position of the skin incision. (b) The forceps are forced outwards through the incision to the external surface. The feeding tube is grasped with the forceps and drawn into the pharynx through the pharyngostomy incision. (c) The tube is redirected down the oesophagus. (d) The pharyngostomy tube in its final position. It should be capped and fixed in place and the neck bandaged.*

Illustrations provided by the Iams Company.

worthy of description. Both procedures require the animal to be anaesthetized.

Percutaneous cervical oesophagostomy (Rawlings, 1993)

1. The animal is placed in right lateral recumbency and the lateral mid-cervical skin is clipped and prepared aseptically
2. A stiff large bore tube with an oblique end (endotracheal tubes are ideal) is advanced until the oblique end is in the mid-cervical oesophagus (Figure 22.31a)
3. The caudal end of the tube is pushed towards the left lateral aspect of the oesophageal wall so that it can be palpated under the skin
4. An 18 gauge over-the-needle intravenous catheter is passed through a small skin incision and into the end of the tube (Figure 22.31b)
5. The needle is removed and the tips of a pair of Carmalt forceps are placed in the end of the catheter
6. Both the forceps and the catheter are forced into the lumen of the guide tube (Figure 22.31c)
7. Once the forceps are within the guide tube, the catheter is released to slide out of the guide tube

which is lowered to help the removal process
8. A large (at least 14 French gauge) tube (tube 1) is passed down the guide tube, until the tube is felt to strike the opened tips of the Carmalt forceps
9. The forceps is closed onto the end of the tube, which is then withdrawn from the oesophagus to outside the skin (Figure 22.31d)
10. The guide tube can now be removed
11. The oesophagostomy tube (tube 2) is cut to an appropriate length for the distal end to lie in the caudal oesophagus and then its distal end is tied to the end of tube 1 (Figure 22.31e)
12. Both tubes are withdrawn back into the oesophagus by retracting tube 1 out of the mouth
13. Tube 1 is removed and a stylet is passed down the oesophagostomy tube from its proximal end at the skin incision site towards its distal end at the mouth (Figure 22.31f)
14. The tube is slowly withdrawn from the skin incision site while applying lateral pressure on the tip, forcing it toward the right side (Figure 22.31g)
15. When the tube is perpendicular to the surface of the skin, the tube is then directed in a caudal direction to lie within the oesophagus
16. The stylet can now be withdrawn and the tube

secured to the skin (Figure 22.31h)

17. The tube should capped when not in use and the skin wound should be regularly inspected and cleaned (the neck should be bandaged to keep the site clean and to prevent self-interference)

18. On removal, the wound is allowed to heal by second intention.

The tube can be placed on either side, and has only been described on the left side for clarity.

Oesophagostomy tube catheterization

An oesophagostomy tube catheterization set is available, which makes the process of mid-cervical oesophagostomy very straightforward (Figure 22.32). Two oesophagostomy tube sizes are available: either a 12 French or a 14 French.

1. The animal is placed in lateral recumbency and the lateral mid-cervical skin is clipped and prepared aseptically

2. The introduction tube is inserted via the mouth into the mid-cervical oesophagus (Figure 22.32a)

3. The bulb of the introduction tube is angled laterally to tent the skin

4. The opening of the bulb can be palpated with a gloved finger, and a small nick in the skin over the bulb is made using a no. 11 blade

5. The needle and sheath of a peel-away sheath needle is inserted through the skin nick

6. It is advanced through the wall of the oesophagus and into the opening of the introduction tube bulb

7. The assembly is carefully advanced in a cranial direction into the oesophageal lumen

8. The needle is removed and the sheath firmly grasped and immobilized while the introduction

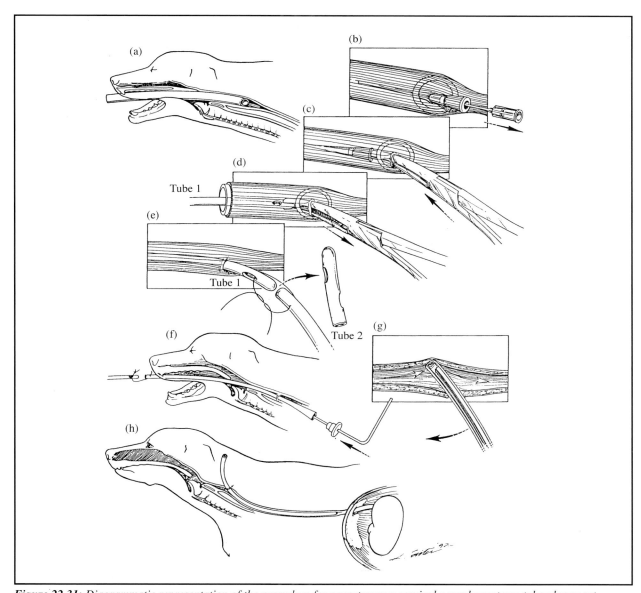

Figure 22.31: *Diagrammatic representation of the procedure for percutaneous cervical oesophagostomy tube placement.*

Reproduced from Rawlings (1993) with the permission of the Journal of the American Animal Hospital Association.

tube is removed from the mouth (Figure 22.32b)

9. The sheath is now carefully redirected caudally by flipping it 180° in that direction (lateral pressure should be applied to ensure that the sheath remains within the oesophageal lumen)
10. The sheath can now be advanced easily into the distal cervical oesophagus
11. The feeding tube is inserted into the oesophagus through the sheath (Figure 22.32c)
12. Once the feeding tube is in place, the sheath can be peeled away by pulling on the tags (Figure 22.32d)
13. The tube is secured to the skin and capped when not in use
14. The skin wound should be regularly inspected and cleaned (the neck should be bandaged to keep the site clean and to prevent self-interference)
15. On removal, the wound is allowed to heal by second intention.

Naso-oesophageal and nasogastric catheterization

Naso-oesophageal and nasogastric catheterization are both considered to have an advantage over other enteral feeding systems in that the technique can be undertaken without general anaesthesia in the majority of individuals. They both have the disadvantage of only being able to place a comparatively narrow feeding tube, making the administration of food materials both more difficult and more expensive. Figure 22.33 shows how to select the correct diameter of tube.

Remember, placement of the distal end of enteral feeding tubes within the stomach predisposes to vomiting, reflux oesophagitis and gastric ulceration. Therefore, it is recommended that the distal end of all oesophageal feeding tubes terminate in the caudal oesophagus. It is not recommended that this system of enteral feeding is utilized in individuals with compromised distal oesophageal function (e.g. megaoesophagus).

1. Infuse local anaesthetic (proxymetacaine) into the nare and elevate the muzzle
2. The length of tube to be inserted into the caudal oesophagus is determined by measuring the distance from the tip of the nose to the 9th/10th rib (this length should be marked onto the tube in some way)
3. The length of tube to be inserted into the stomach is determined by measuring the distance from the tip

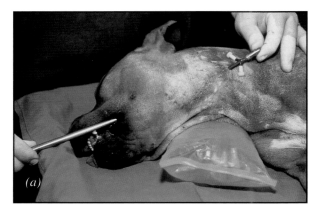

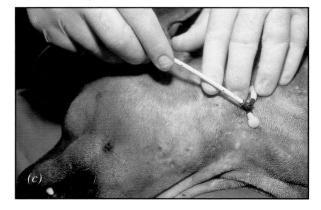

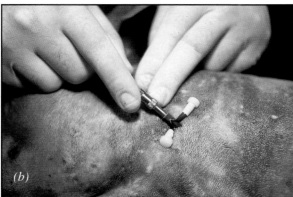

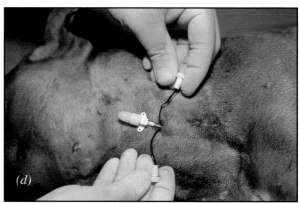

Figure 22.32: *Mid-cervical oesophagostomy. (a) Introduce the introduction tube via the mouth into the mid-cervical oesophagus and angle its bulb to tent the skin. A small nick is made over the bulb of the tube. Insert the needle and sheath through the skin into the bulb and carefully advance the assembly. (b) Remove the needle and grasp the Peel-away® sheath firmly and remove the introduction tube. Redirect the sheath caudally by flipping it 180°. It should now advance easily in the distal oesophagus. (c) Insert the feeding tube into the oesophagus through the sheath. (d) Peel the sheath away by pulling on the tags.*

Courtesy of Cook Veterinary Products.

Animal size	Tube diameter	Use of guidewire/stylet
Puppies/kittens	3.5 Fr	No
Cats <4.5 kg	5 Fr	No
Cats >4.5 kg	5–8 Fr	No
Dogs <7 kg	5 Fr	Yes
Dogs 7–15 kg	5–8 Fr	Yes
Dogs >15 kg	8 Fr	Yes

Figure 22.33: Selection of nasogastric and naso-oesophageal tubes. Data modified from Abood and Buffington (1992).

of the nose to the caudal rib margin

4. Lubricate the tip of the catheter
5. Insert the catheter into the ventromedial aspect of the nare (below the alar fold) and advance it aborally in the ventral meatus to the pre-determined length (this may be aided by pushing the external nares dorsally as the tube is advanced beyond the external nares)
6. To avoid tracheal intubation, the animal's head should be held at the normal angle of articulation
7. Placement is assessed by infusion of 3–5 ml of sterile saline through the tube and presence or absence of coughing or gagging following this procedure
8. The position of the tube should routinely be confirmed radiographically
9. Once the catheter is positioned appropriately, it is secured to the face between the eyes by means of adhesive glue or butterfly tapes and suturing, thereby avoiding the whiskers (Figure 22.34)
10. Secure a more proximal portion of the catheter to the skin on the forehead
11. An Elizabethan collar should be placed to prevent inadvertent removal of the tube.

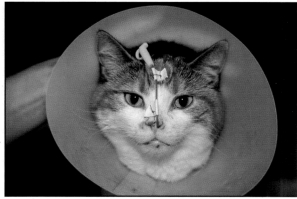

Figure 22.34: A naso-oesophageal catheter may be secured in place by using butterfly tapes and skin sutures. In the cat, securing the catheter between the eyes avoids interference with the whiskers. The use of an Elizabethan collar is recommended to prevent patient interference.

Gastrostomy

Gastrostomy tubes are ideal for the long-term enteral feeding of an animal. They are generally well tolerated, but they should not be used in animals with uncontrolled vomiting, gastric paresis or gastric outflow obstruction.

Percutaneous endoscopic gastrostomy (Matthews and Binnington, 1986; Twedt and Wheeler, 1990)

The procedure of percutaneous endoscopic directed gastrostomy tube placement (PEG) was first reported in small animals by Bright and Burrows in 1985. The procedure requires heavy sedation or light anaesthesia and carries a low morbidity in small animals. Many commercially available systems are available for PEG in small animals. The mushroom-tip catheter is the most commonly used, although the system available from Fresenius (Freca®) is probably the safest ultra long term system available.

1. The animal is ideally anaesthetized or, at the very least, heavily sedated and placed in right lateral recumbency
2. A 10 cm x 10 cm area just caudal to the last rib on the left side is clipped and prepared aseptically
3. With a mouth gag in place, the endoscope is advanced to the stomach, which is insufflated until there is notable distension of the gastric viscus against the abdominal wall (often, in thin walled individuals, the light beam from the endoscope will be visible percutaneously)
4. An area that is away from the pylorus and antral region of the stomach should be selected for tube placement
5. Depending on the tube system being placed, a small skin incision is made at the site of tube entry
6. An over-the-needle catheter (in general, 18 gauge), is placed through the skin incision and into the lumen of the stomach (this procedure is aided by gastric insufflation) (Figure 22.35a)
7. Once accurate placement is confirmed with the endoscope, the stylet is removed and a strong thread or suture is passed through the catheter into the lumen of the stomach
8. A snare or grasping forceps is used to grasp the thread or suture, and the endoscope, with the trailing thread, is withdrawn through the mouth
9. The catheter is then removed from the body wall
10. Depending on the tube system being used, the thread or suture exiting the mouth is attached in some manner to the gastrostomy tube
11. When using many of the commercially available mushroom tip catheters, it is important to remove a short portion of the catheter (2–3 cm) to be used as a 'T-bar' at the level of the mushroom tip to help prevent premature escape of the catheter from the gastric lumen
12. The catheter assembly is then advanced into the stomach and through the abdominal wall to the exterior by gentle traction on the thread or suture

exiting the abdominal wall (Figure 22.35b)

13. The catheter assembly is pulled until it is seated firmly against the stomach wall

14. The endoscope is then re-introduced to confirm correct positioning

15. The gastrostomy tube can then be capped and secured to the skin with sutures, butterfly tapes or a commercially available retention disc.

The tube can safely be removed after 7 days. Depending on the tube system used, removal can be achieved by either cutting the tube off close to the abdominal wall and the remaining tube pushed into the stomach lumen to be passed in the faeces, or by simply applying traction to the tube and pulling the mushroom tip through the body wall. The Fresenius system requires the oral retrieval of the gastric portion of the tube with the aid of an endoscope. The gastrocutaneous fistula can be allowed to heal by second intention.

The tube should not be removed until 5–7 days after placement to ensure that adequate adhesions occur around the tube and the body wall.

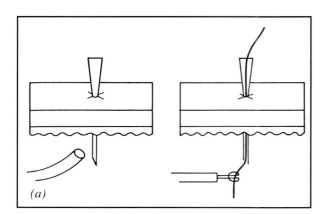

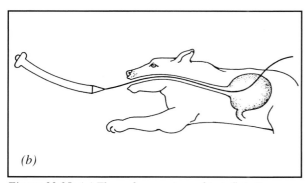

Figure 22.35: *(a) The endoscope is used to inflate the stomach so it comes into direct contact with the abdominal wall. The light from the endoscope can be viewed at the left costal arch where an intravenous catheter is introduced into the stomach. After removal of the stylet, nylon suture is threaded down the catheter and into the stomach. Endoscopic forceps are now used to pick up the suture and retrieve it back through the mouth. (b) Once the catheter assembly is attached to the suture, it is pulled back down into the stomach and out through the incision in the abdominal wall.*

Reproduced from the BSAVA Manual of Canine and Feline Gastroenterology.

Percutaneous non-endoscopic gastrostomy

There are a number of commercially available systems that are designed to allow the percutaneous placement of a gastrostomy tube without the need for endoscopic guidance. All of these systems utilize a reusable introduction tube that is long enough to be passed from the mouth into the stomach (Figure 22.36). Each available system differs very slightly in placement technique required, but a general description of this useful technique is as follows.

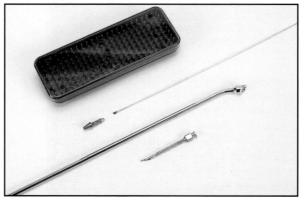

Figure 22.36: *Equipment required for percutaneous non-endoscopic gastrostomy.*
Courtesy of Cook Veterinary Products.

1. The animal should be anaesthetized or heavily sedated and placed in right lateral recumbency

2. The introduction tube is passed orally via the oesophagus to lie within the stomach (Figure 22.37a)

3. Air can be insufflated down the tube (Figure 22.37b) to confirm the gastric placement (in fact, by manually manipulating the tube, its distal end can be palpated cutaneously on the lateral abdominal wall just caudal to the left costochondral arch)

4. A wire introduction needle is passed percutaneously at this lateral abdominal wall site so that its point enters the distal opening of the introduction tube (Figure 22.37c)

5. Firm manipulation of the proximal end of the introduction tube at the mouth will ensure that the tip of the introduction needle remains within the distal introduction tube lumen

6. A wire or strong thread is passed down the introduction needle and introduced until it protrudes from the proximal, oral end of the introduction tube (Figure 22.37d)

7. The introduction needle and introduction tube can now be removed leaving the wire or thread only (Figure 22.37e)

8. The wire or thread can now be attached to the gastrostomy tube (a threaded wire system makes this process very simple and robust) (Figure 22.37 f, g)

9. The wire or thread and the attached gastrostomy tube are now pulled from the abdominal wall (Figure 22.37h)

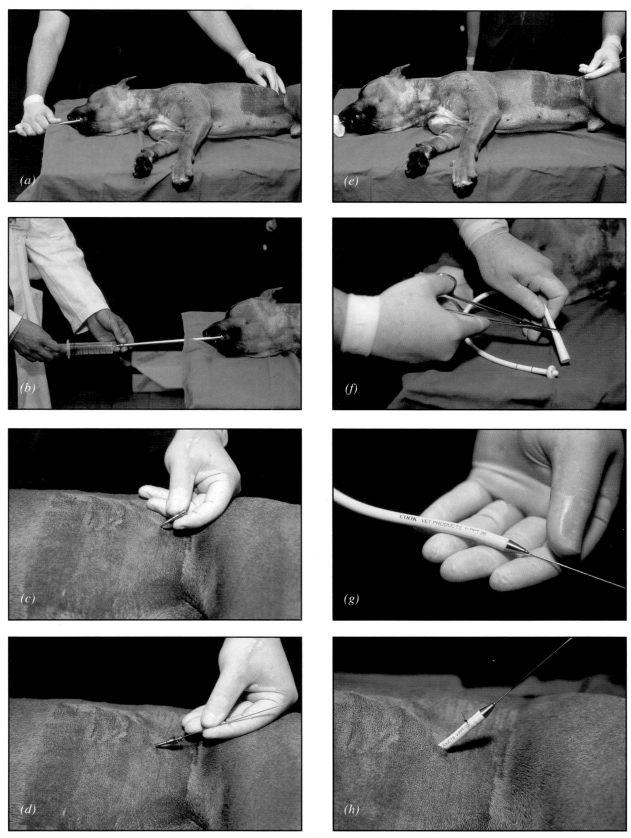

Figure 22.37: *(a) Non-endoscopic gastrostomy. (a) Introduce the tube into the stomach. (b) Insufflate with air to confirm position. (c) Pass the needle percutaneously into the tube's distal end. (d) Introduce threaded wire down the needle. (e) Remove the tube and needle to leave only the wire. (f) Remove the fitting on the tube and insert the adaptor. (g) Screw the adaptor on to the threaded wire. (h) Pull the tube through the tract and out of the flank.*

Courtesy of Cook Veterinary Products.

(Continued over page)

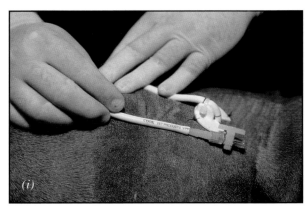

Figure 22.37: *(i) Secure the tube at the skin and fit a stopcock.*
Courtesy of Cook Veterinary Products.

10. The gastrostomy tube is now in place; it should be capped and secured to the skin with butterfly tapes, sutures or a commercially available retention disc. (Figure 22.37i)

Surgical placement

Surgical placement of gastrostomy tubes is generally considered less desirable than percutaneous placement, but under certain circumstances, for example, lack of relevant equipment or the decision to place a gastrostomy tube intraoperatively, surgical placement becomes a necessity. The use of silicone catheters has the advantage that silicone is resistant to degradation by stomach acid.

In cats and small dogs, 18–24 French tubes should be used. In larger dogs, 26–30 French tubes will be required. In all cases, a 5 ml balloon-tipped catheter should be used. The description that follows assumes the decision to place a gastrostomy tube has not been taken intraoperatively:

1. The animal is anaesthetized and placed in right lateral recumbency
2. The left paracostal area is clipped and prepared aseptically
3. A 2–3 cm incision is made through the skin and subcutaneous tissues just behind a parallel to the last rib (the dorsal limit of the incision should be just below the ventral edge of the paravertebral epaxial musculature)
4. A grid incision is bluntly made through the external and internal oblique and transverse muscles of the abdominal wall
5. Inflation of the stomach with 10–15 ml/kg of air via a stomach tube will allow the stomach wall to be easily located via the surgical incision
6. Temporary stay sutures (2–0 polypropylene) are placed in the greater curvature of the stomach (these sutures are placed such that the portion of the stomach between them is the chosen site of the gastrostomy)
7. Two concentric full-thickness purse-string sutures

of 2–0 polypropylene or nylon are placed through all layers of the gastric wall (it is helpful if double needle suture is used)
8. The gastrostomy tube is prepared by cutting the tip of the Foley catheter (taking care not to damage the balloon – the balloon should be checked prior to placement)
9. A small stab incision is made into the stomach wall at the centre of the purse-string ligatures
10. The tube is passed through the incision into the gastric lumen
11. The innermost purse-string suture is tightened and tied
12. The outermost purse-string suture is then tied while the stomach region adjacent to the tube is inverted
13. The needles on the outer-purse suture can now be used to approximate the stomach wall to the abdominal wall and to close the abdominal muscle layers (a small piece of omentum may be wrapped around the gastrostomy site to further minimize the risk of local peritonitis)
14. The subcutaneous and skin layers are closed in a routine manner
15. The tube should be capped and secured to the skin with sutures (finger trap), butterfly tapes or a commercially available retention disc.

Complications of surgically placed gastrostomy tubes include pyloric obstruction, peritonitis and cellulitis. Pyloric obstruction is more likely if 30 ml balloon catheters are used. Securing the stomach gastrostomy site to the peritoneal wall makes the occurrence of peritonitis unlikely. The presence of the omentum is likely to ensure that any peritonitis that should develop will remain localized.

The tube may be removed by deflating the balloon after 7 days, by which time strong adhesions should have developed between the stomach wall and the peritoneum. The gastrocutaneous fistula that is formed after gastrostomy tube removal spontaneously heals in 3–7 days. Antibiotic cover may be required with tube placement to reduce the risk of localized abscess formation.

Jejunostomy

Jejunostomy tubes may be indicated in individuals undergoing proximal gastrointestinal tract surgery. The surgical procedure may make the use of nasogastric or gastrostomy enteral feeding systems impossible. The jejunostomy enteral feeding system, on the other hand, only requires the gastrointesinal tract to be intact from the duodenum onwards. The placement procedure requires a coeliotomy. The system is most elegantly placed using the Peel-away® sheath needle technique.

1. The animal is anaesthetized and a cranial midline coeliotomy performed
2. A Peel-away® sheath needle (Cook®) is used to pass the jejunal feeding tube (8 French gauge closed end catheter with distal side holes) percutaneously

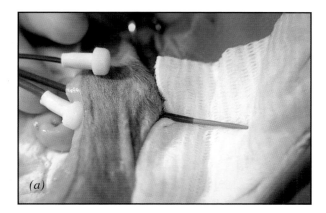

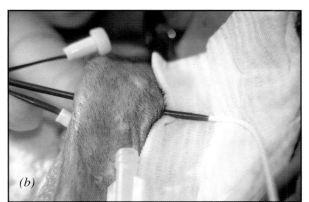

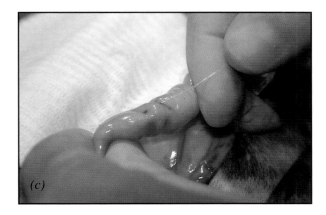

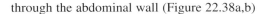

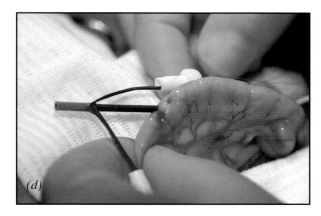

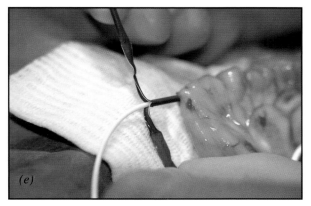

Figure 22.38: *(a) A Peel-away® (Cook®) sheath needle has been passed through the right abdominal wall. (b) The catheter can be used to pass the jejunal feeding tube percutaneously through the abdominal wall. (c) A purse-string suture has been placed in the antimesenteric border of an isolated loop of proximal jejunum. (d) A Peel-away® sheath has been passed in an aboral direction through the purse-string suture and into the lumen of the intestine. (e) The feeding tube is passed via the Peel-away® sheath into the lumen of the intestine. Once in place, the sheath is removed by peeling its two halves apart.*

through the abdominal wall (Figure 22.38a,b)

3. A loop of the distal portion of the duodenum or the proximal jejunum is located and surgically packed-off with abdominal swabs
4. A purse-string suture of 3-0 or 4-0 polydioxanone or polyglyconate is placed in the antimesenteric border of the isolated loop of intestine (Figure 22.38c)
5. A second Peel-away® sheath needle is used to pass the jejunal feeding tube through the purse-string suture and into the lumen of the intestine (Figure 22.38d,e)
6. The feeding tube should be advanced 20–30 cm aborally from the enterostomy site
7. The purse-string suture is tightened and tied
8. The enterostomy site is advanced towards the exit site of the tube through the abdominal wall (excess tube is fed through the abdominal wall penetration site during this manoeuvre)

9. The enterostomy site is sutured to the abdominal wall using four 3–0 or 4–0 interrupted polypropylene sutures (omentum may be wrapped around the enterostomy wound prior to suture ligation)
10. The feeding tube is capped and secured to the abdominal skin using sutures, butterfly tapes or a commercially available retention disc
11. The celiotomy wound is closed in a routine manner.

Removal of the feeding tube can be performed after 7 days and is accomplished by removing the skin securing device and slowly withdrawing the tube. Complications of jejunostomy feeding are similar to those described for feeding via a gastrostomy tube.

Gastric lavage

Gastric lavage is best performed in the lightly anaesthetized individual. Obviously, the potential for aspiration is increased in this situation and measures to guard against this should be instigated. It is imperative that a cuffed endotracheal tube is placed as part of these measures. It is also advisable to keep the animal's head lowered during the lavage procedure.

1. The animal should be unconscious or lightly anaesthetized and a well fitting cuffed endotracheal tube should be placed
2. A large-bore stomach tube (same diameter or bigger than the endotracheal tube) is passed into the stomach via the gagged mouth (egress tube)
3. A second smaller bore stomach tube is also passed into the stomach (fluid ingress tube). Alternatively, a commercially available gastric lavage tube may be used, which incorporates a dual lumen (both ingress and egress) in a single tube
4. The length of tube to place can be pre-determined as the distance from the nose to just beyond the 13th rib
5. The stomach may be lavaged with either saline or water
6. The lavage is instilled through the ingress tube and returning gastric contents should pass through the egress tube (the stomach should not be over-distended and gastric filling should be monitored by watching and feeling for evidence of gastric distension)
7. The lavage should be repeated until the lavage fluid runs clear (the lavage process may be helped by moving the animal into both right and left lateral recumbencies during the lavage procedure)
8. Once complete, the smaller ingress tube is removed, secure endotracheal tube placement is ensured, and the large bore tube is kinked-off and removed.

Abdominocentesis

- Ideally, the four quadrants of the abdomen should be tapped
- Right cranial and caudal quadrants should be tapped with the animal in the standing position or in right lateral recumbency
- Left cranial and caudal quadrants should be tapped with the animal in the standing position or in left lateral recumbency
- Local anaesthetic infiltration of the skin can be performed if necessary, but this is rarely the case in the emergency situation.

1. Using an aseptic technique, insert a 18–20 gauge needle or intravenous cannula through the skin 2–3 cm lateral to the midline on the right and left sides in both the cranial and caudal halves of the abdomen (catheter placement may require a small skin incision with a blade)
2. The needle or catheter are attached to a three-way

tap and syringe
3. Slight negative pressure is applied to the syringe as the needle or catheter are advanced into the peritoneal cavity
4. Care should be taken not to penetrate the urinary bladder, spleen or viscera
5. Any free peritoneal fluid should be aspirated as the needle penetrates the peritoneal cavity.

Peritoneal lavage

1. The animal is positioned in lateral recumbency
2. A wide area around the umbilicus is clipped and aseptically prepared
3. A large bore (10–14 gauge) over-the-needle catheter, which has been multi-fenestrated, or a trocar peritoneal catheter can be used
4. A small skin incision is made in the midline with a blade 1–2 cm caudal to the umbilicus
5. The peritoneal catheter is passed through the skin incision and into the peritoneal cavity in a caudal direction
6. Care should be taken not to penetrate the urinary bladder
7. The needle or trocar is removed and the catheter is advanced to lie against the ventral peritoneal wall in the midline
8. Secure the catheter firmly to the skin with sutures and tapes
9. Instil approximately 20 ml/kg of warm normal saline or Hartmann's solution into the peritoneal cavity
10. Gently roll the patient from side to side to distribute and mix the fluid
11. Wait several minutes and then drain the fluid into a syringe or sterile bag for analysis.

GENITOURINARY SYSTEM TECHNIQUES

The technique of urethral catheterization varies between the sexes and between dogs and cats. Most dogs can be catheterized without chemical restraint but cats, especially males, usually require sedation or anaesthesia.

Many catheters are commercially available for the urethral catheterization of small animals. The majority of catheters are manufactured from polyurethane, red rubber or silicone. Metal catheters cannot be recommended because of the increased likelihood of trauma to the urethra and/or bladder. Silicone has certain advantages for the patient which include softness, flexibility and biological inertness. These allow for atraumatic placement, minimal epithelial irritation and long-term patient comfort.

Urethral catheters for use in cats will generally be sized between 3 and 4 French. There are a number of urethral catheters specifically designed to be used as in-dwelling catheters in the cat. The most well recognized of these is the Jackson's catheter. Narrow gauge catheters manufactured from silicone often require a wire guide stylet to assist their introduction.

Catheters for use in small dogs and bitches will be sized between 3 and 5 French. Catheters for use in medium to large/giant sized dogs and bitches will be sized between 6 and 10 French. Softer material catheters may require a wire guide stylet. A selection of urethral catheters is available that have a detachable Luer lock fitting, allowing the catheters to be trimmed to any length. This is of considerable use when these catheters are used as indwelling systems.

In the larger dog and the majority of bitches, Foley catheters can be utilized as indwelling catheters. Their introduction requires the use of a stylet. Sizes are similar to those described for standard catheters above.

Indwelling catheters should ideally be connected to a sterile closed urine collecting system. This can often be constructed in an aseptic manner from an intravenous fluid giving-set and bag. Commercially available systems are also available.

Urethral catheterization techniques are well reviewed by Holt (1994).

Urethral catheterization in the dog

1. Grasp the caudal os penis with one hand and retract the prepuce caudally with the other hand, exposing the glans penis
2. One of the fingers of the hand grasping the os penis, is used to keep the prepuce retracted and the glans exposed
3. The catheter to be inserted should be lubricated with a water-soluble jelly
4. The catheter is then inserted into the urethra under aseptic conditions (either by wearing a sterile glove or by handling the catheter through its sterile polythene bag)
5. Once the catheter is inserted to the level of the caudal os penis, the grip of the hand holding the penis is relaxed allowing further unobstructed passage of the catheter
6. As soon as the catheter tip enters the bladder and urine appears in the catheter hub, passage of the catheter is discontinued
7. The catheter may be sutured to the cranial preputial skin using butterfly tapes, and maintained as an indwelling catheter
8. An Elizabethan collar should be fitted to prevent self-removal of the catheter.

Urethral catheterization in the bitch

1. The bitch is positioned in dorsal or lateral recumbency with the pelvic limbs flexed cranially by an assistant (right lateral recumbency if right handed, left lateral recumbency if left handed)
2. A vaginal speculum is inserted into the vestibule/vagina taking care not to enter the ventrally placed clitoral fossa
3. The slit of the speculum is positioned ventrally allowing the raised external urethral orifice to be identified on the floor of the cranial vestibule
4. Visualization of the external urethral orifice is often made easier if an assistant pulls the ventral vulva caudally
5. The catheter is then inserted into the urethra in an aseptic manner (when using soft rubber or silicone catheters it may be advantageous to stiffen the catheter with a stylet)
6. The catheter is advanced until urine is seen to flow
7. The catheter may be sutured to the perivulval skin using butterfly tapes, and maintained as an indwelling catheter
8. An Elizabethan collar should be fitted to prevent self-removal of the catheter.

Urethral catheterization in the tom

1. The tom is positioned in lateral recumbency
2. In the right-handed operator, the thumb and index finger of the left hand are used to push the prepuce cranially and expose the glans penis
3. The tip of the catheter is inserted into the penile urethra (lubrication of the catheter tip with a water-soluble lubricant may prove advantageous)
4. To allow the safe advancement of the catheter, the prepuce is grasped with the left hand and pulled in a caudal direction (this aligns the penile and membranous urethrae, making further catheter passage possible)
5. As soon as the catheter tip enters the bladder and urine appears in the catheter hub, passage of the catheter is discontinued
6. When the Jackson's catheter is used, it may be sutured to the preputial skin using the holes in the catheter flange, and maintained as an indwelling catheter
7. An Elizabethan collar should be fitted to prevent self-removal of the catheter.

Urethral catheterization in the queen

The anatomy of the queen is such that the external urethral orifice is found as a depression on the vaginal floor. This anatomical situation allows 'blind' urethral catheterization in the queen.

1. For the right-handed operator, the queen is positioned in right lateral recumbency
2. The left hand is used to grasp the vulval lips allowing the right hand to pass the catheter along the vestibular floor in the midline
3. This passage of the catheter will commonly result in entrance to the urethra

4. As soon as the catheter tip enters the bladder and urine appears in the catheter hub, passage of the catheter is discontinued

5. When the Jackson's catheter is used, it may be sutured to the preputial skin using the holes in the catheter flange, and maintained as an indwelling catheter

6. An Elizabethan collar should be fitted to prevent self-removal of the catheter.

If 'blind' catheterization fails, an otoscope may be used as a vaginoscope to identify the external urethral orifice, allowing urethral catheterization.

Cystocentesis

The technique of cystocentesis will allow a urine sample to be obtained without contamination from the urethra, the genital tract or the skin. It will also reduce the risk of producing an iatrogenic urinary tract infection. The technique may also be required to decompress a severely over-distended bladder in an individual suffering from a urethral obstruction when urethral catheterization is not possible. In the non-obstructed individual, the bladder must contain a reasonable volume of urine so that it can be safely identified and immobilized. Ultrasonography may be used to help guide the needle into the bladder of an obese individual.

1. The skin of the caudoventral abdomen (from umbilicus to pelvic brim) is clipped and prepared aseptically

2. In the cat and small dog, the technique is most readily performed with the animal in either lateral or dorsal recumbency (Figure 22.39)

3. In the larger dog, the procedure may be performed with the animal in either lateral recumbency or in the standing position (Figure 22.40)

4. In all instances, an assistant is required to restrain the subject

5. The operator's free hand is used to palpate and stabilize the bladder by pushing it in a caudal direction against the pelvic brim

6. The needle (21 or 23 gauge, 1–2 inches in length) is attached to a 5 or 10 ml syringe and inserted through the abdominal wall, in the midline, 5–10 cm cranial to the pelvic brim

7. The ideal site of bladder penetration is a short distance cranial to the junction of the bladder with the urethra (this will permit removal of urine and decompression of the bladder without the need for re-insertion of the needle into the bladder lumen)

8. The needle is inserted in a caudal direction at a 45° angle, and once the needle is within the abdominal wall slight negative pressure should be applied to the syringe

9. Once the bladder lumen is penetrated, urine will be seen to fill the syringe.

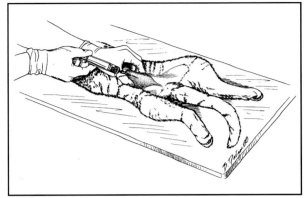

Figure 22.37: Technique for cystocentesis in the cat and small dog. (From the MediClip Veterinary Anatomy Collection, 1997, Williams & Wilkins, A Waverly Company)

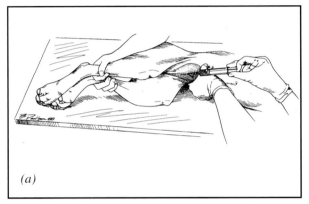

(a)

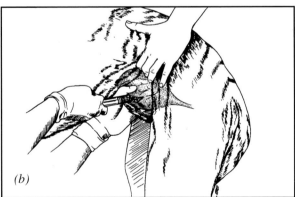

(b)

Figure 22.40: (a) Technique for cystocentesis in the larger dog, which is restrained in lateral recumbency. (b) Technique for cystocentesis in the larger dog, which is restrained in a standing position. (Both from the MediClip Veterinary Anatomy Collection, 1997, Williams & Wilkins, A Waverly Company)

OPHTHALMIC TECHNIQUES

Schirmer tear test

The Schirmer tear test uses standardized strips of filter paper to quantify aqueous tear production. When a tear production test is suggested, it should be undertaken prior to any drops or irrigants being used on the eye.

The Schirmer I test measures aqueous production in the unanaesthetized eye and is therefore a measurement of basal and reflex tear production. The Schirmer II test measures aqueous production in the topically locally anaesthetized eye and, therefore, measures basal tear production only.

1. The test strip should be bent slightly at the point of the notch on the strip prior to its removal from the pack
2. The strip should ideally not be touched with fingers so as to maintain sterility and to avoid depositing cutaneous lipid on the paper, which might interfere with aqueous tear absorption
3. The short end of the strip is placed in the lateral half of the lower conjunctival sac so that the notch is at the level of the lid margin and the strip is in contact with the lower lid margin and the cornea
4. In the majority of animals, the examiner will need to keep the lids closed so that the strip is retained in position
5. At the end of 1 minute, the strip is removed and the flow of aqueous measured against the template on the box
6. The process is then repeated on the other eye.

The Schirmer II test is performed in a similar manner to the Schirmer I test, although the eye is locally anaesthetized with 1 or 2 drops of a local anaesthetic agent (proxymetacaine) several minutes before the test is undertaken.

Intraocular pressure measurement (Renwick, 1993)

The measurement of intraocular pressure is termed tonometry. Two types of tonometer are available to the veterinary profession; the Schiøtz tonometer and applanation tonometers.

The Schiøtz tonometer is readily available and relatively cheap. This device estimates intraocular pressure by the use of a weighted plunger, which indents the eye to a degree that is roughly dependent upon the intraocular pressure.

1. A topical anaesthetic agent is applied to both eyes (proxymetacaine)
2. After several minutes, and once the anaesthetic agent has taken effect, measures can be made
3. The patient is restrained with the head back so that the cornea lies in the horizontal plane
4. The plunger of the tonometer is placed vertically on the central cornea on several occasions until three similar readings have been obtained (care must be taken to keep the footplate away from the third eyelid)
5. In cases of doubtful accuracy the measurement can be repeated using a different weight and the values compared
6. The procedure is then repeated in the other eye.

Limitations of the Schiøtz tonometer are listed below:

- Indentation tonometry is inherently subject to a degree of inaccuracy
- The tonometer should not be used after recent intraocular surgery
- Corneal oedema may render the reading inaccurate
- Difficulty in restraining some patients may artefactually increase intraocular pressure
- A dirty instrument can be highly inaccurate.

Applanation tonometers operate on the principle of measuring the force required to flatten or applanate a given, small area of cornea. These instruments tend to be the most accurate in clinical use, but are expensive to purchase. They can be used with the animal in a normal standing position, and following intraocular surgery. Numerous applanation tonometers are commercially available but their specific use is beyond the scope of this text.

NEUROLOGICAL TECHNIQUES

Cerebrospinal fluid collection (Wheeler and Sharp, 1994)

General anaesthesia is required for cerebrospinal fluid (CSF) collection. Animals should be intubated and, ideally, an armoured endotracheal tube should be used. It is most common to use the cerebellomedullary cistern (CMC) collection site. There is a theoretical advantage in using the lumbar spine; CSF flows in a cranial to caudal direction making a diagnostically abnormal CSF more likely to be sampled at a caudal collection site. Unfortunately, the collection of CSF from the lumbar site is more difficult and blood contamination occurs more often. The technique of CMC collection is described:

1. The animal should be placed in either right or left lateral recumbency depending on whether the operator is right or left handed (e.g. right lateral recumbency for a right-handed individual)
2. An area of skin on the dorsal aspect of the neck and caudal head is clipped and prepared aseptically
3. The head is held by an assistant in 90° flexion with the nose parallel to the table top and the dorsum of the neck close to the edge of the table
4. An armoured or kink-proof endotracheal tube should be used, and respiratory pattern and reservoir bag movement should be monitored
5. An imaginary line is drawn between the wings of the atlas vertebra, and the puncture site is on the midline of the patient, half way between the occipital protuberance and the imaginary line joining the wings of the atlas (Figure 22.41)
6. A commercial spinal needle is preferred because it possesses a stylet, a shallow bevel and a notch in

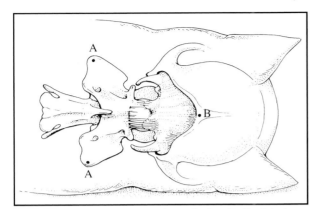

***Figure 22.41:** A: Prominent wings of atlas. B: Occipital protuberance.*

Reproduced from the BSAVA Manual of Small Animal Neurology, 2nd Edition.

the hub, which indicates the position of the bevel
7. The needle is inserted perpendicular to the skin, and the stylet is removed once the tip of the needle is in muscle
8. The needle is then advanced until the dura mater is penetrated and CSF appears in the hub of the needle (a slight pop can sometimes be felt when the needle enters the subarachnoid space)
9. Fluid is generally collected passively by letting it drop into a sterile vial.

Complications of CSF collection are:

• Sudden movement of the patient is generally a result of spinal cord damage; remove the needle, ventilate the animal and administer methylprednisolone (30 mg/kg i.v.)
• No CSF flows, although an apparently normal tap has been achieved; the needle may be off the midline, the brain may have herniated or the spinal cord may have been penetrated. Treat as a potentially serious complication until physiological parameters suggest otherwise

• A blood-contaminated tap is obtained; penetration of the dural vessel or the venous plexus. Repeat tap with a fresh needle, although a second contaminated tap is probably more likely now to occur.

REFERENCES

Abood SK and Buffington CAT (1992) Use of nasogastric tubes: indications, technique and complications. In: *Kirk's Current Veterinary Therapy XI — Small Animal Practice*, eds. RW Kirk and JD Bonagura, pp. 32–35. WB Saunders, Philadelphia

Böhning RH Jr, DeHoff WD, McElhinney A and Hofstra PC (1970) Pharyngostomy for maintenance of the anorectic animal. *Journal of the American Veterinary Medical Association* **156**, 611–615

Bright RM and Burrows CF (1985) The use of percutaneous endoscopic tube gastrostomy in the dog. *Veterinary Surgery* **14**, 49

Crowe DT and Downs MO (1986) Pharyngostomy complications in dogs and cats and recommended technical modifications: experimental and clinical investigations. *Journal of the American Animal Hospital Association* **22**, 493–503

Fitzpatrick RK and Crowe DT (1986) Nasal oxygen administration in dogs and cats: experimental and clinical investigations. *Journal of the American Animal Hospital Association* **22**, 293–300

Holt PE (1994) Other diagnostic aids. In: *Color Atlas of Small Animal Urology*, pp. 33–54. Mosby-Wolfe, London

Matthews KA and Binnington AG (1986) Percutaneous incisionless placement of a gastrostomy tube utilizing a gastroscope: preliminary observations. *Journal of the American Animal Hospital Association* **22**, 601–610

Melker R (1988) *Insertion of the Melker Emergency Cricothyrotomy Catheter. Videotape.* Shands Hospital, University of Florida, Gainsville, Florida USA (available from Cook Critical Care, PO Box 489, Bloomington, Indiana, USA)

Rawlings CA (1979) Pharyngostomy. In: *Small Animal Surgery — an Atlas of Operative Techniques*, eds. WE Wingfield and CA Rawlings, pp. 65–67. WB Saunders, Philadelphia

Rawlings CA (1993) Percutaneous placement of a midcervical esophagostomy tube: new technique and representative cases. *Journal of the American Animal Hospital Association* **29**, 526–530

Renwick PW (1993) Glaucoma. In: *Manual of Small Animal Ophthalmology*, eds. SM Petersen-Jones and SM Crispin, pp. 193–212. BSAVA, Cheltenham

Seldinger (1953) Catheter replacement of the needle in percutaneous arteriography. *Acta Radiologica* **38**, 368–376

Twedt DC and Wheeler SL (1990) Percutaneous endoscopic gastrostomy tube placement. In: *Small Animal Endoscopy*, ed. TR Tams, pp. 291–295. CV Mosby, St Louis

Wheeler SJ and Sharp NJH (1994) Diagnostic aids. In: *Small Animal Spinal Disorders — Diagnosis and Surgery*, pp. 34–56. Mosby-Wolfe, London

CHAPTER TWENTY THREE

Imaging Techniques for the Critical Patient

Frances Barr

INTRODUCTION

Imaging techniques should be used with care in critically ill patients, as manipulation and restraint of the patient may be a source of added stress, while existing injuries may inadvertently be exacerbated. It is therefore important to keep the number of procedures to a minimum by selecting the appropriate techniques for a given situation, and to carry out each examination carefully to minimize the need for repeat examinations. At all times, the patient should be handled gently, paying due regard to the existing clinical problem.

PLAIN RADIOGRAPHY

Plain radiography is an invaluable imaging technique, which may be used to define the problem(s) in an individual patient and to monitor progress over a period of time. Detailed descriptions of radiographic positioning for different parts of the body are available elsewhere, but it may be useful to bear the following points in mind:

- If general anaesthesia is deemed inappropriate, then adequate positioning and restraint can usually be achieved using foam or plastic troughs, foam wedges and floppy sandbags. Manual restraint is only allowed under 'exceptional clinical circumstances' (Ionizing Radiations Regulations, 1985) and is in fact rarely required
- In some clinical situations, it may be preferable to use a horizontal X-ray beam to obtain an orthogonal projection rather than re-positioning the patient (e.g. in extreme dyspnoea, when lateral recumbency may not be tolerated; in suspected spinal fracture/dislocation, when it is important to minimize patient manipulation). If a horizontal X-ray beam is used, due regard must be paid to radiation safety
- Ideally, select a fast film-screen combination so that exposure time may be kept to a minimum. This reduces the risk of movement blur impairing the sharpness of the image
- Examine the resulting images in a careful and systematic fashion, under appropriate viewing conditions, to minimize the risk of missing abnormalities. If manual processing is used, a final evaluation of the radiographs should not be made until they are dry.

Thorax

A minimum of two radiographic projections is required for evaluation of the thoracic cavity — dorsoventral and lateral. A dorsoventral projection is generally tolerated well by the patient and is usually preferred to a ventrodorsal projection in critical cases. A recumbent lateral projection may not be tolerated by an animal with dyspnoea, in which case a lateral projection can be achieved using a horizontal X-ray beam with the patient standing or in sternal recumbency. In some situations, it may be advisable to take radiographs with the animal in both right and left lateral recumbency. Small masses or areas of consolidation may be seen more clearly in the uppermost lung, where they are surrounded by air-filled alveoli, than in the lower lung, which tends to undergo partial collapse.

It is important to include the whole thoracic cavity on each radiograph, and the X-ray beam should be centred and collimated accordingly. The exposure should be made, wherever possible, at peak inspiration, so that the lungs are maximally aerated. Occasionally, an exposure may be made deliberately at end expiration to check that the lungs are able to deflate and there is no evidence of air trapping.

Abnormalities of the ribs, spine, sternum and soft tissues of the thoracic wall

It is important to check the soft tissues of the thoracic wall for swelling, emphysema or radiodense foreign material. The thoracic spine should be evaluated for evidence of fracture and/or dislocation and, if necessary, further radiographs should be taken centred on the thoracic spine. The sternum should also be assessed. It is important to bear in mind that congenital anomalies of the sternum are not uncommon in dogs and cats (e.g. pectus excavatum) and these must be differentiated from traumatic sternal disruption (Figure 23.1). Fractures of the ribs are not always easy to identify and a meticulous check should be made along the length of each rib on each radiograph. If several adjacent ribs

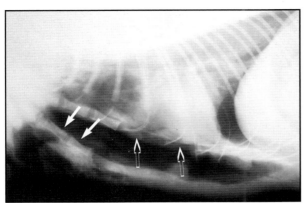

Figure 23.1: Lateral thoracic radiograph of a cat with dog bite injuries. Two sternal segments (closed arrows) have been displaced ventrally and cranially, leaving a sternal defect (open arrows). There is extensive associated subcutaneous emphysema and a small pneumothorax.

have multiple fractures, it is wise to check the patient for evidence of 'flail chest'.

Abnormalities of the diaphragm

Rupture of the diaphragm is most clearly demonstrated by the passage of abdominal viscera into the thoracic cavity. This results in an overall increase in radiopacity in the thorax and displacement of intrathoracic structures, together with a corresponding absence of some normal structures from the abdominal cavity (Figure 23.2). In some instances, the diagnosis is evident on plain radiography; in other cases, contrast radiography or ultrasonography may be needed to confirm the diagnosis.

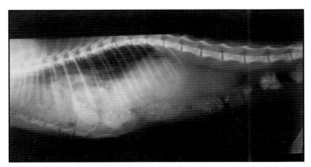

Figure 23.2: Lateral radiograph of the thorax and abdomen of a cat after a road traffic accident. Gas-filled small intestinal loops and part of the faeces-filled colon are visible in the ventral thorax, obscuring the cardiac outline and the ventral part of the diaphragmatic line. The radiographic diagnosis is traumatic rupture of the diaphragm.

The outline of the diaphragm may become partially obscured by free thoracic fluid or adjacent intrathoracic masses.

Abnormalities of the pleural space

Pneumothorax: A small amount of free air in the thoracic cavity is most clearly seen on the recumbent or erect lateral radiograph. On the recumbent lateral projection, the heart apex appears raised from the sternum

and, as the quantity of free air increases, the caudal lung lobes start to collapse and retract from the thoracic spine and diaphragm. On the erect lateral projection, the air accumulates in the dorsocaudal thorax, with retraction of the lung margins at this site (Figure 23.3). This projection may be useful in providing a semi-quantitative evaluation of the amount of free air. Collapse and retraction of the lung lobes is visible on the dorsoventral projection if moderate or large quantities of free air are present. If a tension pneumothorax is present, the ribs will be maximally spread and the diaphragm flattened. Intrathoracic structures may be displaced to one side if the problem is unilateral.

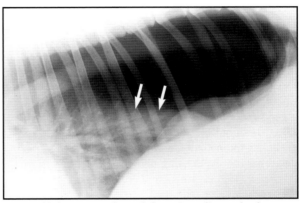

Figure 23.3: An erect lateral thoracic radiograph of a German Shepherd Dog with bilateral pneumothorax. Free air has accumulated in the dorsocaudal thorax and the edges of the retracted caudal lung lobes are visible (arrows).

It is important to recognize that collapsed or partially collapsed lung lobes will be of increased radiopacity, even if they are otherwise normal. It may be useful to repeat thoracic radiography after drainage of free air and re-expansion of the lungs to check for evidence of lung pathology (e.g. bullae, pulmonary haemorrhage).

Pleural fluid: A small amount of free fluid in the thoracic cavity is most clearly seen on the dorsoventral radiograph, as a band of soft tissue separating the margins of the lung lobes from the thoracic wall and running between individual lung lobes (Figure 23.4). On the recumbent lateral projection, fluid often lies in the ventral thorax, with partially retracted lung lobes apparently 'floating' on top. As the quantity of fluid increases, the caudal lung lobes become separated from the thoracic spine and diaphragm by fluid. Since most soft tissues and fluid have a similar radiopacity, the presence of an intrathoracic mass may be masked by surrounding fluid. Ultrasonography is the imaging modality of choice in such instances as it will allow ready differentiation of fluid and soft tissue.

Abnormalities of the mediastinum and structures running within the mediastinum

Air may track within the mediastinum ('pneumomediastinum'), outlining the trachea, oesophagus, heart base

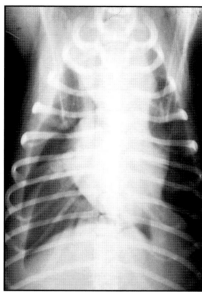

Figure 23.4: *A dorsoventral thoracic radiograph of a dog with warfarin poisoning. A soft tissue opacity separates the lung lobes on the right from the thoracic wall. There is also marked widening of both the cranial and caudal mediastinum. The radiographic diagnosis is free pleural fluid on the right and mediastinal fluid, in this case blood.*

and major vessels with abnormal clarity. This may be a consequence of dyspnoea or blunt thoracic trauma, but may also result from jugular venepuncture or penetrations of the pharynx, oesophagus or trachea.

Fluid within the mediastinum may result in radiographic widening of the mediastinum and 'reverse fissure' formation as fluid insinuates between the lobes of the lung at the hilus (Figure 23.4).

The lumen of the trachea should be carefully checked throughout its cervical and thoracic length. Foreign bodies are generally easily seen, as they are outlined by air. Localized narrowing of the lumen may be a consequence of a static lesion (e.g. a stricture, granuloma or neoplasm) or a dynamic lesion (e.g. tracheal collapse). Generalized narrowing of the lumen may be a result of tracheal hypoplasia, mucosal oedema or haemorrhage, or severe tracheal collapse. Tracheal penetrations result in extensive pneumomediastinum, subcutaneous emphysema and sometimes disruption of the visible tracheal outline. Intrathoracic tracheal rupture is typically associated with the formation of a thin-walled bullous structure in place of the normal tracheal walls (Figure 23.5).

The oesophagus must also be carefully checked throughout its cervical and thoracic length. A little gas within the oesophagus is not unusual, especially in an animal with dyspnoea or under general anaesthesia, but large quantities of gas suggest either gas accumulation proximal to an oesophageal obstruction, or a motility disorder (e.g. megalo-oesophagus). Penetration of the oesophagus usually results in air and/or fluid within the mediastinum. Contrast studies are often required for a full evaluation of the oesophagus.

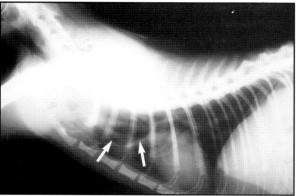

Figure 23.5: *A lateral thoracic radiograph of a cat with inspiratory dyspnoea following a road traffic accident 11 days previously. No clear tracheal outline is visible between the lower cervical region and the 4th rib, and a thin-walled 'bullous' structure is apparent in this region (arrows). The radiographic diagnosis is tracheal rupture.*

Abnormalities of the lungs

- Well defined soft tissue nodules or masses within the lung are generally indicative of primary or metastatic neoplasia, although granuloma or abscess formation may also be seen. Gas shadows within a mass can indicate cavitation, either within an abscess or necrotic tumour. Bullae or cysts usually contain air or air and fluid and have thin well defined walls
- Flooding of the alveoli with blood, inflammatory fluid or oedema fluid, or filling of the alveoli with neoplastic cells, result in areas of increased opacity within the lung. Small ill-defined areas which blur the normal pulmonary vascular pattern may coalesce to form large areas of opacity with air-filled bronchi running through them ('air bronchograms') (Figure 23.6). The distribution of such changes may help narrow the list of differential diagnoses. For example, cardiogenic oedema in the dog often begins with a peri-hilar distribution, while aspiration pneumonia

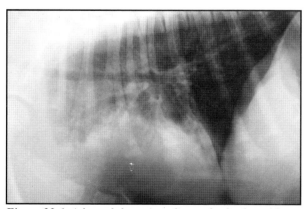

Figure 23.6: *A lateral thoracic radiograph of a dog with aspiration pneumonia. There is consolidation of the ventral parts of the cranial and middle lung lobes. Branching radiolucent tracts within the consolidated regions represent air bronchograms.*

characteristically affects the ventral portions of the cranial and middle lobes

- Collapse of a lung lobe may result in a similar radiographic appearance to alveolar filling. While lobar collapse (atelectasis) may be a consequence of disease processes, such as air or fluid in the pleural cavity or a space-occupying lesion, it may also be a consequence of prolonged recumbency. If the increase in lung opacity is due to recumbency collapse, it is often associated with radiographic evidence of a loss of lung volume on that side (e.g. raising of the hemidiaphragm on that side and/or shifting of the heart to that side). This is important to remember when dealing with critically ill patients, who may spend much of their time lying down
- The walls of the major bronchi are usually visible radiographically as thin tapering radiodense lines and rings. The bronchial markings may become more prominent if the bronchial walls become thickened, calcified, or if there is peribronchial cellular infiltration. Some increase in the bronchial markings is to be expected as the animal ages, but may also be associated with airway disease.

Abnormalities of the heart

The normal shape and size of the cardiac silhouette in the cat and dog is well established. In the dog, there is marked variation with breed and conformation. On a lateral radiograph, for example, a deep-chested dog normally has a narrow upright heart, while a barrel-chested dog normally has a rounded heart with marked sternal contact. There is far less variation among breeds of cat. Assessment of the shape and size of the heart should be made using lateral and dorsoventral radiographs, taking into account breed and conformation.

- If the heart is smaller than normal, this may indicate hypovolaemia (e.g. blood loss, dehydration, Addison's disease)
- If the heart is larger than normal, this may indicate enlargement of one or more chambers of the heart. Changes in the shape of the heart may help suggest which chambers or great vessels are involved. For example, an increase in the height of the heart on the lateral radiograph, with bulging of the dorsocaudal angle, indicates left chamber enlargement. An increase in the craniocaudal diameter of the heart is often seen with right chamber enlargement
- A round, globular heart on both radiographic projections is often seen in association with pericardial fluid (Figure 23.7). Once again, ultrasound is the technique of choice for confirming the diagnosis and for searching for any underlying causes (Figure 23.8).

Abdomen

A minimum of two radiographic projections is necessary for evaluation of the abdominal cavity — ventrodorsal

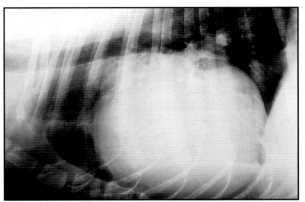

Figure 23.7: *A lateral thoracic radiograph of a German Shepherd Dog with a pericardial effusion. The cardiac silhouette is generally enlarged, with an unusual globular shape.*

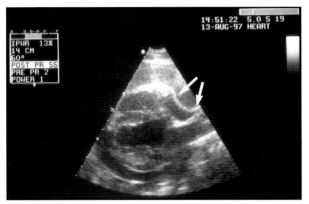

Figure 23.8: *A long axis view taken during ultrasonographic examination of the heart of a Golden Retriever. The heart is seen contained within a sac of pericardial fluid. Note the collapse of the right atrial wall (arrows), indicating cardiac tamponade.*

and lateral. A ventrodorsal projection is preferred to a dorsoventral projection, because the abdomen is stretched out and the hindlimbs are not superimposed on the area of interest. However, there may be situations (e.g. dyspnoea) where it is not desirable to turn the animal on to its back, in which case a dorsoventral projection of the abdomen may be all that can be achieved. If clinically appropriate, the animal should be starved for 12 hours prior to radiography and given the opportunity to defaecate, so that food/faecal material does not obscure other structures in the abdomen.

It is important to include the whole abdominal cavity. In large breed dogs, it may be necessary to take two separate radiographs centred on the cranial and caudal abdomen respectively. This may also be advisable in very narrow-waisted dogs when different exposures will be required for the thick cranial abdomen and the thin caudal abdomen. Make the exposure at end expiration, when the abdominal thickness and respiratory movement are minimized. When the abdominal thickness exceeds 10 cm, the use of a grid will improve image quality by reducing the amount of scattered radiation reaching the film.

Abnormalities of the abdominal wall

Check the soft tissues of the abdominal wall for integrity, swelling, emphysema or radiodense foreign bodies. The lumbar spine should be assessed for evidence of trauma, bone proliferation or destruction. If necessary, further radiographs should be taken centred on this area.

Abnormalities of the abdominal cavity

- Detail in the abdominal cavity, allowing differentiation of the various soft tissue structures, is normally provided by fat. Consequently, poor abdominal detail may be seen in very young or very thin animals. However, the presence of free fluid in the abdominal cavity will also obscure detail; a small or moderate amount of fluid blurs fine detail, while larger quantities result in a homogeneous opacity throughout the abdomen, relieved only by gas/food/faecal material in the gastrointestinal tract
- Peritonitis results in blurring of abdominal detail, either throughout the abdomen or in a localized area, due to the production of exudate (Figure 23.9). There may also be a mottled effect due to the formation of adhesions and pocketing of fluid. Intestinal loops in the area may be dilated and static due to paralytic ileus, corrugated due to irritation, or abnormally bunched due to adhesions.
- Free air in the abdominal cavity ('pneumoperitoneum') may be seen as irregular accumulations of gas which cannot be localized within bowel, sometimes accumulating between the liver and the diaphragm. If there is no penetrating wound of the abdominal wall, or recent laparotomy, a pneumoperitoneum is highly suggestive of perforation of the gastrointestinal tract.

Abnormalities of the gastrointestinal tract

- The stomach is a naturally distensible organ and so varies greatly in size. Excessive distension of the stomach may be an acute phenomenon (as part of the gastric dilatation volvulus syndrome) or may be more chronic. Acute gastric distension is usually due to food or gas accumulation. When volvulus is present, transposition of the fundus and pylorus may be recognized, and soft tissue bands may be seen compartmentalizing the stomach. Chronic distension due to gastric outflow obstruction or motility disorders is usually associated with fluid and sometimes the collection of particulate 'gravel' in the pyloric region
- The small intestine normally contains a mixture of gas and fluid. The diameter of small intestinal loops does not normally exceed the depth of a lumbar vertebral body. Undue fluid or gaseous distension of small intestinal loops may be seen in cases with generalized paralytic ileus (e.g. after a laparotomy; due to hypokalaemia) or secondary to a mechanical obstruction. In cases of chronic partial intestinal obstruction, particulate material may accumulate proximal to the obstruction — a so-called 'gravel sign' (Figure 23.10). The cause of an obstructive process may be apparent on plain radiographs (e.g. radiodense foreign body), but in other cases contrast studies or ultrasonography may be required
- The normal large intestine may contain gas or faecal material. If an enema has been given, or if the patient has diarrhoea, the contents may be fluid
- Displacement of any part of the gastrointestinal tract may be useful evidence of other disease processes. For example, movement of sections of the gastrointestinal tract into the thoracic cavity or into the subcutaneous tissues indicates loss of

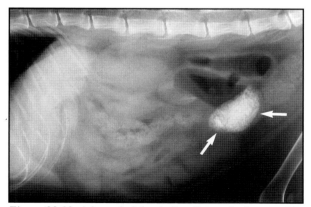

Figure 23.9: *A lateral abdominal radiograph of a cat presented with vomiting and abdominal pain. There is a generalized loss of detail, which is particularly apparent in the mid-ventral abdomen. There are also small accumulations of free gas, especially evident craniodorsally. The diagnosis was peritonitis secondary to intestinal rupture.*

Figure 23.10: *A lateral abdominal radiograph of a cat with a history of chronic vomiting. The radiograph shows a dense accumulation of mineral material (arrowed) superimposed on the faeces-filled colon. Dorsal to this are some distended gas-filled small intestinal loops. The diagnosis was a chronic partial obstruction of the distal small intestine, leading to gravel accumulation.*

integrity of the abdominal boundaries. A change in shape and size of the liver often results in gastric displacement. Any abdominal mass can push aside the small intestine. The descending colon may be displaced dorsally by an enlarged prostate and ventrally by enlarged sublumbar lymph nodes
- The normal pancreas is not visible radiographically, but detection of a mass or evidence of a localized peritonitis in the right cranioventral abdomen should lead to the suspicion of pancreatic disease.

Abnormalities of the liver and spleen

- Symmetrical hepatic enlargement results in extension of the ventral lobes well beyond the last rib, and often the tips of these lobes become rounded. The pyloric region of the stomach is pushed caudally and dorsally, resulting in an unusually horizontally positioned stomach. With focal asymmetric enlargement, the normal triangular shape of the liver is lost
- When the liver is unusually small, the ventral lobes lie well within the costal arch and lose their normal triangular shape. The stomach is displaced cranially and becomes unusually upright. The spleen may also move cranially to lie within the costal arch. It should be remembered that the liver has a large functional reserve, and the radiographic detection of a small liver is not necessarily of clinical significance
- The spleen is a very mobile organ, which is extraordinarily variable in both size and position. However, it is usually smooth in outline, with a triangular or elongated shape, and departures from this may be considered abnormal.

Abnormalities of the urogenital tract

- Renal enlargement may be smooth and symmetrical (e.g. hydronephrosis, amyloidosis) or irregular (e.g. renal neoplasia, polycystic disease). The accumulation of fluid between the kidney and its capsule may mimic renal enlargement. Reduction in renal size may be associated with renal dysplasia, hypoplasia or chronic parenchymal disease. Renal calculi may be recognized if they are radiodense. Further information about renal architecture and the ureters requires the use of contrast studies and/or ultrasound
- The adrenal glands lie medial to the cranial pole of each kidney. In the dog, the presence of calcification or a mass in this region is often indicative of adrenal neoplasia. In the cat, adrenal calcification may be a normal finding
- The bladder normally lies in the caudoventral abdomen, but is naturally very variable in size. Identification of a bladder shadow does not preclude a small tear in the bladder or urethra, and

confirmation or exclusion of these possibilities requires the use of contrast studies (Figures 23.11 and 23.12). Radiodense calculi may be identified on plain radiographs, but for further information, proceed to contrast studies and/or ultrasound
- The prostate gland lies at the neck of the bladder in the male dog and cat. Enlargement of the prostate in the dog results in cranial displacement of the bladder and sometimes dorsal displacement of the rectum/descending colon. While a degree of enlargement is normal in entire dogs as they age, enlargement may also be associated with prostatic disease
- The normal non-gravid uterus is not usually visible radiographically, except in very fat animals. Enlargement of the uterus may result in separation of the bladder from the descending colon by a soft tissue tubular structure and the identification of coiled, distended loops cranial to the bladder (Figure 23.13). Until fetal skeletal mineralization is detectable in the last trimester of pregnancy, it may be difficult to differentiate uterine enlargement due to pregnancy and that due to disease, but ultrasound is useful in this respect.

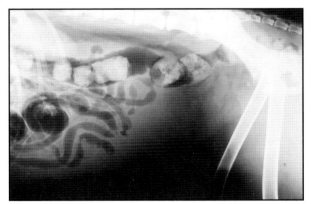

Figure 23.11: *Lateral abdominal radiograph of a cross bred bitch with a traumatic bladder rupture. The plain radiograph shows a generalized loss of detail due to the presence of fluid in the abdominal cavity.*

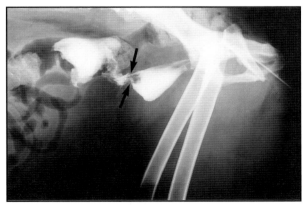

Figure 23.12: *Same animal as Figure 23.11. Water-soluble iodinated contrast medium has been introduced into the bladder and can be seen leaking into the peritoneal cavity (arrows).*

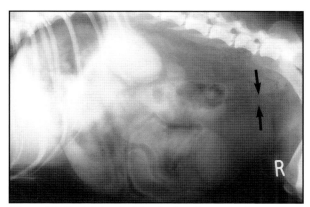

Figure 23.13: *A lateral abdominal radiograph of an entire Jack Russell Terrier bitch with a closed pyometra. A distended, fluid-filled tubular viscus is visible in the mid-ventral abdomen. The uterine body and cervix lie between the bladder and descending colon (arrows).*

Head

Accurate positioning of the patient is particularly important when undertaking radiography of the head and pharynx. Even slight rotation can result in confusion, since the anatomy of the area is relatively complex. Therefore it is preferable to have the patient positioned under general anaesthesia. Occasionally, radiographs may be taken under sedation only, but it should be appreciated that positioning is likely to be suboptimal and all but gross lesions may be missed.

A number of specialized projections are described for different regions of the skull, such as the frontal sinuses, temporomandibular joints and tympanic bullae. It will be necessary to plan the examination carefully so that all areas under suspicion from the clinical examination or standard radiographic projections are fully evaluated. Non-screen film can be useful for intra-oral radiography of the maxilla/nasal chambers, the mandible and individual teeth.

- Check the soft tissues of the head for swelling, emphysema and radiodense foreign material
- Evaluate the bony contours of the skull for disruption (usually traumatic), or bone destruction or proliferation (usually associated with neoplasia or infection)
- Check that the oro- and nasopharynx, the larynx and the cervical trachea are air filled and of a normal calibre.

Spine

As with the head, accurate positioning of the spine is vital if the maximum amount of diagnostic information is to be gleaned from the radiographs. Therefore, general anaesthesia is usually required. If fracture/dislocation of the spine is suspected, survey radiographs may be taken with the animal conscious for a preliminary assessment of the site of the lesion and degree of damage.

The principles behind accurate positioning of the spine for radiography are:

- To keep the spine parallel to the cassette. This may involve padding areas which naturally sag (typically the neck and the lumbar region)
- To avoid any axial rotation
- To avoid bending of the spine to one side and undue flexion or extension. Specific stressed projections in hyperflexion or hyperextension may be used after the standard projections have been assessed, depending on the precise problem suspected.

A minimum of two projections are required for evaluation of the spine — lateral and ventrodorsal. It is important to include only a small section of the spinal column on each radiograph, with accurate centring and collimation. This is because divergence of the X-ray beam towards the periphery of the X-ray film results in a slightly oblique projection of the vertebrae and intervertebral disc spaces, which is not ideal for interpretation.

The radiographs should be checked for:

- The number and alignment of the vertebrae. Remember that a minor malalignment does not necessarily reflect minor spinal cord damage, as the displacement at the time of the injury may have been far greater (Figures 23.14 and 23.15)
- The shape of the vertebrae. Some changes in shape may be due to developmental anomalies (such as block vertebrae, hemivertebrae) while others may be associated with disease processes (e.g. compression fractures)
- Fractures of the vertebrae, including the dorsal spinous and transverse processes and the articular facets as well as the vertebral bodies

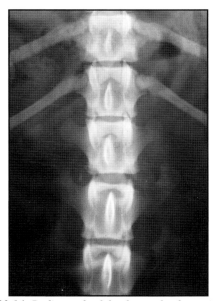

Figure 23.14: *Radiograph of the thoracolumbar spine of a dog with a traumatic vertebral luxation. The ventrodorsal projection shows slight asymmetric widening of the intervertebral disc space between L1 and L2 and slight malalignment of the dorsal spinous processes of L1 and L2.*

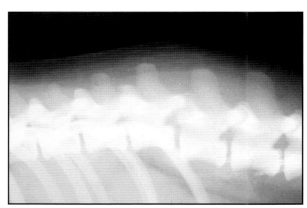

Figure 23.15: Same animal as Figure 23.14. On the lateral projection, a subluxation is clearly visible, with widening of the facet joint and a step between the vertebral bodies at this site.

- Bone proliferation (e.g. associated with trauma, infection, neoplasia, nutritional disorders) or bone destruction (e.g. infection, neoplasia)
- Evidence of intervertebral disc disease (i.e. narrowing of the intervertebral disc space and/or intervertebral foramen; calcification of disc material with or without displacement).

It may be necessary to proceed to contrast studies after studying the plain radiographs, in order to demonstrate the site and severity of any spinal cord compression.

CONTRAST RADIOGRAPHY

Contrast radiography is indicated in the following situations:

- When plain radiographs do not demonstrate a lesion, but the clinical examination and other diagnostic tests suggest that a lesion is present
- When plain radiographs do show a lesion, but further information is required in order to allow a rational treatment to be instituted and an informed prognosis given.

It is important that a good plain radiographic examination precedes the contrast study. This ensures that the appropriate exposure factors are used for the contrast examination, confirms that the contrast technique is indeed necessary and appropriate, and that no lesions are visible on the plain radiographs which may subsequently be masked by contrast medium. Make sure that everything you may require is ready at the beginning of the procedure and that the examination is carried out carefully and thoroughly.

Detailed descriptions of recommended protocols for contrast examinations may be found in standard texts and may differ from the procedures given here, as a result of personal preference. It is very important to note the additional factors listed below.

Oesophageal contrast studies

It is important to note the following:

- General anaesthesia is contraindicated because of the risk of regurgitation and inhalation. In addition, the normal oesophagus may appear dilated during general anaesthesia
- Oesophageal contrast studies are usually contraindicated in very dyspnoeic or collapsed patients because of the risk of aspiration
- Some authorities argue that a water-soluble iodinated contrast medium should be used in preference to barium if an oesophageal perforation is suspected, as barium is inert and will persist in the thoracic cavity. If a water-soluble iodinated contrast medium is chosen, it should be remembered that they tend to be very bitter (so may not be accepted as readily as barium) and are also hypertonic (so that inadvertent inhalation may lead to pulmonary oedema)
- Liquid contrast medium is useful for outlining abnormalities of the oesophageal wall (e.g. ulceration, neoplasia, diverticula), intraluminal masses or foreign bodies, or for demonstrating a perforation
- It may be useful to use contrast medium mixed with food to show a partial oesophageal obstruction or to fill a dilated oesophagus completely.

A procedure for oesophageal contrast studies is shown in Figure 23.16.

Gastrointestinal contrast studies

- Preparation of the patient is important in order to ensure that the stomach is empty and the colon contains minimal faecal material. Food and faeces will result in filling defects in the contrast column or pool, and thus mimic foreign bodies or masses
- General anaesthesia should not be used, as it interferes with gastrointestinal motility and increases the risk of inhalation
- Water-soluble iodinated contrast media may be used in cases of suspected perforation. Arguments for and against its use are outlined above. The hyperosmolarity of the iodinated contrast media tends to draw fluid into the lumen of the gastrointestinal tract, resulting in progressive dilution of the contrast and exacerbation of any existing dehydration
- It is possible to evaluate the large intestine by following the barium through from the stomach. If a large intestinal lesion is specifically suspected, it may be quicker and more efficient to perform a barium enema instead, although endoscopy is usually the technique of choice in such situations
- Normally, contrast begins to leave the stomach

1. The patient should be conscious, not under general anaesthesia.

2. Administer orally 5–40 ml liquid barium sulphate, depending on the size of the patient and the site and nature of the lesion suspected. Alternatively, barium may be mixed with food and the animal allowed to eat this naturally. This technique may be used to demonstrate a partial oesophageal obstruction or to fill a distended oesophagus completely.

3. Take lateral radiographs of the neck and thorax 2–3 minutes after administration. A VD or VD view is occasionally helpful. If contrast medium is retained, further radiographs may be useful to show its subsequent progress.

Figure 23.16: Oesophageal contrast study.

within 30 minutes but may be delayed up to 1 hour in nervous animals. Emptying of the stomach is usually complete within 4–6 hours. A delay in gastric emptying may occur in the presence of systemic illness (e.g. renal failure, peritonitis) or due to gastric outflow obstruction. In most animals, the time between onset of gastric emptying and appearance of barium in the large intestine is between 30 minutes and 1 hour, although this is very variable. Delayed transit may result from systemic illness, or from paralytic or obstructive ileus

- Check the contrast pool or column for persistent filling defects, which may represent foreign material or masses projecting into the lumen (Figure 23.17). Since an apparent defect may be caused by a peristaltic or segmental contraction, it is important to be able to demonstrate that an abnormality is consistently found on successive radiographs
- Evaluate the walls of the gastrointestinal tract for persistent areas of thickening or irregularity
- Check for evidence of perforation and consequent barium leakage.

A procedure for upper gastrointestinal contrast studies is given in Figure 23.18.

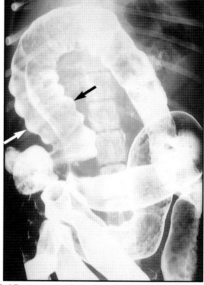

Figure 23.17: A ventrodorsal radiograph of the abdomen of a Golden Retriever taken 2 hours after oral administration of liquid barium. Distended small intestinal loops are visible in the caudal abdomen. In the right cranial abdomen, a corrugated section of intestine (arrows) with a streak of barium running centrally represents an ileo-colic intussusception.

1. Starve the patient overnight, but allow access to water. Administer an enema or allow the animal an opportunity to evacuate the bowel naturally before beginning the procedure.

2. The patient should be conscious or sedated.

3. Administer 1–2 ml/kg liquid barium sulphate (the higher dose rate for smaller animals) either orally or by stomach tube.

4. Take a lateral projection immediately, centred on the cranial abdomen, followed by a ventrodorsal view of the same area.

5. If a gastric lesion is suspected, additional films should be taken at approximately 15 and 30 minutes. If any thing suspicious is seen (e.g. a filling defect or an area of irregularity), the same view should be repeated as soon as possible to confirm or rule out the suspected problem. It can be useful in some cases to take four views of the stomach (right lateral recumbency, left lateral recumbency, ventrodorsal and dorsoventral) as the barium and any gas in the stomach will occupy different parts of the stomach in each view.

6. For the small intestine, radiographs should be taken at 30 minutes and thereafter at hourly intervals until a lesion is seen or passage of barium into the colon has been demonstrated and the stomach is empty.

Figure 23.18: Upper gastrointestinal contrast study.

Upper urinary tract contrast studies

- The study is best carried out under general anaesthesia unless this is clinically contraindicated, as the intravenous administration of the contrast material may result in nausea or vomiting
- A ventrodorsal projection of the abdomen immediately after injection of the contrast agent should show opacification of the renal parenchyma. A complete lack of opacification on this and subsequent radiographs may reflect disruption of the renal blood supply or a non-functional kidney. If the kidneys are opacified, then their size, shape and position should be evaluated
- After about 5 minutes, excretion of the contrast agent should be apparent, with contrast visible in the renal pelvis and ureter on each side. 'Renal shut down' is a recognized but uncommon idiosyncratic reaction to the contrast medium, resulting in initial renal opacification but no visible excretion. Excretion usually begins a short while after administration of intravenous fluids and diuretics, and the animal should be treated for acute renal failure (see Chapter 6). Other reasons for delayed visualization of the renal pelvis include pelvic/ureteral dilation or obstruction, or severely impaired renal function (Figure 23.19).
- Once excretion of the contrast agent is apparent, any distension of, or filling defects within, the ureters can be seen. Loss of integrity of a ureter with consequent spillage of contrast medium into the retroperitoneal space may be seen. Occasionally, the ureters may be seen to be intact but displaced by a mass or haemorrhage within the retroperitoneal space.

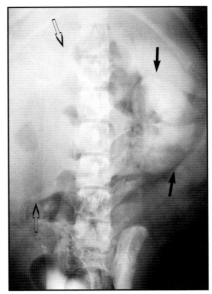

Figure 23.19: *A ventrodorsal abdominal radiograph of a young Rottweiler taken 10 minutes after intravenous injection of a bolus of water-soluble iodinated contrast medium. The left kidney has opacified (closed arrows) and contrast medium is visible in the left renal pelvis and ureter. There is a large soft tissue mass in the region of the right kidney (open arrows), but no excretion of contrast is apparent. The final diagnosis was an enlarged and non-functional right kidney due to a renal abscess.*

A procedure for intravenous urography is given in Figure 23.20.

Lower urinary tract contrast studies

- It is preferable to ensure that the colon and rectum are empty before beginning lower urinary tract

---

1. Except in an emergency, starve the patient overnight but allow access to water. Administer an enema and wait for evacuation of the bowels before premedication.

2. Use general anaesthesia unless clinically contraindicated.

3. If the distal ureters are to be examined, catheterize the bladder to empty it of urine and introduce air before administering the contrast medium.

4. Use water-soluble iodinated contrast medium with a high iodine concentration (ideally 300–450 mg/ml). Administer 1 ml/kg contrast medium intravenously, rapidly as a bolus.

5. For optimum delineation of the kidneys take a VD view of the abdomen centred over the kidneys immediately after injection of the contrast medium. A VD view 5 minutes later will show opacification of the renal pelvis and ureter on each side.

6. Further films centred on the areas of interest are taken as and when required, depending on the indications for the examinations. Excretion normally continues for at least one hour, and bladder filling may be seen 10–15 minutes after the intravenous injection. If renal function is grossly impaired, opacification of the renal pelvis and ureter may not occur or may be delayed for several hours. For examination of the distal ureters and the vesico-ureteric junction, oblique views of the pelvic area may be helpful in addition to the standard lateral and VD views.

Figure 23.20: *Intravenous urography.*

1. Encourage normal evacuation of the bowel or administer an enema.

2. General anaesthesia is usually required except in very sick or placid animals.

3. Catheterize and empty the bladder.

4. (a) Positive contrast cystography: Inject 10–50 ml water-soluble iodinated contrast medium through the urinary catheter – a high level of iodine is not essential for this technique. Withdraw the catheter.
(b) Double contrast cystography: Following a positive contrast cystogram, aspirate as much of the contrast medium as possible. Roll the patient over so the residual contrast medium is spread over the bladder mucosa. Inject 30–200 ml of air according to the size of the animal. Inject the air until moderate resistance to injection is felt, or until distension of the bladder is felt on palpation of the caudal abdomen. Withdraw the catheter.

5. Take a lateral radiograph of the caudal abdomen as soon as possible after introduction of the contrast medium. VD and oblique views may be useful on occasions.

Figure 23.21: Cystography.

contrast procedures, as faecal material may compress and obscure the bladder and prostate. If possible, catheterize and empty the bladder once plain radiographs have been taken
- A positive contrast urethrogram (in the male) or vaginourethrogram (in the female) should allow evaluation of virtually the entire length of the urethra. Check for any irregularity of the urethral wall (e.g. due to neoplasia, inflammation or stricture formation), filling defects within the contrast column (e.g. due to calculi, blood clots, or masses), or leakage of contrast into the surrounding soft tissues. In the male dog, the path of the urethra through the prostate should be assessed, as an asymmetrical path is suggestive of focal prostatic disease (e.g. neoplasia, abscessation, cysts)
- Cystography allows evaluation of the bladder wall and lumen, If bladder rupture is suspected, positive contrast cystography is the preferred technique (Figure 23.21). Otherwise, double contrast cystography allows accurate assessment of the wall for thickening and irregularity and of free structures within the lumen, such as calculi or blood clots.

Spinal contrast studies

- General anaesthesia is mandatory for such procedures
- It is important that only non-ionic water-soluble iodinated contrast media are used. The ionic forms are too irritant for use around the spinal cord
- Plan the procedure carefully before beginning, deciding on the preferred site of puncture and the required dose of contrast medium. These decisions will be influenced not only by the site of the suspected lesion, but the probable stability (or otherwise) of the vertebrae in the region
- Once the contrast has been injected, follow its path from the site of injection to the region of interest, looking carefully for any deviation or thinning of

the contrast columns which may allow localization of any spinal cord compression and differentiation between extradural, intramedullary and extramedullary/intradural lesions (see Figure 23.22). Once a lesion has been identified, it is important to take radiographs in at least two planes (usually lateral and ventrodorsal).

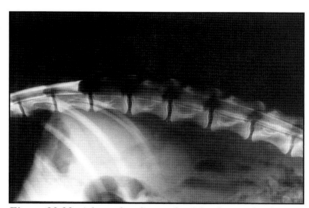

Figure 23.22: A lateral radiograph of the thoracolumbar spine of a young Springer Spaniel taken during cisternal myelography. The dorsal contrast column flares and stops abruptly at the caudal end of T13, outlining the cranial end of an extramedullary/intradural mass.

A procedure for spinal contrast studies is given in Figure 23.23.

ULTRASONOGRAPHY

Diagnostic ultrasonography is an imaging technique which is a very useful complement to radiography. Ultrasonography is a safe non-invasive technique which produces cross-sectional images of the soft tissues of the body. Therefore, information regarding the internal architecture of organs may be obtained. In addition, these images are continuously updated, so that movement of structures may be seen. Consequently,

1. General anaesthesia is essential.

2. A water-soluble non-ionic iodinated contrast medium should be selected and warmed to approximately body temperature.

3. Dosage of the contrast medium will depend on both the size of the animal and the level of the suspected lesion. A dose rate of 0.3 ml/kg up to a maximum of 10 ml has been suggested, but this should be reduced if the suspected lesion is close to the site of injection.

4. (a) Cisternal puncture: Place the animal in lateral recumbency. Clip the site of puncture and prepare aseptically. With the head flexed and held steadily by an assistant, palpate the occipital crest and the two wings of the atlas. Place a sterile spinal needle, with the bevel facing caudally, perpendicular to the skin on the midline in the centre of the triangle formed by these landmarks. Advance the needle slowly until a 'pop' is felt as the needle enters the cisterna magna. Withdraw the stylet and wait for the flow of CSF, which indicates correct needle placement. If the tap is bloody, then withdraw the needle and repeat the procedure with a clean needle.
   (b) Lumbar puncture: The animal may be placed in either lateral or ventral recumbency, and the site of puncture clipped and prepared aseptically. Palpate the dorsal spinous processes of the caudal lumbar vertebrae. Introduce a spinal needle in the midline, just in front of the dorsal spinous process of L6. Slowly advance the needle until it impinges on bone, then slowly 'walk' the tip of the needle forwards along the bone until it passes through the intervertebral space. The needle passes for a short distance, coming to a stop on the floor of the spinal canal. Often a twitch of the hindlimbs or tail is noted as the needle passes through the cauda equina. CSF is not invariably obtained, even if the needle is correctly located, so a test injection of contrast medium may be required to check the position of the needle tip.

5. Inject the required dose of contrast medium slowly, then withdraw the needle.

6. Following contrast medium injection, lateral radiographs are taken, starting at the site of injection, and working progressively down (in the case of cisternal injection) or up (in the case of lumbar injection) the spinal column to follow the flow of contrast medium. If it fails to flow, then it may help to tilt the animal head up (if the contrast medium was given cisternally), or to apply traction to the spinal column. If a lesion is found, then a VD view of the region should also be taken.

Figure 23.23: Myelography.

ultrasound examination is an extremely valuable imaging tool in critical patients.

It does, however, have limitations. The ultrasound beam is blocked by bone or gas, so that the information gleaned from imaging skeletal structures, or gas-filled organs such as the lung or, on occasions, the gastro-intestinal tract, is often minimal.

It may be useful to bear in mind the following principles when planning an ultrasonographic examination.

- Select the scanning site carefully by choosing an area of the body surface overlying the organ or tissue of interest, but avoiding intervening bone or gas
- Clip hair from the skin of the scanning site, clean the skin carefully and apply liberal quantities of acoustic gel to ensure good acoustic contact
- When a choice is available, select as high a frequency of sound as you can while still achieving an adequate depth of tissue penetration. In general, high frequency sound (e.g. 7.5 MHz) will penetrate less far but provide better image resolution than lower frequency sound (e.g. 5 MHz)

- Once an image is obtained, optimize the detail by adjustment of gain controls, such that there is an even brightness throughout the depth of the image. Too dark an image will result in loss of visible detail, whereas too bright an image may obscure detail with background 'noise'
- Ensure that a thorough ultrasonographic examination is carried out, sweeping the sound beam through the entire area of interest, in at least two planes of section
- Colour flow and spectral Doppler techniques may be useful in some cases in order to define blood flow (in terms of direction, nature and velocity) within the cardiac chambers and great vessels.

Thorax

The most common reason for ultrasonographic examination of the thoracic cavity is to evaluate the heart. While radiography enables an assessment of the shape and size of the cardiac silhouette only, ultrasound will allow visualization of the separate chambers, great vessels and valves. For a full description of the recommended protocol for ultrasonographic examination of the heart and the abnormalities which may be found, the reader is referred to texts cited under 'References and further reading'. However, the following points may be helpful in assessing the critical patient.

- Pericardial fluid appears as an echolucent (black) band around the heart. It is important to evaluate the regions of the heart base and the right atrium carefully for evidence of hypoechoic (grey) masses, which when present are usually neoplastic and the underlying cause of the effusion. Collapse of the right atrial wall during systole is evidence of cardiac tamponade (see Figure 23.8) and is an indication for immediate drainage of the pericardial fluid
- The thickness of the myocardium should be assessed. The myocardium may be thickened as a physiological response to a cardiovascular abnormality (e.g. right ventricular hypertrophy in response to pulmonic stenosis) or as part of the primary disease process (e.g. hypertrophic cardiomyopathy). It may sometimes appear thinner than normal, usually in association with chamber dilation (e.g. a dilated thin-walled left ventricle is often a feature of dilated cardiomyopathy)
- Chamber size should be evaluated. Ventricular dilation may be seen as a consequence of volume overload (e.g. a left-to-right shunting ventricular septal defect will result in pulmonary overcirculation and dilation of the left atrium and ventricle). Atrial dilation may occur in response to pressure or volume overload (e.g. reduced ventricular compliance as in hypertrophic or restrictive cardiomyopathy; atrioventricular valve insufficiency)
- The leaflets of each of the major valves should be assessed. Thickening and irregularity of valve leaflets may be seen in congenital (valvular dysplasia) or acquired disease (endocardiosis, endocarditis). An abnormal motion may also sometimes be seen (e.g. rupture of chordae tendinae)
- Myocardial contractility may also be evaluated. It is useful to view overall myocardial movement on both long and short axis sections, in order to detect regions of myocardium with abnormal or reduced movements. M mode measurements may then be made in an attempt to quantify contractility — a number of different measurements may be made, but the potential limitations of each should be appreciated. For a full discussion of this complex area, the reader is referred to the texts listed under 'References and further reading'. Myocardial activity may be reduced (e.g. due to myocardial disease) or increased (e.g. in association with atrioventricular valve incompetence).

The remaining structures in the thoracic cavity are not usually visualized in the normal animal, as they are obscured by air-filled lung. However, the presence of free thoracic fluid will act as an acoustic window, outlining and separating thoracic structures. If sufficient fluid is present, the great vessels may be followed in the mediastinum, partially collapsed lung lobes can be identified and any solid masses lying within the fluid identified. The fluid itself usually appears echolucent (black), although the presence of particulate matter, gas bubbles or a highly cellular content may result in echoes swirling within the fluid.

Abdomen

The presence of free abdominal fluid, as in the thoracic cavity, enhances ultrasonographic visualization by outlining and separating structures. If only a small amount of free fluid is present, it will tend to accumulate in dependent parts of the abdomen.

Liver and spleen

It is preferable to starve the patient before imaging the liver, as a food-filled stomach will obscure part of the liver. It is acceptable to give the patient a drink, as fluid within the stomach does not impair image quality and indeed may act as a useful landmark.

Evaluation of the hepatic and splenic parenchyma may reveal irregularity of the surface of the organ, and focal or diffuse disturbances of the parenchymal architecture (Figure 23.24). Such changes are usually indicative of disease, but are non-specific. For example, circumscribed nodules in the hepatic or splenic parenchyma may be neoplastic, hyperplastic, abscesses, infarcts, haematomas or granulomas. Equally, a normal ultrasonographic appearance does not preclude disease. Therefore, a fine needle aspirate or tissue core biopsy may be required for a definitive diagnosis.

The vascular supply can also be assessed. In the spleen, major vessels are only visible in the hilar region. In the liver, the caudal vena cava and portal veins can be identified, as well as their intrahepatic branches and tributaries. Thus venous congestion can be recognized, as well

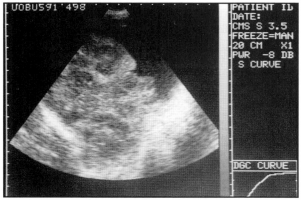

Figure 23.24: *An ultrasonogram of the liver of a Wire Haired Fox Terrier with ascites. The fluid is anechoic and thus outlines the irregularly rounded liver lobes. Multiple hypoechoic nodules are scattered throughout the liver parenchyma. The final diagnosis was lymphosarcoma.*

as intraluminal thrombi or neoplastic invasion. Vascular anomalies, such as portosystemic shunts and arteriovenous fistulation, may also be recognized by the presence of single or multiple tortuous anomalous vessels.

Within the liver, the gall bladder is readily seen, but the intrahepatic bile ducts are not usually visible. Distension of the common bile duct and subsequently the intrahepatic bile ducts can be detected in cases of obstructive jaundice.

The kidneys and adrenal glands

Ultrasound provides a clear demonstration of the renal cortex, medulla and pelvis. Blurring or distortion of the normal architectural pattern is indicative of renal parenchymal disease but, once again, many of the changes seen are non-specific. In the critical patient, ultrasound may be useful in differentiating between renal failure due to an acute renal insult or pre-renal causes, when the kidney often appears ultrasonographically normal, and renal failure due to established

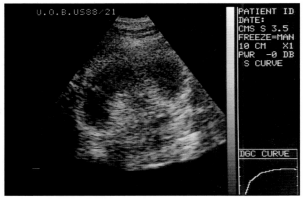

Figure 23.25: An ultrasonogram of the right kidney of a young Bassett Hound with renal dysplasia. The renal cortex is thin and irregular and intensely hyperechoic due to a combination of fibrosis and calcification.

underlying renal disease, when ultrasonographic changes can often be seen (Figure 23.25).

Dilation of the renal pelvis (e.g. due to ureteral obstruction, or ascending urinary tract infection) is readily detected. Dilation of the proximal ureter as it leaves the kidney and of the distal ureter as it approaches the bladder may be detected, but the middle section is often difficult to distinguish.

The adrenal glands may be identified medial to the cranial pole of each kidney in close apposition to the aorta, providing the patient is not too obese. The adrenals are normally hypoechoic elongated structures. Enlargement of the gland, with loss of the normal elongated shape and even echotexture, may be seen with either adrenal hyperplasia or neoplasia. Remember to check the adjacent great vessels for evidence of invasion or thrombus formation if an adrenal mass is found.

The bladder and prostate

Ultrasonographic examination of the bladder allows careful evaluation of the wall for regions of thickening or irregularity or for discrete masses projecting into the lumen. It may be helpful in treatment planning to determine the precise location of any mass relative to the bladder neck and the points of entry of the ureters, as well as the size of the mass. It is difficult to differentiate between a polypoid or neoplastic mass and a blood clot adherent to the bladder wall. Sequential examinations over a period of time may be required to clarify the situation. Calculi, irrespective of their mineral composition, are seen as echogenic structures lying in the dependent part of the bladder. Hypoechoic masses floating freely within the lumen of the bladder are likely to be blood clots.

The prostate gland is located caudal to the bladder and may be predominantly intra-abdominal or intra-pelvic in location. It should be smooth in outline, with an evenly granular hypoechoic appearance. Small fluid foci measuring <1 cm in diameter are considered normal findings. Larger fluid foci may represent intraprostatic cysts, haematocysts, abscesses or tumours with necrotic centres. Disturbance of the normal parenchymal architecture may occur with either inflammatory or neoplastic disease. Therefore, fine needle aspiration of fluid foci and tissue core biopsies of disturbed parenchyma may be necessary for a definitive diagnosis.

The uterus

Ultrasound is the imaging modality of choice for differentiation between uterine enlargement due to pregnancy and that due to disease. From 3–4 weeks gestation onwards, fetal structures may be clearly recognized within the uterus, and fetal viability assessed in terms of generalized fetal movements and fetal cardiac activity. Cessation of fetal movements and subsequent loss of fetal structure is indicative of fetal death. In the absence of fetal structures, accumulation of fluid within the uterus is abnormal and usually indicates pyometritis.

The gastrointestinal tract and pancreas

The gastroinstestinal tract is amenable to ultrasonographic examination provided it does not contain excessive gas. If a high frequency transducer is used to obtain images of optimal quality, then a distinct layered appearance of the wall of the stomach and small intestine is seen. The alternating hyperechoic and hypoechoic layers correspond exactly to the histological layers of mucosa, submucosa, muscularis and serosa. The lumen may be collapsed, with a central hyperechoic streak representing residual mucus and ingesta, or may be fluid filled. In the normal animal, peristaltic and segmental contractions can be seen.

Gross thickening of the wall may be detected, either with retention of the normal layered structure (usually hypertrophy or inflammation) or loss of normal architecture (severe inflammation or neoplasia). If abnormal fluid distension of the stomach or small intestinal loops is seen, it is useful to determine whether peristaltic and segmental contractions remain, or whether they are reduced or absent. If fluid is present within the gastro-intestinal lumen, then foreign material or intraluminal masses may become evident.

The pancreas is difficult to image ultrasonographically, partly because of its awkward location and partly because of its poorly defined margins. It lies in the right cranial quadrant of the abdomen, with the right limb closely apposed to the descending loop of the duodenum. In acute pancreatitis, the pancreas becomes enlarged, often with hypoechoic regions representing necrosis and haemorrhage. The adjacent duodenum may be dilated and static, with a thickened wall.

REFERENCES AND FURTHER READING

Anon (1988) *Guidance Notes for the Protection of Persons against Ionising Radiations Arising From Veterinary Use.* National Radiological Protection Board and the Health and Safety Executive

Burk RL and Ackerman N (1986) *Small Animal Radiology: a Diagnostic Atlas and Text.* Churchill Livingstone, New York

Lee R (1995) *Manual of Small Animal Diagnostic Imaging, 2nd edition.* BSAVA, Cheltenham

Nyland TG and Mattoon JS (1995) *Veterinary Diagnostic Ultrasound.* WB Saunders, Philadelphia

Suter PF (1984) *Thoracic Radiography of the Dog and Cat.* Wettswil, Switzerland

Thrall DE (1994) *Textbook of Veterinary Diagnostic Radiology.* WB Saunders, Philadelphia

Index